Metabolic and Endocrine Physiology

FIFTH EDITION

PHYSIOLOGY TEXTBOOK SERIES

These volumes may be purchased individually.

PHYSIOLOGY of the DIGESTIVE TRACT,
Fifth Edition HORACE W. DAVENPORT, PH.D., D.SC. (OXON.)

PHYSIOLOGY of the NERVOUS SYSTEM,
Second Edition CARLOS EYZAGUIRRE, M.D., *and* SALVATORE J. FIDONE, PH.D.

PHYSIOLOGY of the KIDNEY and BODY FLUIDS,
Third Edition ROBERT F. PITTS, PH.D., M.D.

METABOLIC and ENDOCRINE PHYSIOLOGY,
Fifth Edition JAY TEPPERMAN, M.D., *and* HELEN M. TEPPERMAN, PH.D.

COMROE'S PHYSIOLOGY of RESPIRATION,
Third Edition *(in preparation)* NORMAN C. STAUB, M.D.

METABOLIC AND ENDOCRINE PHYSIOLOGY

An Introductory Text

JAY TEPPERMAN, M.D.
Emeritus Professor of Experimental Medicine
Department of Pharmacology
State University of New York Health Sciences Center at Syracuse
Syracuse, New York

HELEN M. TEPPERMAN, Ph.D.
Emeritus Professor of Pharmacology
Department of Pharmacology
State University of New York Health Sciences Center at Syracuse
Syracuse, New York

FIFTH EDITION

YEAR BOOK MEDICAL PUBLISHERS, INC.
Chicago • London • Boca Raton

2 3 4 5 6 7 8 9 K C 89, 88, 87

Library of Congress Cataloging-in-Publication Data

Tepperman, Jay, 1913-
  Metabolic and endocrine physiology.
  Includes bibliographies and index.
  1. Endocrinology. 2. Metabolism. I. Tepperman, Helen M.
II. Title [DNLM: 1. Endocrine Glands—physiology.
2. Hormones—physiology. 3. Metabolism. WK 102 T314m]
QP187.T42 1987   612'.4   86-19086
ISBN 0-8151-8757-2

Sponsoring Editor: Stephany S. Scott
Manager, Copyediting Services: Frances M. Perveiler
Copyeditor: Francis A. Byrne
Production Project Manager: R. Allen Reedtz
Proofroom Supervisor: Shirley E. Taylor

For our children (and our grandchildren):
JEAN (CAROLYN *and* SARAH L.)
KATHY (ELIZABETH *and* SARAH H.)
JIM (SAM)

Preface to the First Edition

The time has long since gone when anyone could presume to say to the beginning student: "Here are the facts of physiology which you must learn in order to prepare yourself to be a physician." Every attempt to describe the state of development of a field of physiology at present must involve arbitrary selection of material, emphasis colored by the personal experience and limitations of the author, and the occupational risk of offending the sensibilities of one's colleagues and fellow authors. This is not to be regarded as a plea for sympathy, since my choice to write a review of endocrine physiology was a free one, but the reader should reflect, for a moment, about the problems involved in constructing such a review.

In the first place, the preparation or (in the educationist's patois) the "readiness" of our first-year medical students in this area is quite variable. I have seen students who have been exposed to excellent undergraduate courses in endocrinology on the one hand and some who were quite virginally innocent of any knowledge about the glands of internal secretion on the other. The future application of this information by individual students may be equally variable; some of our students have elected to become specialists in this field and have devoted their lives to study, teaching and research in it, while others have chosen to work in some branch of medicine which they manage to visualize as nonmetabolic (although it is difficult to understand how they contrive to do this). In the intermediate zone there is a whole spectrum of professional activities, which range from internal medicine and gynecology through general practice to psychiatry, in which the facts and concepts of endocrinology and metabolism are not merely pertinent but crucial in the diagnosis of disease and the management of sick people.

These variations in educational origin and professional destination of our students are confusing enough, but when one adds to this the nature of the material to be presented, the confusion is compounded. The rate at which new knowledge is accumulating in the field of endocrinology cannot be appreciated by anyone who has not been obligated to try to keep up with some of it. These essays are beads drawn on rapidly moving targets.

This, then, is one author's account of the current state of knowledge of endocrinology as he understands it, and it is directed to an imaginary undifferentiated, totipotential first- or second-year medical student (I would not be desolate, however, if a colleague or fellow-teacher were to experience an occasional "shock of recognition" in these pages). Some students, like the little girl who wrote the review of a book on penguins, may find more here than they care to know. Others may find much less, and for them I have included key references (mainly to monographs, symposia and recent review articles) which were selected to guide the reader back to original sources. I intend to indicate, wherever possible, how the physiological idea is applied in the clinic, for I do not subscribe to the view that a physiological insight that has practical application is necessarily less interesting or beautiful than one for which there is as yet none. This is not to be construed as a promise to omit mention of concepts which may not yet have been applied to the practice of medicine or public health, or to refrain from discussing certain theories and speculations. It seems to me that the fantasies and daydreams of physiology are an important part of the art, and that they do no harm if they are clearly identified. The good ones will one day be validated by experiment and the bad ones will be punctured and discarded in due time.

It is assumed that by the time the student attempts to read this account he will have acquired some information about the gross and microscopic anatomy and embryology of the endocrine glands, and that he is familiar with the broad outlines of carbohydrate, fat and protein metabolism. No attempt will be made here to recapitulate in detail material which is readily available in any standard textbook of histology or biochemistry.

The selection of illustrative experiments from our own experience is not intended to convey the impression that the data cited have any special significance or originality. It often indicates merely that the material was more readily available to me than other similar data would have been. It is obviously impossible to give more than a very small sample of the kinds of data on which statements made in the text are based. In fact, it would be unfair to both the reader and the data to attempt too broad a reporting of more or less original information. Therefore, in the few examples I have used, I have tried consciously to include samples taken from every wavelength of the biological research spectrum from the molecular to the epidemiological.

There are two widely used methods of drawing diagrams of the endocrine system: in one, the endocrine organs, kidneys, gastrointestinal tract, etc., are represented by more or less faithful cartoons of their gross anatomical structure (the "Giblet School"); in the other, the related structures are rendered simply as engineers' "black boxes" (the "Mondrianesque School"). Many of the diagrams to be presented herein are in the latter category, and they are intended both as guides to and summaries of the discussion. The encircled numbers represent subsections of the text which are identified by the corresponding numbers in the text. These diagrams have been designed to show the structures and hormones to be discussed and some of their interrelationships.

No one can really understand any subject unless he has some knowledge of the historical development of the modern idea. When I have attempted historical accounts of some of the subjects to be covered in this section in lectures, I have noticed a certain restiveness on the part of students who appeared to be impatient to reach topics that seemed more likely than Minkowski's dogs to be included in an examination. While I have been unable to permit myself the luxury of extended historical treatment of the subject, I could not bring myself to present this inventory without giving some indication that the intellectual edifice of

physiology was built over many years by patient and devoted individuals to whom we and those who follow us owe a great debt. Therefore, I have included abbreviated chronologies of some subjects at the beginnings of most chapters. In addition to serving as a small tribute to our professional ancestors, these chronologies illustrate beautifully the interchange of information between clinic and experimental laboratory that has occurred mainly in the past century, and promises to be even more fruitful in the future.

Acknowledgments

There is no doubt that this enterprise could not have been completed without the help of my wife, Dr. Helen Tepperman. In addition to teaching me most of the material in Chapters 5 and 11 and helping in the collection and evaluation of much source information for all other chapters, she read every word of this account in three successive drafts, criticized gently but firmly, and made many valuable suggestions for improving the final product.

I am grateful, too, to Dr. Alfred Farah, Chairman of the department in which I work, for his encouragement and help in many ways. I have requested and received welcome help from each of the following: D. Tapley, R. Barrnett, G. Sayers, M. Karnofsky, J. L. Kostyo, H. Rasmussen, R. C. Haynes, Jr., D. Sabbatini, D. H. P. Streeten, M. Voorhess, L. Gardner, A. Moses, and L. Raisz.

I owe a special debt to Nicolas Apgar and Julia Hammack for the great care and skill with which they prepared the illustrations, and to Shirley Martin for expert secretarial help. I am grateful, too, to the publishers for their understanding cooperation.

JAY TEPPERMAN, M.D.

Preface to the Fifth Edition

When, 26 years ago, one of us (J. T.) participated in a conversation with Julius Comroe, Robert Pitts, Alan Burton, Horace Davenport, and Year Book's Fred Rogers to plan a series of monographs in physiology, he could not have predicted that anyone would be interested in publishing a *fifth* edition of *Metabolic and Endocrine Physiology*. Of our original fellow authors in the enterprise, only Horace Davenport, our great and good friend since 1940, survives. On this occasion, we remember the others not sadly but with pleasure: Comroe, a genuinely witty and wise scholar, investigator, teacher, and administrator; Burton, who was gently funny and extraordinarily literate and articulate in the Old World tradition; and Pitts, decidedly not a comic genius like the others, but a scientist-poet who found his inspiration up and down the renal tubule. To all of them we say, hail and farewell.

The authors of this edition, recently retired from teaching and research, have been privileged to watch the astonishing evolution of modern endocrinology for an aggregate total of 98 people years. When we began our respective graduate school training (J. T. in 1934 and H. M. T. in 1938), endocrinology had only recently achieved a degree of respectability, having been identified previously in the public consciousness primarily with giants, dwarfs, and bearded ladies in circuses. Insulin had only been discovered in 1921, the giants of steroid biochemistry were the avantgarde, and two decades had to pass before anyone knew the structure of a peptide hormone or of DNA. With the massive infusions of money into biomedical research in the 50s and 60s, growth of knowledge in endocrinology, as in all other fields, has been exponential. We and our colleagues have functioned as self-appointed Greek choruses, commenting on the action as we tried to follow new developments. In 39 years of teaching, we have been responsible for introducing over 4,000 medical students, and more than a few Ph.D. candidates, to the study of endocrinology.

Someone once said that all Michelangelo had to do was to find a large piece of marble and chip away everything that was not David or Moses. Michelangelo had the great advantage of knowing precisely how he wanted David and Moses to look. In our case, the block of marble was vast, but we were never sure that we or anyone could chisel from it an introduction that would be both appropriate for students and acceptable to their teachers. Knowing how many demands were placed on our students by other teachers, we wanted to avoid overload; but at the same time, we know modern students too well to presume to condescend to them. We have settled, as in the past, for a narrative style, and we have tried, wherever it was possible, to demonstrate how contemporary ideas have their roots in older ones.

Our procedure was to read current material related to each chapter, to reread what we had written before, and either to preserve or rewrite segments in the fourth edition according to our assessment of need. In every case, we rewrote much that was retained and added a considerable number of new mini-essays. Most of the cyclic AMP chapter was rewritten to emphasize the concept of multiple second messengers, including calcium-calmodulin, and polyphosphatidyl inositol turnover. The prostaglandin chapter was expanded to include more on the leukotrienes. All aspects of neuroendocrinology were reevaluated, and accounts of new hypothalamic hormones, CRF, GHRH and PIF, have been included. There is new information on the mechanism of action of hormones in virtually all chapters. When it was announced that Brown and Goldstein were awarded the 1985 Nobel Prize in medicine, we repaired a longstanding deficiency by writing an entirely new chapter (Chapter 15) on lipoproteins and lipid transport.

We have directed this book to a population of students who have had courses in gross anatomy, histology (including ultrastructure) and biochemistry, but not pathology, immunology, or clinical medicine. While the prerequisite courses are certainly desirable, one of us (J. T.) has used previous editions of this book in one-on-one tutorials with Ph.D. candidates. He has been impressed by how much a conscientious student without prior training in anatomy or histology can extract from the book with the help of a good dictionary.

This is *not* intended to be a textbook of clinical endocrinology. The brief references to endocrine diseases and other clinical matters are included to illustrate the point that in this field, as in so many other areas of modern medicine, application of basic biochemical and physiological information is swift and pervasive.

Many old illustrations have been revised to reflect new knowledge, and we have drawn a large number of new ones. For these, we are grateful for the help of Ellie Carbone. We are also grateful to Chester Carlson, who invented xerography, and to every one

(unknown to us) who made it possible for us to have a word processor in our home. Without them, this revision would have been quite impossible.

We look back with pleasure over a quarter century's association with Year Book Medical Publishers. We thank our Chicago friends for their careful and concerned editing and production.

JAY TEPPERMAN, M.D.

HELEN M. TEPPERMAN, PH.D.

Contents

PART I

Introduction

1

Overview of Hormonal Mechanisms

No multicellular organism can long survive without some sort of internal communications system that can transmit messages from one part to another. In animals there are two major communications systems: (1) *The nervous system,* with all of its projections and arborizations, which is analogous to an elaborate system of telegraphy in which there is a "wire" connection from the source of initiation of the message to the place where reception of the message has its effect; and (2) *the endocrine system* (really a loosely affiliated group of subsystems), which uses the circulatory system to carry messages in the form of highly specialized chemical substances called hormones—a "wireless" system. Hormones are recognized by target cells, which have been preprogrammed by the process of differentiation to respond to their presence by acting in predictable and stereotypical ways. In collaboration, the nervous system and the endocrine system maintain the "constancy of the internal milieu," as Claude Bernard described it with remarkable prescience about a century ago. The features of the internal milieu, whose constancy is vigilantly monitored by the "wired" and "wireless" communications systems of the body, are the concentrations of solutes in the blood, as well as blood pressure and blood flow. Whether we describe regulation of serum glucose concentration, serum free fatty acid, calcium, or blood pressure, the equilibrium state is one in which the forces that tend to elevate the variable under study and those that tend to depress it are in perfect balance so that a steady state exists. A perturbation that displaces the variable (X) upward galvanizes appropriate neural or endocrine cells into action to restore equilibrium. A depression of X may recruit other sentinel cells to defend against downward displacement of X. The history of physiology from Bernard through W. B. Cannon to the present day, when physiologic regulations are often described in terms of computer programs, has been largely a progressively more complex description of this principle. Prominent among the sentinel cells that help to maintain the constancy of the internal milieu are those that synthesize and secrete hormones—cells of the endocrine glands.

At one time, neurobiology and endocrinology were explored by investigators who saw little connection between the two fields. One of the most striking features of the recent history of both enterprises has been the realization that they are in fact closely related to one another and are functionally interdependent. As we shall see, it is possible for a reflex arc to consist of a neural afferent component and an endocrine efferent component (see Chapter 5). In fact, since the recent discovery of morphine-like peptides in the pituitary and in the central nervous system, it is even possible to suggest a Bernardian theory of pain, which may be conceived of as an equilibrium state maintained by pain signals opposed by anti-pain signals—a balance that can be tipped in either direction, with consequent recruitment of the opposing force. Certainly the discovery of a large number of peptides in the central nervous system, some of them long identified as "gastrointestinal" hormones, has provided the neurobiologist and the endocrinologist with parallel problems and shared interests.

Endocrinology then, like neurobiology, is concerned with communication: with messages-as-molecules, which are recognized by discriminators on or in sensitive cells and, by elaborate molecular means, transduced into a response. The response, most of the time, is physiologically advantageous to the whole organism. When a hormone is inappropriately overproduced, as in hyperthyroidism, or by a neoplasm, the response may be maladaptive—in fact, destructive. The remainder of this book contains an account of two observers' understanding of the chemical signals, the cells that produce them and the cells that respond to them.

History of Endocrinology

Endocrinology has its roots in the observations and descriptions of physicians and philosophers in ancient times. References to a disease that must have been diabetes mellitus can be found in Egyptian papyri of 1500 B.C. Allusions to goiter and to the effects of castration in man and animals were among the first clinical descriptions of disorders that later proved to be endocrine in nature. Old clinical descriptions of endocrine diseases were provided not only by western observers but also by ancient Chinese and Indian clinicians.

If one plots the major discoveries in many areas of endocrinology on a time scale, the resulting display represents a mini-course in the history of biology and medicine. After scattered clinical descriptions in ancient times and through the middle ages, progress was very slow indeed. During the last half of the 19th century, a quantum leap forward occurred in many fields, both in the quality and detail of clinical description and in the beginning of our understanding of mechanism. The historical reasons for this acceleration of the pace of discovery are no doubt complex, but we can discern some interesting correlations with the development. In the first place, the industrial revolution resulted in the generation of capital that could be applied to research in many fields, but most impressively in chemistry. The brilliant flowering of organic chemistry in Germany was stimulated by the needs of textile manufacturers who required dyes for their products. Similarly, some of Pasteur's most famous work was done in his capacity as consultant to the wine industry of France. Since endocrinology deals with the interactions of specific chemical substances, the developing sciences of chemistry and physics made possible the description of endocrine mechanisms in molecular terms.

Another revolution occurred in the latter half of the 19th century—one that was basic to the growth of endocrinology as well as to that of all biology and medicine, i.e., the study of experimental animal models. Pioneers such as Claude Bernard and Oscar Minkowski demonstrated that it was possible to make controlled and reproducible observations in the laboratory: in other words, to cross-examine nature. If this activity had been prohibited or proscribed, most of what we now know about endocrinology would have been impossible to learn. All of the substances that we now call hormones began as "substance X" or "factor ?"—as a result of experiments on whole animals, frequently suggested by prior observations in sick people. "Koch's postulates" of endocrinology evolved into the following sequence:

1. Extirpation of putative gland.
2. Description of biologic effects of operation.
3. Injection of extract of gland.
4. Demonstration that injection of extract corrected deficits described in 2.
5. Isolation, purification, and identification of active substance.

By World War II, a lot of information had accumulated in the field of endocrinology, much of it fundamental to later developments. But the availability of a battery of new techniques after that war produced an unprecedented quickening of the tempo of discovery. Concurrently there was an enormous expansion of the research force and research laboratory plant, with the result that the literature of endocrinology, like that of all other aspects of biomedical knowledge, is now growing at an exponential rate. This means that new discoveries are being made constantly, and that old ideas must be reexamined periodically in the light of new facts.

The flow of information and understanding from the physical sciences and from basic biologic insights into hormone research has not been undirectional. In surprisingly many cases, investigators working on endocrine problems have made fundamental contributions to all of biology. An example of this is shown in Figure 1–1.

Some Problems in Definition

Hormones are usually defined as chemical messengers that are secreted directly into the bloodstream by specialized cells capable of synthesizing and releasing them in response to specific signals. A few or many target cells are equipped to detect the hormone and to show a typical response to it. The physiologic concentration range for most hormones is 10^{-7} to 10^{-12}, i.e., they are effective at very low concentrations. Often, hormones are described as exerting their effects over long distances via the bloodstream *(telecrine)*. Substances that are secreted by one cell and exert their biologic effects by local diffusion are called *paracrine*. Substances that act on cells that secrete them are called *autocrine*.

These are difficult distinctions to make since some authentic hormones, especially those of the hypothalamus, travel a very short distance before encountering their target cells. Others, like testosterone and estrogens, have both telecrine and paracrine actions, since they are known to act locally near their cells of origin as well as at a distance after having traveled through the bloodstream. To make definitions even more confusing, at least one hormone, testosterone, is present in high concentration in the seminiferous tubules and

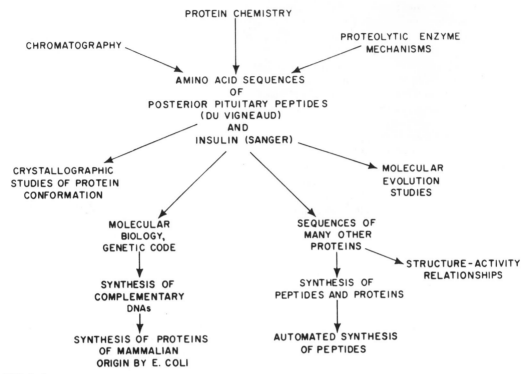

FIG 1–1.
Relationship of studies on hormones to history of biology.

in their efferent duct system and is presumed to affect ductular structures, which are responsible for the transport and maturation of newly formed spermatozoa.

In addition to hormones, there are many other chemical substances that have a regulatory or modulatory role in the control of biologic processes. The *neurotransmitters,* mainly acetylcholine and the catecholamines, are synthesized in nerve cells and released from nerve endings. Other neurotransmitters have been described, among them serotonin, gamma aminobutyric acid (GABA), and histamine. These characteristically exert their effects over very short distances and, typically, for much shorter periods of time than are required for the action of peptide, protein, steroid, and thyroid hormones.

Prominent in the category of chemical compounds that exert their effects near their cells of origin are those called "*autacoids,*" These include histamine, slow-reacting substance (SRS·A), bradykinin, and many compounds generated during inflammatory responses. Later we will examine some of the relationships of hormones with these materials.

Other categories of information-carrying chemical substances function as agents or deputies or "*second*

messengers" for hormones at the intracellular level. Among these are the cyclic nucleotides, cyclic adenosine monophosphate (AMP) and cyclic guanosine monophosphate (GMP), calcium and certain hydrolytic products of the phospholipid, phosphorylated phosphatidyl inositol. It is an arresting thought that examination of the mechanism of action of a hormone in a hormone-sensitive cell and that of a neurotransmitter in a stimulated neuron reveals common thematic patterns and similar biochemical machinery. Similarly, the responses of mast cells to a variety of stimuli and of lymphocytes to mitogens are strikingly like those of some hormone-sensitive cells to their respective hormones.

Another set of compounds cannot easily be classified; perhaps *modulators* of hormone and neurotransmitter action would be most appropriate to describe the effects of a series of substances called *prostaglandins*. These ubiquitous materials will be described in Chapter 4. Their most distinctive feature is that they are often synthesized in response to hormonal and neurotransmitter stimulation, and in some instances they tend to enhance the hormone effect, whereas in others they appear to blunt the effect.

All of these regulatory substances are extremely

potent agents that are effective at low concentrations, but they are not the only sources of information on which cells act or fail to act. *Circulating substrates* (e.g., glucose, free fatty acids, and lipid in other forms) and amino acids constitute an important set of instructions to individual cells and groups of cells. Similarly the circulating levels of calcium, phosphorus, sodium, potassium, iodine, and other ions serve important regulatory functions. Hormones do not circulate as solutions of pure amines, proteins, peptides, and steroids. Hormone-responsive cells live in a complex and continually changing environment of fuels and ions, and the regulations that occur in them are the results of the effects of both the hormonal and nonhormonal information in which they are bathed.

Evolution of Endocrine Systems

Hormones, hormone precursors, and many of the agents that mediate or modulate hormone action (receptors, second messengers, prostaglandins, and other related substances) have been found in bacteria, worms, insects, and plants. It is somewhat startling to learn that protozoa, fungi, and *E. coli* contain a molecule that cross-reacts with anti-insulin antibody and stimulates glucose oxidation in isolated fat cells. Its function in *E. coli* is unknown. What sea coral does with its prostaglandins is equally mysterious.

Some of the functions of the hormone second messenger, cyclic AMP, in primitive forms have been studied intensively. In the slime mold, which is an aggregation of cells that were once dispersed as individual amoebae, cAMP is the primary aggregating stimulus and is secreted into the medium when nutrients are in short supply. Similarly, in glucose-deprived *E. coli*, the same substance causes the derepression of the lac operon which enables the organism to metabolize galactose.

Some hormones acquired different functions as organisms became more complex. Prolactin, for example, is an important osmoregulating hormone in amphibia, but its most prominent function in mammals is in the physiology of lactation. Other hormones may have different functions in different tissues of the same organism, i.e., angiotensin stimulates the production of aldosterone by the adrenal and also plays an important role in the central nervous system as a regulator of thirst. The behavioral effects of antidiuretic hormone and ACTH, in addition to their effects in the kidney and adrenals, respectively, illustrate the same point.

In general, regulatory molecules evolved long before the metabolic processes they were destined to regulate. In Francois Jacob's appealing metaphor, Nature appears to behave like a provident tinker or handyman who hoards molecular tools that acquire new regulatory functions as new and more complex metabolic needs evolve.

Integrative Functions of Hormones

The endocrine glands are involved in all of the important life transactions of the organism.

DIFFERENTIATION

In the developing embryo, hormones play a crucial organizing role, most notably in differentiation of the generative tract (testosterone) and in differentiation of the CNS (thyroxine).

REPRODUCTION

Reproductive functions generally require hormones for their successful accomplishment. Fertilization, implantation, pregnancy, and lactation all involve the actions of many hormones in both male and female. The same hormones act in the male and the female to influence complementary functions, i.e., the differentiation and development of the spermatozoon and the ovum.

GROWTH AND DEVELOPMENT

Hormones are required for growth and development of the maturing individual. Growth hormone, thyroid hormones, and insulin are all required for optimal growth, and the inappropriate presence of insulin antagonists or sex steroids can inhibit growth.

ADAPTATION

Hormones are necessary for adaptation to the quantity and quality of food ingested, both acutely and over a longer time scale. Similarly, hormones are necessary for successful adaptations to changes in fluid and electrolyte availability in the environment.

AGING AND SENESCENCE

The inexorable process of aging is associated with diminished secretion of gonadal hormones in both the female and male, thought this is more obvious in the former than in the latter.

Classification of Hormones

The earliest chemical characterizations of hormones occurred in the early 20th century with the elucidation of the structures of the catecholamines. The golden age of steroid biochemistry, when the structures of the gonadal steroids were proved, took place in the 1930s. Within little more than a decade, the structures of estrogen, progesterone, testosterone, cortisol and adrenal androgen were solved.

Although much basic information about peptide chemistry existed before 1953, the modern era of amino acid sequencing of peptides and proteins began at about that time with reports on the structures of posterior pituitary peptides by du Vigneaud and his school. The first larger peptide for which an amino acid sequence was established was insulin. Sanger's pioneer work on insulin was a landmark not only in endocrinology but in all other subdivisions of biology. As the technology of peptide chemistry became more widely known, the structures of all of the peptides and proteins listed in Table 1–1 were described, and many of these substances have been synthesized.

In Table 1–1, the major sources of the hormones

TABLE 1–1.

Chemical Classification of Hormones

CHEMICAL CLASS	HORMONE (ABBREV.)	MAJOR SOURCE
Amines	Dopamine	CNS
	Norepinephrine	CNS, adrenal medulla
	Epinephrine	Adrenal medulla
	Melatonin	Pineal
Iodothyronines	Thyroxine (T_4)	Thyroid
	Triiodothyronine (T_3)	Peripheral tissues (thyroid)
Small peptides	Vasopressin (antidiuretic h.; ADH)	Post. pituitary
	Oxytocin	Post. pituitary
	Melanocyte-stimulating h. (MSH)	Pars intermedia
	Thyrotrophin-releasing h. (TRH)	Hypothal., CNS
	Gonadotrophin-releasing h. (GnRH, LHRH)	Hypothal., CNS
	Somatostatin (SRIF)	Hypothal., CNS, pancreatic islets
	CRF	Hypothal., CNS
	Somatocrinin (GRH, GRF)	Islet tumor, hypothal., CNS
	Angiotensins (A_2, A_3)	Blood (from precursor), CNS
Proteins	Insulin	β cells, pancreatic islets
	Glucagon	α cells, pancreatic islets
	Growth h. or somatotrophin (GH, STH)	Ant. pituitary
	Placental lactogen (PL)	Placenta
	Prolactin (PRL)	Ant. pituitary
	Parathyroid h. (PTH)	Parathyroid
	Beta lipotropin and enkephalin	Pituitary, CNS
	Calcitonin	C cells, thyroid
	Adrenocorticotrophic h. (ACTH)	Ant. pituitary
	Secretin	Gastrointestinal tract, CNS
	Cholecystokinin (CCK)	Gastrointestinal tract, CNS
	Gastrin	Gastrointestinal tract, CNS
	Gastric-inhibitory peptide (GIP)	Gastrointestinal tract
Glycoproteins	Follicle-stimulating h. (FSH)	Ant. pituitary
	Luteinizing hormone (LH)	Ant. pituitary
	Chorionic gonadotropin (CG)	Placenta
	Thyroid-stimulating h. (TSH)	Ant. pituitary
Steroids	Estrogens (E_2, E_3)	Ovary, placenta
	Progesterone (P)	Corpus luteum, placenta
	Testosterone (T)	Testis
	Dihydrotestosterone (DHT)	T-sensitive tissues
	Glucocorticoids	Adrenal cortex
	Aldosterone	Adrenal cortex
	Cholecalciferol (vit. D) metabolites	Liver, kidneys

listed also are given. However, recent studies on the cellular localization of many hormones have revealed that such peptides as ACTH, the hypothalamic releasing hormones, many gastrointestinal hormones, angiotensin, and enkephalin, all posterior pituitary hormones, occur in extrahypothalamic areas of the brain. These discoveries were made possible by the development of the powerful method of immunofluorescence, by which intracellular hormones can be highly selectively labeled and displayed by covalently binding a fluorescent probe to a specific antibody. Although little is now known about the precise function of CNS peptidergic neurons, there is a strong possibility that they may be important modulators of the functions of CNS neurons. Classification of a substance as a "hormone" is no guarantee that it will not turn up in some other capacity in the future.

The special class of glycoprotein hormones enumerated in Table 1–1 is worth noting. These substances are dimeric proteins, and all of them share an identical alpha subunit. The elucidation of the structures of these glycoproteins has proved to be especially important in the development of radioimmunoassay methods for their detection since discriminating antibodies can be made to their distinctive beta subunits.

Sometimes chemical classification is less useful than another type of classification, e.g., according to *gland of origin*. There are at least six hormones produced by cells of the anterior pituitary gland: prolactin (PRL), LH, follicle-stimulating hormone (FSH), adrenocorticotrophin (ACTH), thyrotrophin (TSH) and growth hormone (GH, or STH). In addition to these, β lipotropin, a precursor of endogenously produced peptides with morphine-like properties, has assumed a prominent place among pituitary hormones.

Specific subgroups that are structurally related are often discussed together, e.g., the catecholamines: dopamine, norepinephrine and epinephrine, or the thyroid hormones, thyroxine (T_4) and triiodothyronine (T_3).

Some hormones play regulatory roles in certain aspects of physiology and therefore are conveniently grouped *according to function*. Examples of these are vasopressin (ADH), aldosterone, and angiotensin, and atrial natriuretic factors (ANF), which collaborate in maintenance of fluid and electrolyte homeostasis. Similarly, hormones secreted by cells of the islets of Langerhans are not chemically related but are closely related functionally: insulin, glucagon, and somatostatin. Parathyroid hormone, calcitonin, and the cholecalciferols (vitamin D derivatives) are all important in homeostatic regulation of body calcium.

Hormone systems may involve diverse hormones of different chemical types. For example, the gonadotrophic system in the female includes the following:

1. One or more CNS neurotransmitters.

2. Peptidergic neurons that secrete gonadotrophin-releasing and -inhibiting factors.

3. Three different types of anterior pituitary cells: one that secretes LH, one that produces FSH and one that is the source of PRL.

4. Steroid hormones produced in specific ovarian cells and in the corpus luteum (estrogen and progesterone).

5. Target tissues in the generative organs, the breast and the brain.

6. An FSH inhibitor produced in the ovary.

Note that this system uses chemical messengers, which are monoamines, small peptides, glycoproteins, and steroids. Similar systems are constructed around the testis, the adrenal cortex, and the thyroid.

Shared Characteristics of Hormones

Certain generalizations may be made about all hormones, whatever their chemical class. Among these are the following:

REACTIONS IN SENSITIVE CELLS

Hormones do not initiate reactions in sensitive cells. This is a restatement of the principle that the capacity of the responsive cell to be stimulated or inhibited by a hormone was built into the cell when it differentiated. The hormone, by interacting with its receptor, initiates a sequence of events, which collectively constitute the response. Often the response is a coordinated one that involves acceleration of some biochemical processes and concurrent inhibition of others. A closer examination of the cellular mechanism of action of hormones will be given in the next section.

SECRETION RATES

Hormones are secreted at variable rates that are determined by circulating substrates, ions, neural transmitters, or other hormones. Some, like pituitary growth hormone and ACTH, show striking diurnal fluctuations that are linked to sleep-awakening cycles. Others (gonadotropins) are secreted in complex patterns that are set by internal "clocks" that function over many time scales: (1) the lifetime of the individual (embryonic life, childhood, puberty, reproductive period, menopause, senescence); (2) pregnancy-lactation cycles; (3) menstrual cycle; (4) pulsatile secretion with a regular periodicity measured in minutes.

METABOLIC INACTIVATION/EXCRETION

Hormones are continually lost from the body by processes of metabolic inactivation and/or excretion. Thus a constant, basal hormone production must be maintained to compensate for loss. It follows that the production rate must be increased to compensate for temporary increases in hormone requirement. Thus the processes of hormone *secretion* and hormone *synthesis,* although they can be dissociated from one another in some experimental circumstances, are closely linked phenomena.

INFORMATION TRANSFER SYSTEMS

Hormones function in closed-loop systems of information transfer. Operationally, this means that when a hormone begins to act on a sensitive cell or system of cells, a "turn-off" signal of greater or lesser strength is also initiated. Feedback inhibition of a stimulated gland may occur as the result of an *increased concentration of another hormone* (e.g., when thyroxine, elicited by an increase in pituitary TSH secretion, feeds back on the pituitary thyrotrophe to prevent its stimulation by TRH from the hypothalamus). Another general mechanism by which an activated gland can be back-inhibited is by *correction of the physiologic disequilibrium that originally activated the gland.* We will examine a number of examples of this paradigm in later sections, which deal with fuel homeostasis, calcium regulation, and electrolyte balance.

TIME SCALES

Hormones act on different time scales. If one arranges chemical messengers according to the time scales over which they work, from seconds to days, the following rank order is apparent:
Neurotransmitters (milliseconds)
Peptides (seconds-minutes)
Proteins and glycoproteins (minutes-hours)
Steroids (hours)
Iodothyronines (days)
This description should be qualified by the observation that a peptide or protein hormone whose effect may be readily detectable in a few minutes may exert its action over a period of hours or days if it is continuously present.

Conceptual Framework for Study of Hormones

In our study of each hormone, we would like to have certain information.

PRECISE CHEMICAL STRUCTURE AND PROPERTIES OF HORMONES

In many cases, a knowledge of the chemistry of a hormone involves not only the naturally occurring substance but also synthetic variants produced by the organic chemist: synthetic analogues often have desirable properties that are absent from the natural hormone. They can be more or less potent than the original hormone or they can display selective effects of the original while eliminating undesirable effects. Sometimes analogues are found to exhibit antihormone actions that are useful both in research and in the clinic. The use of a series of analogues may help to elucidate structure-biologic activity relationships.

BIOSYNTHESIS OF HORMONES

Peptide hormones are synthesized on ribosomes affiliated with the endoplasmic reticulum and packaged into secretory vesicles in the Golgi apparatus. It is now apparent that, in all cases, a peptide larger than the finished hormone is translated from the mRNA presented to the ribosomes. At this stage, the translation product can be described as *pre-pro-hormone.* The *pre* sequence consists of hydrophobic amino acids and is believed to facilitate the extrusion of the protein through the lipid wall of the endoplasmic reticulum into the lumen. The *pre* sequence of amino acids is cleaved from the remainder of the original translation product very soon after it enters the lumen. In the case of insulin, *pro* is split from *hormone* by an enzyme within the secretory granule. The possible functional significance of proinsulin is discussed in Chapter 14.

The special case of synthesis of thyroid hormones will be considered later. However, these hormones are derived from hydrolysis of a high molecular weight glycoprotein, thyroglobulin. This prohormone differs from most in being stored, not in secretory granules within the cells that synthesize it, but as large colloid droplets shared by many epithelial cells that constitute a follicle. Thyroglobulin, as well as the glycoprotein hormones, illustrates the point that post-translational modification of a newly synthesized protein may be an important feature of hormone synthesis. This process, which involves the addition of oligosaccharides to the protein, is presumed to occur in the lumen of the endoplasmic reticulum and in the Golgi apparatus.

In all cases, protein and peptide hormones are stored in secretory vesicles or as hormone precursor (thyroglobulin). The steroid hormone-producing cells in the ovary, corpus luteum, testicular Leydig cell, and adrenal cortical cell do not characteristically store large amounts of prepackaged hormone. Instead they store hormone precursor, cholesterol ester, in the form of lipid droplets. In the case of these hormone-producing cells, the signal for hormone release is very tightly coupled to that for acceleration of hormone synthesis. As the hormone newly synthesized from stored cholesterol is formed, it is promptly detectable in venous blood draining the organ.

Hormone Secretion

Identifiable signals elicit the release of the hormone under study. These may be few and highly selective, as in the case of parathyroid hormone, or many and intricately interrelated, as in the case of insulin, or aldosterone release. As we consider each hormone, we will attempt to assess the relative importance of release signals, since the endocrine gland's response to signals often helps to define the role of its hormonal product in the vital economy of the intact individual.

Inhibition of Hormone Secretion

There are at least two categories of hormone release inhibitors: (1) those that may function physiologically in regulation of hormone release and (2) pharmacologic agents that may be helpful in elucidating the nature of the hormone release mechanism. An example of the first type of inhibitor is the feedback inhibition of ACTH release by cortisol or the inhibition of insulin release by sympathetic nerve stimulation. An example of the second is as follows: if the microtubular system of a cell is believed to be involved in extrusion of hormone from storage vesicles, failure to secrete the hormone on signal by a colchicine-treated cell (colchicine is a microtubule toxin) is taken as circumstantial evidence that unimpaired microtubular function is required for the secretory process.

Circulating Form of the Hormone

Steroid hormones and thyroid hormones are transported by carrier proteins. The hormone bound to the carrier at any instant is biologically inactive; the concentration of *free* hormone determines the effective hormone environment for responsive cells. Since carrier-protein concentrations for both steroids and thyroid hormones are known to fluctuate in some physiologic and pharmacologic circumstances, it is important to examine the biology of hormone-carrier proteins.

Nature of the Hormone Receptor

The response of a cell to a hormone is initiated by the interaction between the hormone and a stereospecific receptor or discriminator. Some recent advances in our understanding of hormone receptors, for peptide, steroid, and thyroid hormones, are presented in the section on hormone action (Chapters 2, 3, and 4).

Cellular Mechanism of Action of Hormones

The responses of hormone-sensitive cells to hormones have been described in a fast and rapidly growing literature. Fortunately it is now possible to discern response patterns, which we can begin to describe in prototypical terms. This is the subject of Chapters 2, 3, and 4.

Relation of Hormone Action to Vital Economy of Intact Organism

How do cellular effects of a hormone fit into the vital economy of the intact organism? This question and its answers pervade our contemplation of the mechanisms involved in hormone action and the physiologic regulation of hormone concentrations. Perhaps the following discussion will help to emphasize the interconnections between and among the levels of organization of the intact person or animal.

Fragmentation and Synthesis: Reductionism and Holism

Metabolic control mechanisms, whether neural or endocrine, operate at many levels of organization, each of which is part of a hierarchical order. In descending order from the most complex to the least, these levels may be represented as follows:
1. Intact person or animal
2. Organ system
3. Organ
4. Cell
5. Cell organelle
6. Enzyme system

7. Individual enzyme
8. Molecule
9. Atom
10. Free radicals and subatomic particles.

HIERARCHY OF LEVELS OF ORGANIZATION

Intact Person or Animal (Holistic Biology)

Hormones have profound effects on behavior and, in fact, are essential for CNS function. Frequently a patient with a disturbance in endocrine function may appear to have "problems in living" and may be seen first by a psychiatrist before the underlying endocrine nature of the difficulty is appreciated. Conversely, some individuals who manifest extreme anxiety and apprehension may resemble patients with hyperthyroidism, though careful laboratory tests reveal no evidence of thyroid dysfunction. The CNS absolutely requires the presence of thyroid hormone for its development. Deficiency of thyroid hormone in the neonatal period has profound behavioral consequences for the individual.

A long and steadily lengthening list of hormones affect behavior, either when inadequate amounts are available or when they are present in excess. Among these are hypothalamic releasing hormones, gonadotrophins (including prolactin), sex steroids, glucocorticoids, insulin, aldosterone, angiotensin, parathyroid hormone, and cholecystokinin. ACTH peptides 4–10 have been shown to accelerate the acquisition of a conditioned response and to delay its extinction in animals. There is a large volume of literature devoted to the subject of the behavioral effects of hormone deficiencies and excesses. The technology of behavioral research has been used effectively by students of these problems. However, all pertinent observations of behavior are not necessarily made at the level of organization of the intact animal: studies on animals with sharply localized lesions in the CNS, or observations on unanesthetized animals with chronically implanted stimulating electrodes, have helped to elucidate mechanisms involved in behavioral changes, particularly those associated with eating and drinking behavior. Behavioral observations have been supplemented by autoradiographic and immunocytologic analyses of CNS distribution of receptors for hormones and drugs.

Historically, useful information at the level of organization of the intact person or animal was obtained by means of the *balance experiment*. The balance idea may be used in relation to total energy intake and expenditure; water and its primary electrolytes, sodium and potassium; calcium and phosphorus; and many other biologically important materials. The principle in all cases is the same: a careful inventory of intake and outgo permits conclusions concerning net loss or gain of the constituent under study. We speak of "positive nitrogen balance" when nitrogen intake exceeds nitrogen loss by all possible routes of elimination. By the same token, "negative nitrogen balance" signifies failure of intake to equal total loss. Important information about hormone deficits, replacements, and excesses can be obtained by this method, since it is possible to do this type of experiment on unanesthetized, unrestrained animals or on patients in suitable metabolic wards.

Organ System

The effects of hormone lack or excess can be studied in diffusely distributed organ systems that do not lend themselves readily to isolation from the whole organism. Examples of these systems are the nervous system, peripheral vascular system, reticuloendothelial system, and hematopoietic system. For example, effects of hormone deprivation and replacement may be reflected in changes in the EEG, in blood pressure, in phagocytic activity of reticuloendothelial cells, and in the blood picture and bone marrow histology.

Organ

When observations are made in the intact individual, it is not always easy to determine what contribution is made to the total effect by a particular organ. For example, elevation of the blood glucose level could be due either to a decreased rate of removal of glucose from the blood by peripheral tissues or to an excessive release of glucose into the blood by the liver. Arteriovenous difference techniques have been used to assess the function of a particular organ. If one measures the concentration of a substance such as glucose in the blood entering an organ and in the venous blood draining it while simultaneously estimating the rate of blood flow, it is possible to calculate either the extent of substrate removal or its addition by the organ. The recent perfection of safe intravascular catheterization techniques in human beings has enabled investigators to perform elegant experiments of this sort in people. Some of these will be described in some detail in Chapter 13.

Another commonly used technique involves the isolation or removal of the *organ* of an experimental animal so that it can be selectively *perfused* with fluids of known composition at flow rates that can be maintained accurately by specially designed perfusion pumps. Many organ perfusion studies have been done, particularly in the heart, liver, and kidney, but other organs such as the pancreas and the fat pad have also been perfused successfully. This technique affords the opportunity to compare the metabolic activity and hormone responsiveness of an organ removed from a hormone-deprived animal with that obtained from an intact control or from a hormone-treated animal.

Much valuable information has been obtained from study of *thinly sliced fragments* of specific organs such as liver and kidney. Although such preparations are useful, the trauma to the tissue involved in preparing them is considerable, and generally their metabolic performance capabilities tend to be less than those of well-perfused organs or dispersed cell preparations (see next section).

One interesting way of studying a mini-organ—the islets of Langerhans of the pancreas—involves the preparation and harvesting of many islets by gently treating the rat pancreas with enzymes that separate them from adjacent exocrine pancreatic tissue. Islets can then be studied either in incubation vessels or by the technique of *perifusion*. In this method, islets are retained on a suitable porous platform and perifusate can be dripped on them continuously and collected. The composition of the perifusate can be changed abruptly, and the minute-to-minute release of hormones (e.g., insulin and glucagon) can be measured. Again the sensitivity of radioimmunoassay methods made possible the performance of experiments of this type.

During recent years, endocrinologists have begun to exploit the techniques of *tissue* and *organ culture* in the analysis of their problems. The advantages of this technique are many, most notably the ability of the experimenter to study a "pure culture" of eukaryotic cells after the manner of the microbiologist observing a pure culture of microorganisms. Later we will see how the introduction of *genetic analysis of hormonal responses in cultured cells* by the Tomkins school, by A. G. Gilman, and by others, has proved to be a powerful tool in elucidation of the cellular mechanisms of actions of hormones.

The Cell

In the tradition of Schleiden, Schwann, and Virchow, the endocrinologist is obsessed by the cell and its hormone responses. The isolated, dispersed adipocyte and its responses to lipolytic and antilipolytic hormones must rank as one of the most intensively studied eukaryotic cells in history. These cells are prepared according to a technique introduced by Rodbell: thin fragments of adipose tissue are gently treated with collagenase, which separates cells from each other. They can be harvested readily because their high triglyceride content makes them float in a centrifuge tube. More recently, similar techniques have been introduced for the study of a variety of dispersed cell preparations, including adrenal, pituitary, bone and pancreatic islet cells, as well as hepatocytes.

There was a time when the morphologic sciences and biochemistry existed independently of one another. However, developments in electron microscopy, autoradiography, histochemistry and immunocytology have brought about an ecumenical union of the two fields. The beginnings of endocrinology in the United States were rooted in histology, and more recently morphologic techniques have been applied to endocrine problems with striking success. For example, the electron microscopist can distinguish among the many secretory cells of the anterior pituitary gland on the basis of their structural characteristics and the appearance of their secretory granules. Central nervous system cells that selectively concentrate certain steroid hormones can be identified readily. Cells that secrete particular hormones can be picked out of a crowd by the technique of immunofluorescence microscopy, in which an antibody to the cell's hormonal product is covalently linked to a fluorescent probe, which can be seen with an appropriate lighting system.

Cell Organelles

In Virchow's day, the cell was the end of the line of the ultimate reductionist. Now, it is a new macrocosm consisting of parts that themselves contain elaborately organized constituents. Each of these parts figures prominently in our attempts to understand the mechanisms of action of hormones.

The *plasma membrane,* at once a barrier between a cell and its environment and its main communication channel to the outside world, is now the central object of attention of regiments of investigators. Some endocrinologists unapologetically specialize in the study of the plasma membrane, and with good reason: this structure contains many hormone receptors, ion and substrate transport channels, enzymes that generate "second messengers," and no doubt much else. What appears to be a collection of inert potatoes in the familiar Singer-Nicholson fluid mosaic model of the plasma membrane turns out to be a dynamic congregation of molecules that exert important control over intracellular events and participate prominently in the adaptations of cells to changing environments. We will have occasion to return to the plasma membrane later.

The *nucleus,* which contains most of the genetic material in the cell, is intimately involved in hormone action. Current theories of the mechanism of action of steroid hormones and of thyroxine focus on nuclear events. Peptide and protein hormones also have prominent effects on the nucleus.

The *mitochondrion,* the main energy generator in the cell, understandably plays an important role in the actions of hormones involved in the control of intermediary metabolism, i.e., insulin and glucagon. It also provides energy necessary for the responses to many other hormones, e.g., those that involve stimulation of secretory processes or of protein synthesis. Alterations in mitochondrial function are prominent features of hyper- and hypothyroid states.

The *ribosomes* and *protein synthetic machinery* are central in many hormone effects that require protein synthesis. This is true not only of steroids and thyroid hormones but also of ACTH, LH, FSH, and many others.

The *endoplasmic reticulum* and its affiliated organelles, the Golgi apparatus, are especially involved in protein hormone biosynthesis, as well as in synthesis of plasma membrane components.

Lysosomes are important in the turnover of macromolecular cell constituents and are also implicated in the inflammatory process. Hormones, prostaglandins, and leukotrienes are intimately involved in the biology of inflammation (see Chapter 11).

Microtubules and *microfilaments* have been implicated both in hormone secretory processes and in the mechanisms of action of hormones.

The technique of *density gradient centrifugation* has been used widely in the study of cell organelles, particularly membranes. By following membrane fractions with marker enzymes—enzymes that occur distinctively in the membrane under study—it has been possible to prepare purified membranes that can be examined by a variety of techniques. In fact, Schwartz and colleagues have prepared luminal and contraluminal plasma membranes from kidney tubular cells and have studied their special characteristics (see Chapter 6).

Enzyme Systems

In addition to the visible subcellular organization of cells, there is an invisible kind of organization in the interrelations of enzymes in functional systems or metabolic pathways. Some, such as those involved in the process of electron transport and oxidative phos-

phorylation, are architecturally articulated with one another within the mitochondrial membrane—an arrangement that Lehninger has called "solid state enzymology." Others have been localized at or near the cell surface. Still others are affiliated with the endoplasmic reticulum. Many enzymes are found in what is operationally defined as the *cytosol,* or that part of a homogenate that remains as supernatant after centrifuging at $100,000 \times$ gravity. Of course this does not mean that enzymes in the extramitochondrial, extramembranous parts of the cell are randomly distributed. For all we know, enzyme arrangements may be elaborately compartmentalized in the cell gel, though we may be accustomed to thinking of them as "soluble."

One of the main consequences of hormone action is to *alter the pattern of substrate traffic through multienzyme systems.* This will become one of the major themes of our discussion of the effects of hormones, particularly insulin and glucagon, on the processes of lipogenesis, gluconeogenesis, and ketogenesis in the liver (see Chapter 14).

Individual Enzyme

The importance of individual enzymes in hormone action will shortly become evident. In the study of endocrinology, the impact of a single enzyme deficiency on the intact organism may be seen in human mutants who lack either an enzyme important for the biosynthesis of a hormone or an enzyme in a cell that is normally responsive to a hormone. Such inborn errors of metabolism have been studied extensively in the thyroid system, the adrenal cortical system, and the parathyroid-cholecalciferol system.

The Molecule

The term "molecular biology" has been largely appropriated by students of the central dogma: DNA → RNA → protein synthesis. Endocrinology is nothing if not molecular, even when hormones may act by affecting events only indirectly related to the genetic apparatus of the cell. Even when it is not yet possible to provide a precise molecular description of a hormone mechanism, our theories are formulated on the basis of properties of individual molecules, both macromolecules and substrate-sized molecules. Our discussion of the cellular mechanisms of action of hormones (Chapters 2, 3, and 4) will represent attempts to come as close as possible to describing hormone action in molecular terms.

Atoms and Ions

It is impossible to describe hormone action, or some of the consequences of hormone deprivation, without stressing the importance of all sorts of atoms, particularly electrolytes and the constituents of water. Sodium, potassium, phosphorus, calcium, and other ions are crucially involved both as regulated quantities and as participants in regulatory processes.

Free Radicals and Subatomic Particles

At least one hormone has, as one of its actions, the effect of stimulating the production of a free radical from an ion: peroxidation of iodide → iodinium, which occurs in the thyroid cell in response to TSH, is fundamental to the action of TSH, since it permits iodination of thyronine groups in thyroglobulin. If this peroxidation fails to occur, as in certain inborn errors of thyroid metabolism, thyroid hormone deficiency results.

Hormones are intimately involved in processes that involve electron transfer (as in the mitochondrion or the P450 hydroxylation system involved in steroid hormone biosynthesis). Many enzymes that participate in systems that generate reducing equivalents for biosynthetic reactions (lipogenesis, gluconeogenesis) are under hormonal control, directly or indirectly.

Some experimenters may begin by making an observation at the level of organization of the whole animal and find themselves asking ever more pointed questions until they are dealing with the original problem at the molecular level. Most of the history of endocrinology describes this sequence of events. Others may begin with a "purely" molecular problem, which turns out to have implications for the whole organism. For example, a variant of hemoglobin, A_{1c}, was first found because its physical characteristics differed from those of hemoglobin. Then it was found to contain glucose, covalently bound. Finally, the concentration of this form of hemoglobin was found to reflect the integrated blood glucose level of diabetic patients over the several weeks preceding the time of sampling. Thus, a primary molecular discovery may become a useful index of the efficacy of blood glucose control in diabetes (see Chapter 14). It is the constant interaction between students of the whole and students of the fragments at all levels of biologic organization that produces interesting and useful new information.

Methods

When powerful new morphologic, chemical, electrophysiologic, immunologic, and other procedures are developed, they are promptly applied to the solutions of endocrine problems. For example, in the 1930s and 40s, sophisticated methods were developed for studying steroids. This resulted in great advances in our understanding of steroid hormone structure and biosynthesis. In the late 40s and 50s, the availability of radioisotopes produced a quantum leap in our understanding of the iodine cycle, many aspects of intermediary metabolism, ion movements, and much else. The far-reaching effects of advances in peptide and protein chemistry have already been mentioned. Most recently, the combination of polyacrylamide gel electrophoresis and autoradiography has been used imaginatively in the study of many proteins, including hormone receptors. Concurrently with all of these impressive advances in chemistry has been an ever more rewarding use of histochemistry, immunohistochemistry, and electron microscopy.

Variations on the theme of chromatography—column, thin layer, paper, multidimensional, gas-liquid (with or without mass spectrometry), high pressure liquid—have been applied by endocrinologists as soon as they became available. Historically, they were important not only in the sequencing of peptides and proteins but also in the study of lipids (notably, the prostaglandins and related substances), carbohydrates, and amines.

As the techniques of molecular biology developed, mostly in prokaryotic organisms, students of hormone action quickly applied them to their problems. Now, recombinant DNA technology is being used not only by investigators of the mechanisms of action of hormones but also in the manufacture of protein hormones (insulin, growth hormone) for use as replacement therapy in deficiency states. In fact, it is difficult to think of a biochemical or physiological method that has *not* been used by explorers of hormone-related problems.

Measurement of Hormones

BIOASSAY

In order to discover hormones, it was necessary to develop reproducible methods of assay for them, and for many years the *bioassay* was the only feasible method of estimating hormone levels. Although these methods were often cumbersome, they were and continue to be extraordinarily effective (witness the recent discovery of somatostatin by Guillemin et al.). The principle of all bioassays is the same: an assay system (whole animal, organ, fragment of tissue, cell, enzyme system) is standardized with known amounts of the hormone under study, and a standard curve is constructed. The activity of the unknown in the system may then be compared with that of known standards, e.g., testosterone stimulates the growth of the prostate gland of an immature or castrate rat in a dose-dependent manner. Therefore it is possible by means of this test to express the androgenic potency of an unknown substance by comparing it with testosterone.

Are bioassay methods out of date now that newer methods of hormone assay (see below) are available? One cannot be aware of recent work by Vane and colleagues on prostaglandins and come to this conclusion (see Chapter 4). Moreover, bioassay methods must continue to be useful, since radioimmunoassay (see below) may measure substances that have no biologic activity. Therefore, it is often necessary to make parallel measurements of radioimmunoassayable and biologic activity.

For many years, *chemical methods* were the major procedures used in the study of hormones. They are still extremely useful, notably for estimating metabolites of hormones such as thyroid hormones, steroids and catecholamines, prostaglandin metabolites, and other small molecules (see "Methods" above).

RADIOLIGAND ASSAY

During the course of studies on the mechanism of insulin resistance in certain diabetic patients, Berson and Yalow discovered that some of their patients had antibodies to insulin when they injected tracer doses of radioactively labeled insulin with increasing amounts of "cold" insulin. They observed that radioactive insulin and nonradioactive hormone appeared to be competing for antibody-binding sites. Realizing that this competition could well provide the basis for a quantitative assay for circulating insulin, they began a systematic study of the interaction of labeled and unlabeled insulin with antibody; this culminated in their brilliant development of the first feasible radioimmunoassay method. This methodologic breakthrough had for modern endocrinology an impact roughly comparable to that of the invention of the telescope for 17th century astronomy. The principles developed by Berson and Yalow have not only been applied to an ever-growing variety of biologically important substances but also underlie many recent discoveries in the field of hormone-receptor interaction. It is now possible to measure with great accuracy as little as 1 $\mu\mu$g or less of a specific hormone in the presence of a several *billion*-fold higher concentration of other proteins and peptides in plasma. Not only can these minute concentrations be detected: *minute-to-minute* changes in concentration can be followed with great accuracy. The best way to appreci-

ate the significance of these methods is to understand that we are talking about accurate measurements of 0.0000000001 gm of hormone in 7.5000000000 gm of protein and that the hormone (if it is a peptide) is composed of combinations of the same amino acids that are found in the total protein. Moreover, with some luck it is possible to produce such potent and specific antiserums that they can be used at dilutions as high as 1:4,000,000, which means that a single antibody-producing animal can yield enough antibody for many millions of assays. In some cases the binding protein for the substance to be measured is not an antibody but a specific protein that has a high affinity for the substance (e.g., a membrane receptor or a carrier protein).

The principle of all radioligand assay (radioimmunoassay or assay by means of nonantibody-binding protein) is the same in that it is necessary to incorporate a method of separating bound (B) from free (F) hormone. In their original method, Berson and Yalow accomplished this by means of paper electrophoresis. The radioactivity was recoverable in two spots, one B and one F, and it was therefore possible to express the ratio of B to F as the integrated activity, one peak divided by that of the other.

Other investigators (Hales and Randle) have found it convenient to separate B from F by a *double antibody method*. It is often true that the antibody-hormone complex, $H \cdot Ab_1$ (B), is comparatively soluble. However, it can be precipitated by a *second* antibody (Ab_2) directed against the first (Ab_1). The separation of B from F then proceeds as follows:

1. $H(F) + H^* Ab_1 (B) \rightarrow H \cdot H^* Ab_1 (B)$ (soluble) + $H^* (F)$
2. $H \cdot H^* Ab_1 (B) + Ab_2 \rightarrow H \cdot H^* Ab_1 \cdot Ab_2 (B)$ (insoluble)

(H = cold hormone; F = Free; H* = radioactive hormone; Ab_1 = guinea pig anti-H; B = bound; Ab_2 = rabbit anti-guinea pig globulin).

The binding sites are saturated with a radioactively labeled form of the substance to be measured. If the hormone under study is a protein, care is taken to insure that the labeled hormone retains its biologic activity. The antibody-radioactive hormone complex is incubated in the cold with the unlabeled or cold hormone to be measured. Although the antibody or other binding protein has a high affinity for the hormone, constant association and dissociation of the antibody-hormone complex occur. The cold temperature prevents denaturation of the reactants. As a result of the competition between radioactive and cold hormone for binding sites, the ratio of antibody-bound *labeled* hormone to antibody-bound *unlabeled* hormone is diminished as the concentration of unlabeled

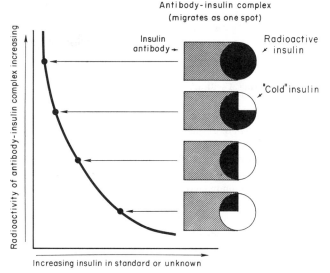

FIG 1–2.
Schematic description of principle of typical Berson-Yalow radioimmunoassay. (From Berson SA, Yalow RS: *Diabetes* 1965; 14:549 [Banting lecture]. Used by permission.)

hormone is increased (Fig 1–2). Solutions containing known amounts of unlabeled hormone are used to construct a standard curve. The concentration in the unknown can then be read on the curve.

If a comparison between only antibody-bound hormone of known and unknown is required, the precipitate can be washed free of F (both H and H*) and counted. Other methods of separating B from F involve covalent attachment of antibody to beads or to the inner surface of test tubes. Sometimes F is selectively adsorbed by adsorbents that do not remove B.

The principle of radioimmunoassay has been extended to some small molecules such as drugs, steroids, cyclic nucleotides, and thyroid hormones, to name a few. These small molecules are covalently bound to protein molecules (haptenes), and an antibody complex of extraordinary discriminative power is produced. For example, antibodies are able to identify 17β-estradiol and reject 17α-estradiol, two compounds that differ only in the planar projection of a single H^+.

One of the main advantages of the availability of radioimmunoassay procedures has been that it is now possible to obtain minute-to-minute measurements of changes in hormone concentration in human subjects with minimal inconvenience and discomfort. When one works with experimental animal models, it is often necessary to extrapolate the results to the human, but if the measurement is initially made in the human being there is no need to extrapolate.

BIBLIOGRAPHY

Alberts B, Bray D, Lewis J, et al: *The Molecular Biology of the Cell.* New York, Garland Publishing Co, Inc, 1983.

Barrington EJW: *An Introduction to General and Comparative Endocrinology,* ed 2. Oxford, Clarendon Press, 1975.

Bloom W, Fawcett DW: *A Textbook of Histology.* Philadelphia, WB Saunders Co, 1968.

Bondy PK, Rosenberg LE (eds): *Diseases of Metabolism,* ed 7. Philadelphia, WB Saunders Co, 1974.

DeGroot LJ (ed): *Endocrinology,* vol 3. New York, Grune & Stratton, 1979.

Felig P, Baxter JD, Broadus AE, et al (eds): *Endocrinology and Metabolism.* New York, McGraw-Hill Book Co, 1981.

Gilman AG, Goodman LS, Rall TW, et al (eds): *Goodman and Gilman's The Pharmacological Basis of Therapeutics,* ed 7. New York, Macmillan Publishing Co, 1985.

Greenspan FS, Forsham PH: *Basic and Clinical Endocrinology.* Los Altos, California, Lange Medical Publications, 1983.

Martin CR: *Endocrine Physiology.* New York, Oxford University Press, 1985.

Wilson JD, Foster DW (eds): *Williams Textbook of Endocrinology,* ed 7. Philadelphia, WB Saunders Co, 1985.

Zubay G (ed): *Biochemistry.* Reading, Massachusetts, Addison-Wesley Publishing Co, 1983.

PART II

The Cellular Mechanisms of Action of Hormones

2

Steroid Hormones

A discussion of endocrinology can begin either at the level of organization of the intact organism or at the cellular level. A description can be given of signals that elicit hormone secretion, fluctuations in blood hormone concentrations, and the overall physiologic effects of hormones without attributing more than "black-box" characteristics to the individual cells. Recent advances in our knowledge of hormone action at the cellular level have revealed recognizable patterns of response in many different types of cells to a variety of hormones. If we can understand certain prototypical mechanisms of hormone action at the outset, the problem of presenting distinctive features of the mechanism of action of each hormone later will be greatly simplified.

The Unstated Assumption

In all discussions of hormone action, there is an _unstated assumption_ that is both a powerful conceptual tool and a confession of ignorance: the assumption that _hormone effects are achieved by means of conformational changes in strategically placed protein molecules in cells._ The proteins may function as hormone receptors; as transducing elements between the receptor and some effector enzyme protein; as enzyme proteins; as activators or inhibitors of enzymes; or as components of membrane transport systems. All hormone actions on all hormone-sensitive cells are conceivable as a complex series of coordinated changes in shape of an array of cell-specific proteins. That we are almost totally ignorant of the precise changes in three-dimensional structure of the proteins involved in hormone action does not detract from the power of the concept of such changes in the construction of hypotheses on the mechanisms of hormone action.

The primary amino acid sequence of each protein contains the information necessary for it to assume its secondary and tertiary structure, i.e., its helical and nonhelical domains and its three-dimensional globular or ovoid structure. The quaternary structure, or the aggregation of subunits, is determined by the shapes of the individual units. The biologic activity of a protein is determined by its tertiary and quaternary conformation. Generally, tertiary and quaternary conformation may be altered by one of the following:

1. _Allosteric modulators,_ which bind noncovalently to a protein at some distance from its active site.

2. _Covalent modulators,_ such as phosphate, which are attached to proteins by kinases and must be detached by phosphatases. (The importance of control by reversible phosphorylation of strategically placed proteins will be discussed more in Chapter 3.) The different activity states usually are represented as reversible, thus:

$$Inactive \rightleftarrows Active$$

$$\square \quad \overset{or}{\rightleftarrows} \quad \bigcirc$$

$$b \quad \overset{or}{\rightleftarrows} \quad a$$

In the case of some enzymes, intermediate states of activity may be inferred from kinetic analyses between the fully inactive state and the fully active one. Much information has accumulated about the structural requirements for biologic activity and receptor binding for both steroid and nonsteroid hormones. Gross changes in the physical characteristics of steroid-receptor complexes have been described. But so far there is no precise information about any of the modifications in three-dimensional or quaternary structure of any protein involved in the action of any hormone. Yet if we were to eliminate the _inference_ of protein conformational change from our consideration of hormone action, there would be very little to discuss.

Time Scales of Regulation

If an enzyme functions at a metabolic switch point in a reaction sequence, its activity can be changed in two ways: (1) the total number of enzyme molecules may be unchanged but the activity may be increased or decreased by an allosteric or covalently bound modulator (such as PO^{4-}), resulting in a change in affinity of the enzyme for a reactant; and (2) there may be an increase in the total number of enzyme molecules, which may be subject to the same kinds of modulator control that prevailed before the increase in enzyme molecular population occurred. We describe the first of these paradigms as *acute* regulation and the second as *long-range* or *chronic* regulation. Obviously, in order for an increase in the population of enzyme molecules to occur, there must either be an increased rate of enzyme synthesis or a decreased rate of enzyme degradation, or some combination of these. In the following discussion we shall encounter many examples of acute and chronic regulation *not only of metabolic pathways but also of components of the regulatory machinery, which are themselves regulated.*

History

On gross anatomical and histologic evidence alone, it was obvious that estrogens and androgens stimulate protein synthesis in target organs. In the 1950s, G. Mueller described accumulation of ribonucleic acid (RNA), protein and deoxyribonucleic acid (DNA) in estrogen-stimulated tissues. Later, Mueller and Gorski performed the first inhibitor analysis of estrogen action and demonstrated that most of the effects of estrogen were blocked by a translation inhibitor (puromycin) and a transcription inhibitor (actinomycin D).

In 1960, Karlson and Clever demonstrated the sequential "puffing" pattern in giant chromosomes of insect larvae following injection of small amounts of a steroid hormone, ecdysone. Autoradiographic studies showed that the "puffs" observed were sites of vigorous RNA synthesis, presumably DNA mediated. Karlson formally stated the hypothesis that was implicit in Mueller's inhibitor studies, i.e., steroid hormones stimulate or activate specific gene sites to produce tissue-specific messenger RNAs (mRNAs), which then participate in the synthesis of a distinctive pattern of proteins. Synthesis of ribosomal and transfer RNAs is also stimulated. This remains a succinct statement of our current hypothesis, though there are coordinate effects of steroid hormones that may not involve transcription (see discussion below).

Shortly afterward, a technologic advance occurred that resulted in a landmark experiment. Tritium-labeled estradiol of very high radioactivity became available. This made it possible for E. V. Jensen and colleagues to administer labeled estradiol to rats in physiologic doses (i.e., microgram quantities) and to follow the tissue distribution of the steroid in tissues and blood. They discovered that the target tissues—uterus and vagina—selectively concentrated the labeled hormone and retained it far longer than did other tissues—indeed, long after the concentration in the blood had fallen to imperceptible levels. They also were the first to demonstrate the binding of labeled estradiol to a specific receptor protein. The introduction of sucrose-density centrifugation in the study of the estradiol receptor by Toft and Gorski gave great impetus to further study. The characterization of steroid receptors according to their position in a density gradient (4S, 5S; S = Svedberg units) became a useful linguistic tool for investigators.

More recently, the theories and methods of molecular biology, pioneered by students of viruses and prokaryotes, have been applied imaginatively to the analysis of mechanisms of hormone action. The development of two areas of research, recombinant DNA technology and monoclonal antibody production, has opened almost limitless possibilities for exploration in this and all other aspects of biology and medicine.

Steroid Hormone Action

Steroid hormones affect differentiation, growth, and adaptation of cells to new metabolic demands. Steroid hormone-sensitive cells are dependent on a continuing maintenance supply of hormone in order to function. The steroids induce the synthesis of a cell-specific battery of proteins that are specified when the cell differentiates. In some target cells (for example, in the oviduct), a small number of hormone-induced proteins may constitute over 70% of the total amount of protein synthesized by the cell, while in others (i.e., liver), glucocorticoid treatment only affects the synthesis (either positively or negatively) of less than 5% of the total number of proteins synthesized. Thus, the problems of the mechanisms of steroid hormone action are a subset of problems in the very difficult field of enzyme regulation in eukaryotes.

The Coordinate Nature of Steroid Hormone Action (Fig 2–1)

Without specifying *where* steroid hormones act, the sequential steps *involved* in the action of a steroid hormone can be summarized as follows:

1. Entry of steroid (S).
2. Formation of S-R complex.

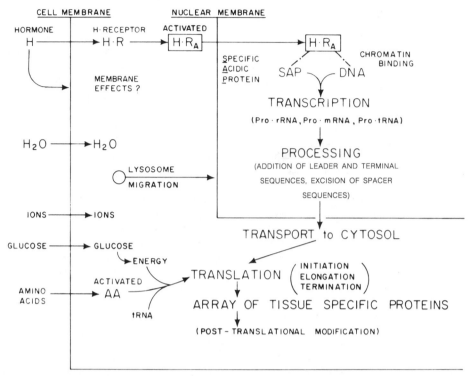

FIG 2–1.
Model for steroid hormone action. See discussion for comments on location of unoccupied receptors.

3. Transformation of S-R to a form that can bind nuclear acceptors [S-R].

4. Binding of [S-R] to chromatin acceptors: specific acidic protein and specific DNA base sequences.

5. Selective initiation of transcription of specific messenger RNAs (mRNAs); coordinate transcription of transfer RNAs (tRNAs) and ribosomal RNAs (rRNAs).

6. Processing of primary RNA transcripts: methylation, polyadenylation, excision of introns, splicing of exons, metabolism of excised introns, etc.

7. Transport of definitive messages to cytoplasm.

8. Translation of influx of new mRNAs on enriched population of ribosomes in an environment that contains increased amounts of metabolic and biosynthetic substrates (glucose, amino acids) and sufficient tRNA to sustain a high level of protein synthesis.

9. Posttranslational modifications of newly synthesized proteins.

Entry of Steroid

Steroid hormones are lipid-soluble substances that circulate bound to carrier proteins. The affinity of each hormone for its carrier protein is such that only a minute amount of hormone is present in the unbound, or free, form; yet, it is the free steroid that is biologically active.

There is some uncertainty about how steroid hormones enter cells. It was long assumed that they simply dissolve in the lipid bilayer of the plasma membrane. However, there is now some evidence that specific plasma membrane receptors may exist for estrogens and glucocorticoids and that these may serve a transport function for their respective hormones. The relationship between these membrane steroid-binding proteins and the interior receptors (to be described below) is not clear.

Receptors and Their Activation

All steroid hormone receptors are elliptical proteins, of approximately the same size, which bind their hormones with very high affinity. This is why hormone-sensitive cells can concentrate their hormones out of an extremely dilute concentration of free hormone in solution. Until recently, most authorities taught that a population of unoccupied receptors in the extranuclear part of the cell promptly captured steroids that entered the cell via the plasma membrane and that the resulting steroid-receptor complexes were translocated to the nucleus where they were bound by chromatin acceptors. Translocation was considered temperature-dependent; i.e., it did not occur at 2° C but did at 37° C. These conclusions were based on differential centrifugation of tissue homogenates (separation of nuclei from cytosol) and on autoradiographic data (visualization of radioactively labeled steroid over nuclei and cytosol in fixed cell populations). Most investigators now believe that the experiments on which they were based were technically flawed. It appears that practically all unoccupied receptors are bound in the nucleus *before* the steroid encounters the cell (see Gorski, et al., 1984 for review). This leaves open the following question: How do steroids, now no less hydrophobic than they were before, traverse the aqueous cytoplasm on their way to the nucleus? In any case, a temperature-dependent process must transform S-R to [S-R] before high affinity binding to nuclear components can take place.

The "classical" steroid mechanism model has been modified by the discovery that estrogen, progesterone, and glucocorticoid receptors are reversibly phosphorylated by a kinase and dephosphorylated by a phosphatase. Moreover, the receptor cannot bind hormone unless it is phosphorylated. In addition, an SH group seems to be required for hormone binding by the glucocorticoid receptor. Thus, some sort of preparation of the receptor has to occur before it is competent to bind the hormone and undergo transformation into a species that can interact effectively with its chromatin acceptors.

Binding of [S-R] to Chromatin Acceptors

Each somatic cell contains all of the genetic information in the fertilized egg from which it was derived. At the time of differentiation, when a cell was destined to be a muscle cell, nerve cell, or secretory cell, most of its DNA was supercoiled into a dense mass in association with the "correct" mix of nuclear proteins that precluded the possibility of transcription. This DNA packing configuration renders the DNA resistant to digestion by the enzyme DNase I. The small amount of the total genome (<10%?) that is sensitive to DNase I consists of three kinds of DNA: (1) transcriptionally "silent" during the cell's lifetime; (2) constitutively expressed; and (3) inducible by hormones or other signal molecules, either directly or indirectly via metabolites or unknown mediators. Nuclear chromatin consists of DNA, arginine, lysine rich (and, therefore, basic) proteins called histones and a variety of nonhistone acidic proteins. Histones play a major role in determining the density of packing of

DNA and therefore its availability for transcription and hormonal induction. Tissue and hormone-receptor-specific acidic proteins have been described, but there is still no hard evidence that they guide [S-R] complexes to specific DNA transcription sites, although this is an attractive possibility. The major mystery in the mechanism of action of all hormones, steroid and nonsteroid alike, is this: how did whatever it was that determined the differentiation of a hormone-sensitive cell instruct the chromatin to assume exactly the correct conformation to render it responsive to a particular hormone?

There is good evidence that treatment of animals or hormone-sensitive tissues with steroids increases the steady state concentration of mRNAs of induced proteins. This was demonstrated by two different methods of measuring mRNA concentration: (1) by isolating an mRNA fraction from stimulated and unstimulated tissues and testing for a specific mRNA in a reconstructed, cell-free translation system in which mRNA was the rate-limiting reagent; and (2) preparing a purified mRNA, using it to synthesize a radioactive complementary DNA (cDNA) via the enzyme reverse transcriptase and then titrating a specific message, by hybridizing it to the cDNA, in control and stimulated tissues. By means of these methods, more than a dozen different hormone-induced mRNAs in a number of target tissues have been shown to be increased in response to androgens, estrogens, glucocorticoids, and ecdysone.

An increase in the steady state concentration of mRNA could be due to an increased rate of transcription of the message, a decreased rate of its degradation, or some combination of these. In the case of some messages, a prolongation of half-life has been observed as a consequence of hormone treatment and, conversely, a shortening of mRNA half-life when the hormone stimulus was withdrawn. In order to assess the relative contributions to the mRNA accumulation of stimulation of mRNA synthesis versus stabilization of mature mRNAs, the rate of elongation of nascent messages was tested in isolated nuclei from hormone-treated animals under conditions in which neither initiation of transcription nor posttranscriptional processing could occur. In all cases, nuclei from hormone-treated cells showed a striking increase (often many thousandfold) in (previously initiated) mRNA synthesis. While there is an undeniable component of mRNA stabilization in the increase in specific mRNAs seen after hormone treatment, *most* of the increase is due to stimulation of the rate of transcription. According to one hypothesis, prolongation of half-life of mRNAs in hormone-treated cells may be due to stabilization of mRNAs by a high ribosome population elicited by the hormone treatment.

In some manner we cannot yet describe, [S-R] does something to specific regions of DNA that permits the enzyme RNA polymerase II to gain access to domains that selectively control rates of mRNA synthesis. Individual genes that are "turned on" by steroids may be arranged linearly (as some are in the chick oviduct) or they may be on different chromosomes. While the nature of the guidance system that directs [S-R] precisely to the positions on the genome where it can perform its function is not known, there have been some interesting advances on several fronts. Older studies revealed the existence of hormone and target tissue specific acidic proteins that were capable of binding preferentially hormone-receptor complexes. For example, one such protein could bind progesterone-receptor but not androgen-receptor, while a similar protein prepared from prostate chromatin behaved in the reverse manner.

In the special case of progesterone, a dimeric receptor has been described that consists of two dissimilar subunits: A, which binds to DNA, and B, which binds to an acidic protein. In theory, B could bind to a protein near a target transcription site where, on dissociation of the subunits, A would be free to bind to a preferred sequence of DNA nucleotides. However, recent evidence for a single steroid-binding progesterone species in the rabbit (Loosfelt) suggests that the asymmetrical progesterone receptor may be peculiar to avian species. It is possible that single receptor molecules may contain both DNA and protein binding domains, and thus incorporate in a monomeric protein the properties attributed to dimeric avian progesterone receptor.

A new development in this field has stimulated great interest. Improbably, it started with the observation that mouse mammary tumor virus (MMTV) replication was stimulated by treating mice inoculated with the virus with adrenal glucocorticoids. By ingenious application of recombinant DNA technology, it was possible to discover a DNA sequence in the viral genome within the long terminal repeat (LTR) sequence upstream from the promoter site which specifies where transcription begins. Purified rat glucocorticoid receptor binds preferentially to this specific adenine-thymine (AT) rich sequence and protects it against nuclease digestion. A chimaeric plasmid containing this sequence of bases upstream from a gene for a protein that is not normally inducible by glucocorticoid renders it inducible by the hormone.

Similar experiments have been done with progesterone and the induction of ovalbumin. In this case, as in that of the MMTV experiments, both the capacity to respond to the hormone and the AT rich preferential DNA binding site for the receptor were found in the same region of the genome. The hormone control site is distinct from the promoter site which specifies where transcription begins (Fig 2–2). From its effect on transcription, it qualifies as an *enhancer* site. However, preferentially binding sequences also occur in *transcribed* regions of the genome and at considerable distances upstream from the transcription "enhancer" site. The functional significance of these binding sites is unknown.

Recently, hormone-receptor binding sites have been found associated with the *nuclear matrix,* a structure that can be visualized as a sort of protein skeleton for chromatin components. There is some evidence that active RNA transcription may occur preferentially in matrix-associated segments of chromatin. The role of the nuclear matrix in hormone-receptor-instigated RNA transcription has not yet been elucidated.

Selective Initiation of Transcription

In spite of demonstrations of binding of [S-R] complexes to specific acidic proteins and defined sequences of DNA, the molecular consequences of the binding are unknown. By analogy with what happens in ecdysone-stimulated salivary gland chromosomes, the major effect of [S-R] may be a disruption of condensed chromatin and its unfolding into a configuration that permits access of RNA polymerase II molecules to it. Indeed, one of the consequences of the action of both estrogens and glucocorticoids is increased DNA sensitivity to DNase I digestion over and above the increased sensitivity that already exists in a region of the genome open for transcription. This does not preclude the possibility that [S-R] or an affiliated protein may also play a catalytic role in the initiation of transcription in addition to a physical, chromomere "unravelling" one.

So far, the primary influence of hormone-receptor complex on RNA synthesis has been limited to *messenger* RNA. At some time in the sequence of events entrained by [S-R], both *ribosomal* RNA and *transfer* RNA synthesis are stimulated. Although little is known about the mechanisms responsible for these events, experiments with estrogens and glucocorticoids suggest that, unlike mRNA synthesis stimulation, protein synthesis is required for stimulation of synthesis of rRNA. Thus, it is reasonable to suggest that some protein product dependent upon primary mRNA synthesis must accumulate *before* the *secondary* effects on rRNA and tRNA can occur.

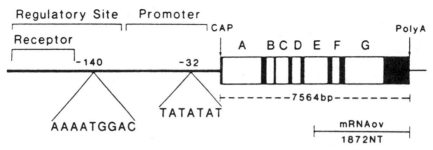

FIG 2–2.
Structural features of the ovalbumin gene. The lettered gene segments are introns. Only the black exons appear in the 1872 base mRNA. [S-R] binds selectively to the region marked "receptor." (From Schrader WT, Compton JG, O'Malley BW, in Eriksson H, Gustafsson JA [eds]: *Steroid Hormone Receptors: Structure and Function.* (Nobel Symposium No. 57.) New York, Elsevier North-Holland, Inc, 1983, p 310. Used by permission.)

Transport of mRNA, rRNA, and tRNA to Cytoplasm: Translation of a Cell-Specific Battery of Proteins

Among the earliest biological effects of estrogen administration are intracellular accumulation of water and electrolytes and increased cellular uptake of glucose and amino acids. Thus, a favorable cytoplasmic environment for protein synthesis is encountered by the various newly synthesized RNA species as they enter the cytoplasm from the nucleus. Two of the primary requirements for *translation* of new message, GTP and amino acids, are abundantly present. In addition, Liao has suggested that androgens stimulate the appearance of a *translation initiation factor* by a mechanism that does not require transcription. While the authors are unaware of similar observations by students of other steroids, the idea that this effect may be a general one is too attractive to remain unexplored.

Posttranslational Modifications of Proteins

Many of the new proteins synthesized in steroid hormone-stimulated cells are glycoproteins—either plasma membrane constituents or secretory products. Components of the metabolic machinery involved in glycoprotein synthesis, specifically those responsible for core sugar transfer (dolichol phosphate pathway), are coordinately stimulated, along with other processes, in steroid hormone-stimulated cells and tissues. According to Lucas et al., one of the most striking examples of this aspect of steroid hormone action occurs in the estrogen-stimulated chick oviduct.

ESTROGEN EFFECTS ON DNA AND THE CELL CYCLE

It has long been known that estrogen induces cellular hypertrophy and increases mitotic activity in uterine cells. By means of ^{3}H-thymidine labeling and autoradiography, large increases in mitotic activity and in number of cells synthesizing DNA have been observed in sensitive cells after estrogen administration. Cell generation time was shortened from 42 to 26 hours, mainly due to a decrease in the G_1 and S stages of the cell cycle. In the immature rat uterus, all cellular elements show peak mitotic activity between 24 and 48 hours after one dose of estradiol, but the effect is most marked in epithelial cells (Kaye et al.).

A recent study (see Walker et al.) has revealed that stimulation of DNA synthesis in immature rat uterus is closely correlated with an increase in activity of one of three known DNA polymerases, α. The major increase in the activity of this enzyme occurs between 12 and 24 hours after administration of estradiol. The time of development of this part of the estrogen response machinery is later than that for early responses, since it is not until the 20th postnatal day that the full DNA polymerase α-stimulatory effect can be elicited.

Two general hypotheses are suggested to explain the connection between the early and late effects of estrogen: (1) the "domino" theory and (2) the "sustained action" theory (Gorski). According to the domino theory, the estrogen-receptor complex first triggers an increased rate of synthesis of a very small number of mRNAs, which are translated into new proteins. This response, in turn, is responsible for another wave of selective protein synthesis. After "n" such waves, the full expression of estrogen action— cell growth and cell division—occurs. The sequential puffing pattern of the salivary gland of the ecdysone-treated fly strongly suggests such a pattern of response. The very early protein, inducible protein (IP), is believed to play an important but unspecified role in initiating the estrogen response.

Many observations are not entirely consistent with the domino theory. For example, estradiol and estriol are equipotent in eliciting the *early* effects of estrogen (RNA synthesis, uterine water imbibition, glucose oxidation), but estriol is only one-third as active as estradiol in stimulating DNA synthesis at 24 hours and uterine weight increase at 24–72 hours. Thus the early responses do not necessarily result in the later ones. Moreover, if estriol is given at 0 time and estradiol six hours later, the late response at 24 hours is the same as if estradiol had been given at 0 time.

Clark et al. have suggested that since estriol is not retained by the uterus as well as estradiol, "sustained action" may be related to the time of residence of the steroid in the nucleus. Estriol is less capable of eliciting a late response because it does not permit nuclear retention of hormone-receptor complex long enough for the response to be initiated and sustained. This time is somewhere between 2 and 10 hours, long before the actual increase in DNA synthesis is detectable. According to the sustained action hypothesis, initiation of later responses requires not only the transcription of RNA and accumulation of specific proteins during the early phase of the response (during the first hour), but also the *continuous presence* of hormone-receptor complex in the nucleus for a critical period beyond the time when the early responses occur.

CAN ALL STEROID EFFECTS BE ACCOUNTED FOR BY STIMULATION OF TRANSCRIPTION?

Many effects of steroids occur too soon to be accounted for by stimulation of gene transcription. For example, Szego and Pietras have pointed out that many estrogen effects can be seen in the uterus within minutes after the administration of estradiol. These include estradiol binding to the plasma membrane, histamine release, calcium efflux, increased transport of glucose and amino acids, micropinocytotic vesiculation of the plasma membrane, release of several lysosomal enzymes, and nuclear translocation of lysosome-like vesicles. These investigators believe that estrogens bind not only to receptors associated with the nucleus but also to plasma membranes, mitochondrial membranes, and lysosomal membranes.

Whether these binding sites are identical with the much studied "interior" receptors is not known.

Although it is hazardous to attempt to distill their 300-page monograph into a laconic statement, they believe that estrogens have rapid effects on all three membranes, and that membrane perturbations produced by instant estrogen binding account for some of the early effects enumerated above. A major feature of their hypothesis is the importance of *controlled release of lysosomal enzymes* as one of the mechanisms by which the estrogen stimulation is propagated to all parts of the cell, including the nucleus. Although they do not specify precise mechanisms, they attribute the histamine release and glucose and amino acid transport effects to local lysosomal enzyme release in what they call "microquanta." The migration of lysosomes to the nucleus may be related to the impending stimulation of gene transcription, since it appears to be necessary for a busily transcribing nucleus to increase selectively its catabolic activities in parallel with its anabolic ones.

These are interesting and provocative ideas that add to and don't diminish the brilliant achievements of the molecular biology school of steroid hormone action analysts. They emphasize that the coordinated, cohesive, and pleiotropic action of estrogen involves immediate and rapidly propagated effects in addition to (and contributory to) the striking effects on the control of gene expression that have engaged many investigators of steroid hormone action for the past 15 years.

Another example of a rapid steroid effect is the immediate inhibition of ACTH release from the pituitary by glucocorticoids. The feedback inhibition of the hypothalamo-pituitary ACTH system occurs on two different time scales: a few minutes and hours to days. An effect at the level of transcription or translation is not required for the first, while the synthesis of proopiomelanocortin, the precursor of ACTH, is inhibited at the level of transcription during the second. The mechanism of the acute inhibition is not known, but it is presumed to be due to an interference with the exocytosis of peptide hormones from the ACTH-producing cell.

In Chapter 3 we discuss mechanisms of action of peptide and amine hormones that are presumed to initiate their biological effects by binding to a receptor in the plasma membrane. At one time, many of us taught confidently that steroids work (over a period of hours to days) by entering cells and selectively stimulating gene transcription while peptide hormones act (in minutes) on the cell surface, stimulate the production of "second messenger" or "deputy" molecules like cyclic AMP, which then disperse throughout the cell and bring about a complex, coordinated response. This was heuristically useful and pedagogically convenient, but in real life, things are much more complicated.

In the first place, both estrogens and androgens cause rapid increases in cyclic AMP in some of their respective sensitive cells. In fact, some of the effects of androgens on enzyme synthesis can be duplicated by cyclic AMP (Singhal). Therefore, we must leave open the possibility that some of the nuclear events that occur after estrogen and androgen administration may be modulated by the action of cyclic AMP-dependent kinases (see Chapter 3). Moreover, another important second messenger that has been implicated in the action of many peptide hormones, Ca^{2+}, clearly must be involved in the actions of androgens and estrogens since it is so prominently featured in the control of cell division.

To blur the distinction between the two workhorse models even more, many peptide hormones (trophic, growth factors, insulin, glucagon, etc.) clearly influence the selective transcription of genes, either positively or negatively. All of them, with their respective receptors, are internalized by pinocytosis, but whether or not hormone-receptor internalization participates in the control of gene expression is presently unknown. The more likely probability is that these hormones affect gene expression by way of intricate combinations of second messengers (see Chapter 3). They not only have striking effects on gene expression in nondividing cells, but some of them also stimulate cell division and therefore resemble steroids in their long-term effects. The two models, once so distinctively different, now appear to overlap, and similar ideas and experimental strategies are being used by steroidologists and peptidologists (not to mention students of the thyroid hormones: see Chapter 10).

HORMONES AND DIFFERENTIATION

In addition to stimulating fully differentiated cells, steroid hormones and thyroid hormones play important roles in the processes of *differentiation*. The fetal development of the male generative tract is stimulated by androgen. Thyroid hormone is essential for the development of the CNS. Estrogen stimulation of differentiation is best seen in the chick oviduct, which produces three distinct types of cell in response to the hormone: tubular gland cells, goblet cells and ciliated cells. The gland cells are the source of ovalbumin. If DNA synthesis is inhibited by hydroxyurea, differentiation in response to estradiol fails to occur.

An example of sequential differentiation is seen in the goblet cell, which differentiates as a result of estradiol stimulation but does not secrete its characteristic protein product, avidin, until it is secondarily stimulated by progesterone. Moreover, estrogen actually induces the appearance of progesterone receptors.

Although these effects of hormones are striking, we cannot construct a plausible theory of the molecular mechanisms involved in them at this time. The exploration of hormonal control of differentiation may one day result in a better understanding of the process of differentiation than we now have.

AN EXAMPLE OF APPLIED BIOLOGY

Basic information about estrogen receptors was quickly applied to the management of patients with breast cancer. It was known that some kinds of cancer cells retain some degree of responsiveness to hormones that had regulated their cells of origin. Depriving breast cancer cells of estrogen, either by surgically removing endogenous sources of estrogen or by administering an estrogen antagonist, frequently results in remission of the disease. When methods became available for measuring estrogen receptor (ER) concentrations in cancer tissue, it was found that (1) the individual tumors showed a wide continuum of ER concentrations (from 10 to 1,000 fmoles per mg of tissue protein) and (2) there was a highly significant correlation between the ER concentration and the probability of remission due to estrogen deprivation. Generally, remissions occurred most frequently in patients with tumors that contained high concentrations of receptors. Since tumors consist of heterogeneous populations of cells, those that are indifferent to estrogen are selected (by estrogen deprivation) for survival and replication. When such cells become dominant, the remission ends (Heuson et al.).

BIBLIOGRAPHY

Anderson JN: The effect of steroid hormones on gene transcription, in Goldberger RF, Yamamoto KR (eds): *Biological Regulation and Development*, vol 3B. *Hormone Action*. New York, Plenum Publishing Corp, 1984, pp 169–212.

Auricchio F, Migliaccio A, Castoria S, et al: Estrogen receptor hormone activity is regulated by phosphorylation-dephosphorylation of the receptor, in Bresciani F (ed): *Progress in Cancer Research and Therapy,* vol 31. New York, Raven Press, 1984, pp 49–62.

Bonner JJ: An assessment of the ecdysteroid receptor of Drosophila. *Cell* 1982; 30:7.

Chambon P, Dierich A, Gaub MP, et al: Promoter elements of genes coding for proteins and modulation of transcription by estrogens and progesterone, in *Recent Progress in*

Hormone Research, vol 40. New York, Academic Press, 1984, pp 1–42.

Compton JG, Schrader WT, O'Malley BW: DNA sequence preference of the progesterone receptor. *Proc Natl Acad Sci USA* 1983; 80:16.

Eriksson H, Gustafsson JA (eds): *Steroid Hormone Receptors: Structure and Function.* (Nobel Symposium No. 57.) New York, Elsevier North-Holland, Inc, 1983.

Goldberger RF, Yamamoto KR (eds): *Biological Regulation and Development: Hormone Action,* vols 3A and 3B. New York, Plenum Publishing Corp, 1984.

Gorski J, Welshons W, Sakai D: Remodeling the estrogen receptor model. *Mol Cell Endocrinol* 1984; 36:11.

Grody WW, Schrader WT, O'Malley BW: Activation, transformation, and subunit structure of steroid hormone receptors. *Endocr Rev* 1982; 3:141.

Gronemeyer H, Pongs O: Localization of ecdysterone on polytene chromosomes of *Drosophila melanogaster. Proc Natl Acad Sci USA* 1980; 77:2108.

Heuson JC, Longeval R, Mattheim WH, et al: Significance of quantitative estrogen receptors for endocrine therapy in advanced breast cancer. *Cancer* 1977; 39:1971.

Heuson JC, Coune A: Hormone-responsive tumors, in Felig P, Baxter JD, Broadus AE, et al (eds): *Endocrinology and Metabolism.* New York, McGraw-Hill Book Co, 1981, pp 1275–1303.

Jensen EV, Greene GL, Closs LE, et al: Receptors reconsidered: A 20-year perspective, in *Recent Progress in Hormone Research,* vol 37. New York, Academic Press, 1981, pp 1–40.

King WJ, Greene GL: Monoclonal antibodies localize oestrogen receptor in the nuclei of target cells. *Nature* 1984; 307:745.

Lee F, Mulligan R, Berg P, et al: Glucocorticoids regulate expression of dihydrofolate reductase cDNA in mouse mammary tumor virus chimaeric plasmids. *Nature* 1981; 228.

Liao S, Chang C, Saltzman AG: Androgen-receptor interaction—An overview, in Eriksson H, Gustaffson JA (eds): *Steroid Hormone Receptors: Structure and Function.* New York, Elsevier North-Holland, Inc, 1983, pp 407–418.

Loosfelt H, Logeat F, Hai MTV, et al: The rabbit progesterone receptor: Evidence for a single steroid-binding subunit and characterization of receptor RNA. *J Biol Chem* 1984; 259:14196.

McGuire WL, Horwitz KB, Zava DT, et al: Hormones in breast cancer: Update 1978. *Metabolism* 1978; 27:487.

Nevins JR: The pathway of eukaryotic mRNA formation. *Ann Rev Biochem* 1983; 52:441.

O'Malley BW: Steroid hormone action on eukaryotic cells. *J Clin Invest* 1984; 74:307.

Renoir JM, Mester J: Chick oviduct progesterone receptor: Structure, immunology and function. *Mol Cell Endocrinol* 1984; 37:1.

Rousseau GG: Control of gene expression by glucocorticoid hormones. *Biochem J* 1984; 224:1.

Spelsberg TC: Chemical characterization of nuclear acceptors for the avian progesterone receptor, in Litwack G (ed): *Biochemical Actions of Hormones,* vol 9. New York, Academic Press, 1982, pp 141–204.

Szego C, Pietras RJ: Lysosomal functions in cellular activation: Propagation of the actions of hormones and other effectors, in Bourne GH, Danielli JF, Jeon JW (eds): *International Review of Cytology,* vol 88. New York, Academic Press, 1984.

Walker MD, Kaye AM, Fridlander BR: Age-dependent stimulation by estradiol 17β of DNA polymerase in immature rat uterus. *FEBS Lett* 1978; 92:25.

Yamamoto KR: On steroid regulation of gene expression and the evolution of hormone-controlled gene networks, in Eriksson H, Gustafsson JA (eds): *Steroid Hormone Receptors: Structure and Function.* New York, Elsevier North-Holland, Inc, 1983, pp 285–306.

3

Intracellular Messenger Systems Involved in Peptide Hormone Action: Cyclic AMP, Calcium, and Phosphatidyl Inositol Metabolites

Peptide hormones, amines and neurotransmitters, unlike steroids, are hydrophilic substances that do not traverse plasma membranes easily. In general they interact with outwardly facing, plasma membrane-limited receptors, and they do not have to be internalized in order to elicit their effects. Hormone-receptor interaction results in a highly coordinated biological response that may involve many individual cellular components, some of them at a distance from the plasma membrane. We address the following questions in this chapter: What do we know about how hormone activation of its receptor is transduced into a complex, coordinated biological response? How is the message that a receptor is occupied by its hormone dispersed throughout the cell?

Cyclic AMP (see below) was first called a "second messenger" by its discoverer, Sutherland. He used that designation because he regarded the hormone itself as the bearer of the "first message" which induced the intracellular production of a second messenger which, in turn, was capable of effecting a biological response. For several years, most attention was focussed on cyclic AMP as *the* second messenger, although it had been known for some time that calcium (Ca^{2+}) plays an important role in muscle contraction and in epinephrine secretion. Rasmussen was among the first to suggest that Ca^{2+} qualifies as a second messenger in the action of several hormones. Meanwhile, Michell and others began to explore the possibility that some effects of hormones via

Ca^{2+} might be linked to phosphatidyl inositol (PI) turnover. Recent discoveries confirm phospholipid as the progenitor of at least two new second messengers that are important in hormone action and neural transmission.

Thus, we now have at least three categories of second messengers: (1) cyclic nucleotides (i.e., cyclic AMP and, possibly, cyclic GMP); (2) Ca^{2+}; and (3) PI metabolites. All of these are intricately connected, and we can predict confidently that there are probably other second messengers waiting to be discovered.

All of these second messenger systems represent means by which a comparatively small number of hormone molecules can bind to receptors and induce the production of many more second messenger molecules. These in turn can affect (either positively or negatively) the activity state of a larger number of protein molecules. Thus, there is a progressive *amplification* of the signal that was originally generated by hormone-receptor binding.

Parenthetically, investigators in this field have demonstrated again that studies of hormone action can have a seminal influence on the development of biological concepts in general. The idea of reversible phosphorylation of key proteins as an important mechanism for metabolic control, which first came into prominence in studies of cyclic AMP, has spread throughout all of biology, including some aspects of cancer research. The importance of GTP as an allosteric regulator of protein function, a central issue in the analysis of hormone-receptor directed cyclic AMP synthesis, has been established in such apparently unrelated fields as retinal biochemistry and the regulation of the process of mRNA translation on ribosomes.

Discovery of Cyclic AMP

Cyclic AMP (3′,5′ adenosine monophosphate) was discovered while Sutherland was attempting to elucidate the mechanism of epinephrine-stimulated glycogenolysis in liver. When his studies began (c. 1950), the reaction sequence for glycogenolysis had been worked out by the Coris and their associates: Glycogen → Glucose 1 PO_4 *(phosphorylase);* Glucose 1 PO_4 → Glucose 6 PO_4 *(phosphoglucomutase);* and Glucose 6 PO_4 → Glucose + P_i *(glucose-6-phosphatase).* The first step (by Sutherland and C. Cori) was the demonstration that the first reaction was rate limiting. Later, Wosilait and Sutherland proved that the enzyme phosphorylase was phosphorylated in its active state and dephosphorylated in its inactive state.

Following the demonstration that phosphorylase was activated in liver slices exposed to epinephrine

and glucagon, the hormones were found to activate the enzyme in a broken cell preparation. This was the first authentic demonstration of hormone action on anything but an intact cell and was therefore a major advance.

When various centrifugal fractions of liver homogenates were tested for their ability to activate phosphorylase on epinephrine addition, it was found that a heavy particulate fraction, on treatment with ATP (adenosine triphosphate) and Mg^{2+}, generated a heat stable substance that was capable of activating phosphorylase in a particle-free supernatant. When this substance X was isolated and purified, it proved to be 3′,5′ cAMP (Fig 3–1). Within a surprisingly short time, the enzyme responsible for the formation of cAMP from ATP + Mg^{2+} was discovered and named *adenylate cyclase.* At about the same time, an enzyme was found that is responsible for inactivation of cAMP by converting it to 5′ AMP, *phosphodiesterase.* Fluoride was found to stimulate adenylate cyclase in broken cell preparations but not in intact cells. Readers who are interested in the process of discovery are referred to Sutherland's Nobel Prize lecture for a reconstruction of the state of the art in the pioneer days of the late 1950s.

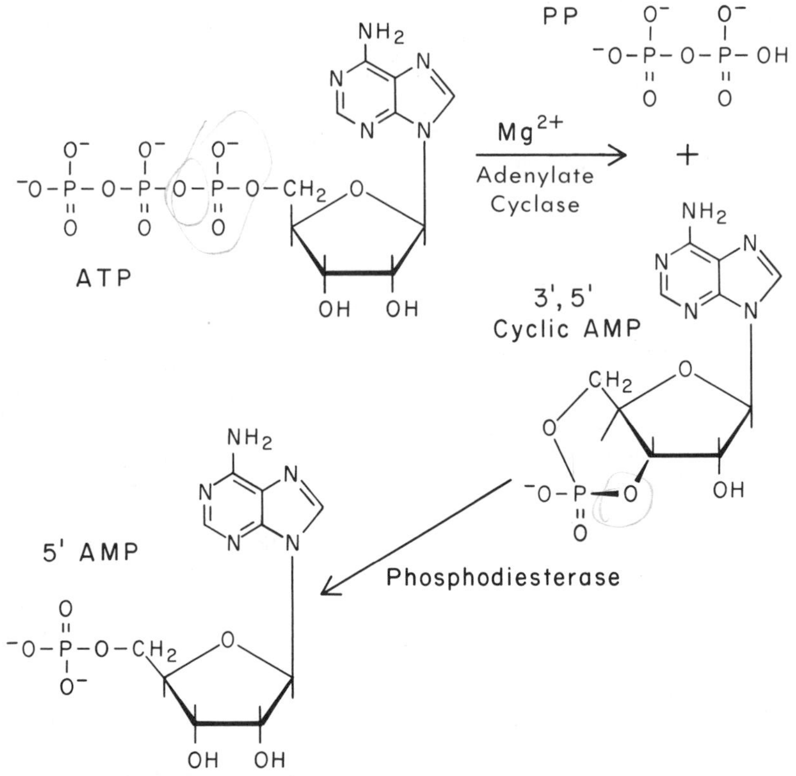

FIG 3–1.
Reactions catalyzed by adenylate cyclase and phosphodiesterase.

Variety of Biologic Processes Affected by Cyclic AMP

Studies on liver glycogenolysis were followed by Haynes and Berthet's demonstration that stimulation of steroid hormone production in the adrenal by ACTH involved Sutherland's "second messenger." Cyclic AMP was found to be involved in one way or another in the action of pituitary LH, antidiuretic hormone (ADH), parathyroid hormone (PTH), thyroid-stimulating hormone (TSH), and the effects of hypothalamic-releasing factors (HRFs). Moreover, glucose-induced insulin secretion was found to be affected by cAMP, and insulin action on certain tissues was accompanied by a *fall* in tissue cAMP concentration. De-repression of the lac operon in glucose-deprived microorganisms proved to be associated with an effect of cAMP.

The variety of *biologic effects* of the many hormones and other agents that use cAMP as a second messenger is impressive. Table 3–1 contains a representative sample of such effects. It is intended to demonstrate that the end product of the response—the biologic effect—may vary widely from cell to cell, although the basic design of the response system may be similar.

Sutherland and coworkers suggested a model for hormone action that is generally applicable. In its simplest form, the "second messenger" hypothesis may be stated as follows:

1. Hormone + stereospecific receptor
2. Activation of adenylate cyclase
3. Production of cyclic AMP
4. Responsibility of cyclic AMP for coordinated response.

Greengard and his colleagues found cAMP-dependent protein kinase activity in many tissues and concluded that the ultimate responses to cAMP involved regulation of structure and function of reversibly phosphorylatable proteins. Krebs, Walsh, and colleagues and many other investigators systematically studied the role of cAMP-activated protein kinases in the phosphorylation of specific proteins. As a result, it was possible to construct a general model of hormone action via cAMP, as illustrated in Figure 3–2. Although the broad outlines of this model are still considered useful, many features of the system are unknown.

Criteria for Implication of Cyclic AMP in Biologic Response

At the beginning of the cAMP era, Sutherland and colleagues established the following criteria for implication of cAMP in the response of a cell to chemical stimulation:

1. The agent must stimulate adenylate cyclase activity in a preparation derived from a sensitive tissue.
2. The tissue concentration of cAMP must increase in response to the agent.
3. Potentiation of a hormone effect by a phosphodiesterase inhibitor is strong circumstantial evidence that cAMP was involved in the response.
4. Reproduction of a coordinated hormone response by cAMP or by its dibutyryl derivative (db cAMP) was taken as evidence of a cyclic nucleotide-mediated effect.
5. The hormone-stimulated rise in tissue cAMP concentration had to *precede* a measurable biologic response (e.g., muscle contraction, glycogenolysis,

TABLE 3–1.

Some Biologic Effects of 3',5'/Cyclic AMP

PROCESS	EXAMPLES
Membrane permeability, ions	Nerve cells, muscle cells, retina, etc.
Membrane permeability, water	Kidney, toad bladder, toad skin
Steroid hormone synthesis	Adrenal cortex, corpus luteum, Leydig cell
Secretory responses	Exocrine glands (pancreas, salivary), thyroid, insulin, gastric HCl, pituitary
Triglyceride and cholesterol ester hydrolysis	Fat cells, liver, steroid-producing cells, muscle
Lipogenesis inhibition	Liver, fat cells
Movements of intracellular structures	Melanophore distribution, sperm motility, cell process maintenance (fibroblast), lysosome migration
Glycogenolysis stimulation; glycogenesis inhibition	Liver, fat cells, muscle
Gluconeogenesis stimulation	Liver, kidney
Gene transcription	Microorganisms (lac operon); enzyme induction, fetal liver
Protein synthesis, translation	Catabolic effect (liver), selective protein synthesis (adrenal cortex)
Motility and aggregation, unicellular organisms	Slime mold aggregation

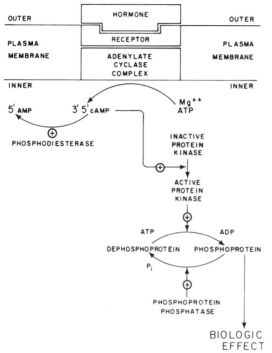

FIG 3–2.
General model of cAMP-mediated hormone response.

lipolysis) in order to qualify as a potential mediator of the response.

Although these criteria are still useful, analysis of some biologic responses (e.g., those of the adrenal cell, testicular Leydig cell, skeletal muscle cells) has revealed that responses to hormones may occur without a measurable change in tissue cAMP concentration but still involve components of the cAMP system. There may be multiple explanations for this, but two are often proposed: (1) local, compartmentalized changes in cAMP concentration may occur that are not reflected in an analysis of the whole tissue; and (2) sensitivity of the cAMP-dependent protein kinase to an unchanging cAMP concentration may be altered in either direction. Thus, if an inhibitor of protein kinase is elicited by a hormone, the biologic response may resemble that expected by decreasing cAMP concentration in the cell. An example of this is presented in Chapter 14.

Molecular Components of cAMP-Mediated System

The plasma membrane is 60–100 Å thick, and those amine and peptide hormones that act by way of

cAMP act on the exterior surface of the membrane. The rest of this chapter will be an attempt to describe how this external event can result in a biologic response. For example, ACTH stimulates adrenocortical cells to synthesize and secrete a steroid hormone. The same hormone stimulates an adipocyte to hydrolyze triglyceride and release free fatty acid. Both processes involve the cAMP machinery. How can one molecule be involved in the responses of so many different cells that are involved in such a variety of biologic effects?

HORMONE-RECEPTOR INTERACTION

The availability of radioactively labeled hormones has advanced our knowledge of hormone binding. The binding of a radioactive hormone either to the exterior surface of an intact cell or to a more or less purified plasma membrane preparation of a hormone-sensitive cell is carried out in the absence and in the presence of a large excess of cold (i.e., nonradioactive) hormone. "Specific" binding is defined operationally as the amount of bound radioactive hormone that is displaceable by cold hormone. The data obtained can be treated in a variety of ways that yield estimates of the number of hormone-binding sites per cell, the density of the receptor population on the surface of the cell and the Km, or concentration of hormone at which the binding sites are half saturated (affinity).

The following criteria have been proposed for receptors:

1. Strict structural specificity.
2. Saturability (i.e., finite number of binding sites).
3. Tissue specificity that parallels target cell responsiveness.
4. Affinity that corresponds to physiologic hormone concentration range.
5. Reversal or prevention of binding that produces a reversal of biologic effect.

Criterion 1, structural specificity, is the first determinant of the specificity of response of a target cell. Obviously, if the cell is not equipped with a discriminator capable of establishing a strong, noncovalent bond with the hormone molecule, no biologic response can be expected. Some analogues of hormones are capable of binding to a hormone receptor but are incapable of initiating the hormone's usual biologic response. Such agents may bind with high affinity and block the hormone effect by denying the receptor to the hormone.

Hormones can be prevented from interacting with their specific receptors not only by man-made analogues but also by antibodies directed against the receptor. Flier and Kahn and colleagues have recently described several patients who had circulating antibodies to their own insulin receptors and therefore exhibited a rare form of insulin-resistant diabetes. The antibodies of these patients have been used in ingenious experiments designed to elucidate problems in receptor biology.

The specificity of plasma membrane receptors and their affinity for their hormones is so great that membrane preparations may be used for measurement of hormone concentration in a radioligand assay (radioreceptor) similar to a radioimmunoassay. This has been accomplished both for measurement of ACTH with adrenal cell membrane concentrates and for LH, or interstitial cell-stimulating hormone (ICSH), with testicular Leydig cell preparations.

Plasma membrane receptors, which participate so centrally in the metabolic regulation of hormone-sensitive cells, are themselves subject to regulation, both acute and chronic. The affinity of a receptor for its hormone may change when the total population of receptors remains unchanged.

Long-range, or chronic, regulation of the total number of receptor units on the cell surface also has been described for insulin, GH, TRH, and β catecholamines. Perhaps the most extensively studied case of chronic regulation of receptor population is that of insulin, which was explored by Roth, Kahn, and colleagues. These investigators found that in both experimental and clinical obesities, which are characterized by high circulating insulin levels, the concentration of insulin receptors on sensitive cells was low. Following weight reduction the hyperinsulinemia disappeared and the number of insulin receptors increased toward normal. A similar *"down-regulation"* of receptor number was observed in a strain of lymphocytes grown in tissue culture, i.e., reciprocal changes were seen in receptor population when the insulin concentration was increased or decreased.

These findings illustrate the fact that membrane components are in a state of dynamic equilibrium; receptors, like other protein and glycoprotein membrane constituents, are continuously being degraded and replaced. The suggestion has been made that continuously high occupancy of receptors by their hormones favors internalization and degradation of the receptors. Although the significance of down regulation is not certainly known, it has been suggested that decrease in receptor number may protect against too intense stimulation by inappropriately high hormone levels. Diminished responsiveness to hormones (particularly in the case of insulin) is not only attributable to decreased numbers of hormone receptors (see Chapter 15). There may be coordinate changes not only in other membrane components (e.g., glucose transport system) but in "interior" or postmembrane metabolic machinery.

The relation between total receptor number and biologic effect of the hormone has been studied extensively in a number of cases. There is general agreement among students of peptide hormones that a *maximal* biologic effect may be seen at concentrations of hormone that can account for only 5%–10% occupancy of the total available specific binding sites. This is generally known as the phenomenon of *spare receptors*. The meaning of the existence of spare receptors is not completely understood. It is possible that some of the binding sites classified as specific receptors may not articulate with an effector complex of molecules which would permit the expression of a biologic effect. It is also conceivable that total receptor number plays a statistical role in facilitating hormone action at low hormone concentrations. It also has been suggested that the spare receptors constitute a local hormone-concentrating mechanism. In any case, the spare receptor phenomenon has become a feature of the action of many amine and peptide hormones.

Distinctive features of individual receptors will be discussed in more detail later, particularly in Chapters 13 and 14.

Activation of Adenylate Cyclase: Embryology of a Model, 1960–1986

Shortly after cyclic AMP was discovered, a simple model was proposed (by Sutherland and Robison):

1. H (Hormone) + R (Receptor) + C (Adenylate Cyclase) $\rightarrow$ ↑ cAMP

The presumption was that occupation of R by H caused a conformational change in R which in turn altered C so that it became active. R and C were visualized as a regulatory subunit in association with a catalytic one.

The first suggestion that the introductory model was inadequate was made by Rodbell, Birnbaumer, and their colleagues who demonstrated, on the basis of kinetic experiments on liver membranes, that GTP is absolutely required for activation of C by H. At first, they suggested that C might contain a GTP allosteric site and a catalytic site, but their data did not permit any conclusions about how GTP worked. With remarkable prescience, however, they suggested (by analogy with electrical circuits) that there might be a *transducing element* interposed between H-R and C. Their model can be described as follows:

2. H-R + Transducer + C $\xrightarrow{\text{GTP}}$ ↑ cAMP

Important advances in this field were made possible by genetic analyses of the adenylate cyclase system in cells in culture by Tomkins and his colleagues. It was known that catecholamine stimulation of lymphocytes causes the death of such cells, and that this event is mediated by cAMP. Mutant cells of a murine lymphoma (S49) were found that survived usually lethal concentrations of catecholamines. One such mutant, cyc⁻, was able to bind hormone normally and to contain a normal complement of C. Hormone binding occurred, but did not result in increased cAMP. It was subsequently discovered that this mutant lacked a third protein component that corresponded to Rodbell's transducer and was variously called N protein or G protein. Such a protein was shown by Pfeuffer to be distinct from both R and C in detergent-solubilized membrane preparations. At this stage, we can describe the model as follows:

$$3. \text{ H-R } + \text{ G } + \text{ C} \rightarrow \uparrow \text{ cAMP}$$

Many converging lines of investigation were proceeding concurrently. Among them were important observations on the mechanism of action of cholera toxin, the agent produced by *cholera vibrio*. It was soon discovered that cholera toxin stimulates fluid and electrolyte loss from the intestinal mucosa by irreversibly activating C. The toxin consists of multiple subunits, one of which, after a time lag of about 60 minutes, can enter the lipid bilayer membranes of cells. Cholera toxin was found to have the ability to elicit cell-specific biological responses in many cells that employ cAMP as a second messenger. Remarkably, it could cause a thyroid cell to secrete thyroid hormone, an adrenal cell to release adrenal hormone, and a fat cell to break down its triglyceride and release free fatty acids.

As a result of the work of Gill and of Vaughan and others, it was discovered that the lipophilic subunit of cholera toxin is an enzyme, an ADP-ribosylase, which covalently binds ADP-ribose to the G protein of the cyclase system and permanently activates it. This property made it valuable in establishing the separate identity of G protein, distinct from R and C, since it made possible the labelling of the protein with radioactively labelled ADP-ribose. Covalently bound ADP-ribose made it possible to track the protein through purification procedures, culminating in polyacrylamide gel electrophoresis and autoradiography.

Radioactively labelled GTP also binds, *noncova*lently, exclusively to G. Thus:

$$4. \text{ H-R } + \text{ G-GTP } + \text{ C} \rightarrow \uparrow \text{ cAMP}$$

It is convenient to think of the proteins of the cyclic AMP-generating system as molecules dissolved in the exterior lipid bilayer of the cell in loose affiliation, interacting according to shape changes imposed on them by the presence or absence of hormone. R is oriented to the exterior of the cell, but G and C are integral proteins that are accessible from the cytoplasm, for GTP (necessary for the action of G) and ATP (precursor of cAMP) are generated there.

The following model, not only for activating C but also for terminating its activation, was generally accepted:

5. a. $\text{H } + \text{ R } + \text{ G-GDP} \rightarrow \text{ H-R-G } + \text{ GDP}$
   b. $\text{H-R-G } + \text{ GTP} \rightarrow \text{ H } + \text{ R } + \text{ G-GTP}$
   c. $\text{G-GTP } + \text{ C} \rightarrow \uparrow \text{ cAMP } + \text{ G-GDP}$

Thus, the hydrolysis of GTP is the "turn off" signal. To restart the cycle, GDP must be split from G by hormone occupation of R, as in 5a. The reason C is irreversibly activated by cholera toxin is the fact that ADP-ribosylation of G prevents GTP hydrolysis.

Elegant purification and chemical characterization studies of G protein have been done by Ross and Gilman, by Birnbaumer and others. The G protein involved in activating C is a trimer consisting of the following:

α subunit, 45,000 D
β subunit, 35,000 D
γ subunit, 8,000 D

The G protein has been inserted into G-deficient membranes (by Schramm and by Ross and Gilman), and a hormonally responsive system has been so reconstructed. Occupation of the receptor by hormone results in the dissociation of α and β subunits. The larger subunit, α, contains the GTP binding site and a cholera toxin-mediated ADP-ribosylation site. It is presumed to be the proximate agent for activation of C. The function of the γ subunit is unknown. A function of the β subunit will be discussed later.

Another facet of the story was unfolding in parallel with the one we have described. Early, it was appreciated by several investigators, notably Rodbell, that some agents exert an *inhibitory* effect on adenylate cyclase and cause a *decrease* in cAMP concentration, particularly after it has been elevated previously. Examples of *cyclase-stimulating* agents are: glucagon, vasopressin (via VP_1 receptors), LH, FSH, TSH, and ACTH. *Cyclase-inhibiting* agonists include opioids (pharmacologic and endogenous), somatostatin, angiotensin II, and acetyl choline (via muscarinic M_1 receptors).

Epinephrine can either stimulate (via β receptors) or inhibit (via $α_2$ receptors). How can we explain this bidirectional control of the cyclic AMP-generating system?

The answer lies in the above discussion of the anatomy of the G subunit. In an awesomely symmetrical series of studies, it was established that the *inhibitory* system contains a trimeric protein that is precisely analogous to the G protein whose biography we have already written. The *stimulatory* G protein has been designated as G_s; the *inhibitory* one is called G_i. Moreover, each has the same subunit structure—α, β, γ. The β subunits of both G_s and G_i are identical, but the α subunits differ. $G_{i\alpha}$ has a molecular weight of 41,000 D (as compared with $G_{s\alpha}$, 45,000 D). Subunits of both are dissociated when receptor is occupied by agonist. We can describe the effect of G_i as follows:

6. a. $H + R + G_i\text{-}GDP \rightarrow H\text{-}R\text{-}G_i + GDP$
    b. $H\text{-}R\text{-}G_i + GTP \rightarrow H + R + G_i\text{-}GTP$
    c. $G_i\text{-}GTP + C \rightarrow \; \downarrow cAMP + G_i\text{-}GDP$

(The reader can now go back to equation 5 and fill in the subscript "s" wherever the G protein appears.)

GTP "activates" both G_s and G_i; that is, it causes G_s to stimulate C and G_i to inhibit the enzyme. How can we account for these effects in molecular terms? According to Gilman, $G_{s\alpha}$ is truly stimulatory to C in its GTP-bound configuration, and GTP hydrolysis probably occurs during the act of stimulation. However, $G_{i\alpha}$ is only weakly inhibitory. Therefore he proposes that

7. a. $H + R + G_i\text{-}GDP \rightarrow H\text{-}R + G_{i\alpha}\text{-}GTP + G_{i\beta}$
    b. $G_{i\beta} + G_{s\alpha} + G_{s\beta} \rightarrow G_{s\alpha}\text{-}G_{s\beta}$

Since the G_s is effective as a stimulator only when the dimer is dissociated, the presence of an excess of the β subunit (identical in both proteins) forces the G_s into its undissociated form by mass action. This hypothesis, though appealing, is not universally accepted as the only possibility.

As if to emphasize the delicate balance between G_s and G_i, elucidation of the function of the latter was aided by the availability of its own distinctive bacterial toxin. Just as the cholera toxin played a significant role in the identification of G_s and in describing its mechanism of action, the toxin of B. pertussis proved to be important in the evolving history of G_i. Cholera toxin permanently turns on C because it prevents GTP hydrolysis by ADP-ribosylating $G_{s\alpha}$. Pertussis toxin also ADP-ribosylates $G_{i\alpha}\cdot G_{i\beta}$, but the effect of this is to prevent dissociation of α and β subunits. This prevents the accumulation of enough $G_{i\beta}$ subunits to back inhibit $G_{s\alpha}$. Thus, there are enough free $G_{s\alpha}$ subunits to stimulate C. In other words, interfering with the action of G_i by pertussis toxin permits G_s to act unopposed.

This is probably not the ultimate model, but the interested reader must agree that it is a considerable advance over equation 1. All things considered, the development of these ideas was not a bad quarter century's work.

The G protein saga represents another example of the development by explorers in endocrinology of an idea that may be widely applicable in biology. Parallel with the events we have described, students of retinal biochemistry have discovered an entirely analogous G_s in the retina. It is a trimeric protein that functions as a transducing element (in fact, it has been named "transducin") in light-stimulated, GMP phosphodiesterase activation. In this system, light is analogous to a hormone, rhodopsin plays the role of a hormone receptor and phosphodiesterase imitates adenylate cyclase. Similar G proteins (i.e., activatable by GTP and dissociable on stimulation) occur in association with initiation, elongation, and termination factors when messenger RNA is translated on ribosomes. One such protein may be involved in the action of insulin.

Although the G proteins have undeniable esthetic appeal, practical applications for this new knowledge have already been found (see Spiegel, et al.). Symptoms of both cholera and pertussis (whooping cough) are attributable to the actions of toxins produced by their etiological agents. Some patients with pseudohypoparathyroidism, a disease in which target organs of a hormone fail to respond to an adequate supply of the hormone, show a genetically determined deficiency or functional inadequacy of G_s. There is some evidence that transducin deficiency may be involved in certain animals with retinal degeneration. There are even structural homologies between G proteins and certain oncogene products. In summary, G proteins are not only important in the mechanism of adenylate cyclase activation, but related regulatory proteins are involved in many other biological mechanisms.

Cyclic AMP-Dependent and Other Protein Kinases

The concept of metabolic regulation by reversible phosphorylation of key proteins had its origins in studies on glycogenolysis by C. and G. Cori in the early 1940s. They demonstrated that phosphorylase, the rate-limiting enzyme of glycogenolysis, exists in two activity states: *a*, highly active and *b*, inactive. In 1956, Sutherland and coworkers, and Fisher and Krebs, all working in the Coris' laboratory, showed (in liver and muscle, respectively) that phosphorylase *a* is a phosphoprotein and phosphorylase *b* is a dephosphoprotein. Shortly thereafter, Friedman and Larner (also in the Coris' group) demonstrated that activated glycogen synthase is a *de*phosphoprotein but that inactivated glycogen synthase is phosphorylated. Krebs, Walsh, and their colleagues and Greengard and his have established protein phosphorylation by cyclic AMP-dependent protein kinase (cAMP-PK) as the major, if not the only, mechanism by which cyclic AMP works in eukaryotic cells.

Cyclic AMP-PK, in its inactive, or occluded, form is a tetrameric protein consisting of two regulatory (R) subunits and two catalytic (C) ones, R_2C_2. The catalytic units are active only when the complex is dissociated by the binding of cAMP to R, thus:

$$R_2C_2 \text{ (inactive)} + 4 \text{ cAMP} \rightleftharpoons (R:cAMP_2)_2 + 2 \text{ C (active)}$$

At low cAMP concentrations, R and C reassociate into the inactive tetramer. Table 3–2 suggests some types of proteins that can serve as substrates for cAMP-PK.

In the early history of cAMP, cAMP-PK from one tissue was found to activate substrates in another. Therefore, PK was not considered a contributor to the specificity of a cell's response to cAMP. Now, however, we think that some degree of specificity of response may be determined by the fact that there are two kinds of cAMP-PK, Type I and Type II, and that these may exist in different proportions in different cells, or even in the same cell at different times.

Type I and Type II PKs have identical C units and therefore affect substrates similarly. Their R subunits differ in at least four ways: (1) they have different molecular weights; (2) they have different peptide maps after partial proteolysis; (3) Type II R undergoes autophosphorylation by its own C partner, an event that inhibits, to some extent, reassociation into the inactive tetramer; and (4) the cAMP binding sites on R_I and R_{II} differ.

Many observers have commented on the fact that Type I PK is especially prominent in cells that have been stimulated to undergo hypertrophy or in those (such as mitogen-stimulated lymphocytes) that are actively dividing. Type I PK is activated at lower cAMP concentrations than Type II, so there is the possibility that part of a cell's response to cAMP might be determined by its Type I:Type II PK ratio.

How could this be accomplished? According to one attractive hypothesis, the R subunits could not only function allosterically as releasers of bound C when they bind cAMP, but also as *determinants of the intracellular localization of the complex* by binding to intracellular organelles. This could create circumscribed compartments where C would be in relatively high concentration, and thus enhance the statistical probability that certain PK substrates would be phosphorylated. One can imagine that individual cells, when they differentiate, not only express the genes for their distinctive PK substrates but also for proteins with special affinities for R_I and R_{II}. This would be a way of conferring a kind of substrate specificity on substrate-indifferent C units.

Another delightful part of the cAMP-PK story is the fact that, in a number of cases, highly purified PK C units have been micro-injected into cAMP-sensitive cells and have duplicated the expected biological response, thereby bypassing increased cAMP synthesis in response to an agonist and cAMP interaction with R.

The importance of these discoveries related to cAMP-PK for biology as a whole is difficult to overestimate, for it turns out that they represent only the tip of a conceptual iceberg. The theme of regulation of biologically important proteins by reversible phosphorylation is now a dominant one in regulatory biochemistry. There are now more than 50 proteins that have been shown to be reversibly phosphorylated in various circumstances. Perhaps half of these show alterations in function associated with altered phosphorylation states; the others, so far, represent "silent" phosphorylations ("silent," perhaps, because we haven't yet learned what they are trying to tell us).

Protein substrates of cAMP-PK are phosphorylated on serine and threonine residues. Often (as in the case of glycogen synthase, for example) they are phosphorylated at multiple sites. Some cases have been described in which biologically antagonistic hormones (for example, epinephrine, via cAMP-PK and insulin, via a cAMP-independent PK) have induced phosphorylation of the same protein at different sites with different consequences for the activity state of the protein.

But cAMP-PK was only the beginning. At first, several other serine-threonine PKs were discovered that are regulated by intracellular second messengers

TABLE 3–2.

Types of Proteins That May Serve as Substrates for Cyclic AMP-Activated Protein Kinase

TYPE	EFFECT OF PHOSPHORYLATION
Membrane constituent	Permeability change
Rate-limiting enzyme	Activated
Rate-limiting enzyme	Inhibited
Ribosomal protein	↑ or ↓ translation
Initiation factor	Inhibited
Nuclear protein	↑ or ↓ transcription
Microtubular protein	Secretory, motor or cell configuration effect

Note: Any cell may have more than one substrate.

other than cAMP. A summary of some of these is given in Table 3–3. In some cases, when we can identify their substrates, they overlap with cAMP substrates, as in the case of $(Ca^{2+})_n \cdot CalM \cdot PK$. In one case, that of cyclic GMP-PK, we cannot identify *any* certain protein substrate. With this available arsenal of potential regulators, the possibilities for subtle control and modulation of biochemical reactions overstimulates our collective imagination.

Nor is this inventory the end of the phosphorylation story. Between 1979 and 1985, another development occurred that promises to pervade many areas of biological thought, including peptide hormone action, growth stimulation, and cancer research, i.e., the discovery of tyrosine protein kinases. In three cases, the interaction of a peptide agonist with its receptor has been found to cause autophosphorylation of the receptor on tyrosine residues (epidermal growth factor, EGF; platelet-derived growth factor, PDGF; and insulin). Tyrosine phosphorylation of other proteins by the agonist-receptor complex has also been demonstrated. How receptor phosphorylation participates in the propagation of the biological effect of the agonist is not known.

To illustrate how far we have come from the Coris' phosphorylase *a* and *b* in 1940, we now know (1) that various oncogenes show tyrosine kinase activity; (2) that one is genetically related to PDGF and another is similarly related to the EGF receptor; and (3) that the molecular biology of normal and abnormal growth is likely to be examined from the vantage point of tyrosine PKs for some time to come.

The tyrosine PKs are summarized in Table 3–4.

THE INTRACELLULAR MESSENGER FUNCTION OF CALCIUM

Students of biology have been interested in the calcium ion for a long time, mainly in its relation to the bony skeleton and to the homeostatic regulation of its concentration within tight limits in body water. It was also appreciated that it plays an essential role in stimulus-contraction coupling in muscle and in stimulus-secretion coupling in the adrenal medulla and other secretory cells. In 1970, Rasmussen indicated its importance as an intracellular mediator of hormone action. He found that parathyroid hormone stimulated gluconeogenesis in kidney tubules in the presence of Ca^{2+} but failed to do so in its absence in spite of the fact that an increase in cyclic AMP was permitted. Later it was shown (by Borle) that parathyroid hormone produced an increase in intracellular Ca^{2+} concentration ($[Ca^{2+}]_c$) in the kidney.

In order to understand how small changes in $[Ca^{2+}]_c$ can be perceived by cellular elements as signals, it is necessary to recall that $[Ca^{2+}]_c$ in an unstimulated cell is only 1/10,000 of the concentration of Ca^{2+} in extracellular fluid. The cell, in fact, must protect itself with vigilance against the potentially lethal concentration of Ca^{2+} in which it is bathed. If too much Ca^{2+} accumulates in a cell, phosphate is precipitated and all production and utilization of ATP comes to a gritty halt. Cells, therefore, pump Ca^{2+} overboard with a Ca:H:ATPase in the plasma membrane. In unstimulated cells, $[Ca^{2+}]_c$ is 0.1 μM or less; in stimulated ones it can rise to 0.6–2.0 μM. When an external signal causes an increase in $[Ca^{2+}]_c$, it can do so by (1) permitting an influx of Ca^{2+} from the exterior, (2) inhibiting efflux, or (3) mobilization of internal stores from sequestered bound Ca^{2+}, from the endoplasmic reticulum and plasma membrane, but also (according to some authorities) from mitochondria as well. It is now possible to record very rapid changes in $[Ca^{2+}]_c$ by means of certain compounds (Quin 2 and aequorin) which can be introduced into the cytosol of resting cells. As $[Ca^{2+}]_c$ rises, a proportional increase in fluorescence indicates the extent and duration of the change. These methods have made it possible to demonstrate a rise in $[Ca^{2+}]_c$ in many types of stimulated cells.

TABLE 3–3.

An Abbreviated List of Serine-Threonine Protein Kinases*

REGULATORY AGENT	REGULATED PROTEIN KINASE
Cyclic AMP	cAMP-dependent PK (Type I,II, heart; Type II, brain)
Cyclic GMP	cGMP-dependent PK
$(Ca^{2+})_n \cdot$ Calmodulin†	Phosphorylase kinase (Glycogen synthase kinase 2)
Ca^{2+}, diacylglycerol, phospholipid†	Protein kinase C

*Adapted from Krebs EG: *Philos Trans R Soc Lond (Biol)* 1983; 302:3.

†This will be discussed in the next section.

TABLE 3–4.

Tyrosine Protein Kinases*

REGULATORY AGENT	REGULATED PROTEIN KINASE
Epidermal Growth Factor (EGF)	Receptor autophosphorylation
Platelet Derived Growth Factor (PDGF)	Receptor autophosphorylation
Insulin	Receptor autophosphorylation
Unknown	Various oncogene products and transforming proteins

*Modified from Krebs EG: *Philos Trans R Soc Lond (Biol)* 1983; 302:3.

Calmodulin

At about the time a second messenger role for Ca^{2+} was proposed by Rasmussen (1970), Cheung discovered a heat stable, Ca^{2+}-dependent activator of brain cyclic nucleotide phosphodiesterase. Within a few years, Cheung's activator was purified and its amino acid sequence described. It is a single-chain protein, consisting of 148 amino acids, with a molecular weight of 16,700 D. A third of its amino acids are either glutamate or aspartate, whose acidic side chains provide the COO^- groups that bind Ca^{2+}. The molecule, like a four-leaf clover, is divided into four symmetrical domains, each of which contains a Ca^{2+} binding site. At low $[Ca^{2+}]_c$, most of the protein is in the cytosol of the cell. When the protein is activated by bound Ca^{2+}, part of it becomes affiliated with plasma and interior cell membranes and other organelles.

By 1978, when Cheung named his phosphodiesterase activator *Calmodulin* (CaM), the Ca^{2+} activatable protein had been found in all eukaryotic cells examined. Apparently, it is a highly conserved protein, since the material isolated from a protozoon can activate mammalian phosphodiesterase. Like cyclic AMP, it was found to be involved in a great variety of biological processes and enzyme regulations. Among them are the following: insulin secretion, thyroid secretion, pituitary secretion, adrenal secretion, neurotransmitter release, intestinal secretion, cell proliferation, cell shape, lysosome release, prostaglandin synthesis, microtubule disassembly, histamine release, ciliary motility, leucocyte phagocytosis, etc.

In all of these cases, Ca^{2+} is necessary for a response to a stimulus. The response is dependent upon the activation of a cell-specific array of proteins that may be enzymes, membrane constituents or organelle components. Just as in the case of cyclic AMP, the thyroid cell, when it differentiated, expressed precisely the "correct" collection of Ca-CaM sensitive proteins to contribute to the coordinate response of the cell to TSH. In the adrenal fasciculata cell, a different but teleonomically appropriate set of Ca-CaM-sensitive gene products are produced. (No doubt, the reader had observed that we have used two cell types as examples that use cyclic AMP as a second messenger. We will discuss interrelationships among messengers below.)

How does Ca-CaM act to change the activity state of an enzyme? Although some details are still in dispute, one appealing model (Huang et al.) is as follows:

Let E = Enzyme in low activity state and
E* = Enzyme in high activity state, then
$$(Ca^{2+})_2 + E = (Ca^{2+})_2 \cdot E$$

That is, the binding of Ca^{2+} to two of the four available CaM binding sites is sufficient to cause binding to E without activating E. But, in this condition, the remaining two unoccupied sites bind Ca^{2+} much more avidly. Thus,

$$(Ca^{2+})_2 \cdot E + (Ca^{2+})_2 = (Ca^{2+})_4 \cdot E^*$$

Other models have been proposed, and the reaction sequence may not be the same for every CaM-sensitive molecule. For discussion and documentation of this field, see the review by Rasmussen and Barrett.

Ca-CaM can affect the activity state (either positively or negatively) of many proteins in one of two ways: (1) by direct interaction between the Ca-CaM complex and the target enzyme, or (2) via a Ca-CaM-activated protein kinase. The effects of this protein kinase are entirely analogous with those of cyclic AMP-dependent protein kinase; the target proteins may be different. In some cases (e.g., phosphorylase kinase), both kinases phosphorylate the same enzyme. The two kinases, therefore, can exert a much more disseminated effect throughout the hormone-sensitive cell than can either alone.

We have described *two* elegant messenger systems capable of transmitting the message that the receptor is occupied to every interested molecule throughout the cell. However, the responsive cell's resources go even beyond this.

Phosphatidyl Inositol, Diacylglycerol, Inositol Triphosphate, and Protein Kinase C

Molecules involved in metabolic control mechanisms are often products of ubiquitously abundant precursors. Cyclic AMP is made from ATP; calcium is readily available in almost unlimited amounts in extracellular fluid and intracellular stores; the steroid hormones can be synthesized from cholesterol; catecholamines and thyroid hormones from tyrosine; tryptophane is the precursor of serotonin; and prostaglandins and other autocrine and paracrine regulators are derived from arachidonic acid, which is a readily available constituent of membrane phospholipids. As a result of discoveries that began in 1953 but have come to rapid fruition only since 1975, a metabolite of the membrane phospholipid phosphatidyl inositol has been identified as a precursor of two important second messengers for certain hormones, neurotransmitters, platelet activators and other agonists, including photons acting on photoreceptors and sea urchin spermatozoa fertilizing their eggs!

The point of departure for this exciting journey of discovery was the finding by Hokin and Hokin (1953) that ^{32}P incorporation into phospholipids was stimulated by acetyl choline. In 1969, Durell et al. suggested that this phenomenon might be related to receptor function. Michell, in a seminal review published in 1975, proposed that phosphoinositol turnover may be stimulated by those agonists that increase $[Ca^{2+}]_c$.

In 1977, Nishizuka and coworkers described a new protein kinase that they called protein kinase C since it was activated by Ca^{2+} in the presence of phospholipids. Later they found that diacylglycerol (DG), a primary hydrolysis product of the membrane phospholipid, phosphatidyl inositol polyphosphate, greatly increased the affinity of Ca^{2+} for the enzyme. (This is a direct Ca^{2+} action that does not involve CaM.) They also discovered that certain tumor-promoting phorbol esters (structural analogues of DG) mimic the effect of DG in their system. C kinase phosphorylates many proteins on serine and threonine residues, and it shares some substrates, but not others, with cyclic AMP-dependent protein kinase.

Biological effects of C kinase activation were demonstrated in isolated platelets, which respond to certain agonists by releasing serotonin and lysosomal enzymes that can be conveniently measured. When platelets are stimulated by thrombin, selective phosphorylation of two proteins can be seen, one of 40,000 D (40K) and one of 20,000 D (20K). When $[Ca^{2+}]_c$ is increased not by thrombin but by the Ca^{2+} ionophore, A23187 (a widely used maneuver for increasing cytosol Ca^{2+} concentration), only the 20K protein is phosphorylated and the biological response is markedly impaired. Similarly, when C kinase is activated by a DG analogue (phorbol ester), only the 40K protein is phosphorylated and the biological response is minimal. However, if the platelets are treated with both agents, both proteins are phosphorylated and the biological response is equal to that produced by thrombin. Similar synergistic effects between Ca^{2+} and DG analogues have been noted in at least seven different cell types.

Contemporaneous studies on inositol triphosphate (see Berridge review) indicate that this agent, the other primary hydrolysis product of inositol polyphosphate, increases $[Ca^{2+}]_c$ by mobilizing the ion from intracellular stores, primarily from the endoplasmic reticulum. Another degree of complexity is added by the fact that the number 2 carbon of DG is usually arachidonic acid, which is the precursor of prostaglandins and many other related biologically active molecules (to be described in Chapter 4).

Figure 3–3 represents a graphic summary of the ways in which hydrolysis of phosphatidyl inositol 4,5P$_2$ (PIP$_2$) can participate in control mechanisms in cells stimulated by hormones or other agonists. Within this large design, each individual cell type contains its own cell-specific set of regulatable com-ponents; therefore, cells have distinctive patterns of responses. Again, the precursor for the two new second messengers, DG and IP$_3$, is readily available on the cytosolic side of the plasma membrane, waiting to be hydrolyzed on a signal generated at the receptor by the hormone. The effect of hormone receptor occupation on phospholipase C is transduced by a G protein.

INTERRELATIONS OF SECOND MESSENGERS

We have now developed a considerable inventory of second messengers: cyclic AMP, Ca^{2+}, Ca-CaM, diacylglycerol, and inositol triphosphate—an embarrassment of riches. Having seen ways in which DG and inositol triphosphate can act cooperatively to produce a biological effect, we are left with the problem of relating Ca^{2+} to cyclic AMP.

In the first place, as we saw in the history of calmodulin, Ca^{2+} has a *stimulating* effect on cyclic AMP phosphodiesterase; therefore, it could function as a governor of cAMP-mediated responses by inhibiting the accumulation of cAMP. In some cells (brain, for example), Ca-CaM *stimulates* adenylate cyclase, which would have the effect of potentiating a cAMP-mediated response. In other cells, Ca-CaM *inhibits* adenylate cyclase, which would have the opposite effect. Obviously, it is difficult to make sweeping generalizations about cAMP and Ca^{2+} beyond the one that each has effects on the other's system.

Rasmussen's conceptualization of the problem is useful. One can think of five different circumstances in which the ultimate, integrated biological response is affected by the simultaneous presence, either together or sequentially, of cAMP and Ca^{2+}: (1) an even *partnership;* i.e., both are necessary for the full expression of the biological effect; (2) one or the other messenger is the major one, but the response is *aided* or *facilitated* by the effect of the other; (3) they may act *sequentially;* i.e., Ca^{2+} release may enhance cAMP production and both then collaborate, or vice versa; (4) the dual control may represent *redundant,* or backup, or fail-safe control; and (5) they may act *antagonistically;* i.e., one may act as a brake, or turn-off signal, for the effect of the other. The interested reader can find experimental evidence in support of all of these paradigms in Rasmussen's book.

Finally, different messengers may act on different time scales, as is seen in the stimulation of insulin secretion by glucose, or the stimulation of aldosterone secretion by angiotensin II. In these examples, an increase in cytosolic $[Ca^{2+}]$ occurs immediately after the stimulatory signal, but it disappears in a few min-

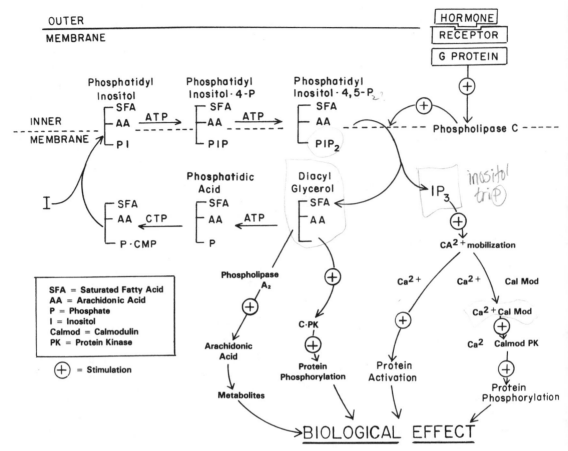

FIG 3–3.
A composite view of the origins and actions of the polyphosphatidyl phosphate metabolites, *diacylglycerol* and *inositol triphosphate*. (Adapted from Nishizuka (*Science,* 1984), Berridge (*Biochem J,* 1984), and Rasmussen (*Physiol Rev,* 1984). See bibliography for complete references.)

utes in spite of the continuing presence of the agonist. The response, however, continues for an hour or more. Ca^{2+} is involved in both the early and the late responses: the responses over the first few minutes are associated with calmodulin-mediated events, while the sustained response is due mainly to events entrained by the activation of C kinase. The total response is represented by the sum of the two.

Ca^{2+} is also important as a signal for releasing arachidonic acid from membrane phospholipids—not only from phosphatidyl inositol-derived diacylglycerol (see Fig 3–3), which, quantitatively, is a minor phospholipid component of membranes, but also from phosphatidyl choline and other more abundant membrane phospholipids. The significance of this fact will become more apparent when we discuss arachidonic acid metabolites in the next chapter.

Coordination of Cyclic AMP-Mediated Responses

Responses of cells to hormones are highly coordinated. Some cell functions may be stimulated, others inhibited. The character of the response ultimately depends on the particular array of PK substrates found in the responsive cell. For example, in the liver cell, the enzyme phosphorylase b kinase is a substrate for cAMP-activated PK. Thus, when cAMP increases (in some species), glycogenolysis is stimulated via the Krebs cascade. If glycogen synthesis persisted at a high level, phosphorylase activation would simply be part of a "futile cycle." However, the enzyme glycogen synthase is also a substrate for cAMP protein kinase, but in this case the phosphoprotein is the inactive form of the enzyme. Thus, phosphorylation of these two enzymes, which have physiologically opposing effects, results in stimulation of glycogenolysis and inhibition of glycogen synthesis. Under these conditions the liver cell secretes glucose into the hepatic vein.

Another example of synchronous phosphorylation is found in the adrenocortical cell stimulated by ACTH. In this instance, at least *three* proteins are phosphorylated by cAMP PK: (1) a cholesterol ester hydrolase (which provides cholesterol for steroid hormone biosynthesis); (2) a ribosomal protein, which may have a role in the translation of a specific protein required for hormone synthesis; and (3) phosphorylase, which promotes glycogenolysis.

Even when we cannot identify PK substrates with certainty, or when we can demonstrate them we do not know their biologic function, these examples are conceptually useful. They suggest that each responsive cell has its own distinctive complement of PK substrates that play important regulatory roles in that cell's vital economy. Examples of some of these are given in Table 3–2. Thus, the cell can generate its characteristic response in spite of the fact that many of the molecular components of the response system may be shared with other cells that are programmed to yield *their* characteristic responses by the nature and distribution of *their* PK substrates.

Cyclic GMP

Cyclic GMP was first found in urine of rats in 1963. It has been extensively investigated ever since, but so far it has been implicated in one physiologic process, 'vision (see below). Although many hormones have been shown to activate adenylate cyclase in cell-free systems and even in purified plasma membrane preparations, attempts to activate guanylate cyclase under similar conditions have met with indifferent success.

The most extensively studied biologic effect involving cGMP is the increase in tissue concentration of the nucleotide that occurs in heart muscle and in other tissues in response to acetylcholine and its congeners. This increase is time- and dose-dependent, is blocked by atropine, is magnified by phosphodiesterase inhibitors, and requires Ca^{2+}. It is not always possible to attribute a second messenger role to cGMP in the responses under study, since in some cases (e.g., smooth muscle contraction, salivary gland amylase secretion) the increase in cGMP concentration occurs *after* the biologic response, and in others (negative inotropic effect in heart muscle) it may occur at the same time as does the biologic effect.

Since Ca^{2+} is necessary for the demonstration of increased tissue cGMP concentration and since Ca^{2+}

can stimulate the soluble guanyl cyclase, some investigators believe that the changes in cGMP observed in many tissues may be indicating increases in cytosolic calcium ion concentration.

One of the most interesting areas of cGMP research is in the retina, where a cGMP phosphodiesterase is believed to be involved in light-induced hyperpolarization of the rod membrane (see Clack et al.).

Hormone activation of guanylate cyclase in a cell-free system has now been demonstrated. Waldmann et al. have described activation of particulate guanylate cyclase, in crude membranes prepared from homogenates of rat kidney by atrial natriuretic factor (ANF). This experiment will no doubt rekindle interest in cyclic GMP. (See also Atlas SA: *Recent Prog Hormone Res* 1985; 42:207.)

BIBLIOGRAPHY

Atlas SA: *Recent Prog Hormone Res* 1985; 42:207.

Berridge MJ: Cellular control through interactions between cyclic nucleotides and calcium, in Greengard P (ed): *Advances in Cyclic Nucleotide and Protein Phosphorylation Research,* vol 17. New York, Raven Press, 1984, p 329.

Berridge MJ: Inositol triphosphate and diacylglycerol as second messengers. *Biochem J* 1984; 220:345.

Birnbaumer L, Codina J, Mattera R, et al: Regulation of hormone receptors and adenyl cyclases by guanine nucleotide binding N proteins. *Recent Prog Horm Res* 1985; 41:41.

Cherrington AD, Assimacopoulos FD, Harper SC, et al: Studies on the alpha adrenergic activation of hepatic glucose output. *J Biol Chem* 1976; 251:5209.

Cheung WY: Calmodulin plays a pivotal role in cellular regulation. *Science* 1980; 207:19.

Clack JW, Oakley B, Stein PJ: Injection of GTP-binding protein or cyclic GMP phosphodiesterase hyperpolarizes retinal rods. *Nature* 1983; 305:50.

Cohen P: The role of protein phosphorylation in neural and hormonal control of cellular activity. *Nature* 1982; 296:613.

Fain JN: Hormones, membranes, and cyclic nucleotides, in Cuatrecasas P, Greaves M (eds): *Receptors and Recognition,* vol 6. London, Chapman and Hall, 1979, Chapter 1.

Friedman DL, Johnson RA, Zeilig CE: The role of cyclic nucleotides in the cell cycle. *Adv Cyclic Nucleotide Protein Phosphorylation Res* 1976; 7:69.

Gill DM: Cholera toxin catalyzed ADP-ribosylation of membrane proteins, in Hayaishi O, Ueda K (eds): *ADP-Ribosylation Reactions in Biology and Medicine.* New York, Academic Press, 1982, pp 593–621.

Gilman AG: Guanine nucleotide-binding regulatory proteins and dual control of adenylate cyclase. *J Clin Invest* 1984; 73:1.

Hildebrandt JD, Codina J, Risinger R, et al: Identification of a gamma subunit associated with the adenylyl cyclase regulatory proteins N_s and N_i. *J Biol Chem* 1984; 259:2039.

Hughes SM: Are guanine nucleotide binding proteins a distinct class of regulatory proteins? *FEBS Lett* 1983; 164:1.

Insel PA: Membrane-active hormones: Receptors and receptor regulation, in Rickenberg HV (ed): *Biochemistry and*

Mode of Action of Hormones, II, vol 20. Baltimore, University Park Press, 1978, pp 1–43.

Krebs EG: Historical perspectives on protein phosphorylation and a classification system for protein kinases. *Philos Trans R Soc Lond (Biol)* 1983; 302:3.

Lohmann SM, Walter U: Regulation of the cellular and subcellular concentrations and distribution of cyclic nucleotide-dependent protein kinases, in Greengard P, Robison GA (eds): *Advances in Cyclic Nucleotide Research,* vol 18. New York, Raven Press, 1984, pp 63–117.

Michell RH: Inositol phospholipids and cell surface receptor function. *Biochim Biophys Acta* 1975; 415:81.

Miller WH: Physiological evidence that light-mediated decrease in cyclic GMP is an intermediary process in retinal rod transduction. *J Gen Physiol* 1982; 80:103.

Nishizuka Y: The role of protein kinase C in cell surface signal transduction and tumour promotion. *Nature* 1984; 308:693.

Nishizuka Y: Turnover of inositol phospholipids and signal transduction. *Science* 1984; 225:1365.

Pfeuffer T: GTP-binding proteins in membranes and the control of adenylate cyclase activity. *J Biol Chem* 1977; 252:7224.

Rangel-Aldao R, Rosen OM: Effect of cAMP and ATP on the reassociation of the phosphorylated and nonphosphorylated subunits of the cAMP-dependent protein kinase from bovine cardiac muscle. *J Biol Chem* 1977; 252:7140.

Rasmussen H: Cell communication, calcium ion and cyclic adenosine monophosphate. *Science* 1970; 170:404.

Rasmussen H: *Calcium and cAMP as Synarchic Messengers.* New York, John Wiley & Sons, 1981.

Rasmussen H, Barrett PQ: Calcium messenger system: An integrated overview. *Physiol Rev* 1984; 64:938.

Rodbell M, Birnbaumer L, Pohl SL, et al: The glucagon-sensitive adenylcyclase system in plasma membranes of rat liver. V. An obligatory role of guanyl nucleotides in glucagon action. *J Biol Chem* 1971; 246:1877.

Ross EM, Gilman AG: Biochemical properties of hormone-sensitive adenylate cyclase. *Ann Rev Biochem* 1980; 49:533.

Schulman H, Greengard P: Ca^{2+}-dependent protein phosphorylation system in membranes from various tissues and its activation by "calcium-dependent regulator." *Proc Natl Acad Sci USA* 1978; 75:5432.

Spiegel AM, Gierschik P, Levine MA, et al: Clinical implications of guanine nucleotide binding proteins as receptor-effector couplers. *N Engl J Med* 1985; 312:26.

Sutherland EW: Studies on the mechanism of hormone action (Nobel lecture). *Science* 1972; 177:401.

Tomchik KJ, Devreotes PN: Adenosine $3'5'$ monophosphate waves in *Dyctyostelium discoideum:* A demonstration by isotope dilution-fluorography. *Science* 1981; 212:443.

Tomlinson S, Macneil S, Walker SW, et al: Calmodulin and cell function. *Clin Sci* 1984; 66:497.

Ui M: Islet activating protein, pertussis toxin: A probe for functions of the inhibitory guanine nucleotide regulatory component of adenylate cyclase. *Trends Pharmacol Sci* 1985; 5:277.

Waldman SA, Rapoport RM, Murad F: Atrial natriuretic factor selectively activates particulate guanylate cyclase and elevates cyclic GMP in rat tissues. *J Biol Chem* 1984; 259:14332.

Walsh DA, Cooper RH: The physiological regulation and function of cAMP-dependent protein kinases, in Litwack G (ed): *Biochemical Actions of Hormones,* vol 6. New York, Academic Press, 1979.

4

Prostaglandins, Thromboxane, and Leukotrienes

In the early 1930s, two apparently unrelated observations were made: (1) that fresh human semen added to human uterine strips in vitro could cause either contraction or relaxation of smooth muscle (Kurzrok and Lieb), and (2) that a deficiency of polyunsaturated fatty acids in the diet could produce a variety of pathologic changes in experimental animals (Burr, Evans). It is now possible to look back over half a century and see the confluence of the two streams of investigation that had their sources in these early studies.

Kurzrok and Lieb's experiments were quickly confirmed by Goldblatt in England and von Euler in Sweden, who discovered that lipid-soluble extracts of seminal fluid were capable of stimulating various kinds of smooth muscle and, in addition, of lowering blood pressure in intact animals. However, the chemical technology for pursuing the problem did not exist until Bergstrom, in 1947, launched an attempt to purify and identify what von Euler had already named "prostaglandin" activity, so called because especially potent extracts were made from sheep prostate glands.

With newly available chromatographic techniques and solvent extraction procedures, Bergstrom was able to isolate two pure crystalline compounds and, 15 years after the beginning of his search (1963), he was able to assign definitive structures to two prostaglandins, PGE_1 and PGE_2. Many similar compounds have been found. Some of these have proved to be among the most potent biologically active materials known. For example, 1–2 $\mu g/kg$ can lower the blood pressure in a hypertensive person.

More recently, Hamberg, Samuelsson, and their collaborators discovered the existence of extremely evanescent compounds, which they called PGG_2 and PGH_2. These proved to be endoperoxides with a half-life of only five minutes in aqueous solution. The substances provided a clue to the biosynthetic pathway for all known prostaglandins from their common precursor, arachidonic acid (C20:4 double bonds). Later, it was found that the endoperoxides are precursors not only of the known prostaglandins but of two new substances, which have been given the names *prostacyclin* (PGI_2) and *thromboxane* (TxA_2). These remarkably potent materials, like the endoperoxides, also have very short half-lives in aqueous solution, but fortunately they leave tracks in the form of stable metabolic transformation products (TxB_2 for TxA_2 and 6-keto-PGF_1 for PGI_2). Thus the activity of the prostacyclin-forming system or the thromboxane-forming system may be assessed by measuring the accumulation of stable metabolites following administration of arachidonic acid to a tissue or cell system (Fig 4–1). A summary of the chemistry and nomenclature of prostaglandins is given in Figure 4–2.

All of the arachidonic acid metabolites discussed so far are generated via a *cyclooxygenase* enzyme complex that catalyzes the formation of endoperoxides from arachidonic acid (Fig 4–3). The prostaglandins, thromboxane, and prostacyclin are all derived from the endoperoxides.

The synthesis of another family of arachidonic acid metabolites, known as *leukotrienes,* is catalyzed initially by *lipoxygenase* enzymes. Since the elusive slow-reacting substance of anaphylaxis (SRS-A, see below) was identified as one or more of these metabolites in 1979, much literature about them has accumulated. Collectively, *all* arachidonic acid metabolites, whether products of the cyclooxygenase or lipoxygenase pathways, are known as *eicosanoids.*

All of these substances are in the category of *autocrine* or *paracrine* agents, i.e., they can act back either on cells that synthesize them in response to stimuli or on neighboring cells. They may have either

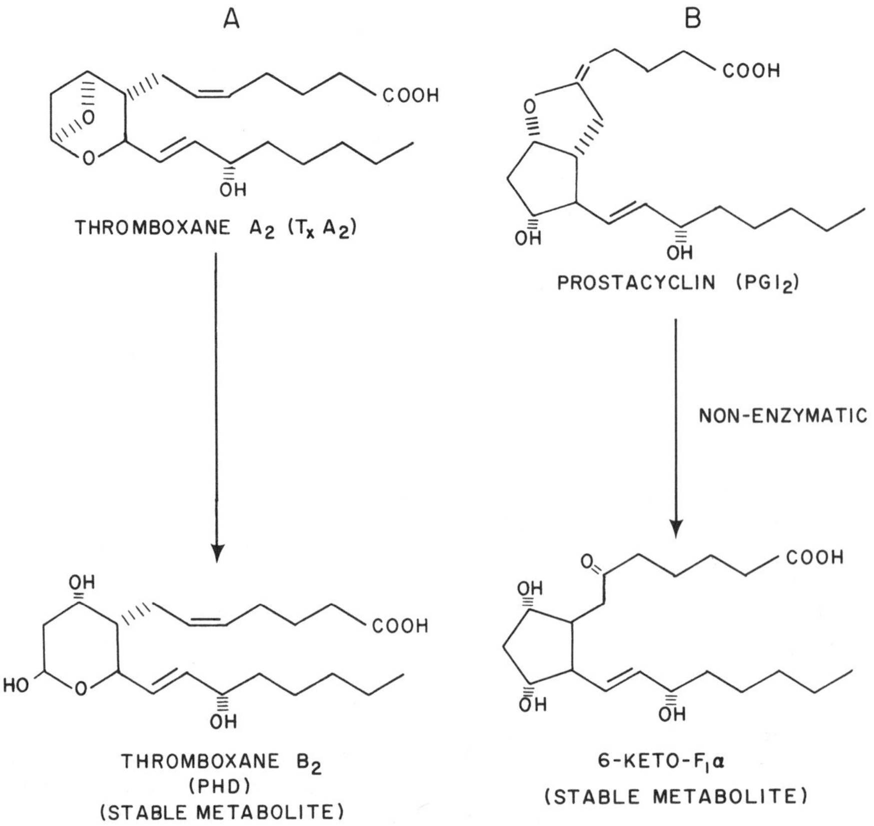

FIG 4–1.
A, thromboxane, **B,** prostacyclin, and their stable metabolites.

an enhancing or inhibitory effect on the actions of hormones or other agonists that elicit their synthesis and release. Thus, to the many second messengers described in Chapter 3 we must now add another extensive collection of information-carrying molecules, all derived from arachidonic acid, which may exert their effects by means of those very messengers.

We plan to recapitulate history by first describing the cyclooxygenase products, then the lipoxygenase metabolites.

Cyclooxygenase Products: Prostaglandins, Prostacyclin, Thromboxane

Nomenclature, Chemistry, and Biosynthesis

The *chemistry* of the prostaglandins and some conventions of their nomenclature are given in Figure 4–2. When arachidonic acid is written in the "hairpin"

configuration, it is easy to see how cyclization between carbons 8 and 12 can produce prostanoic acid. The letter designation following PG refers to the configuration of the 5-membered ring. The numerical subscript denotes the number of double bonds in the molecule. The designation α or β refers to the stereoisomeric form of the compound.

The *biosynthesis* of the prostaglandins is summarized in Figure 4–3. In the first place, the immediate precursor of the endoperoxide intermediates is arachidonic acid, which is liberated from membrane phospholipids in many cells when they are stimulated by hormones, neural transmitters, immunologic stimuli, or physical or chemical noxious stimuli. The rate-limiting step in PG synthesis is the supply of arachidonic acid. It has recently been appreciated that part of the anti-inflammatory effect of adrenal glucocorticoids is due to an inhibiting effect of pharmacologic doses of these steroids on phospholipase A_2, the arachidonic-acid-mobilizing enzyme. This anticipates one of the main achievements of prostaglandin investigators:

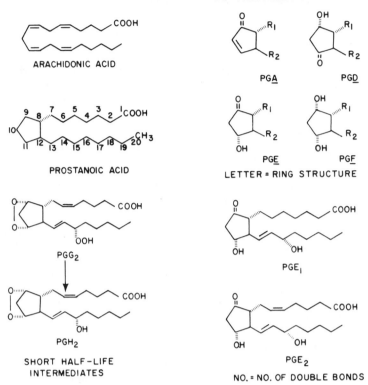

FIG 4–2.
Chemistry and nomenclature of prostaglandins.

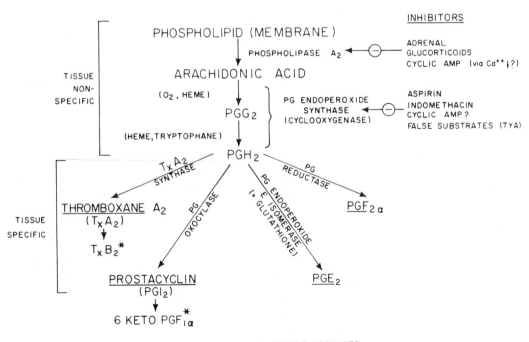

FIG 4–3.
Biosynthesis of prostaglandins.

i.e., demonstration of the importance, indeed, the necessity of prostaglandin formation to occur in order that inflammation can proceed.

The second stage of PG biosynthesis is the cyclooxygenase, or endoperoxide synthetase, step. This step was shown by Vane and colleagues to be inhibitable by nonsteroid anti-inflammatory agents (NSAID) such as aspirin and indomethacin. Acetylsalicylic acid has been ingested in huge quantities by vast numbers of people, but this is the first plausible explanation of its mechanism of action. The first and second stages—through the endoperoxides—are initial common pathways in all tissues that can form PGs.

PGH_2 endoperoxide may have a variety of fates depending on the tissue in which it is generated. It is useful to think of the PG-synthesizing complex as similar to the biochemical machinery used in synthesis of steroid hormones (see Chapter 11). The basic enzymatic equipment is very similar from one steroid-producing cell to another, but the *enzyme emphasis* differs from cell to cell so that each cell makes its distinctive complement of steroids. Similarly, cell A might be differentiated to produce thromboxane, whereas cell B might specialize in producing prostacyclin. We shall examine an important example of this specialization later.

The "steering" of PGH_2 over one or another of the four routes shown in Figure 4–3 may not only be related to the prominence of a particular enzyme in a tissue (e.g., TxA_2 synthetase or PG oxocyclase). If large amounts of glutathione were generated in a cell, PGE_2 would be preferentially synthesized at the expense of the production of other compounds.

BIOLOGIC EFFECTS OF PROSTAGLANDINS

The effects of prostaglandins are summarized in Table 4–1. Since the phospholipids of the membranes in all cells contain arachidonic acid, the potential for prostaglandin production is everywhere in the body. Most of the vast literature on this subject that had accumulated prior to 1975–1976 was concerned with effects of stable PGs, especially PGEs, PGFs, and, to a lesser extent, PGAs. These compounds produced effects in almost every system and, in general, PGEs and PGFs were found to have opposite effects in most test circumstances. More recently, with the discovery of prostacyclin and thromboxane, we are beginning to appreciate that the newer compounds have about the same relationship to each other that PGE and PGF had.

Prostaglandins can be tested for their effects on cells and tissues, but even if an effect is observed, one cannot assume that these compounds are physiologically important in cell regulation. Even if the capacity to produce PGs is demonstrable, it is often difficult to evaluate their physiologic role. Accordingly, indirect evidence of the participation, or lack of participation, of prostaglandins in a particular biologic process is often inferred from inhibitor experiments: a biologic response (e.g., secretion, contraction, hormone response) is measured and then remeasured after the animal or tissue is treated with a PG synthesis inhibitor such as acetylsalicylic acid or indomethacin. If the response is modified by the inhibitor, this is taken as circumstantial evidence that PG production is an essential feature of the reaction.

Prostaglandin effects have often been observed in hormone-responsive cells in which cAMP functions

TABLE 4–1.
Summary of Effects of Prostaglandins

PROCESS	TISSUE	EFFECT
Smooth muscle contraction or relaxation	Lungs	Bronchodilation
	Uterus	Contraction
	Gastrointestinal tract	Contraction
	Blood vessels	Vasodilation
Steroidogenesis	Adrenal cortex	Stimulation
	Corpus luteum	Stimulation
Salt and water movement	Kidney	Natriuresis; increased free water clearance
	Toad bladder	Na transport; alters effect of ADH on water transport
Thyroid hormone release and biosynthesis	Thyroid	Mimics TSH
Lipolysis	Adipocyte	Inhibits lipolysis
Blood clotting	Platelets*	Inhibits or promotes aggregation
Acid secretion	Gastric mucosa	Inhibits

*See text.

as a second messenger. In general, PGEs and prostacyclin alter cAMP by effects on adenylate cyclase.

Cardiovascular-Renal

There have been many studies on the effects of PGs in cardiovascular-renal physiology and pathophysiology. For example, Terragno and Terragno have found that prostacyclin is quantitatively the most important PG derivative in blood vessel walls in both mother and fetus. In the latter, prostacyclin concentration is especially high in aorta and pulmonary artery. In this connection it is pertinent to observe that the PGs may be extremely important in the development of the fetal and neonatal vascular system. Heymann et al. have demonstrated closure of an inappropriately patent ductus arteriosus in premature infants who were treated with a PG synthetase inhibitor, thus accomplishing with a drug a process that had been amenable only to surgery. This observation suggests that one of the functions of prostacyclin in the fetus is to maintain the configuration of the circulatory system in its prenatal condition.

PGAs and PGEs have been shown to have blood pressure-lowering effects in normotensive animals as well as antihypertensive effects in hypertensive patients. The mechanisms of these effects are not entirely clear, but the two evidently do not lower blood pressure in precisely the same way. In addition, PGA especially proved to be diuretic and natriuretic (sodium-excreting) in hypertensives—both highly desirable features in an antihypertensive agent. One popular hypothesis (see Lee) links renal production of PGs with homeostatic regulation of blood pressure by suggesting that these compounds are the long-sought "antihypertensive endocrine agent" of the kidneys. It is difficult to evaluate the many experiments on the relation of PGs to cardiovascular-renal function, since investigators have only begun to explore the participation of the evanescent PGs, prostacyclin and thromboxane, in cardiovascular function. It seems clear that prostacyclin is the major PG metabolite in the vascular system (see Moncada and Vane; Sivakoff et al.). It is also interesting that the same compound is apparently a powerful renin releasing stimulus (see Oates et al.).

REPRODUCTIVE SYSTEM

The chemically stable PGs have powerful effects on the reproductive system in both male and female. Historically, high PG activity has been associated with seminal fluid since the time of PG prehistory. Its

function in that fluid is still unknown, though some have suggested that PGs stimulate smooth muscle of the female generative tract and may therefore play a role in sperm migration to the fallopian tube where fertilization occurs.

The best documented action of PGs in the female is *stimulation of uterine smooth muscle*. This has led to the use of $PGF_2 \alpha$ as a midtrimester abortifacient drug and as a labor-inducing agent (see Karim and Filshei). That PGs play a role in initiating labor and delivery is suggested by the fact that treatment of either experimental animals or women with PG synthesis-inhibiting drugs results in a significant delay in onset of labor.

In certain species (e.g., sheep) PGs produced by the uterus are responsible for the *involution of the corpus luteum*. There is no convincing evidence that uterine PGs have a luteolytic role in women whose corpora lutea involute normally even in the absence of the uterus. However, PGs produced elsewhere may be shown to be involved in the process of luteolysis.

PGs probably are physiologically involved in the process of *ovulation,* since the ovulatory response to LH is blocked in the presence of PG synthesis inhibitors. This is a PG effect that has not so far been linked with the cAMP system.

PGs are involved in the etiology of *dysmenorrhea.* The uteri of women who suffer from this recurrent pain overproduce PGs, and there is widespread use of nonsteroidal cyclooxygenase inhibitors in this condition.

There is evidence that the pattern of PG production varies not only from cell to cell but also in the same cell at different times and under different conditions. For example, Murota et al have shown that estrogen increases prostacyclin in cultured vascular cells and that aging diminishes it. Thus, the ratio of prostacyclin synthesis to that of other PGs varies widely over the life span of the female animal. This observation may help to explain the apparent resistance to degenerative vascular disease in premenopausal women.

PLATELETS AND BLOOD CLOTTING

The effects of PG compounds on platelets have proved to be among the most interesting that have yet been described. This aspect of the problem may yield some of the most important therapeutic and disease-preventive results of prostaglandin research. A knowledge of platelet function is necessary for understanding not only thromboembolic disease but also the cause of atherosclerosis and its sequelae.

When only the stable PGs were available, much

work was done on platelets, which may be summarized as follows:

1. Platelets are prevented from aggregating and releasing the contents of their dense granules (ADP, serotonin) by *increases* in cAMP.
2. Aggregation and release occur when cAMP is low.
3. PGE_1 increases cAMP by stimulating adenylate cyclase (and inhibiting phosphodiesterase?).
4. PGE_2 decreases cAMP by inhibiting cyclase, thereby promoting aggregation and release.
5. Prostaglandin synthesis inhibitors prevent platelet aggregation and granule release.

Thus, PGEs that differ only to the extent of one double bond had antagonistic effects on a biologic process.

With the discovery of prostacyclin and thromboxane, a reexamination of the PG-platelet problem was undertaken by a number of investigators (see Gorman). Their results are summarized briefly in Figure 4–4. The blood vessel wall (intima) was found to be enzymatically specialized to produce prostacyclin, whereas the platelets were equipped with the enzyme that catalyzes the production of thromboxane. The two agents have precisely opposite effects on two crucial processes: prostacyclin relaxes vascular smooth muscle and inhibits platelet aggregation; thromboxane constricts vascular smooth muscle and promotes aggregation. Since the two structures are contiguous, materials may diffuse from one to the other in small quantities (suggested by the dotted lines in the diagram). Moreover, Moncada and Vane have shown that prostacyclin resists inactivation in the lung and actually circulates, thus providing a tonic anticoagulatory signal to intravascular platelets.

The beauties of this formulation are many. The clotting process may be regarded as a classic physiologic regulatory mechanism that is maintained in balance by clotting and anticlotting forces. The balance may be tipped in either direction by a pathologic process or by a drug that affects selectively one or the other force. In addition, this model extends our previously presented concept of cell regulation based on an interaction between calcium and cAMP to include the intracellular modulators, prostacyclin and thromboxane. The major effect of thromboxane is the mobilization of intracellular Ca^{2+} stores, which in turn is primarily responsible for the release reaction and stimulation of contractile protein in platelets. Prostacyclin, by increasing cAMP, prevents both Ca^{2+} mobilization and thromboxane synthesis.

ENDOCRINE SYSTEM

In the endocrine system, the interplay between PGs and the cAMP system is most striking. In the case of some hormones (TSH, ACTH, LH, PTH), PGs increase cAMP levels and to some extent mimic the hormonal effects. In others (lipolytic hormones in adipose tissue, ADH in the kidney), PGs act antagonistically to the hormonal stimulus and decrease cAMP. Again, the process of reexamining the extensive literature on which these statements are based has begun. For example, the antilipolytic effects of PGEs

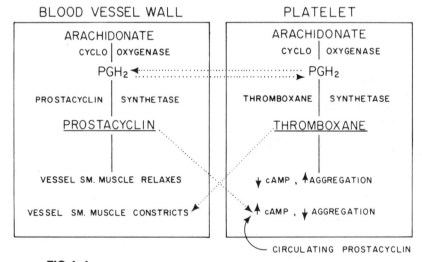

FIG 4–4.
Effects of thromboxane and prostacyclin on platelet aggregation.
Dotted lines represent possible interactions.

were well recognized, but no effects of PGEs on adenylate cyclase were demonstrable. However, Gorman has found that PGH_2 has a direct inhibitory effect on adenylate cyclase.

The effects of the prostaglandins on adenylate cyclase are mediated by the G_s and G_i proteins discussed in Chapter 3 (Aktories et al.). Apparently each prostaglandin has its own stereospecific receptor which is entirely analogous with a hormone receptor, i.e., the PG-receptor complex can affect the activity state of G_s or G_i.

GASTROINTESTINAL SYSTEM

The gastrointestinal system has been a central preoccupation of students of PGs. PGEs, in fact, appear to have many of the characteristics of an ideal peptic ulcer remedy: they decrease gastric HCl secretion and protect against experimental peptic ulceration. Prostaglandin synthesis inhibitors (e.g., acetylsalicylic acid) increase acid secretion and produce or enhance experimental peptic ulceration. Inhibition of gastric acid secretion by PGs occurs whether the stimulus is histamine, pentagastrin, or ingested food.

The PGs, particularly $PGF_2\alpha$ used in gynecology, have been demonstrated to have powerful stimulatory effects on intestinal motility. It has been suggested that they may play a role in the modulation of normal peristalsis.

CENTRAL AND PERIPHERAL NERVOUS SYSTEMS

There are well-documented effects of the stable PGs in the central and peripheral nervous systems. Various responses (stupor, catatonia, excitement) have been described in some species of animals. PGE is a powerful pyrogen and it potentiates the febrile response to administration of other pyrogens. We must therefore conclude that PGs may have some role in the thermoregulatory function of the CNS. Fever can be prevented or attenuated by prostaglandin synthesis-inhibiting drugs such as aspirin. The pulsating headaches that have been observed following the administration of PGEs in man may more properly be categorized as vascular than CNS responses.

SKIN

There is not much information about PG effects in skin other than those associated with increased vascular permeability associated with inflammatory responses. However, it is appropriate here to recall one interesting experiment that unites investigators in the 1930s who had no way of knowing that they were collaborators. Some investigators had attempted to cure the skin manifestations of essential fatty acid deficiency with prostaglandins administered by a number of parenteral routes, all without success. Hsia and colleagues reasoned that the compounds were too quickly metabolized to produce an effect when given subcutaneously or intraperitoneally. They therefore produced essential fatty acid deficiency in the rat and treated the scaly skin and hair loss of one paw with prostaglandin in an unguent vehicle by inunction. The contralateral paw was used as a control. The result was that the skin lesion of the treated paw disappeared. This was a clear demonstration that at least one manifestation of essential fatty acid deficiency disease is due to inadequate synthesis of prostaglandins.

Lipoxygenase Products: Leukotrienes

HISTORY

Just as the discovery of the prostaglandins had its odd origin when seminal fluid stimulated a uterine muscle strip to contract, the discovery of the leukotrienes began with an experiment on the effect of cobra venom on dog lung. In 1938, when the stimulatory effect of histamine on bronchial smooth muscle was well known, Feldberg and Kellaway found that dog lung perfused with cobra venom released a potent bronchoconstrictor agent whose effect lasted much longer than that of histamine. They also found that a similar substance was released from sensitized guinea pig lung during challenge with antigen, and they named their factor *slow reacting substance* (SRS) (to distinguish it from histamine, which was a fast reacting substance).

In the early 1940s, Brocklehurst added the A to SRS (i.e., SRS-A, A = Anaphylaxis) when he found that a similar factor was produced by human lung tissue from asthmatic patients when the tissue was exposed to pollen. Since antihistamine drugs were generally ineffective in the treatment of human asthma, it was widely agreed that SRS-A is the agent responsible for bronchoconstriction in that disease. This agreement provided the major stimulus for attempts to identify the material.

During the 1970s, there were several attempts to determine the chemical nature of purified SRS-A. Near the end of that decade, the substance was found to be fat soluble and to comigrate near arachidonic acid on two-dimensional chromatography. Its synthesis was enhanced by the addition of cysteine to peritoneal macrophages stimulated to produce it by the calcium ionophore, A23187. Accumulating evidence suggested that SRS-A is a metabolite of arachidonic acid.

BIOSYNTHESIS AND NOMENCLATURE

This line of investigation, which began with the 1938 snake poison experiment, was pursued in parallel with studies on arachidonic acid metabolism and prostaglandin synthesis (see above) by Samuelsson and his colleagues in Stockholm. The Karolinska investigators were aware of the fact that not all arachidonic acid metabolites were derived from the cyclic endoperoxides, but little was known about the potential biological importance of the "linear" (i.e., noncyclic) metabolites. Using murine mastocytoma cells propagated in the peritoneal cavities of mice (known to produce SRS-A on incubation with the calcium ionophore, A23187), they proved that the radioactivity of both ^{35}S-labeled cysteine and tritium-labeled arachidonic acid was incorporated into biologically active SRS-A. Again, the availability of a powerful, new method, high-pressure liquid chromatography and an appropriate bioassay (so important in studies on the cyclooxygenase metabolites) enabled them to do these experiments. In yet another awe-inspiring demonstration of organic chemical virtuosity, the biosynthetic pathway of the leukotrienes was elucidated (Fig 4–5).

The first product of arachidonic acid in the lipoxygenase pathway is 5-HPETE (5-hydroperoxyeicosatetranoic acid). (Hydroperoxidation can occur on other carbon atoms of arachidonic acid, but little is known about the biological significance of metabolites other than the 5-HETE series). 5-HPETE is the precursor of LTA_4 which in turn is transformed into either LTB_4 or the SH-containing peptide and amino acid conjugates, compounds LTC_4, LTD_4, and LTE_4. The last three together constitute SRS-A; they are secreted by mast cells that participate in hypersensitivity reactions. LTB_4 has been studied most as a product and agonist of leukocytes.

BIOLOGICAL EFFECTS

Lung

Histamine is a potent stimulator of smooth muscle in the tracheobronchial tree, but the SRS-A compounds are 4,000 times more powerful. The mast cell is an example of a cell that responds to stimuli much

the way other cells respond to peptide hormones: it has an adenylate cyclase response mechanism, a polyphosphatidyl inositol turnover system capable of generating diacylglycerol and inositol triphosphate, and an arachidonic acid response system. In this case, the plasma membrane receptor is IgE, an immunoglobulin that has been precoded to recognize "not self." Standing guard at cutaneous and mucosal surfaces the mast cell can take immediate action against any antigen to which it has been sensitized by secreting the contents of its granules and by releasing SRS-A when the "hormone" antigen binds to its "receptor" IgE. The SRS-A released near bronchiolar smooth muscle cells is powerfully stimulatory; in a human asthmatic, the resulting bronchoconstriction can seriously impair the tidal movement of air. Leukotriene stimulation of bronchial mucus secretion compounds the problem. We will come back to this subject in subsequent comments on the pharmacology of arachidonic acid metabolism.

Cardiovascular

Effects of LTC_4 and LTD_4 have been described in microvessels, large vessels, and in the heart. The SRS-A compounds have been found to increase small vessel permeability as well as to stimulate arterial smooth muscle in some species. A negative inotropic effect on cardiac muscle contraction in association with diminished coronary blood flow has also been described. The decreased contractile power of the heart is greater than can be accounted for by diminished coronary flow alone. The pathophysiological significance of these effects has not yet been evaluated.

Gastrointestinal

The SRS-A group stimulates gastrointestinal smooth muscle, but not as powerfully as it does bronchiolar smooth muscle. In the lung, LTC_4 and LTD_4 were equipotent, but in the GI tract, the latter was more potent. They effect an increase in intracellular $[Ca^{2+}]_c$, but the mechanism(s) by which they do this are unknown to us.

Stimulation of Prostaglandin Synthesis

The metabolic products of one route of eicosanoid synthesis can stimulate synthesis and release of compounds generated in the other pathway. In some cell types, SRS-A has been found to stimulate the production of prostaglandins. This may be related to their ability to increase $[Ca^{2+}]_c$, for phospholipase A_2 is activated by the calcium ion.

Inflammation, Leukocytes, and LTB₄

The inflammatory response represents a complex local response to injury. Much of the phenomenology of inflammation at the morphological level has been known for over a century. The response is characterized by increased permeability of microvessels, local vasodilation and a gathering of leukocytes. This stereotypical response is induced by different kinds of challenge, including bacterial infection, mechanical trauma, local hypoxia, chemical or thermal injury, allergic reactions, etc. Clotting factors and the complement system are importantly involved, as are many locally produced mediators, including histamine, bradykinin, serotonin, catecholamines, and others.

Although the inflammatory process had long been studied, two historical events together produced a quantum leap in our understanding of its mechanisms. These were (1) the discovery of the anti-inflammatory effect of the adrenal glucocorticoid steroid hormones in 1949 by Hench and Kendall and (2) the discovery that aspirin, a very effective anti-inflammatory drug, works by blocking the synthesis of prostaglandins (see Vane Nobel lecture). After the second discovery, adrenal steroids were also found to block prostaglandin synthesis. Thus, prostaglandin formation was established as a necessary feature of the inflammatory process.

Prostaglandins, especially PGE_2, are produced in large amounts at the site of inflammation. They can in fact induce an inflammatory response. They potentiate the effects of histamine, bradykinin, and other short-term mediators of inflammation. Inflammation induced by PGs can be demonstrated even when the effects of histamine and serotonin are eliminated by appropriate pharmacologic blocking agents.

With the discovery of the leukotrienes, a new dimension was added to the importance of arachidonic acid metabolites in inflammation. Inflammation cannot occur without leukocytes. This can be demonstrated readily in dogs treated with agents that inhibit leukocyte development and maturation in the bone marrow. Therefore, we can conclude that attraction of

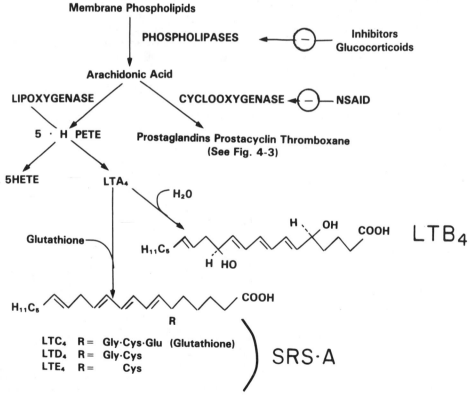

FIG 4–5.
Biosynthesis of leukotrienes.

leukocytes to the inflammatory site and stimulation of leukocytes to phagocytose foreign material and tissue debris and secretion of lysosomal enzymes are integral parts of the inflammatory process. Again, the leukocyte responds to a large variety of stimuli with its own repertory of reactions in much the way a hormone-sensitive cell responds to a hormone. Moreover, it uses many of the same biochemical strategies in its responses. Polymorphonuclear leukocytes can be stimulated to spring into action by bacteria (alive or dead), polystyrene particles, complement 5a, the tripeptide fMet·Leu·Phe (a chemotactic peptide), the calcium ionophore, A23187, and phorbol esters. From the last two stimuli, we can infer that leukocyte stimulation involves an increase in cytosolic $[Ca^{2+}]_c$ and that polyphosphatidyl inositol turnover is probably involved in the response in some way. To make the similarity of the leukocyte response to a hormone response even more striking, several of these stimuli cause an increase in cellular cyclic AMP.

LTB$_4$ (see Fig 4–5) has now been revealed to be the most potent chemoattractant for polymorphonuclear leukocytes known. Moreover, it can duplicate most of the metabolic effects of other leukocyte stimulants, including degranulation and release of lysosomal enzymes. Treatment of leukocytes with LTB$_4$ enhances their tendency to stick to endothelial surfaces. Also, they have been shown to increase $[Ca^{2+}]_c$ of leukocytes. Apparently, different categories of cells are able to regulate the amounts of lipoxygenase products they produce according to their individual needs, as shown by the following LTB$_4$:LTC$_4$ ratios:

Neutrophils, monocytes and macrophages, HIGH
Eosinophils and mast cells, LOW

(We will discuss the anti-inflammatory action of adrenal glucocorticoids in Chapter 11.)

SOME PRACTICAL APPLICATIONS

Figure 4–3 indicates that aspirin, indomethacin, and other nonsteroidal anti-inflammatory agents block at the cyclooxygenase step but do not block at the phospholipase A$_2$ step. Figure 4–5 shows that adrenal glucocorticoids deny arachidonic acid to both pathways. Arachidonic acid availability limits the rate of synthesis of products via both pathways.

These facts provide a plausible explanation for the phenomenon of salicylate-induced asthmatic attacks in people with bronchial asthma. If the cyclooxygenase pathway is blocked, a stimulus to phospholipase A$_2$ in the form of SRS-A may be exaggerated due to the availability of an excessively large pool of arachidonic acid precursor with only one way to go.

The potential pharmacological implications of these developments have been and will be explored extensively. The agents under development fall into two categories: eicosanoid analogues as agonists and eicosanoid analogues and other agents as antagonists. In the first category, PGs have been used as midtrimester abortifacients and, in a few clinics, as inducers of labor. Other analogues are under testing as potential antipeptic ulcer agents and as antihypertensives. In the second category, vigorous attempts are now being made to discover substances that would either inhibit the release of SRS-As or inhibit their biological effect. Obviously, such agents would be valuable in the management of human bronchial asthma.

Nonsteroidal anti-inflammatory drugs, which work by inhibiting cyclooxygenase, are among the most widely used drugs in the world, both as prescription drugs and over-the-counter products.

It is in the field of prevention of platelet aggregation that we are likely to see the most important results of the discoveries we have described. Platelets are importantly involved, not only in thromboembolic disease, but also in the etiology of atherosclerosis and, consequently, in the natural history of strokes and heart attacks. There are encouraging data that suggest that chronic ingestion of an anticlotting agent may prevent or delay the onset of cerebral vascular accidents or coronary thrombosis. A long-acting prostacyclin analogue would be ideal for this purpose since it would not only inhibit platelet aggregation but would also have a desirable vessel dilating effect. There are reports of the beneficial use of prostacyclin analogues in patients undergoing open heart surgery which involves extracorporeal circulation.

The scientific importance of the discoveries we have described in this chapter was recognized by the Nobel Prize committee in 1982. Practical applications of this knowledge cannot fail to be made over many years to come.

BIBLIOGRAPHY

Aktories K, Schultz G, Jacobs KH: Inhibitory regulation of adenylate cyclase by prostaglandins. *Adv Prostaglandin Thromboxane Leukotriene Res* 1983; 12:283.

Chakrin LW, Bailey DM: *The Leukotrienes: Chemistry and Biology.* New York, Academic Press, 1984.

Ford-Hutchinson AW: Leukotrienes: Their formation and role as inflammatory mediators. *Fed Proc* 1985; 44:25.

Goetzl EJ: Oxygenation products of arachidonic acid as mediators of hypersensitivity and inflammation. *Med Clin North Am* 1981; 65:809.

Gorman RR: Modulation of human platelet function by prostacyclin and thromboxane A$_2$. *Fed Proc* 1979; 38:83.

Hammarström S: Leukotrienes. *Ann Rev Biochem* 1983; 52:355.

Heyman MA, Rudolph AM, Silverman NH: Closure of the

ductus arteriosus in premature infants by inhibition of prostaglandin synthesis. *N Engl J Med* 1976; 295:530.

Johnson M, Carey F, McMillan RM: Alternative pathways of arachidonate metabolism: Prostaglandins, thromboxane and leukotrienes. *Essays Biochem* 1983; 19:40.

Karim SMM, Twissell RR: Induction of labor with PGF_2. *Br Med J* 1968; 4:621.

Karim SMM, Filshei GM: Therapeutic abortion using PGF_2. *Lancet* 1970; 1:157.

Kennedy I, Coleman RA, Humphrey PA, et al: Studies on the characterization of prostanoid receptors. Adv Prostaglandin Thromboxane Leukotriene Res 1983; 11:327.

Krilis S, Lewis RA, Corey EJ, et al: Specific binding of leukotriene C_4 to ileal segments and subcellular fractions of ileal smooth muscle cells. *Proc Natl Acad Sci USA* 1984; 81:4529.

Lewis GP, Piper PJ: Inhibition of release of prostaglandins as an explanation of some of the actions of anti-inflammatory corticosteroids. *Nature* 1975; 254:308.

Lewis RA, Austen KF: The biologically active leukotrienes: Biosynthesis, metabolism, receptors, function and pharmacology. *J Clin Invest* 1984; 73:889.

Marcus AJ: The eicosanoids in biology and medicine. *J Lipid Res* 1984; 25:1511.

McGiff JC, Wong PY-K: Compartmentalization of prostaglandins and prostacyclin within the kidney: Implications for renal function. *Fed Proc* 1979; 38:89.

Moncada S (ed): Prostacyclin, thromboxane and leukotrienes (series of essays). *Br Med Bull* 1983; 39:208.

Murota S, Chang W-C, Koshihara Y, et al: Importance of cyclooxygenase induction in the biosynthesis of prostacyclin. Adv Prostaglandin Thromboxane Leukotriene Res 1983; 11:99.

Murphy RC, Hammarstrom S, Samuelsson B: Leukotriene C: A slow reacting substance from murine mastocytoma cells. *Proc Natl Acad Sci USA* 1979; 76:4275.

Oates JA, Whorten AR, Gerkeus JF, et al: The participation of prostaglandins in the control of renin release. *Fed Proc* 1979; 38:72.

Piper PJ: Formation and action of leukotrienes. *Physiol Rev* 1984; 64:744.

Samuelsson B: Prostaglandins, thromboxanes, and leukotrienes: Formation and biological roles. *Harvey Lect* 1981; 75:1.

Samuelsson B: Leukotrienes: Mediators of immediate hypersensitivity reactions and inflammation (Nobel lecture). *Science* 1983; 220:568.

Terragno NA, Terragno A: Prostaglandin metabolism in fetal and maternal vasculature. *Fed Proc* 1979; 38:75.

Vane JR: Adventures and excursions in bioassay: The stepping stones to prostacyclin (Nobel lecture). *Br J Pharmacol* 1983; 79:821.

Vane JR: Prostaglandins and the cardiovascular system. *Br Heart J* 1983; 49:405.

PART III

Neuroendocrinology

5

Adenohypophysis

Until about four decades ago, the adenohypophysis (or anterior pituitary) was widely believed to be a comparatively autonomous organ, which, having developed from an outpouching of the primitive foregut, came to rest in the sella turcica, where it functioned as the "conductor of the endocrine orchestra." Repeated attempts to demonstrate neural connections between the brain and the adenohypophysis had failed. In retrospect, it is easy to find many recorded observations, made in both clinic and experimental laboratory, that suggested the existence of a communication link between the CNS and the anterior pituitary. Now, the hypothalamus and the adenohypophysis are considered components of an integrated functional unit, an informational relay system. The pituitary is now more properly called the "concertmaster of the endocrine orchestra."

The missing link between the brain and the anterior pituitary was, of course, the hypophyseal portal system of blood vessels, which begins in the median eminence of the hypothalamus and drains downward into the sinusoids of the anterior hypophysis. These vessels, discovered independently by Popa and by Wislocki, provided the conceptual basis for our present understanding of the control of pituitary secretion.

The two main divisions of the hypophysis, the neurohypophysis (posterior pituitary) and the adenohypophysis, can be described functionally only in relation to the hypothalamic structures with which they interact. In the case of the posterior pituitary, two discrete constellations of neurons, the supraoptic and paraventricular nuclei, clearly have neuronal connections with the secreting gland. Two specific peptides, oxytocin and vasopressin, are synthesized in the cell bodies of these neurons, travel the length of their axon fibers bound to their respective carrier proteins and are discharged into the bloodstream at the nerve ending. These are peptidergic neurons, which secrete their hormonal products directly into the general circulation. The posterior pituitary will be discussed in Chapter 6.

Effects of Hypophysectomy

The effects of hypophysectomy may be inferred from the general functions of known hypophyseal hormones outlined in Table 5–1. The pituitary is necessary for *differentiation, postnatal growth, for adaptation to starvation and many stresses and for reproductive behavior and function.* Although the hypophysis is not essential for the life of the individual, it is indispensable for the propagation of the species.

Growth failure that occurs when hypophysectomy is performed in young, rapidly growing animals is due to deficiencies in a number of hormones, all of which are essential for normal growth. These include growth hormone, adrenocortical hormone, thyroid hormone, gonadal hormones.

Atrophy of the adrenal cortices is the result of deficiency of corticotrophin, which is essential for maintenance of the *zona fasciculata* of the adrenal cortices. The *zona glomerulosa,* which produces the powerfully salt-retaining mineralocorticoids of the adrenal, has some degree of independence from ACTH stimulation. It is for this reason that untreated adrenalectomy is fatal, whereas hypophysectomy is not. Death in the bilaterally adrenalectomized animal, or in the human being with bilateral adrenocortical destruction, is due ultimately to the consequences of sodium loss and potassium retention.

Secondary hypothyroidism, which is due to TSH deprivation, has many of the features of primary hypothyroidism (see Chapter 10). A continuing supply of TSH is necessary for maintenance of the thyroid hormone-producing follicular cell, and the capacity to adapt to cold exposure requires an intact hypothalamo-hypophyseal response system.

Secondary hypogonadism is the result of hypophysectomy in both sexes. If the operation is performed in sexually immature animals of either sex, the gonads fail to develop. If pituitary failure occurs after sexual maturation has occurred, gonadal function regresses.

Breast development and *function* require the collaboration of many hormones, most of which are either directly (prolactin) or indirectly (estrogen, adrenocortical hormones) dependent on hypophyseal activity.

Maintenance of skin pigmentation depends on a continuing supply of the intermediate lobe hormone intermedin (MSH). In amphibia and certain fishes, this hormone has a far more important adaptive function than it does in human beings, although it does participate in adaptive darkening of the skin in response to sun exposure in people.

It is practically impossible to discuss the adenohypophysis and its hormones as an isolated functional unit because it is centrally involved in the physiology of many other endocrine glands. Although we cannot examine the general features of the hypothalamo-hypophyseal mechanism without referring to the adrenals, the thyroid and the gonads, most of our discussion of the pituitary hormones related to those target glands will be deferred. This chapter is restricted to a description of the brain-pituitary interphase with emphasis on hypothalamic-releasing hormones, growth hormone and some reference to corticotrophin-related peptides.

Cellular Origins of Pituitary Hormones

The adenohypophysis, or anterior pituitary, is not one gland: it is a community of six glands, each con-

TABLE 5–1.

Hormones of Adenohypophysis and Their Functions

HORMONE	FUNCTION
Growth h. (GH) = somatotrophin	Somatic growth; compensatory hypertrophy; carbohydrate and lipid metabolism; renal function
Corticotrophin (ACTH)	Adaptation to starvation, traumatic and other stress; redistribution of body nutrients. Behavioral effects?
Thyrotrophin (TSH)	Maintenance of metabolic rate; adaptation to cold; CNS development
Luteinizing h. (LH) Interstitial cell-stimulating h. (ICSH)	♀, oogenesis and ovulation; steroidogenesis ♂, testosterone secretion; spermatogenesis Both?, Behavioral effects?
Follicle-stimulating h. (FSH)	♀, oogenesis and follicular growth ♂, spermatogenesis
Prolactin (PRL)	♀, lactogenic hormone ♂, ?
Intermedin, melanocyte-stimulating h. (MSH)	Increases skin pigmentation on exposure to sunlight in some people

sisting of a distinctive cell type and each individually controlled. Histochemical, immunofluorescence and electron microscopic methods have been used to assign secretory products to each recognizable cell type (Table 5–2). The cells of the anterior pituitary share many characteristics:

1. Since they receive no innervation from the hypothalamus, signals that control secretion are delivered by way of the hypophyseal portal system of blood vessels.

2. All pituitary cells secrete either protein or glycoprotein hormones from distinctive storage granules, which on appropriate signal discharge their contents by exocytosis.

3. With the possible exception of dopamine, histamine and norepinephrine, all of the known stimuli and inhibitors of pituitary hormone release are peptides.

4. Stimulus-secretion coupling probably involves calcium in all cases. In some cells, at least part of the secretory response is mediated by way of cAMP.

Chemical Classification of Pituitary and Related Placental Hormones

An interesting feature of the chemistry of pituitary hormones is that the *placenta* synthesizes and secretes some protein and glycoprotein hormones that are homologous in many amino acid sequences with those of the pituitary materials. This fact and the discovery of the morphine-like peptides, the endorphins and enkephalins, suggest the chemical classification of pituitary and placental hormones shown in Table 5–3.

This classification is based on the following facts:

1. Group I peptides are proteolytic products of a common 31,000 D glycoprotein precursor, proopiomelanocortin, but the hormones themselves are not glycoproteins.

2. The somatomammotrophins (group II) show striking homologous amino acid sequences as well as intrachain disulfide bridges; GH and hPL are especially closely related structurally, but all three appear to have evolved from a common molecular ancestor. The structural similarities between prolactin and growth hormone explain both the limited lactogenic activity of GH and the difficulty encountered by peptide chemists in establishing the independent existence of PRL in the human being.

3. The glycoprotein hormones (group III) are closely related. Each consists of two peptide chains, both of which are essential for biologic activity. Amino acid sequence analysis has revealed that the α chains of hormones in this group are virtually identical, but that distinctive sequences are found in the β subunits. It is possible to dissociate subunits from one another and then recombine them in homologous or heterologous pairs. The results of such recombination experiments are as follows:

TSH α + TSH β = active TSH
LH α + LH β = active LH
hCG α + hCG β = active hCG
LH α or hCG α + TSH β = active TSH
TSH α or hCG α + LH β = active LH
TSH α or LH α + hCG β = active hCG.

Thus the α subunits appear to be functionally interchangeable. This discovery of the subunit character of the glycoprotein hormones has made possible the development of exquisitely discriminating antibodies to the β subunits for radioimmunoassay purposes.

Hypothalamic Hormones of Known Structure

PHYSIOLOGIC METHODS OF STUDY

Our knowledge of neuroendocrinology has evolved from many different but complementary experimental approaches:

TABLE 5–2.

Cell Sources of Pituitary Hormones

CELL TYPE	PRODUCT	LIGHT MICROSCOPE	SECRETORY GRANULES (EM)	REMARKS
Lactotrophes	PRL	Acidophil	50–400 μ	In pregnancy
Somatotrophes	GH (somatotrophin)	Acidophil	300–400 μ	
Thyrotrophes	TSH	Basophil	50–100 μ	Hypertrophy p̄ thyroidectomy
Corticotrophes	ACTH β LPH*	Basophil	Variable size and density	
LH gonadotrophes	LH†	Basophil	Sparse	
FSH gonadotrophes	FSH†	Basophil	Sparse	Large; vacuoles on castration
Nonsecretory (stem)	—	Chromophobe	Small, variable	

*β LPH = β lipotrophin.
†Both of these hormones have been found in the same cell by immunofluorescence microscopy (EM). Other cells appear to contain one or the other.

TABLE 5–3.

Relationships of Pituitary and Placental Hormones

GROUP	HORMONE	AMINO ACIDS	APPROX. MW	CARBOHYDRATE
I. Corticotrophin related (all from common 31,000 MW precursor, proopiomelanocortin)	MSH	13 (ACTH 1–13)	1,650	0
	ACTH (chorionic ACTH)	39	4,500	0
	β LPH	91	9,500	0
	Endorphins (from β LPH)	31		0
II. Somatomammotrophins (Single peptide chain; 2–3 S–S bridges)	Prolactin (PRL)	198	23,000	0
	Growth h. (somatotrophin; GH)	191	22,000	0
	Chorionic somatomammotrophin (hPL)	191	22,000	0
III. Glycoproteins (2 peptide chains; α similar, β variable)	FSH	236	32,000	+
	LH (Also ICSH)	98, β119	30,000	+
	Chorionic gonadotropin (hCG)	92, β139	57,000	+
	Thyrotrophin	96, β113	28,000	+

1. Studies of hypophysectomized animals bearing well-vascularized grafts in sites remote from the median eminence.

2. Eliciting of adenohypophyseal hormone secretion by *stimulating* discrete regions in the hypothalamus by stereotactically placed electrodes.

3. The blocking of certain anterior pituitary responses (e.g., ACTH release, ovulation or thyroid hypertrophy following inhibition of thyroid hormone synthesis by thiouracil) by stereotactic placement of electrolytic *lesions* in the hypothalamus.

4. Inhibition of release of hormones by placement in the hypothalamus either of very small target organ grafts or pellets of target organ hormone.

5. Analysis of effects of selective destruction of nerve fiber tracts leading to and from the hypothalamus.

6. Mapping of the hypothalamic region for neurotransmitter substances and hormone receptors.

7. Analysis of effects of many agonist and antagonist drugs on pituitary secretory function.

8. Isolation, purification, structural analysis and synthesis of hypothalamic peptides. This has been accomplished recently for five of the postulated hypothalamic peptides (see below). (Structures of posterior lobe peptides were discovered in the 1950s.)

Hypothalamic mapping for peptidergic neurones has been done by means of immunohistochemical methods. In some cases, fairly discrete clusters of neurones containing a single releasing hormone can be found in certain regions of the hypothalamus, but these are not as neatly circumscribed as are those for the posterior pituitary hormones that will be discussed in the next chapter. Often, a variety of peptidergic neurones can be found in the same place. The following summary suggests concentration zones for specific releasing hormones and for dopamine: TRH: Dorsomedial nucleus (weak). LHRH: Anterior—septal, preoptic, suprachiasmatic region; More rostral—medial basal tubercinarium. CRH: Paraventricular nucleus, arcuate, and ventromedial nuclei. Somatostatin: Widely distributed and interspersed with others. Dopamine (PIF): Tuboinfundibular dopaminergic system.

In the case of LHRH, the anterior zone has been associated with cyclic release of gonadotropins, as in the estrus and menstrual cycles, while the more rostral zone controls tonic secretion. The important concept here is that all of these peptidergic neurones have complex connections within the CNS (see later section) and that, for their secretory products, all roads lead to the median eminence through which the peptides are literally funneled into the hypophysial portal blood for delivery to the pituitary.

On the basis of many ingenious physiologic and pharmacologic experiments of the sort enumerated above, evidence for the existence of the regulatory factors listed in Table 5–4 was obtained. (The convention is to designate as *hormones* substances of known chemical structure; *factors* have not yet been chemically identified. We have tried to adhere to this convention, but most authors continue to use the designations GRF and CRF in spite of the fact that these substances have been characterized and synthesized.)

TABLE 5–4.

Nomenclature of Hypothalamic Regulatory Hormones and Postulated Factors*

TRIVIAL NAME	DESCRIPTIVE NAME (HORMONE/FACTOR)	ABBREV.
Vasopressin	Antidiuretic *h.*	ADH, VP
Oxytocin	Milk let-down *h.*	OT, OXT
Thyroliberin	TSH-releasing *h.*	TRH
Gonadoliberin	LH/FSH-releasing *h.*	LHRH, LH/FSHRH, GnRH
Somatostatin	GH (somatotrophin) release-inhibiting *h.*	GHRIH, SRIH
Somatocrinin	GH-releasing *h.*	GRH (GRF)
Prolactostatin	PRL release-inhibiting *f.* (?dopamine)	PIF, PRIF
Prolactoliberin	PRL-releasing *f.*	PRF
Corticoliberin	ACTH-releasing *h.*	CRH (CRF)
Melanostatin	MSH release-inhibiting *f.*	MIF, MSHRF
Melanoliberin	MSH-releasing *f.*	MRF, MSHRF

*Hormone (h.) signifies known chemical structure; factor (f.) = structure unknown, existence suggested by physiologic experiments.

THYROTROPHIN-RELEASING HORMONE (TRH)

TRH is a tripeptide with the amino acid sequence shown in Figure 5–1. It has been synthesized, and the synthetic material has been found to have all of the biologic activity of the naturally occurring peptide. TRH is an extremely potent biologic material, being effective in nanogram amounts. Although it is a tripeptide, it can be absorbed from the gastrointestinal tract in biologically active form.

Before TRH became available, it had been assumed that each hypothalamic factor would prove to be cell specific and that it would affect secretion of only one pituitary hormone. TRH, however, not only stimulated release of TSH but also that of prolactin. (Many investigators believe, however, that TRH cannot be "the" PRF because there are circumstances in which the secretion of TSH and prolactin is clearly dissociable.) Furthermore, TRH appears to stimulate growth hormone release in acromegalic patients. Similarly, more than one cell type responds to LH/FSH RH, and somatostatin inhibits secretion of TSH as well as that

TRH (3)

pyroGlu-His-ProNH2

GnRH (LHRH) (10)

pyroGlu-His-Trp-Ser-Tyr-Gly-Leu-Arg-Pro-GlyNH2

oCRH (CRF) (41)

HSer-Gln-Glu-Pro-Pro-Ile-
Ser-Leu-Asp-Leu-Thr-Phe-His-
Leu-Leu-Arg-Glu-Val-Leu-Glu-
Met-Thr-Lys-Ala-Asp-Gln-Leu-
Ala-Gln-Gln-Ala-His-Ser-Asn-
Arg-Lys-Leu-Leu-Asp-Ile-AlaNH2

hpGHRH (44)

HTyr-Ala-Asp-Ala-Ile-Phe-Thr-
Asn-Ser-Tyr-Arg-Lys-Val-Leu-
Gly-Gln-Leu-Ser-Ala-Arg-Lys-
Leu-Leu-Gln-Asp-Ile-Met-Ser-
Arg-Gln-Gln-Gly-Glu-Ser-Asn-
Gln-Glu-Arg-Gly-Ala-Arg-Ala-
Arg-LeuNH2

SOMATOSTATIN (SRIH, GHRIH) (14)

HAla-Gly-Cys-Lys-Asn-Phe-Phe-Trp-Lys-Thr-Phe-Thr-Ser-CysOH
        └————————————S–S————————————┘

FIG 5–1.
Known structures of hypothalamic peptides.

of growth hormone. The biologic significance of these overlapping effects of hypothalamic hormones is not yet clear.

TRH has proved to be a useful diagnostic agent in differentiation of primary, secondary, and tertiary hypothyroidism. A diagrammatic summary of its use in this way is given in Figure 5–2, although isolated TRH deficiency is a rare form of hypothyroidism.

A major advance in our understanding of feedback control mechanisms was made when thyroid hormone (TH) was found to inhibit the response of the thyrotrophe to TRH. Thus, thyrotrophe responsiveness is maximal in TH deficiency, which helps to account for the high levels of circulating TSH seen in that condition. The inhibitory effect of TH on thyrotrophe sensitivity to TRH occurs only after a lag period and requires protein synthesis to develop. The molecular basis for TH-induced TRH resistance is not known.

GONADOTROPIN-RELEASING HORMONE, LHRH (LH/FSH RH; GNRH)

The second releasing hormone to be identified chemically and synthesized is LHRH, a decapeptide with the structure shown in Figure 5–1. Like TRH, it has a pyroglutamic acid residue at the amino terminal. Again, the synthetic peptide was shown to have full biologic activity. A radioimmunoassay developed for LHRH made possible the observation that the material is detectable even in peripheral blood of women at midcycle, i.e., at the time of the ovulatory LH surge. From much evidence in experimental animals and in women, there is no doubt that the wide cyclic fluctuations in gonadotropin output seen in the estrus and menstrual cycles are mediated in part by way of changes in LHRH secretion by the hypothalamus. In fact, it is possible to induce ovulation both in experimental animals and in women by intravenous injection of synthetic LHRH. Antibodies to LHRH can disrupt gonadotropin secretion.

A whole spectrum of functional disorders of gonadotropin secretion, from psychogenic amenorrhea to pseudopregnancy, is conceivable in terms of disruption of LHRH secretion by messages originating in the cerebral cortex and other parts of the brain. An attempt will be made shortly to demonstrate how such disruption might occur.

The elucidation of the structure of LHRH provides an opportunity to introduce a recurring theme in endocrinology, i.e., the attempt to invent compounds with desirable characteristics by synthesizing variants of the naturally occurring hormone. Chemists have synthesized a large number of LHRH analogues, and many of these have been tested in a variety of biologic systems. Most of the interesting compounds have involved substitutions at the 2 and 6 carbons and the elimination of glycine[10]. Several "super LHRH" substances have been synthesized, one of which, desgly[10],ethyl-pro[9]-D-trp[6], is 144 times as potent as naturally occurring LHRH. Others (e.g., D-Phe[2] substi-

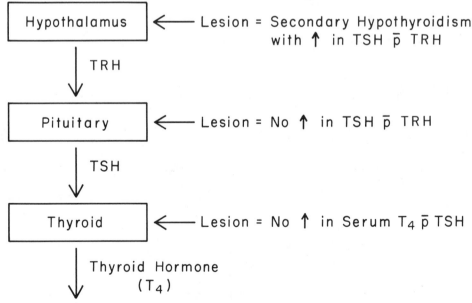

FIG 5–2.
Diagnostic use of TRH and TSH in localizing defect in thyroid function. $\bar{p}$ = after

tuted for His[2]) are very powerful *anti*-LHRH materials. This area is of intense interest to people who are concerned with problems of infertility or with improved chemical methods of contraception. (See section below on pulsatile, diurnal, and cyclic hypophysial hormone secretion.)

SOMATOSTATIN (SRIF)

While searching for a GH-releasing factor, Guillemin, Brazeau, Vale, and colleagues discovered a GH or somatotrophin release-*inhibiting* factor, which they called SRIF. Since previous physiologic experiments by McCann and colleagues had suggested the existence of such a factor, the La Jolla group isolated and purified SRIF, determined its amino acid sequence, synthesized it and demonstrated full biologic activity of the synthetic material. In a remarkably short time since the announcement of the discovery of SRIF, a cascade of research and symposium reports has appeared.

Naturally occurring somatostatin (see Fig 5–1) is a 14 amino acid peptide, which exists as a loop bound by an S–S bridge between cystine 3 and cystine 14. The synthetic molecule is the reduced, or linear, form. The two forms have equal biologic activity.

Although somatostatin is found in high concentration in the hypothalamus and although its initial discovery was based on its GH-release-inhibiting activity, it soon became obvious that it had been named prematurely. Again, on the basis of the unanticipated finding of transient hypoglycemia in somatostatin-treated baboons, it was found first to inhibit glucagon secretion and, later, insulin secretion as well. Although it had no effect on the secretion of prolactin or gonadotrophins, it inhibited both basal and TRH-stimulated TSH secretion. In quick succession this remarkable peptide was found to suppress secretion of all of the following as well:

> Gastrin
> Secretin
> Gastric inhibitory peptide (GIP)
> Vasoactive intestinal peptide (VIP)
> Cholecystokinin
> Calcitonin
> Parathyroid hormone
> Immunoglobulins
> Renin

Not incidentally, it was also found to suppress gastric acid secretion, secretion of bicarbonate and digestive enzymes and intestinal absorption of glucose. Gastrointestinal motility is inhibited by somatostatin, as is splanchnic blood flow.

The peptide also has striking effects on CNS function, including behavioral and electric changes as well as alterations in motor coordination. In human beings, infusion of somatostatin causes sedation, and in experimental animals, microiontophoresis directly into the brain decreases neuronal activity.

Development of specific antibodies, which permitted immunocytochemical localization of somatostatin in cells, led to further surprises. Not only was the peptide present in high concentration in nerve endings of the median eminence, it was also found in the cortex, midbrain, brain stem, spinal cord and sensory ganglia. Moreover, somatostatin-producing cells were identified in the D cells of the islets of Langerhans, in specific endocrine secretory cells in gastric and intestinal epithelium as well as in parafollicular cells in the thyroid. Since the substance is not easily detectable in blood, it is presumed to be paracrine; i.e., when it is released from its cells of origin, it influences adjacent cells by local diffusion except in the case of the pituitary, which it reaches after a very short passage from the median eminence. That somatostatin has a tonic effect on pituitary hormone secretion was shown by Unger and colleagues, who demonstrated *increases* in pituitary and intestinal hormone secretions after administration of anti-somatostatin antibody. In the same experiment, no increase in pancreatic hormone secretion was demonstrable.

Cellular mechanisms involved in somatostatin's enormous repertory of biologic effects are under intensive study, but no satisfactory umbrella theory can yet be advanced. The only common feature of the secretion-inhibiting, smooth muscle-depressing, neuronal-depressing effects catalogued above is the involvement of calcium ion in all of them. Somatostatin is believed to affect calcium flux in an unspecified way and thus influence a wide variety of cell types.

Somatostatin has been used as an investigative tool in the analysis of problems in the metabolism of nutrients, and for a while there was some enthusiasm for its potential as an adjunctive treatment of diabetes mellitus. Some account of this use of the peptide will be given in Chapter 14. For the present it is sufficient to comment that the variety and ubiquity of its biologic effects make it unlikely that the compound will be used therapeutically in the near future, though it is conceivable that some molecular modification with more selective actions may prove to be a valuable agent some day.

Somatostatin is the *first biologic product of a mammal to be produced by a microorganism* (see Itakura et al.). (For the role of somatostatin in the feedback regulation of GH secretion, see section on GRH below.)

PROLACTIN-INHIBITORY FACTOR

The cloned complementary DNA sequence for the precursor protein of GnRH was used to construct an expression vector for a 56 amino acid GnRH-associated protein (GAP) (Nicolics et al.). GAP was found to be a highly potent inhibitor of prolactin secretion and a powerful stimulator of gonadotropin release in cultured rat pituitary cells. Although there have been some editorial reservations expressed about the physiological significance of GAP, we are impressed by the fact that active immunization of rats with GAP peptides (i.e., stimulation of formation of anti-GAP antibodies) leads to greatly increased prolactin secretion. Moreover, the material has been demonstrated immunologically in the hypothalamus and elsewhere in the brain and in the placenta in association with GnRH. Often, but not invariably, gonadotropin and prolactin secretion are reciprocally related. It is appealing, therefore, to imagine that the cosecretion of GnRH and GAP by the same cells may represent one level of coordinated control of secretion of the two pituitary hormones.

CORTICOTROPIN-RELEASING HORMONE (CRH, or CRF, or CORTICOLIBERIN)

The search for pituitary-stimulating substances of hypothalamic origin began with a postulated ACTH-releasing factor (corticotropin-releasing factor, CRF). The existence of CRF was inferred from the experiments of G. Harris and others who showed that pituitary stalk section caused adrenal atrophy; that electrical stimulation of certain discrete zones in the hypothalamus caused release of ACTH; and that pituitary implants under the hypothalamus were more effective in restoring adrenal function than were similar implants elsewhere in the body (Nikitovitch-Winer). Much of this work was done before 1950. In 1955, Porter demonstrated CRF activity in pituitary portal blood of stressed hypophysectomized dogs when carotid arterial blood from the same dogs showed no such activity.

In 1955, Guillemin and Rosenberg and Saffran and Schally independently described the release of ACTH by pituitary fragments coincubated with pieces of hypothalamus in vitro. Although much effort and an unimaginable number of hypothalami harvested in many slaughterhouses were expended over the next quarter century, CRF defied isolation and chemical characterization (see Wade for a fascinating account of "the years in the wilderness"). The search for CRF yielded important byproducts; however, for TRH, somatostatin and GnRH were all purified, characterized and synthesized, and, for these accomplishments, Guillemin and Schally were awarded Nobel Prizes in 1977.

In 1981, Vale et al. isolated, purified, and synthesized a 41 amino acid (AA) peptide from sheep hypothalami that stimulated release of ACTH from pituitary cells in concentrations as low as 0.1 nM. Rat CRH was purified and sequenced by Rivier et al., and the amino acid sequence of human CRH was deduced by Numa and his colleagues from the DNA sequence of the cloned CRH genome. In this case, people resemble rats more than they do sheep, for the human and rat sequences are identical, while that of the sheep differs from both at 7 of the 41 residues. The mammalian peptides show considerable amino acid homology with certain phylogenetically ancient fish and amphibian peptides with which they share an ability to lower blood pressure, although at doses so much greater than those required for ACTH release that they have no apparent physiologic significance.

That purified or synthetic CRH is indeed a physiological agonist is demonstrated by the fact that animals injected with antibodies to the peptide (or with synthetic CRH antagonists) show a markedly diminished increase in ACTH on exposure to a standard stress.

For many years we have known that several well-known neurotransmitters and hormones have weak CRH action. These include epinephrine, norepinephrine, antidiuretic hormone (ADH), oxytocin, and angiotensin II. All of these have been shown to augment the pituitary response to CRH both in vivo and in vitro. All of these agents have been shown in other systems to be capable of increasing intracellular Ca^{2+} concentration. Thus, they can act synergistically with a secretory stimulant. The complex neural and endocrine response to stress is discussed in Chapter 11.

Mechanism of Action

CRH causes a rapid accumulation of cyclic AMP in pituitary cells and in certain pituitary tumor cell lines. Desensitization has been observed with prolonged exposure to CRH. Since adrenal glucocorticoids can inhibit ACTH secretion elicited by either CRH or dibutyryl cyclic AMP, the major inhibitory effect of the steroids is believed to be at the level of the exocytotic process of granule release. All evidence points to the participation of Ca^{2+} in this as in most other secretory processes.

Applications in Humans

Studies on the effects of CRH 41 on people have been done by several groups of investigators (see Chrousos for references). Remarkably, the intravenous injection of as little as 0.03 µg/kg of body weight in human subjects causes a significant increase in immunoassayable ACTH in blood. The concentration of the material at the pituitary after an intravenous bolus of this amount is almost incredibly small.

The most prominent use of the peptide is in the differential diagnosis of pituitary from hypothalamic causes of ACTH deficiency in a manner entirely analogous with the use of TRH illustrated in Figure 5–2. Immunoassay for CRH will certainly be helpful in the diagnosis of ectopic ACTH excess. It is possible that analogue inhibitors of the action of CRH may prove useful in the treatment of patients with certain adrenal hyperfunctional states. There is promise that a single injection of TRH, GnRh, CRH, and GRH (see next section) will be useful as a combined anterior pituitary (CAP) function test (Sheldon et al.).

GRH (GRF, SRF, Somatocrinin)

About two decades ago, the discovery of the structure of GRH was announced and we cheerfully included the published amino acid sequence in an early edition of this book. Sadly, "GRH" turned out to be an artifact, a fragment of hemoglobin, and the search was resumed. Somatostatin was a byproduct of this endeavor, but GRH activity was present in such low concentrations in hypothalamic extracts that it eluded identification until 1982, when two teams of investigators, those of Guillemin and of Rivier, simultaneously announced the purification, characterization, and synthesis of highly potent GRHs.

The breakthrough was made possible by an experiment of nature. For many years, clinicians have been interested in the phenomenon of *ectopic hormone production* by a variety of tumors. For example, a carcinoma of the lung can produce enough AGTH to cause Cushing's disease while others may secrete antidiuretic hormone inappropriately (see next chapter). Although the precise molecular biology involved in the production of hormones by tumors is unknown, it is convenient to attribute it to a dysdifferentiation (see Baylin and Mendelsohn) that occurs when a cell is designated as a progenitor of a line of tumor cells. A segment of DNA that is normally "occluded" is unaccountably "open" for transcription and expressed constitutively; it transcribes mRNA for a particular hormone continuously and is not restrained by feedback inhibition.

One such (rare) tumor of the pancreas produced the syndrome of acromegaly (excessive growth hormone [GH] production) in an individual who showed no evidence of pituitary enlargement. The Guillemin and Rivier teams obtained samples of such tumors and soon demonstrated that tumor extracts were 5,000x as potent (on a per mg wet wt basis) as rat hypothalamus in stimulating the release of RIA assayable GH from primary cultures of rat pituitary gland. Both groups were able to purify, characterize, and synthesize highly active GRH from their respective tumor samples. The Guillemin product is a 44 amino acid (AA) peptide (see Fig 5–1, hpGRH 44). The predominant peptide in the Rivier yield was a 40 AA substance that was identical with the first 40 amino acids of GRH 44, but there was also an active 37 AA fragment. Subsequently, *hypothalamic* GRH was isolated from six species including the human, and five of these were shown to be 44 AA peptides. The exception was the rat, whose hypothalamic GRH proved to be a 43 AA peptide. Human hypothalamic and pancreatic tumor GRH are identical. The amino acid sequences of hypothalamic GRH in nonhuman species vary from that of the human by 3–12 amino acid residues. The 44 AA human peptide is more potent than hGRH 40 on in vitro testing, but the two are equipotent when given as an intravenous bolus. The 44 AA form is probably the native hypothalamic hormone, and the smaller peptides are thought to be preparative artifacts.

GRH is structurally related to the glucagon-secretin family of what are commonly called gastrointestinal peptide hormones, although that designation no longer seems sensible in view of the fact that they are found all over the central nervous system and elsewhere in the body (see Krieger review). Among these peptides are VIP (vasoactive intestinal peptide), GIP (gastric inhibitory peptide), and PHI (peptide histidine isoleucine). VIP is present in the hypothalamus and may work synergistically with GRH to stimulate GH release in much the way we have described the synergistic action of ADH and CRH above.

GRH, like the other known hypothalamic hormones, is an extremely powerful agonist. In the in vitro pituitary cell test system, it is active in a dose-dependent manner over a concentration range of 0.003 to 1.0 nM. In people it can increase the basal level of serum GH 10-fold in an intravenous dose of 1 µg/kg.

Regulation of Somatotrope Response to GRH

Adrenal glucocorticoids increase and adrenalectomy decreases the GH secretory response to GRH. The thyroid hormone, triiodothyronine (T_3), also enhances the response to GRH. In fact, dexamethasone, an adrenal steroid, and T_3 have been shown to act synergistically by stimulating the transcription of GH mRNA in a GH-producing pituitary tumor cell line.

The major *inhibitor* of pituicyte responsiveness to GRH is *somatostatin*. In fact, somatostatin is the central actor in the feedback inhibition of GH secretion by the pituitary, for it is now generally accepted that the feedback inhibition of GH on its own secretion is accomplished via *somatomedin*, whose production is stimulated by GH (see discussion below). *Somatomedin C* has been shown to be a powerful stimulator of the release of *somatostatin* from the basal hypothalamus in vitro. This beautiful in vitro model correctly predicted what would happen in *people*, for somatomedin C has now been shown to stimulate somatostatin release in the intact human being.

Cellular Mechanism of Action of GRH and Somatostatin

GRH stimulates both GH release and GH synthesis. It does this by binding to its plasma membrane receptor and activating the three messenger systems described in Chapter 3. Cyclic AMP and GH secretory response increase in a dose-dependent manner in pituitary cells treated with GRH. GH secretion is also stimulated either by dibutyryl cyclic AMP or by the Ca^{2+} ionophore. GRH action requires Ca^{2+}, and the involvement of phosphatidyl inositol turnover in the action of the releasing factor has been demonstrated. Stimulation of GH mRNA synthesis following GRH administration has been shown. Presumably, all of these effects are mediated by phosphorylation and dephosphorylation of a distinctive population of protein kinase substrates, but none of these has been identified.

Incubation of pituitary cell cultures with somatostatin for 24 hours completely abolishes the ability of either GRH *or* dibutyl cyclic AMP to stimulate GH secretion. Thus, although there is evidence that somatostatin can lower cyclic AMP, the major secretion-inhibiting event induced by somatostatin occurs at some point in stimulus-secretion coupling *beyond* the production of cyclic AMP. The precise molecular mechanism by which somatostatin interferes with Ca^{2+}-mediated exocytotic processes is unknown.

Clinical Applications

GRH, like the other hypothalamic hormones, can be used as a diagnostic tool for testing the competence of the pituitary to respond to a specific stimulus. The peptide has already been used successfully to stimulate growth in short children who were GH-deficient but who responded to a GRH challenge with satisfactory increases in serum GH. Interestingly, the releasing hormone was administered by means of a programmable pump that delivered a bolus of GRH at regular intervals in imitation of the physiologic episodic stimulation of the pituitary. This may prove to be the treatment of choice in the subset of GH-deficient children who have GRH-responsive pituitaries.

Organization and Neural Connections of Hypothalamic-Hypophysial System

A large collection of experimental facts suggests a design something like that shown in Figure 5–3. If we begin by considering a single hypophyseal secretory cell 5, which secretes one hormone, we see that the rate of secretion represents a vector of positive and negative forces 6. Secretion can be increased by increasing + or decreasing −; it can be inhibited by the reverse. Thus, the major determinant of the rate of secretion of the cell is the balance between stimulatory and inhibitory signals. Another important determinant of the cell's secretory response is its *sensitivity* to stimulation by hypothalamic peptides. For example, the sensitivity of the pituitary to LHRH stimulus is markedly increased at the time of the midcycle LH surge. Similarly, the sensitivity of the thyrotrophe to TRH is strikingly decreased by thyroid hormone. Since the secretory cells of the hypophysis have no innervation, they are stimulated or inhibited by hypothalamic peptides, which are carried in the portal system.

The peptidergic neuron 3, whether it secretes a stimulatory or inhibitory peptide, takes its direction from a complex set of monoaminergic neurons. At least three monoamines (dopamine, norepinephrine, serotonin) are known to be involved in the control of hypothalamic peptidergic neurons, and another, gamma aminobutyric acid (GABA), may be. When we realize that norepinephrine exerts its effects by way of at least two different receptors, α and β, we add another dimension of complexity. Whether a monoaminergic neuron sends a positive or negative signal to one or more peptidergic neurons depends on information it receives from near or remote neurons in the CNS 1. These arise in midbrain or brain stem nuclei and are themselves monoaminergic pathways. Figure 5–4 is intended to make the point that the medial hypothalamus is connected with all parts of the CNS. Thus, a tract that carries sleep-related information may arise in a different place and use a different monoaminergic transmitter from one associated with extreme fright. Yet both tracts may carry a stimulatory message to a peptidergic neuron.

Even without attempting to understand the details of these connections, it is easy to imagine how it is possible for anxiety over an examination to elicit

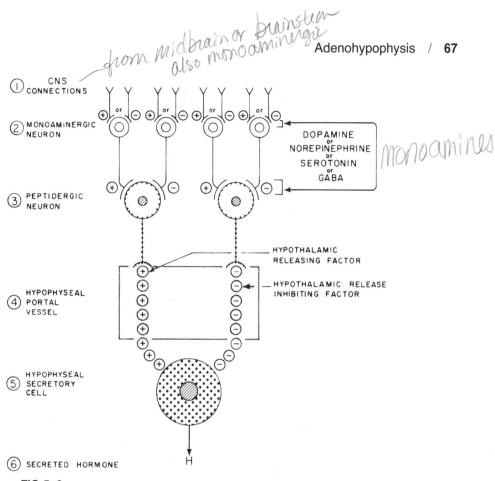

from midbrain or brainstem also monoaminergic

monoamines

FIG 5–3.
Concept of design of control system for single anterior pituitary cell.
GABA = gamma aminobutyric acid.

ACTH secretion or how the aerial bombing of a European city could have resulted in epidemics of menstrual disturbances by interfering with the control of gonadotropin secretion.

We have traced controlling influences for *one* hypophysial cell into the deepest recesses of the brain, but the pituitary gland is not a single gland. In order to appreciate the complexity of control of the individual cell types in the pituitary, it is necessary to inspect Figure 5–3 and multiply it by, at least, six. For each of the hypophysial cells is controlled by a system no less intricate than the one suggested in the diagram. Each cell has its own characteristic secretory response to the mix of hypothalamic peptides by which it is perfused. In addition, each hypothalamic peptidergic neuron is part of its own, distinctive neuronal circuit pattern in the CNS. *It is the combination of wiring diagram and chemical signal that results in the remarkably selective manner in which the hypophysis discharges individual hormones.* To add an additional layer of complexity to an already unimaginably complex subject, the cells of the paraventricular and su-

praoptic nuclei, which are peptidergic neurons responsible for synthesis and secretion of antidiuretic hormone and oxytocin, bear a close resemblance to the hypothalamic peptidergic neurons. Humoral and neural mechanisms that control secretory function of the posterior pituitary are just as complicated as are those depicted in Figure 5–3.

In both in vivo and in vitro experiments (coincubation of hypothalamus and pituitary), it is possible to assess the effectiveness of various monoamines in provoking secretion of pituitary hormones. Table 5–5 contains a summary of data from a number of sources. Consistent changes in secretion rates of some pituitary hormones may be observed when dopamine, norepinephrine, or serotonin is given. The same monoamine may stimulate release of two or more hormones, or it may stimulate one and inhibit another. In the case of growth hormone, which is elicited by a variety of signals (sleep, insulin hypoglycemia, arginine), the CNS pathways involved may use different neural transmitters (see next section).

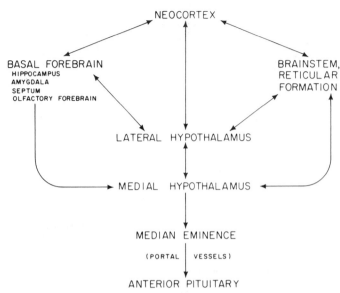

FIG 5–4.
CNS connections of medial hypothalamus.

Selective Control of Individual Pituitary Functions

Many attempts have been made to address the difficult problem of *differential* control of individual functions. These attempts, all of which involve radioimmunoassay for individual pituitary hormone products, are based on a variety of techniques used in a number of different species: (1) in vitro tests involving coincubation of hypothalamic and pituitary tissue or cells; (2) in vivo tests involving microinjection of agents directly into the hypothalamus or intraventricularly; (3) the use of drugs or neurotransmitter analogues, either agonists, which mimic the effects of neurotransmitters, or *antagonists,* which oppose their effects.

Some idea of the difficulties involved in interpret-

ing results of these kinds of experiments can be gained from the observation that, occasionally, the administration of the same agonist (for example, norepinephrine) can result in opposite effects on pituitary secretion depending on whether it is given directly into the hypothalamus or intraventricularly. Some, like dopamine, histamine, and norepinephrine, can have direct effects on the pituitary cell. It is not surprising that, in many cases, precisely opposite results are reported.

Table 5–5 represents an oversimplification of a complex set of control mechanisms studied by the uncertain methods described above. In addition to the difficulties in interpretation already mentioned, each of the neurotransmitters interacts with at least two different receptor complexes. Moreover, if these control mechanisms are like most of the others we know

TABLE 5–5.

Composite Summary of Some Effects of Neural Transmitters and Opioid Peptides on the Secretion of Pituitary Hormones*

AGONIST	GH	TSH	LH, FSH	ACTH	PRL
NE	+	+	+	−	−
AcCh			+	+	+
DA	+	−	+	−	+
5 HT	+	−	−	+	+
GABA	+	−	+	−	−
H		+	+	+	+
Opioids	+		−		−

*Modified from D.T. Krieger, S. Reichlin, and others. Key: + = hormone stimulation by agonist; − = inhibition. Open spaces may indicate either conflicting data or lack of information. NE = norepinephrine; AcCh = acetylcholine; DA = dopamine; 5 HT = serotonin; GABA = gamma aminobutyric acid; H = histamine; opioids = enkephalins and endorphins.

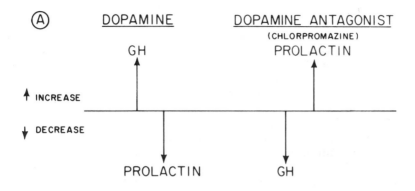

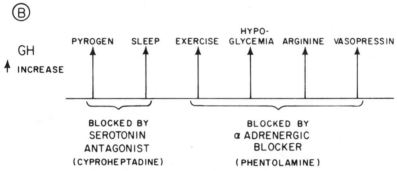

FIG 5–5.
A and **B,** monoamine control of growth hormone *(GH)* and prolactin release.

about, there are probably reciprocal controls in operation, i.e., if a pituitary cell is under the control of both a stimulatory and an inhibitory hypothalamic hormone, when one is elicited via a neural network above it in the CNS, the other is coordinately suppressed.

Figure 5–5,A illustrates the way in which this information was collected. GH secretion is stimulated by dopamine, whereas PRL secretion is depressed, probably by a direct effect of the amine at the level of the pituitary cell. The dopamine antagonist, chlorpromazine, has exactly the opposite effect.

Figure 5–5,B illustrates the point that each hormone may be controlled by *multiple* mechanisms. GH secretion is stimulated by a variety of stimuli that may impinge on the peptidergic neurons that secrete GRH by way of completely different neuronal circuits. These may use different neurotransmitters. Thus, GH secretion stimulated by bacterial pyrogen or by deep sleep is blocked by a serotonin antagonist, while that stimulated by a number of other stimuli is blocked by an α catecholamine blocker.

This brief account is enough to suggest the *possibilities* for differential control of secretory activity of

the major cell types of the anterior pituitary. With six different secretory cell types stimulated or inhibited by perhaps a dozen different peptides secreted by peptidergic neurons controlled by a mix of at least six neurotransmitters and modulated by an unknown number of peptides (including opioids), the hypothalamo-hypophysial relay system is a microminiaturized conduit for information of amazing versatility.

Feedback Control of Hypophysial Function

Hormones secreted by glandular targets of pituitary hormones (sex steroids, thyroid hormones, adrenal glucocorticoids) participate in the feedback regulation of their trophic hormones. Both the hypothalamus and the hypophysis may be sites of feedback regulation; each hormone system has its distinctive pattern of back regulation.

TSH secretion is elicited by the tripeptide TRH and, in turn, stimulates thyroid follicular cells to secrete thyroxine (T_4). As we have seen, T_4 and its metabolite, triiodothyronine (T_3), render the thyrotrophe in the pituitary gland refractory to the stimulatory effect of TRH.

LHRH is under complex control in women. At one stage of the menstrual cycle, estrogen stimulates production of LHRH and makes gonadotrophes more sensitive to the action of LHRH. At other stages, estrogens and progesterone inhibit LHRH production. Both the hypothalamus and the pituitary are involved in both positive and negative feedback effects of estrogen.

FSH is under multiple control systems. Since LHRH, or GnRH, stimulates secretion of both LH and FSH and since LH and FSH do not necessarily appear at the same time to the same extent, some differential control mechanism must exist. According to one hypothesis, the pattern of circulating steroid hormones could have different effects on the sensitivity of FSH trophes and LH trophes in the pituitary, and this could cause quantitatively different responses of the two cell types to the same LHRH stimulus. (Evidence that a change in pulse frequency of LHRH secretion may affect differential release of FSH and LH is a possibility that will be discussed in Chapter 9.) Another possibility involves a substance known as *inhibin,* originally described as a product of the seminiferous tubule of the testis but recently demonstrated in ovarian follicular fluid as well (Channing). This substance selectively inhibits FSH production. Although the specific locus of inhibition is not yet known, far more FSH is produced in its absence than in its presence. It is probably a deficiency in ovarian production of inhibin that causes the high level of production of FSH in postmenopausal women.

GH (somatotrophin) secretion is elicited via CNS stimulation. Although GH administration can inhibit GH secretion, it is now known that the inhibition is by way of somatomedin, which is produced in the body as a result of GH injection (see above).

PRL secretion, like that of GH, is elicited via neural afferent stimuli. The suckling stimulus represents the afferent neural component of a classic neuroendocrine reflex. The efferent part of the reflex is humoral: discharge of PRL from the pituitary and its transport by the blood to the breast. Removal of the repetitive suckling stimulus constitutes an inhibitory message to the PRL secretion control system. Prolactin secretion appears to be under tonic inhibitory control. It is the only pituitary hormone whose secretion is *increased* by pituitary stalk section. The positive stimulus for PRL secretion involves overcoming an inhibition, either by interfering with secretion of PIF (prolactin-inhibiting factor) or by stimulating production of PRF—possibly by both. Many investigators now suspect that one PIF may be dopamine, since dopamine administered directly into the pituitary portal circulation can inhibit PRL secretion (see p. 64).

ACTH secretion is inhibited by cortisol, probably acting both at the pituitary and hypothalamic levels.

Recent work on feedback inhibition at the level of the hypothalamus has suggested the possibility that the peptidergic neurons that secrete regulatory peptides may be controlled not only by target organ hormones (steroids, thyroid hormone, adrenocortical hormone) but also by pituitary trophic hormones, such as gonadotropins, ACTH and growth hormone ("short-loop" feedback). Moreover, the peptidergic neurons may be back-inhibited by their own products ("short, short" or "ultra short-loop" feedback). It is difficult to give a coherent account of the biologic importance of these types of feedback mechanisms. Receptors for steroid hormones and for thyroxine are demonstrable in and near the hypophysiotrophic zone of the hypothalamus, and local implantation of steroid hormone pellets in that zone support the view that target organ hormones must play an important part in feedback inhibition (Fig 5–6).

Pulsatile (Episodic), Diurnal, and Cyclic Rhythms of Hypophysial Hormone Secretion

Growth hormone, prolactin, ACTH and gonadotropins all show sleep-related surges in secretion. Growth hormone blood levels peak in association with deep sleep during the early hours. More than half the daily output of GH may occur during sleep. Prolactin secretion also increases during early deep sleep, but the level stays high longer than that of GH. ACTH, on the other hand, begins to increase just before awakening and peaks at about the time of awakening.

Nocturnal surges in secretion of gonadotropins are seen only during puberty in both sexes. Before puberty the levels are low, and at maturity, day and night levels are not strikingly different. Cyclic secretion of gonadotropins will be discussed in Chapter 9.

Recently an increase in the frequency of sampling has revealed that all pituitary hormones studied so far show the phenomenon of *pulsatile episodic secretion*. This consists of regularly repeated bursts of secretion, a sort of periodic quantal discharge. The diurnal fluctuations include a great many periodic "squirts" of hormone. Each episode of secretion appears to be an all-or-none response to a threshold stimulus that requires a fairly uniform time to accumulate. There is as yet no satisfactory explanation for the phenomenon of episodic secretion, but it appears to be a general property of pituitary hormone-secreting cells.

Pulsatile, or episodic, secretion of pituitary hormones has added a new dimension to our understand-

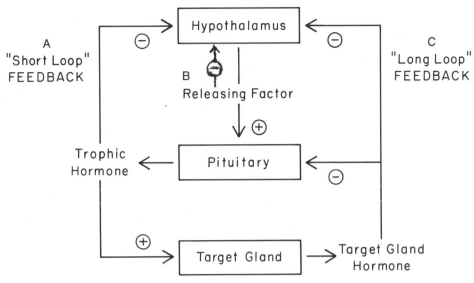

FIG 5–6.
A, "short-loop," **B,** "short-short loop," and **C,** "long-loop" feedback mechanisms.

ing of how chemical messengers can affect the function of cells sensitive to them. For the response of cells to hormones may include not only the ability to recognize a precise stereochemical configuration but also to respond to the *time pattern* of exposure to the agonist. If the hormone is present *continuously* in a sufficiently high concentration, thus:

———————————————————

the response of the cell may be to become refractory, or unresponsive to the stimulus. This may be due, in part, to down-regulation of the hormone receptor, but it no doubt involves components of the message transduction system that can fail to react before down regulation occurs. On the other hand, pulsatile, episodic, or rhythmically intermittent hormone exposure, thus:

•　　•　　•　　•　　•　　•

may produce a certain level of secretory response to the hormone. In at least two cases, and perhaps in all, *increased pulse frequency,* thus:

•　•　•　•　•　•　•　•　•　•

results in an *enhanced* secretory response of the target cell. Thus, *pulse frequency* is an integral part of the information that is received, decoded, and acted upon by the responding cell.

The idea of the biological importance of pulse frequency, pioneered by Knobil and his colleagues in their studies of gonadotrophin function in monkeys,

has had surprisingly swift practical applications in people. (We have already referred to the treatment of GH-deficient children by the injection of GRH in pulsatile fashion by way of a programmable, portable minipump.) In the case of LHRH, gonadotrophin secretion has been either decreased or increased, depending on whether the releasing hormone was administered continuously in high doses or via a pump programmed to mimic the secretory pattern of the normal hypothalamus. Continuous administration of a long-acting LHRH agonist virtually shuts off gonadotrophin output, while pulsatile administration has corrected functional defects in males and females with hypogonadism of hypothalamic origin. For example, a man with gonadotrophin deficiency following head trauma sustained in an automobile accident was able to father a normal baby as a result of pump-administered LHRH (Hoffman and Crowley).

Growth Hormone

Growth hormone is a 191 amino acid single chain peptide containing two disulfide bridges (Fig 5–7). It shows marked amino acid sequence homology with PRL and human placental lactogen (hPL) with which it shares 161 of 191 identical amino acid sequences. Bovine, porcine, and ovine growth hormones are ineffective in man and monkey; the hormone prepared from human pituitaries collected at autopsy is an effective growth-promoting agent in GH-deficient children and subhuman primates.

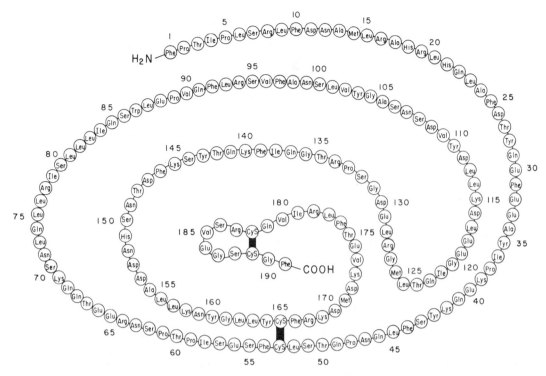

AMINO ACID SEQUENCE of HGH

FIG 5–7.
Growth hormone. (Courtesy of J. Kostyo.)

ASSAY.—GH is assayed by measuring weight gain in hypophysectomized rats. Carcass analyses of GH-treated rats reveal that the increase in weight produced by GH represents protein deposition. Fat content is often relatively diminished.

The width of epiphyseal cartilage has been used traditionally in a bioassay for GH. In the hypophysectomized animal, the cartilage at the ends of long bones is very narrow. It widens on treatment with GH in a dose-dependent manner. The stimulatory effect of GH on cartilage growth was the basis for the discovery of somatomedin (see p. 74).

CIRCULATING GH.—Recent studies of GH are dependent on a *radioimmunoassay* first introduced by Berson, Yalow, Glick, and Roth. The availability of this method has made it possible to observe rapid fluctuations of plasma GH levels in a variety of physiologic circumstances. Even in nongrowing, adult individuals, striking increases in GH are seen in the following:

1. During deep (slow wave) sleep, early in sleep period.

2. After treatment with pyrogens and in association with trauma.

3. Following muscular exercise.

4. In hypoglycemia.

5. After arginine injection.

6. After vasopressin injection.

7. Following administration of morphine and other drugs.

The "resting" level of plasma GH is less than 3 ng/ml. Stimulated levels are characteristically 30–100 ng/ml. Women show a greater response to GH-provocative stimuli than do men, and the response of men to arginine, for example, is exaggerated by prior treatment with estrogen.

Like all other pituitary hormones, GH is secreted episodically in periods of 20–30 minutes. The large diurnal fluctuations represent the integrations of many small, episodic secretory episodes.

Provocative tests of GH secretory reserve are used clinically. Insulin hypoglycemia, arginine infusion, and measured exercise have all been used in this way. Borderline states of GH deficiency may be detected by such tests, and inappropriate overresponses may also be seen. In the latter category, persons with uncontrolled diabetes show abnormally and persistently high increases in level of serum GH after exercise, increases that are not suppressible by glucose infusion. In normal individuals, on the other hand, procedures that normally evoke GH secretion (exercise, arginine infusion) fail to do so if a continuous intravenous infusion of glucose is maintained. Evidently, perception of hyperglycemia by glucoreceptors in the head can *prevent* GH release. By the same token, in animals GH release can be elicited by infusing a competitive inhibitor of glucose transport—2 deoxyglucose. Thus, inhibition of glucose oxidation by sensor cells constitutes a call for GH secretion. The glucoreceptors responsible for this effect may be either in the hypothalamus or in other parts of the CNS that communicate with hypothalamic peptidergic neurons.

Mechanisms of Action of GH

The most striking effect of somatotrophin, stimulation of cartilage growth, is associated with increased uptake of SO_4 for incorporation into chondroitin sulfate, with increased uptake of amino acids and incorporation into protein and, finally, with mitogenesis and cell replication. Contemporary hypotheses concerning these effects will be discussed under ''somatomedins'' (see p. 74).

Metabolic effects of GH are complex and still poorly understood. Acutely, GH has an insulin-like effect in muscle, facilitating the uptake of glucose. Its continued presence, however, results in insulin insensitivity, and it is therefore one of several physiologic antagonists to insulin. GH, in association with adrenal glucocorticoids, has effects on lipolysis in fat cells. Although this effect was observed many years ago, it is still impossible to describe it in molecular terms. We can only say that it is perceptible only after a lag period, that it involves protein synthesis and that it probably increases the sensitivity of the adipocyte to its tonic lipolytic stimuli. In any case, it is expressed in the whole animal as triglyceride hydrolysis, increase in circulating free fatty acids, fatty infiltration of the liver and increase in ketone body production by the liver. It is possible that these effects contribute to the insulin resistance seen in the intact organism. Experiments with fragments of growth hormone suggest that the metabolic effects and growth-promoting effects may reside in different parts of the molecule.

Growth hormone is also necessary for compensatory hypertrophy of a kidney after the contralateral one has been removed. It is also involved in hypertrophy of other tissues. Whether these effects are directly due to GH or to a change in the internal environment induced by GH (somatomedin?) is not now known.

The *cellular mechanism of action* of GH on cartilage is mediated by way of somatomedin. Although

stimulation of growth in other tissues such as liver and muscle may ultimately be shown to involve a similar mechanism, direct effects of GH on muscle in vitro are readily demonstrable (see Kostyo et al.). These include a fast, protein synthesis-independent insulin-like effect on glucose transport, i.e., a stimulation. After a latent period, GH-treated muscle becomes resistant to the action of insulin, but there is an enhanced transport of amino acids that *is* dependent on the synthesis of new protein. Kostyo et al. suggest that the growth stimulation phase is associated with a *decrease* in concentration of free cAMP in the muscle cell. This would be consistent with many other circumstances in which growth stimulation is associated with decreases in cAMP concentration.

The hepatic effects of GH are still in their descriptive phase. The hormone stimulates protein synthesis after a lag period, stimulates RNA synthesis and stimulates polysome aggregation and ultimately DNA synthesis, as indicated by a shift in the direction of polyploidy in hepatocytes. Specific, saturable GH receptors are readily demonstrable in purified hepatic plasma membrane preparations. However, the connection between hormone binding and stimulation of protein synthesis and cell replication has not yet been explained. Growth hormone is bound by a plasma membrane-limited receptor, but its effects are generally similar to those produced by steroid hormones.

The most important unresolved issue about GH is the question of how many of its actions are achieved by way of its stimulation of somatomedin production and how many are brought about by either the GH molecule itself or a critical fragment of the molecule. Somatomedin C production is increased in a bone organ culture system in the presence of GH (Stracke et al.). Van den Brande and Van Buul-Offers reported clear-cut growth effects, including increases in body weight and length, in growth-hormone deficient dwarf mice injected with human somatomedin (see Wallis).

Growth Hormone and Recombinant DNA Technology

The gene for human growth hormone, like those for somatostatin and insulin, has been inserted into plasmids and the hormone has been produced in E. coli. The hormone produced in this manner has been successfully tested in GH-deficient children, and it will soon be possible to produce enough of it to meet the demand.

In another historic adventure in recombinant DNA research, Palmiter et al. constructed a fusion gene consisting of the promoter region of a mouse gene (inducible by cadmium or zinc) coupled to the structural gene for human GH. After these fusion genes were *microinjected into fertilized mouse eggs,* 70% of the mice that incorporated them into their genetic material showed elevated levels of serum GH and significantly greater growth than their controls—some of them grew to more than twice normal size. Synthesis of even greater amounts of GH was induced by injecting the mice with cadmium or zinc which normally "turn on" the promoter region of the fusion gene. The abnormally high levels of serum GH were accompanied by increased serum somatomedin levels (see next section). The fusion genes were variably expressed in all tissues, and the excessive GH could have been synthesized and secreted by any of them. Histological examination of the pituitary showed atrophy of the cells that normally produce GH.

SOMATOMEDINS AND OTHER GROWTH FACTORS

Studies on the mechanism of action of growth hormone, on circulating insulin and on the growth requirements of cells in culture have revealed the existence of a family of circulating peptides that share certain characteristics: (1) their concentration in serum is GH dependent; (2) they show insulin-like actions in nonskeletal tissues (i.e., they stimulate glucose utilization); and (3) they show similar stimulatory effects on cartilage in vitro. A knowledge of these substances is essential, at least for evaluation of growth disturbances in children. It is possible that they may be centrally important in wound healing, compensatory hypertrophy following removal of one of a pair of organs, organ regeneration, aging and neoplasia.

In 1957 Salmon and Daughaday, in an attempt to improve on existing bioassay methods for GH, demonstrated that purified GH did not stimulate incorporation of $^{35}SO_4$ into the chondroitin sulfate of cartilage explants in vitro. Whereas serum from untreated hypophysectomized rats was without effect, GH-treated hypophysectomized rat serum was as effective as normal serum. These experiments were the basis for postulating the existence of a GH-dependent "sulfation factor," which was later named *somatomedin,* since it was postulated to be a mediator of growth hormone's action on cartilage.

Meanwhile, parallel studies were being done on an insulin-like material in plasma, which could not be neutralized by anti-insulin antibodies. This material came to be known as NSILA (nonsuppressible insulin-like activity) and has recently been resolved into two peptide components called insulin growth factor (IGF) I and IGF II. It was subsequently found that IGF conforms to the somatomedin-family definition given above.

Studies by other investigators who were mainly interested in "multiplication stimulating activity" of various constituents of media in which eukaryotic cells were cultured resulted in the isolation and characterization of a number of mitogenic substances, at least one of which, Temin's MSA (multiplication stimulating activity), bears all the marks of a somatomedin. Somatomedin C and IGF I are identical, as are MSA and IGF II.

Since the somatomedins are not stored in any tissue, they have been isolated from very large volumes of outdated blood plasma (in regrettably small amounts). There are at least three identifiable circulating somatomedins, but somatomedin C, a 63 amino acid peptide, has been studied most extensively, by both radioimmunoassay and radioreceptor assay by use of a plasma membrane preparation of human placenta.

A *site of production* is believed to be the liver, though stimulation of somatomedin production by the isolated perfused liver requires excessively high concentrations of GH. Partial hepatectomy results in a 75% fall in circulating somatomedin levels, and higher concentrations are found in hepatic vein blood than in peripheral circulation.

The half-life of injected, labeled somatomedin is 2–4 hours, much longer than that of other peptide hormones, which half-disappear in 20–30 minutes. The reason for the long half-life of somatomedin is that it circulates bound to serum proteins by specific and saturable binding sites. In the hypophysectomized animal the half-life is only eight minutes, which has suggested to some investigators that GH may control primarily not somatomedin synthesis but somatomedin protein carrier synthesis.

The concentration of somatomedin C (Som C) varies with age. In cord blood (neonate), it is about 0.3 units/ml, and at two years 0.4–0.5. The adult level is 1–2 units/ml. These numbers suggest either that, in the period of most rapid growth, tissues are more sensitive to somatomedin or that the turnover of somatomedin may be accelerated at those ages. Van Wyck and colleagues have demonstrated a strong positive correlation between serum Som C levels and growth rate in 31 hypopituitary children treated with hGH over a long period.

The *biologic effects* of somatomedins in cartilage include the following:

1. Stimulation of $^{35}SO_4$ incorporation into proteoglycans
2. Stimulation of thymidine → DNA
3. Stimulation of RNA synthesis
4. Stimulation of protein synthesis

The mechanisms postulated for these effects include stimulation of amino acid transport, but it is not clear how this entrains DNA synthesis and mitosis. While cAMP-lowering has been suggested as a component of the response, the data on this point are not clear.

Somatomedin C is not only mitogenic in cartilage cells; it stimulates mitosis in many other cell types in tissue culture as well. In this it resembles a growing number of peptide growth factors: fibroblastic growth factor (FGF), platelet growth factor (PGF), epidermal growth factor (EGF), nerve growth factor (NGF), erythropoietin, and thymosin. Most of these have some insulin-like activity and some, like NGF, share substantial amino acid sequences with insulin.

Cross-reactivity of Som C and insulin for receptors has revealed that the two substances have their own distinctive receptors and that each can feebly inhibit specific receptor binding of the other. Insulin is 1,000 times less active than Som C in inhibiting Som C binding, and Som C is 50 times less active than insulin in inhibiting insulin binding.

Clinical applications of these findings have been made and will no doubt continue. Acromegalics show 2–4 times the normal adult plasma levels of Som C, and untreated hypopituitary children have levels below 0.1 units/ml. GH treatment of hypopituitarism results in a restoration of Som C levels toward normal in 1–3 days.

In protein-calorie malnutrition (kwashiorkor), circulating GH levels are high and somatomedin levels, assayed by all three methods, are low. Similarly in human mutants known as Laron dwarfs, high plasma GH levels are seen in association with low somatomedin levels. These dwarfs do not grow in response to GH treatment, nor do their somatomedin levels improve on this treatment. These studies, like those on protein-calorie malnutrition, are consistent with the evidence that somatomedin may play a role in feedback inhibition of GH secretion.

Whether all of the growth-promoting activity of GH is mediated by way of somatomedin is an unsettled question. It is clear that GH has direct effects on amino acid transport and lipolysis, which do not require somatomedin production.

Corticotrophin-Related Peptides

BETA LIPOTROPHIN, ENKEPHALINS, AND ENDORPHINS

Corticotrophin (ACTH) will be discussed in the context of hypothalamo-hypophysial-adrenal relationships in Chapter 11. Recent discoveries of a pro-ACTH molecule and of some of its relationships with other biologically interesting compounds warrant a brief review of this subject.

The discovery of specific binding sites in the brain for morphine and structurally related compounds suggested the possibility that the body may produce an "endogenous opiate." After extensive searches, Hughes and colleagues (1975) reported amino acid sequences for two remarkable pentapeptides, methionine-enkephalin and leucine-enkephalin:

Tyr·gly·gly·phe·MET and
Tyr·gly·gly·phe·LEU

These peptides bind to morphine receptors and produce morphine-like responses in animals. Moreover, like morphine, their biologic effects are antagonized by naloxone and other antimorphine drugs (see Chapter 3).

In 1976 Goldstein reported that pituitary extracts contained opioid activity in a molecule larger than a pentapeptide. The metenkephalin sequence was observed to occur in amino acids 61–65 of a pituitary product known as β lipotrophin, or β LPH, whose structure had been worked out by C. H. Li. Investigative interest in β LPH, which had originally been described as a fat-mobilizing hormone, had not been high, but research on "endogenous opiates" stimulated Li, Guillemin and others to reexamine the molecule and its relation to other biologically active substances.

The results of their studies may be seen in Figure 5–8. A large precursor (MW 31,000) glycoprotein is synthesized by the specialized basophil previously known to be the source of ACTH. This prohormone is the precursor of *both* ACTH (39 amino acids) and β LPH (91 amino acids). These molecules may themselves be precursors of other substances with important biologic functions. However, they are not found exclusively in the pituitary: ACTH, β LPH and the endorphins (presumably derived from β LPH by proteolysis) also are found in the brain. Enkephalins, which occur in the brain, cannot be isolated from the pituitary. The persistence of brain peptides after hypophysectomy suggests that they are synthesized in the brain. The relationship between hypophysial and brain peptides of similar structure is not yet known.

The discovery of morphine-like peptides was a major advance in neurobiology. The enkephalins and α endorphin are, mole for mole, as potent analgesics as morphine, whereas β endorphin is actually 5–10 times as potent as morphine on a molar basis. Since these compounds do not penetrate the blood-brain barrier, their effects in animals have been seen following injections into the CNS. They are analgesics, like morphine, and they produce behavioral effects such as those produced by morphine. These include

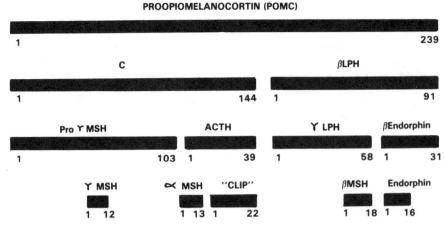

FIG 5–8.
Peptides derived from proopiomelanocortin *(POMC)*.

muscular rigidity and an absence of spontaneous movement, all of which are quickly reversed by the morphine antagonist naloxone.

Discovery of these compounds has led to a new theory of the mechanism of pain perception in which "nonpain" is perceived as an equilibrium between incoming pain signals and tonic "antipain" signals generated by mechanisms involving the endogenous opiate-like peptides. It is interesting, for example, that the analgesic effect of acupuncture can be blocked by naloxone, which suggests that endogenous release of endorphins or enkephalins may occur during this procedure.

It is possible that the endorphins and enkephalins may modulate the secretion of pituitary hormones. Since the stimulatory effect of morphine on growth hormone, prolactin and ACTH secretion was well established, the morphine-like peptides were shown to have similar effects. Since no consistent effects of these substances can be demonstrated directly on the pituitary, they probably exert their influence at the hypothalamic level by way of peptidergic neurons. It is not known whether they are neural transmitters or axo-axonal modulators of nerve endings.

The concentration of endorphins and enkephalins in the blood after stimulation of ACTH secretion is very low, but the peptides are clearly demonstrable by immunohistochemical methods in the brain, gastrointestinal tract, pancreatic islets and elsewhere. Both MSHs are important products of the intermediate lobe of the pituitary gland. The nature of the control exerted by different cell types over the *ratio* of the different POMC derivatives produced by each is unknown. The gene for prepropromC has been cloned by Numa et al. (see Imura). All of the components

are neatly arranged in linear fashion, and must therefore be transcribed coordinately. There may well be cell to cell differences in the processing either of the prepromRNA or its translation products (see MSH below).

Melanocyte-Stimulating Hormone (MSH)

In 1916, Smith and Allen described loss of skin color in tadpoles after hypophysectomy. Three years later, Atwell demonstrated darkening of tadpole skin in solutions containing crude pituitary extracts. In 1938 Zondek described the darkening effect in amphibian skin of extracts of the pars intermedia. He named the putative substance responsible for this effect *intermedin,* but it has since been known most frequently as *melanocyte-stimulating hormone,* or MSH. In some mammalian species (rat, rabbit, sheep, cattle, etc.), the pars intermedia is a well-defined structure between the anterior and posterior lobes of the pituitary and it contains large amounts of α MSH and CLIP (see Fig 5–8), but in human adults and other mammals it is practically vestigial; only a few MSH-producing cells are scattered through the anterior segment of the posterior lobe, and the gland contains insignificant amounts of α MSH and CLIP. At one stage in the development of the human fetus, the pars intermedia is just as prominent as it is in rats, rabbits, etc., and it contains large amounts of α MSH and CLIP. The lack of these products in the adult pituitary suggests that, though MSH-producing cells and ACTH-producing cells contain the gene for POMC, each cell has its own way of processing the peptide. The pituitary lacks the enzyme necessary for splitting ACTH to produce α MSH. Thus, each type of cell controls the fate of translated POMC by packaging its own preferred proteolytic enzymes with the large precursor protein.

CHEMISTRY

There are five known substances with MSH activity: (1) α MSH, (2) β MSH, (3) γ MSH, (4) ACTH, and (5) β LPH. They are all derived from the common precursor, POMC, and their relationships are shown in Figure 5–8. The following heptapeptide, which appears in all of the substances enumerated above, is responsible for MSH activity:

Met·Glu(Gly)·His·Phe·Arg·Trp·Gly

MSH is the major MSH peptide in species that have a distinct pars intermedia. As we have noted, it is practically absent from human pituitaries postnatally and it does not appear in the circulating body fluids. β MSH is now believed to be an artifactual breakdown product of β LPH. While MSH is about 30× as potent as ACTH as a darkening agent, sufficient amounts of ACTH and β LPH are secreted in some circumstances to account for hyperpigmentation in humans (see below). Whether γ MSH is physiologically significant is unknown.

POMC is a glycoprotein, and there has been some interest in the role of the carbohydrate which is attached near the N terminal end of the molecule. Loh has studied the fate of POMC in circumstances when the protein can be synthesized, but glycosylation is inhibited by the drug tunicamycin. He discovered that the carbohydrate protects the molecule from the rapid destruction that occurs when the carbohydrate-free protein is made.

ASSAY

At one stage of evolution, MSH mediated a protective adaptation, i.e., camouflage in the dark, or when a threatened individual was exposed on a dark background. The major bioassay for MSH, which is capable of detecting MSH with great precision over a range of 20–50 pcg, is based on the darkening of amphibian skin under standardized conditions. Melanocytes in such skin contain many fine pigment granules called melanosomes. The intracellular distribution of melanosomes determines the color of the skin; when they are tightly clustered near the nucleus, the skin appears light in color, and when they are dispersed throughout the cell, the skin appears dark. MSH causes melanosome dispersion, while catecholamines and melatonin (see Chapter 7) cause lightening (melanosome concentration).

In addition to bioassay, radioimmunoassay is used extensively for measuring MSH concentration in body fluids and tissues. Immunofluorescence microscopy has been used for the localization of MSH-containing cells in the pituitary and central nervous system.

CONTROL OF SECRETION

Most studies on the control of MSH secretion have been done in species with a well-developed pars intermedia and, therefore, do not apply to humans. In the rat, MSH release is tonically inhibited, probably by α catecholamine neurones as well as by an MSH inhibitory substance, MIF. A candidate for MIF is the tripeptide side chain of oxytocin (Fig 5–9). The ring structure of oxytocin is said to contain melanocyte-stimulating factor, MSF. Many sensory stimuli, including sound, touch, suckling, and trauma, evoke MSH secretion in the rat, but the neural pathways involved are not known.

PIGMENT CELLS IN MAMMALS

Mammalian skin does not show immediate darkening on MSH administration. Mammalian cells in culture, however, do show increased pigmentation about 16 hours after exposure to MSH. This is due entirely to increased synthesis of melanin in specialized pigment cells, the melanocytes. The pigment melanin is a complex material consisting of protein and a polymer of indole 5,6 quinone. It is formed as follows:

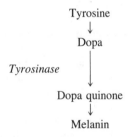

MSH increases the synthesis of melanin by inducing synthesis of *tyrosinase,* the rate-limiting enzyme in the synthetic pathway. This effect, which involves transcription, has been demonstrated in both normal skin cells and melanoma cells in culture.

Hyperpigmentation in humans may be seen in (1) *primary adrenocortical insufficiency* (Addison's disease), (2) *secondary adrenal hyperactivity* (Cushing's disease), and (3) in association with ectopic ACTH-producing tumors. ACTH, βLPH and pro-γMSH are all secreted together by the pituitary, placenta, and tumor cells, and they are overproduced in all of the

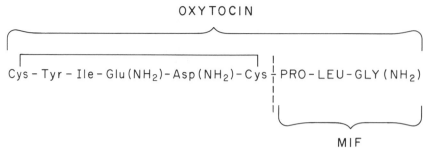

FIG 5–9.
Relationship of melanocyte-inhibitory factor *(MIF)* to oxytocin.

conditions enumerated above. In (1), this is due to failure of feedback inhibition, while in (2) and (3) there is continuous uninhibited secretion of POMC products.

In pregnancy, darkening of the color of all previously pigmented areas occurs; in skin around the nipples, the vulva and the mucous membranes. This could be due to the secretion of large amounts of POMC products by the placenta, as well as to direct effects of estrogen on melanin synthesis.

Other (Nonpigmentary) Actions of MSH

Since MSH clearly does not play a camouflage role in hairy and hairless mammals, is it possible that the highly conserved peptide, like many other substances, was put to different uses as the evolutionary process proceeded? Many interesting extrapigmentary functions have been assigned to MSH.

One of the most interesting hypotheses was suggested by the fact that hairy mammals (rat, rabbit, ox, etc.) have a well-defined pars intermedia while hairless ones (human, whale, armadillo) do not. When one adds to this the observation that MSH stimulates sebaceous gland activity (which coevolved with hair) and pheromone production (a function of modified sebaceous glands), it is at least entertaining to reflect that these functions of the peptide may be very important in species that rely heavily on olfaction when they participate in reproductive activities.

The prominence of the pars intermedia in the human fetus, coupled with the observation that the N-terminal pro-γMSH peptide stimulates the release of glucocorticoids and aldosterone from the adrenals, has suggested to some that the hormone may have a steroidogenic effect in the fetal adrenal. Some observers attribute a generalized fetal growth and development function to MSH.

Finally, the peptide MSH 4–10 (also ACTH 4–10)

has figured prominently in DeWied's well-known studies on the enhancement of memory by a variety of peptides. MSH has been found to be widely distributed in rat and human brain. In the rat, its highest concentration is in the arcuate nucleus, which projects to the anterior hypothalamus, the preoptic nucleus, and the amygdala. The arcuate nucleus may be the origin of much of the other CNS MSH, for if it is destroyed either by electrolytic lesions or by neonatal administration of monosodium glutamate, the MSH content of other parts of the brain diminishes sharply. We have no idea what, if anything, these observations have to do with the postulated role for MSH in storage and retrieval of remembered information, but we suspect that this peptide may prove to be adaptively beneficial in the CNS as it is in anuran skin.

Cellular Mechanism of Action

Melanocytes and melanoma cells have receptors for MSH. All of the phenomena we have described in frog skin, as well as the induction of tyrosinase in mammalian skin, are associated with an increase in intracellular cyclic AMP. Microtubules and microfilaments are involved in melanosome dispersion; therefore, Ca^{2+} must be involved in the action of the hormone.

Peptidergic Neurons of the CNS

The development of powerful immunocytologic methods has revealed the existence of a whole new interface between endocrinology and neurobiology. Substances that were identified first as hypothalamic-releasing, or release-inhibiting, hormones suddenly began to appear in unexpected places. For example: *TRH* and *somatostatin* may be found widely distributed in the brain and spinal cord (somatostatin is absent from the cerebellum). *Endorphins* and *enkephalins,* the opiate-like peptides, are widely distributed in the brain as well as in the pituitary gland. Since they occur in the brain even in hypophysectomized animals, they appear to be synthesized in situ. Other peptides, long associated with the gastrointestinal tract or with other parts of the body outside the CNS, have now been identified in CNS cells. These include gastrin, substance P, and cholecystokinin; the last has been implicated in the process of food intake regulation. Similarly *renin* and *angiotensin II,* key substances in the renin-angiotensin-aldosterone system associated with fluid and electrolyte homeostasis, have now been found in the brain and angiotensin II has been shown to participate in the control of drinking behavior, as well as in that of blood pressure and ADH regulation. It is unlikely that the angiotensin II in the brain was carried there and concentrated, since all of the enzymatic equipment necessary for its synthesis is demonstrable in the brain.

Pearse, on the basis of developmental analysis, suggests that all of the cells that produce similar peptides, whether in the gastrointestinal tract or in the brain, are descendants of the same cluster of neuroectodermal cells. He calls this system of cells the APUD system, for amine precursor uptake decarboxylase. In his view, the endocrine system and the nervous system are subsystems of a larger enterprise. Although this hypothesis is an interesting one, little is known about potential functions of any of the peptidergic neurons in the CNS, with the possible exception of those that make cholecystokinin and angiotensin II. Do these substances function as neural transmitters or are they axo-axonal modulators of monoaminergic nerve endings? Surely the discovery of the opiate-like peptides and of gastrointestinal hormones improbably within CNS neurons represents the beginning of a new era in neurobiology and an additional bond between students of the nervous and endocrine systems (see Krieger).

BIBLIOGRAPHY

Baylin SB, Mendelsohn G: Ectopic (inappropriate) hormone production by tumors: Mechanisms involved and the biological and clinical implications. *Endocr Rev* 1980; 1:45.

Bloom F, Segal D, Ling N, et al: Endorphins: Profound behavioral effects in rats suggesting new etiological factors in mental illness. *Science* 1976; 194:630.

Carpenter G, Cohen S: Epidermal growth factors, in Litwack G (ed): *Biochemical Actions of Hormones,* vol 5. New York, Academic Press, 1978, pp 203–245.

Chrousos GP (Moderator): Clinical applications of corticotropin-releasing factor (NIH conference). *Ann Intern Med* 1985; 102:344.

Collu R, Barbeau A, Ducharme JR, et al (eds): *Central Nervous System Effects of Hypothalamic Hormones and Other Peptides.* New York, Raven Press, 1979.

Conn PM: Molecular mechanism of gonadotropin releasing hormone action, in Litwack G (ed): *Biochemical Actions of Hormones,* vol 11. New York, Academic Press, 1984, pp 68–92.

Daughaday W: Prolactin and growth hormone in health and disease, in Ingbar SH (ed): *Contemporary Endocrinology,* vol 2. New York, Plenum Publishing Corp, 1985, pp 27–86.

DeWied D: Hormones and behavior, in Schmidt FW, Worden FG (eds): *The Neurosciences Third Study Program.* Cambridge, Massachusetts, MIT Press, 1974, pp 653–666.

Eipper BA, Mains RE: Structure and biosynthesis of pro-adrenocorticotropin/endorphin and related peptides. *Endocr Rev* 1980; 1:1.

Guillemin R: Endorphins, brain peptides that act like opiates. *N Engl J Med* 1977; 296.

Guillemin R, Brazeau P, Bohlen P, et al: Somatocrinin, the growth hormone releasing factor. *Recent Prog Horm Res* 1984; 40:233.

Harwood JP, Grewe C, Aguilera G: Actions of growth-hormone-releasing factor and somatostatin on adenylate cyclase and growth hormone release in rat anterior pituitary. *Mol Cell Endocrinol* 1984; 37:277.

Hayward JN: Functional and morphological aspects of hypothalamic neurones. *Physiol Rev* 1977; 57:574.

Hoffman AR, Crowley WF: Induction of puberty in men by long-term pulsatile administration of low-dose gonadotropin-releasing hormone. *N Engl J Med* 1982; 307:1237.

Hughes J, Smith TW, Kosterlitz HW, et al: Identification of two related pentapeptides from the brain with potent opiate agonist activity. *Nature* 1975; 258:577.

Imura H (ed): *The Pituitary Gland.* New York, Raven Press, 1985.

Itakura K, Hirose T, Crea R, et al: Expression in *Escherichia Coli* of a chemically synthesized gene for the hormone somatostatin. *Science* 1977; 198:1056.

Jeffcoate SL, Hutchinson JSM (eds): *The Endocrine Hypothalamus.* New York, Academic Press, 1978.

Krieger DT: Neuroendocrine physiology, in Felig P, Baxter JD, et al (eds): *Endocrinology and Metabolism.* New York, McGraw-Hill Book Co, 1981, pp 125–149.

Krieger DT: Brain peptides. *Vitam Horm* 1984; 41:1.

Krieger DT: Neuroendocrinology, in Ingbar SH (ed): *Contemporary Endocrinology,* vol 2. New York, Plenum Publishing Corp, 1985, pp 1–26.

Labrie F, Belanger A, Dupont A (eds): *LHRH and Its Analogues.* Amsterdam, Excerpta Medica, 1984.

McCann SM: Physiology and pharmacology of LHRH and somatostatin. *Ann Rev Pharmacol Toxicol* 1982; 22:491.

Nicolics K, Mason AJ, et al: A prolactin-inhibiting factor within the precursor for human gonadotropin-releasing hormone. *Nature* 1985; 316:511.

Palmiter RD, Norstedt G, Gelinas RE, et al: Metallothionein-human growth hormone fusion genes stimulate growth of mice. *Science* 1983; 222:809.

Pearse AGE: Peptides in brain and intestine. *Nature* 1976; 262:92.

Phillips LS, Vassilopoulou-Sellin R: Somatomedins (two parts). *N Engl J Med* 1980; 302:371.

Reichlin S: Neuroendocrinology, in Williams RH (ed): *Textbook of Endocrinology,* ed 6. Philadelphia, WB Saunders Co, 1981, pp 589–645.

Reichlin S: Somatostatin (two parts). *N Engl J Med* 1983; 309:1495.

Rivier J, Spiess J, Thorner M, et al: Characterization of a

growth hormone-releasing factor from a human pancreatic islet cell tumor. *Nature* 1982; 300:276.

Schally AV, Coy DH, Meyers CA: Hypothalamic regulatory hormones. *Ann Rev Biochem* 1978; 47:89.

Schulte HM, Chrousos GP, Oldfield EH, et al: Ovine corticotropin-releasing factor administration in normal men. *Horm Res* 1985; 21:69.

Sheldon WR Jr, de Bold CR, Evans WS, et al: Rapid sequential intravenous administration of four hypothalamic releasing hormones as a combined anterior pituitary function test. *J Clin Endocrinol Metab* 1985; 60:623.

Stracke H, Schulz A, Moeller D, et al: Effect of growth hormone on osteoblasts and demonstration of somatomedin C/IGF I in bone organ culture. *Acta Endocrinol* 1984; 107:16.

Streeten DHP, Anderson GH Jr, Dalakos TG, et al: Normal and abnormal function of the hypothalamic-pituitary-adrenocortical system in man. *Endocr Rev* 1984; 5:371.

Terry LC, Martin JB: Hypothalamic hormones: Subcellular distribution and mechanisms of release. *Ann Rev Pharmacol Toxicol* 1978; 18:111.

Thorner MO, Reschke J, Chitwood J, et al: Acceleration of growth in two children treated with human growth hormone-releasing factor. *N Engl J Med* 1985; 312:4.

Unger RH, Dobbs RE, Orci L: Insulin, glucagon, and somatostatin in the regulation of metabolism. *Ann Rev Physiol* 1978; 40:307.

Vale W, Rivier C, Brown MR, et al: Chemical and biological characterization of corticotropin releasing factor. *Recent Prog Horm Res* 1983; 39:245.

Vale W, Greer M (eds): Corticotropin-releasing factor (Kroc Foundation Conference). *Fed Proc* 1985; 44:1–203.

Van Wyck JJ, Underwood LE: The somatomedins and their actions, in Litwack G (ed): *Biochemical Actions of Hormones,* vol 5. New York, Academic Press, 1978, pp 102–148.

Wade N: Guillemin and Schally: The years in the wilderness. The three-lap race to Stockholm, and a race spurred by rivalry. *Science* 1978; 200:279.

Wallis M: Pituitary GH. *Nature* 1979; 281:633.

Weiner RI, Ganong WF: Role of brain monoamines and histamine in regulation of anterior pituitary secretion. *Physiol Rev* 1978; 58:905.

6

Neurohypophysis

SOME LANDMARKS IN NEUROHYPOPHYSEAL CHRONOLOGY

DATE		INVESTIGATOR(S)
1794	Diabetes insipidus distinguished from diabetes mellitus	Frank
1894	Pressor effects of pituitary extracts	Oliver and Schaffer
1897	Pressor substance localized in posterior lobe	Howell
1901	Discovery of antidiuretic action of posterior lobe extract	Magnus and Schaffer
1906	Action of posterior pituitary extracts on uterus	H. H. Dale
1910	Action of posterior pituitary extracts on mammary gland	Ott and Scott
1913	Control of diabetes insipidus by injections of posterior pituitary extracts	Von den Velden; Farini
1928	Separation of vasopressin and oxytocin	Kamm
1949	Isolation of pure oxytocin	Livermore and Du Vigneaud
1953	Synthesis of posterior lobe hormones	Du Vigneaud et al.

As its name signifies, the neurohypophysis, or posterior pituitary, is a physical extension of the nervous system rather than a gland physically separated from the nervous system. Neurons, which have their cell bodies in the supraoptic and paraventricular nuclei of the anterior hypothalamus, extend by way of the pituitary stalk to the posterior lobe where their terminals are organized into a secretory apparatus that discharges directly into the blood. *Arginine vasopressin* (AVP, ADH) plays an important regulatory role in water conservation and maintenance of body fluid osmolality, blood volume and pressure. It may also play a role in memory consolidation and in the release of CRH (Chapter 5). *Oxytocin* is a regulator of lactation and of uterine smooth muscle contraction.

Antidiuretic hormone (ADH, AVP) is only one component of a complex set of neuronal, endocrine and behavioral mechanisms that together preserve fluid and electrolyte homeostasis. Figure 6–1 illustrates some of the factors involved in maintaining or disturbing fluid and electrolyte homeostasis. Although the complexity of the control mechanisms represented in the figure is formidable, this representation is admittedly a gross oversimplification. The constancy of the internal fluid and electrolyte environment is tenaciously defended not by a collection of independent mechanisms but by the coordinated operation of all of

them. The interrelations among the ADH system, the renin-angiotensin system, and thirst and drinking behavior are especially striking.

Although it is inappropriate to review all of the entries in Figure 6–1 at this time, some comment is indicated. The ADH system, the renin-angiotensin-aldosterone system, thirst and drinking behavior and, of course, the kidneys are the front line of defense of fluid and electrolyte homeostasis. Other hormones participate more or less directly in maintaining water balance either by way of renal effects or by affecting the storage of intracellular water. The dietary reference is to the antidiuretic effect of feeding a high carbohydrate diet after a period of starvation. Other factors will be mentioned in context.

The disease *diabetes insipidus* (DI) is characterized by the production of large volumes of urine of low specific gravity and compensatory thirst, which results in drinking large amounts of fluid. The disease can be congenital or acquired and the syndrome as originally described is known as central, or neurogenic, DI. This form of the disease is due to a relative lack of ADH. The symptoms may be controlled by replacement therapy with either the natural hormone or a synthetic substitute (to be discussed).

Nephrogenic diabetes insipidus is due not to a lack of ADH but to the failure of cells in the distal neph-

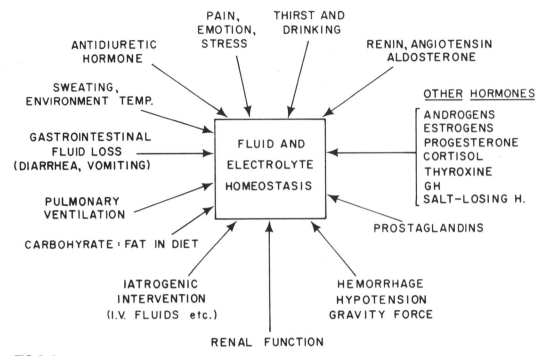

FIG 6–1.
Factors involved in fluid and electrolyte homeostasis.

ron to respond to the hormone. This, too, may have a variety of causes, which will be described below.

In addition to these deficiency states, *too much ADH* can be secreted in various circumstances. This is known as *s*yndrome of *i*nappropriate *anti*diuretic *h*ormone (SIADH). ADH excess is seen in a large number of conditions, among which are (1) *tumors* in many sites, which secrete ADH; (2) *CNS disorders,* which produce malfunction of central regulatory mechanisms for ADH; (3) various *pulmonary diseases* and (4) as a side effect of many *drugs*.

In order to understand these disease states, it is essential to examine the design of the body's water, salt and fluid volume conservation systems.

Figure 6–2 represents an attempt to describe many of the physiologic mechanisms that control the secretion of ADH from the posterior pituitary. AVP secretion is tonically inhibited by an α adrenergic-(norepinephrine-)mediated pathway that originates in the brain stem (Fig 6–2). Decrease in blood pressure or blood volume and signals from the thalamus and vomiting center all may stimulate AVP secretion by opposing the tonic inhibitory effect. Whether or not they coordinately stimulate AVP secretion by acting directly on the neurones of the supraoptic nucleus (SON) is not known. The many question marks in Figure 6–2 indicate uncertainties about the microneuroanatomy of the system.

At one time it was suggested that the peptidergic neurons themselves were osmostats and barostats. We are now reasonably sure that they are not. The osmotic regulation of AVP secretion and thirst are tightly coupled, i.e., both are triggered by only a 1%–2% change in plasma osmolality. Although it is not absolutely certain that both AVP secretion and thirst are controlled by the same osmoreceptors, this is a likely possibility.

There is a close connection among the three major mechanisms involved in fluid, electrolyte and volume defense: the ADH mechanism, renin-angiotensin-aldosterone system, and thirst and drinking behavior. The ADH and renin-angiotensin systems both respond to hypovolemia. Moreover, angiotensin stimulates ADH release, aldosterone secretion (for salt conservation) and also thirst and drinking behavior.

Pain, certain forms of stress, and emotion have traditionally been considered to enhance ADH secretion as part of a nonspecific stress response. However, some so-called stresses do not elicit ADH secretion and others may work by way of the baroreceptor system.

Another important control mechanism operates through the vomiting center, since nausea causes massive release of ADH. It has been suggested that traction and manipulation of the intestines, as during an operation, may elicit massive ADH release, pos-

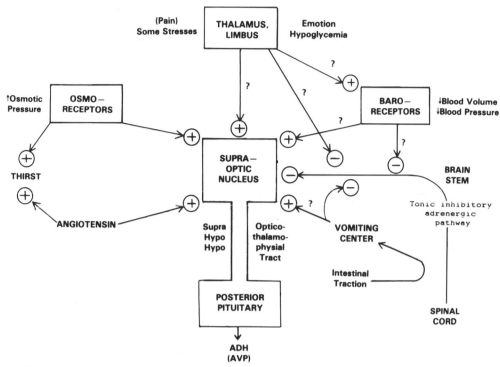

FIG 6–2.
Controls of ADH (AVP) secretion. Inhibition ⊖ of an inhibitory pathway ⊖ is equivalent to stimulation ⊕.

sibly by way of a mechanism that involves the vomiting center. This may account to some extent for the postoperative antidiuresis that sometimes occurs following abdominal surgery.

Chemistry of Posterior Lobe Peptides

The elucidation of the structure of the peptides oxytocin and vasopressin and their subsequent synthesis by Du Vigneaud and his collaborators was one of the most important events in modern biochemistry. The substances are very similar octapeptides in which an amino acid ring structure is formed by the closure of an S-S bond between no. 1 and no. 6 cysteine molecules to form cystine (Fig 6–3). Oxytocin is found in practically all bony vertebrates. The comparative

activities of these compounds in several assays are shown in Table 6–1.

Arginine vasopressin has been found in man, horse, sheep, and other species, but lysine vasopressin (position 8) is characteristic of the pig and hippopotamus.

An intriguing example of the discovery of a biochemically important compound *before* it was isolated from its natural source is the story of arginine vasotocin. During a study of structure activity relationships by Katsoyannis and Du Vigneaud, the side chain of arginine vasopressin was attached to the ring structure of oxytocin as shown in Figure 6–3. The resulting compound, arginine vasotocin, had about equal oxytocic and vasopressin or ADH activities in mammals, unlike the starting materials. But when it

TABLE 6–1.

Comparative Potencies of Neurohypophyseal Hormones in Different Assays*

HORMONE	UTERINE STIMULATION (rat, in vitro)	MILK EJECTION (rabbit)	PRESSOR (rat)	ANTIDIURETIC (dog)
Oxytocin	500	500	7	3
Vasopressin	30	100	600	600

*Data of Van Dyke et al.: *Recent Prog Hormone Res* 1955; 11:1.

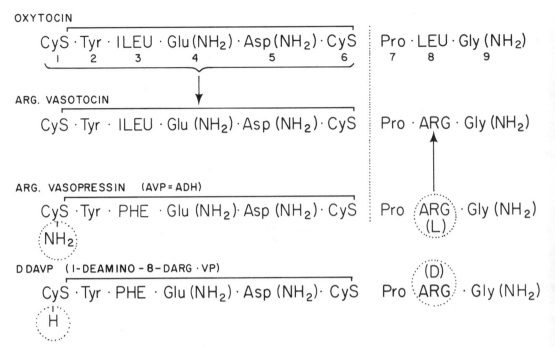

FIG 6–3.
Chemistry of posterior peptides and DDAVP.

was tested in nonmammalian vertebrate systems (frog bladder and isolated frog skin), it was many times more powerful than mammalian ADH. Meanwhile other investigators had postulated the existence of a specific "amphibian water balance principle" or "natriferin." The experience with the synthetic hybrid hormone stimulated a search for the material in amphibia with the result that arginine vasotocin is now known to be the naturally occurring water balance principle of those forms. In 1969, Vizsolyi and Perks described the transitory presence of the amphibian hormone in mammalian embryos. More recently Perks has discovered that, at one stage of development of a *mammal* (rat), neurohypophyseal peptides are capable of affecting water movements through fetal skin and bladder much as they do in the frog!

Many synthetic variants of the posterior lobe peptides have been prepared and studied. The interested reader is referred to the monograph by Berde for a detailed account of the results.

The molecular weight of arginine vasopressin is about 1,100. A perceptible antidiuretic effect can be produced in man with only 2 mμg of pure material; less than 0.1 μg produces a maximal antidiuresis.

One important result of the work on synthetic neurohypophyseal peptides was the development of the compound known as DDAVP (1-Desamino · 8 D-Arg-VP) shown in Figure 6–3. This is not only a pure

antidiuretic hormone (i.e., its pressor activity is only 1/4,000 that of AVP); it also resists degradation. Thus, when administered by the same route as AVP, DDAVP generally produced a higher maximal response and, more importantly, a much longer sustained response. DDAVP is one of many examples of man-made hormone analogues that is superior to the naturally occurring hormone for the replacement of a deficiency.

Hormone Measurement

Bioassays for ADH were and are very useful, but they were not sufficiently sensitive to measure circulating ADH very accurately, since those most commonly used relied on the vasopressor capability of the hormone. More recently, several exquisitely discriminating radioimmunoassays for posterior lobe hormones have been used successfully. Similar RIAs are available for the neurophysins (see next section).

Functional Unity of the Posterior Lobe and Its Hypothalamic Nuclei

The supraoptic and paraventricular nuclei are connected by a bundle of nonmyelinated nerve fibers with endings in the neural lobe of the hypophysis. The nerve endings are in close approximation to capillaries, and a venous effluent drains from the gland. The supraoptic nucleus (SON) and paraventricular nucleus (PVN) differ both in neuronal input and fiber destination. The SON has a high content of AVP cell bodies that project almost exclusively to the posterior pituitary gland. The PVN is much more complicated; it is said to contain eight distinct zones of cell bodies. Among these, in addition to a minority of AVP neurones, are oxytocinergic neurones and others that contain CRH, somatostatin, enkephalins, and other pro-opiomelanocortin products. It has a greater variety of connections from different regions in the CNS, and its terminals are found not only in the posterior lobe but also in the median eminence. The latter fact lends credence to the idea that it may participate with CRH in regulating the release of ACTH.

The posterior lobe peptides are synthesized in the SON and PVN as constituents of much larger prohormones. *Propressophysin* (20,000 D) is the precursor of AVP and its companion protein, neurophysin II. *Prooxyphysin* (15,000 D) is the precursor of oxytocin and neurophysin I. The prohormones are "packaged" in neurosecretory granules that contain enzymes capable of splitting the prohormones into their constituent peptides and neurophysins. Each type of neurone produces one prohormone, one peptide, and one characteristic neurophysin. The neurophysins have no known biological function, but they are secreted stoichiometrically with their respective peptides. Since they have a somewhat longer half-life in serum than their hormones (which disappear from the circulation in a few minutes), measurement of neurophysins represents an integrated record of posterior lobe peptide secretion over a period of hours.

The granules migrate down the nerve fibers and accumulate at the nerve endings in the posterior lobe. The migration of the granules has been observed in the living animal, and they have been timed at the rate of about 3 mm/day. When a stimulus that elicits a discharge of ADH is given, a sharp decrease in the number of granules can be seen in the posterior lobe. If the pituitary stalk is cut, no granules can be seen distal to the cut, but a piling up of granules occurs immediately above the cut and resembles granule aggregation in the "resting" posterior lobe (Fig 6–4). In fact, there can be a vascular reorganization above such a cut, with the development in time of a reconstituted release system for the hormones. If ^{35}S-labeled (radioactive) cysteine is injected into the subarachnoid space, the supraoptic nuclei of rats incorporate the label very actively, and several hours later labeled protein is detectable in the posterior lobe. The release of the active peptides into the bloodstream is accomplished by transmission of a message down the nerve fiber over which the secretory granules migrated to the posterior lobe. The peptides are split from their carrier proteins and enter the capillary circulation.

Some stimuli, notably hemorrhage, elicit a predominantly vasopressin discharge, whereas others (anesthetics, nicotine) stimulate the release of both vasopressin and oxytocin, the latter in larger amounts. Assays of the supraoptic and paraventricular nuclei reveal that the latter has more oxytocic activity and the former more vasopressin. This suggests that different types of signals arising in the nervous system may evoke a hormone mixture rich in one or the other hormone.

Physiologic and Other Stimuli for Release of ADH

If hypertonic saline is injected directly into the carotid artery, evidence of ADH release (antidiuresis) and oxytocin release (milk ejection and uterine contraction) may be seen. Conversely, if an animal or a man is water loaded, one of the mechanisms involved in the establishment of water diuresis is inhibition of ADH release. Although several possible signals for these responses have been described, it is impossible to assess the quantitative importance of each.

There are specific osmoreceptors in the brain that are capable of responding to fluctuations in the osmotic pressure of plasma by signaling either for a discharge of posterior pituitary hormones or for an inhibition of their release. Dehydration is presumed to evoke ADH release by this mechanism, and water diuresis could also set up an inhibition signal via osmoreceptor activity.

The *osmotic threshold* is defined as the plasma osmolality at which ADH release is initiated. This value is controlled with extraordinary precision in each person, and although there is some variation in osmotic threshold from one individual to another, it is remarkably constant in each individual, and nearly the same in identical twins. Figure 6–5 illustrates the determination of osmotic threshold in 73 normal human subjects. Following an oral water load, plasma osmolality fell to a mean value of 281.7 mOsm/kg. During subsequent infusion of hypertonic saline (5%), plasma osmolality gradually rose until it reached 287.3 mOsm/kg, when the release of ADH was initiated, as manifested by a fall in urine volume and in free water clearance (C_{H_2O}).

There has been some discussion about whether the osmotic threshold is a true threshold—i.e., a point in the continuum of changing osmolalities at which the

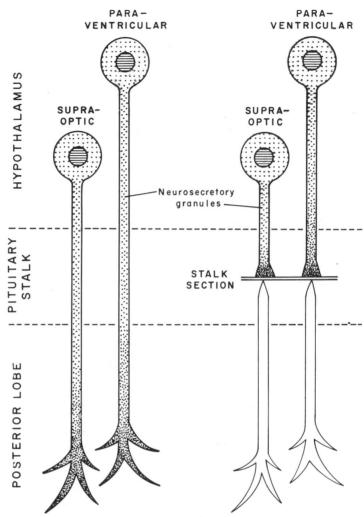

FIG 6–4.
Diagrammatic sketch of migration of neurosecretory granules down hypothalamohypophyseal tract and of the effect of stalk section. Granules contain either vasopressin or oxytocin, each with its neurophysin. Suggested by the studies of Bargmann and Scharrer. (See Sawyer WH: *Pharmacol Rev* 1961; 13:225 for many references.)

system suddenly begins to produce ADH—or a continuous, exponential change in response to increasing plasma osmolality. While the latter view may very well be technically correct, the final effect appears to us to be, operationally, something that looks very much like a threshold.

Hemorrhage is one of the most powerful known stimuli of ADH release. It would be difficult to see how the osmoreceptors could participate in this response, since hemorrhage results in hemodilution rather than hemoconcentration. Certain baroreceptor cells associated with blood vessels appear to be able to monitor continuously a signal that reflects blood volume. When there is a critical fall in this volume, afferent nerves from these "volume receptors" carry an alert to the CNS. There the neuroendocrine reflex arc is completed when the message is received by the cells of the supraoptic and paraventricular nuclei, which then "call" promptly for ADH. The likeliest location for these baroreceptors is in association with the vessels of the neck and thorax, and a similar mechanism is believed by some investigators to be operative in the case of the salt-retaining hormone of the adrenal cortex, aldosterone (see Chapter 12). Many of the clinical conditions associated with secondary aldosteronism (edema, ascites) are also asso-

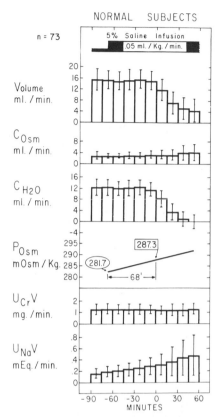

NORMAL SUBJECTS

n = 73

5% Saline Infusion
.05 ml. / Kg. / min.

Volume
ml. / min.

C_{Osm}
ml. / min.

C_{H_2O}
ml. / min.

P_{Osm}
mOsm / Kg.

287.3

281.7

68'

$U_{Cr}V$
mg. / min.

$U_{Na}V$
mEq. / min.

-90 -60 -30 0 30 60
MINUTES

FIG 6–5.
Osmotic threshold determination in 73 normal subjects. Volume = urinary volume; C_{Osm} = solute clearance; C_{H_2O} = free water clearance; P_{Osm} = plasma osmality; $U_{Cr}V$ = creatinine clearance; $U_{Na}V$ = sodium clearance. (From Moses AM, Miller M, in Conn HF, Conn RB, Jr [eds]: *Current Diagnosis,* ed 3. Philadelphia, WB Saunders Co, 1971. Reproduced by permission.)

ciated with the appearance of large amounts of ADH activity in the urine. From a teleologic point of view, both ADH and aldosterone would offer a great survival advantage following hemorrhage in an animal or a man whose fluid intake had been interrupted, for one hormone would conserve water and the other one sodium chloride for the critically depleted body fluids.

The AVP response to hemorrhage is quantitatively much larger than that to osmotic stimuli, and it used to be taught that this is the only known circumstance in which AVP plays a significant role as a vasoconstrictor. More recent studies suggest that AVP is important in the tonic regulation of blood pressure (see McNeill). Increases in circulating AVP within the physiologic range (much below those seen after hem-

orrhage) cause vasoconstriction in muscle, skin, and intestinal vascular beds, but this is not apparent as an increase in blood pressure because it is obscured by a concomitant fall in cardiac output.

There is another whole group of neurogenic stimuli that elicit ADH release. In Chapter 11 participation of the ACTH-adrenal axis is the nonspecific response to a variety of insults, and stresses will be considered in some detail (alarm reaction). Trauma (questionably), pain, even the anxiety incident to taking an examination, can cause ADH release from the posterior pituitary just as they cause ACTH release and adrenal cortical excitation. In cold exposure, on the other hand, ACTH is elicited, but *inhibition* of ADH has been described, so that the two materials apparently are not invariably released together. Presumably, nerve impulses either arising in the periphery (pain) or by way of special sense organs (frightening sight or sound), or recalled stored information within the brain (anticipation of a difficult experience) can trigger the release of these substances and often of aldosterone as well. The significance of the increased availability of these hormonal materials for adaptation or survival will be discussed in Chapter 11.

INTERACTIONS AND RELATIONS OF OSMORECEPTOR AND BARORECEPTOR MECHANISMS

The two regulatory systems for ADH secretion differ in important respects. First, osmoregulation is accomplished within narrow limits: a 1% change in plasma osmolality is capable of eliciting a corrective secreting of ADH. On the other hand, a 7%–15% fall in blood volume is required to trigger an ADH-release response. When the system receives conflicting signals (e.g., blood loss in the presence of hyponatremia), the volume-regulating stimulus overrides the osmoregulation mechanism.

The two systems interact in interesting ways. If an osmotic stimulus is administered to an individual in the prone position, the setting of the "osmostat" is shifted to the right; i.e., a higher plasma osmolality is required to produce a given plasma concentration of ADH. If the same person stands up and fluid accumulates in the lower extremities (perceived as a volume change in the thorax), the setting of the osmostat is shifted to the left, i.e., increase in plasma ADH occurs at a *lower* plasma osmolality. In this connection it is interesting to recall that astronauts experiencing weightlessness had increased urine volumes, presumably because the absence of gravity prevented the pooling of fluid in the lower extremities.

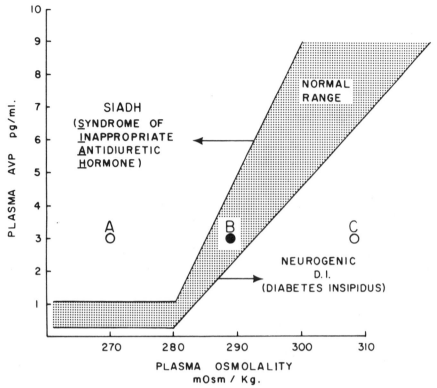

FIG 6–6.
Simultaneous measurement of a hormone and a variable regulated by the hormone.

An Illustration of Limitations of Blood Hormone Measurement

The availability of discriminating radioimmunoassay methods has greatly improved diagnosis of disturbances in water and electrolyte balance. This has been accomplished in spite of the fact that concentrations of AVP from 0.5 to 5 pg/ml cover the entire range from maximal diuresis to maximal antidiuresis. Measurement of plasma AVP is not sufficient by itself to give much information, since it is the *plasma concentration of hormone in relation to the prevailing osmolality of the blood* that is important. In Figure 6–6, the sharp inflection in plasma concentration of AVP (osmotic threshold) is shown as a range for normal individuals. All of the determinations of plasma AVP for persons *A, B,* and *C* are the same, but it is only by making simultaneous measurements of plasma osmolality that we can see that these three people are very different. Subject *B* falls within the normal range (though this does not necessarily mean that he is normal: he might, for example, have either nephrogenic diabetes insipidus or ''psychogenic'' overdrinking). The plasma AVP of *A* is much too high for his plasma osmolality; hence, he is likely to have SIADH. Subject *C*'s plasma AVP is much too low for his ambient plasma osmolality and he is therefore characterized as having neurogenic or central DI. This designation covers a whole spectrum of AVP insufficiencies from practically complete (when no increase in plasma AVP occurs even at very high plasma osmolalities) to nearly normal. The general principle of endocrinology illustrated here recurs in many other circumstances, e.g., measurement of circulating hormone concentration acquires additional meaning when it is *combined with a measure of the variable supposedly controlled by the hormone*. One thinks of high circulating insulin levels in spite of hypoglycemia (insulinoma); high parathyroid hormone (PTH) levels in spite of high serum calcium (PT adenoma); or high glucagon levels in spite of high blood glucose (diabetes).

Cellular Mechanisms of Action of AVP

AVP acts on three main cell types: (1) tubular cells in the kidney; (2) vascular smooth muscle cells; and (3) liver cells. In the *kidney,* its effect is to conserve water by causing its reabsorption from the hypotonic urine that traverses the distal part of the distal convoluted tubule and the collecting ducts. In the smooth muscle cells of *blood vessels,* as we have seen, AVP defends against hypotension when hemorrhage occurs and participates in the homeostatic maintenance of blood pressure. In the *liver,* AVP has effects similar to those of glucagon, i.e., it stimulates glycogenolysis and gluconeogenesis. In fact, in one species, the rat, AVP performs the functions ascribed to cyclic AMP-inducing hormones in other species.

Like other agonists (acetyl choline, catecholamines, histamine, opioids, etc.), AVP produces different results in different types of cells by interacting with different receptors. We have already seen that some synthetic analogues of AVP are purely antidiuretic and not at all vasoactive. The renal tubular effects and the vascular effects involve different parts of the peptide molecule. AVP receptors in the kidney are known as V_2 receptors, while those in blood vessels and hepatocytes are called V_1 receptors. As is the case with all other hormones and neurotransmitters that act by way of multiple receptors, the different receptor types activate different effector systems and thereby entrain distinctive biological effects.

The V_2 receptors in the AVP-sensitive *renal* tubular cells are on the *contraluminal,* or blood-lymph, side of the tubule. Within the contraluminal membrane they articulate with the G protein-adenylate cyclase complex to stimulate the production of cyclic AMP. The most striking biological effect of the increase in cyclic AMP is seen on the *luminal* membrane which is across the cell and in contact with the tubular contents. In the absence of AVP the luminal membranes of the cells that are capable of responding to it are virtually impermeable to water, though the (modified) glomerular filtrate with which they are in contact is hypotonic at this level of the nephron. As a result, markedly hypotonic urine is produced, that is, the ion-concentrating ability of the kidney is lost. When AVP acts through its receptor to increase cyclic AMP, unspecified proteins are phosphorylated, and certain protein particles, readily visible in freeze-fracture electron micrographs (Kachadorian et al.), are translocated from the interior of the cell to the luminal membrane where they cluster in aggregates. These remarkable particles confer on the previously water-proof luminal membrane the capacity to transport ion-free water into the cell. The water flows down its concentration gradient, since the tubular urine from which it is abstracted is hypotonic with respect to intracellular water. That the water traverses the cell on its way back into the extracellular fluid can be seen at the light microscope level (Fig 6–7). These effects can be duplicated by dibutyryl cyclic AMP, but it is now apparent that, in addition to cyclic AMP, Ca^{2+}-calmodulin is also involved, since the biological ef-

fect can be attenuated by calmodulin inhibitors. Although the protein kinase substrates involved in the elaborate movement of H_2O transporters from inside the cell to the luminal membrane have not been identified, some of them probably involve microtubules, since agents that cause disaggregation of microtubules (colchicine, vinca alkaloids) also inhibit the action of AVP.

AVP stimulates renal tubular cells to synthesize prostaglandins and other eicosanoids. PGE_2 antagonizes the effect of AVP and drugs that interfere with PG synthesis (example, indomethacin) enhance the effect of AVP. This suggests that PG synthesis is a component of the AVP response, and that PGE_2 may act as a brake, or governor, in the response.

The *vascular* (V_1) response is that of smooth muscle contraction and it must therefore involve an increase in $[Ca^{2+}]_c$. Calmodulin participates in the response, but there is no definite implication of the phosphatidyl inositol turnover mechanism in this action of AVP.

In the rat liver, (V_1) AVP shares with other hormones (catecholamine, angiotensin II) the ability to stimulate glycogenolysis and gluconeogenesis by mechanisms that do not involve cyclic AMP. These effects are brought about by increases in $[Ca^{2+}]_c$, via both mobilization from a subpopulation of endoplasmic reticular membranes and an increased Ca^{2+} influx from outside the cell. Polyphosphatidyl inositol turnover is stimulated, and IP_3 is mainly responsible for mobilizing Ca^{2+} from interior stores. Ca^{2+} acts by way of Ca^{2+}-calmodulin-stimulated protein kinase and direct actions on enzymes. The role of C kinase, if any, in these complex responses is not yet apparent (Williamson).

AVP has striking CNS and behavioral effects, but little is known about the cellular mechanisms involved in these. V_1 receptors have been demonstrated in certain parts of the brain. AVP has positive effects on both consolidation of memory and retrieval of stored information; oxytocin has the opposite effect, i.e., it is an amnesic peptide. These facts suggest the possibility that AVP may act in the CNS via V_1 receptors and that it may be competitively inhibited by oxytocin.

A summary of cellular mechanisms involved in AVP action via V_1 and V_2 receptors is given in Table 6–2.

Nephrogenic Diabetes Insipidus

Failure of cells of the distal nephron to respond to ADH is the basis of some conditions known as *nephrogenic diabetes insipidus.* This is an example of a growing number of circumstances in which the hor-

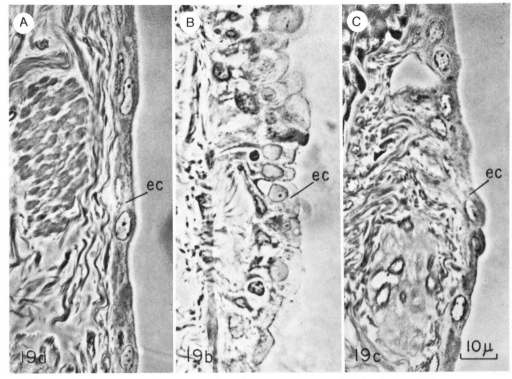

FIG 6–7.
Phase micrographs of toad bladders. **A,** control. **B,** fixed while exposed to antidiuretic hormone. **C,** fixed after effect of hormone had disappeared. *ec* = epithelial cell. (From Peachey LD, Rasmussen H: *J Biophys Biochem Cytol* 1961; 10:529. Reprinted with permission.)

mone response failure is not due to an inadequate supply of hormone but to an inability of the target cell to respond to it. Nephrogenic DI may be hereditary, acquired, or pharmacologically induced. Hereditary nephrogenic DI has been studied in the human being as well as in experimental animal models (see Dousa).

In the experimental animal model (mouse), the *inborn error* appears to be in the transducing element–adenylate cyclase system, since the binding of ADH to its receptor was not impaired but cAMP formation in response to ADH was diminished. Fluoride-stimulated adenylate cyclase was unchanged. Concentrating ability was not improved by ADH in these polyuric animals.

Nephrogenic DI in the human being is more difficult to study. People with this condition fail to respond to ADH by increasing urinary cAMP concentration. But in addition, they fail to respond to intravenously administered cAMP by concentrating their urine as do normal subjects and patients with central, or neurogenic, DI. Although these observations are difficult to interpret, they suggest a complex deficit of the response machinery of the distal tubular cells.

TABLE 6–2.
A Summary of the Effects of AVP in the Kidney, Blood Vessels, and Liver

Tissue	Renal tubule	Vascular small muscle	Liver
Receptor type	V_2	V_1	V_1
Messengers	cAMP	Ca^{2+}-CalMod	Ca^{2+}-CalMod
	Ca^{2+}-CalMod	IP_3 ?	IP_3
Biological effect	Translocation, aggregation of luminal membrane H_2O transporters	Contraction	Glycogenolysis, gluconeogenesis

Pharmacology of the ADH System

DRUGS AND IONS THAT AFFECT RESPONSIVENESS OF THE KIDNEY TO ADH

Impaired responsiveness to ADH may result from the administration of a number of *drugs*.

Lithium

Lithium inhibits noncompetitively ADH-stimulated adenylate cyclase in renal medulla of rabbit and man. Basal activity of the enzyme is not inhibited. It may also interfere with steps beyond cAMP formation. The overall result is a relative failure to respond to ADH and an impairment of concentrating ability. This is of some importance, since lithium is widely used in management of manic psychoses.

Demethylchlortetracycline (DMC)

DMC is an antibiotic that appears to have a rather selective effect on the concentrating function of the kidney without influencing other kidney functions. The drug inhibits basal, fluoride-stimulated, and ADH-stimulated adenylate cyclase activity of human renal medulla. Moreover, it inhibits protein kinase as well. This drug is so effective at blocking the end-organ response to ADH that it is being tested as a possible treatment of inappropriate ADH syndrome.

Vasopressin Analogues

Vasopressin analogues (e.g., vasopressinoic acid) prevent the action of ADH by competing with it for the plasma membrane receptor. This is one of many examples of hormone analogues that are capable of binding to the receptor but incapable of initiating a biologic response.

Impaired responsiveness to ADH may also result from various alterations in the *ionic environment* of the renal epithelial cell. Two examples are hypokalemia and hypercalemia.

Hypokalemia

In patients and experimental animals with chronic potassium deficiency, a concentrating defect occurs. The mechanism of this is not understood, but it is probably related to the cell's response to cAMP rather than to defective ability to generate cAMP in response to ADH.

Hypercalcemia

This may cause unresponsiveness to ADH. As we saw in Chapter 3, calcium has an important regulatory role in the operation of the cAMP-protein kinase system. In concentrations readily attainable in extracellular fluid (ECF) (10^{-3} M), it can inhibit both basal and ADH-stimulated adenylate cyclase. Although intracellular calcium concentration is about two orders of magnitude lower than ECF concentrations, a high ambient Ca^{2+} concentration can inhibit cyclase activation in kidney slices. Moreover, it also may interfere with microtubular aggregation. The overall effect is impairment of ADH responsiveness and interference with free water retrieval.

DRUGS THAT ALTER RELEASE OF ADH

In many circumstances, drugs may either stimulate or inhibit release of ADH and thus cause either fluid retention or diuresis. Although most of these drugs are used for their effects on the CNS, some are not usually associated with CNS effects. Table 6–3 is a summary of drug effects on ADH release. Acetylcholine (AcCh) and drugs that either mimic or potentiate the action of AcCh are stimulatory, as is nicotine. In fact, a heavy cigarette smoker is likely to maintain a high level of ADH output.

Experiments with catecholamine agonists and specific receptor antagonists have established the β catecholamine agonist effect (isoproterenol) as stimulatory, and the effect of receptor antagonists as inhibitory on ADH release.

We have seen that angiotensin, a stimulator of aldosterone biosynthesis, releases ADH as it causes thirst, thus coordinating the functions of water conservation, salt retention and volume repletion (see Chapter 12). Glucocorticoids have complex effects on water balance: they are essential for excreting a large water load promptly and they decrease the sensitivity of the osmostat to its usual osmotic stimulus, thus shifting the osmotic threshold to the right.

Another layer of complexity is added by the fact that glucocorticoids, by inhibiting prostaglandin production in the renal tubular target cells of ADH, increase their sensitivity to the hormone (see above—Cellular Mechanisms of Action of AVP). It is no wonder that the overall in vivo effect of glucocorticoid on the ADH system is not exactly predictable.

Before 1979, there was a general consensus in favor of calling morphine a *stimulator* of ADH release. Since then, experts in the field have been equally unanimous in describing morphine as an *inhibitor* of ADH release. The confusion was related to difficul-

TABLE 6–3

Drugs That Affect ADH Release*

DRUG CATEGORY	STIMULATE ADH RELEASE	INHIBIT ADH RELEASE
Neurotransmitter	Isoproterenol (β-adrenergic)	Norepinephrine (β-adrenergic)
	Acetylcholine	
	Nicotine (nicotinic AcCh† agonist)	
Hormone	Angiotensin	Adrenal glucocorticoids
Narcotic, sedative, etc.		Ethanol
		Morphine
	Ether	
	Phenobarbital	
Tranquilizer	—	Reserpine, chlorpromazine
Anticonvulsant	Carbamazepine	Diphenylhydantoin
Hypoglycemic	Chlorpropamide	—
Hypolipidemic	Clofibrate	—
Antineoplastic	Vincristine	—
	Cyclophosphamide	

*Modified slightly from Arnold Moses.
†AcCh = acetylcholine.

ties with experimental design in the earlier studies.

Ethyl ether and phenobarbital continue to be stimulators of ADH release. The best known inhibitor of ADH release is the most widely used drug in the world, ethyl alcohol. Morphine, ethyl alcohol, ethyl ether, and phenobarbital are all central nervous system depressants, but their actions on the ADH secretory mechanism must involve selective effects on system components that cannot be specified by us.

The drug *chlorpropamide* is an oral hypoglycemic agent of the sulfonylurea class (see Chapter 14). It is used in management of maturity-onset diabetes mellitus, although less widely so than a decade ago. Its effect was discovered by a patient with DI who misdiagnosed his disease and prescribed chlorpropamide for himself. His polyuria disappeared while he was taking the drug. His physician diagnosed the illness correctly and confirmed the antidiuretic effect of chlorpropamide. These observations were soon confirmed and a considerable amount of work on the mechanism of the effect was done. The drug was found to be ineffective when the neurogenic DI condition was complete. When some ADH secretory capacity was present, however, chlorpropamide enhanced secretion in response to a standard osmotic challenge. In addition, it potentiates the effect of exogenously administered vasopressin, both in patients with DI and in a strain of rat (Brattleboro) that has hereditary hypothalamic DI.

Clofibrate, the blood lipid-lowering drug, also stimulates ADH release by an unknown mechanism. The antitumor drugs vincristine and cyclophosphamide are also release stimulants.

Thus, drugs may affect the ADH-renal cell system either by influencing the secretory rate of the hormone or by modifying the response of the target cell to a given amount of hormone.

Oxytocin

The general pattern of oxytocin synthesis—axonal migration in association with its neurophysin, storage in the posterior pituitary and secretion—is similar to that of vasopressin, or ADH. The best evidence suggests that the two neuropeptides are under independent control, and each can be elicited by stimuli that do not cause secretion of the other.

PHYSIOLOGIC FUNCTIONS

Milk Ejection

Milk let-down, or milk ejection, is the major biologic effect of oxytocin. This peptide is released in response to neural signals that arise in the nipple stimulated by suckling—a classic neuroendocrine reflex. It is also released in *anticipation* of nursing, i.e., when a mother hears her baby cry. After milk is secreted, it accumulates in the lumina of alveoli and ducts of small internal diameter. Milk let-down occurs because oxytocin stimulates a population of highly specialized cells (myoepithelial) to contract, thereby expressing accumulated milk into large ducts and collecting cisterns. The effect of oxytocin in the mammary gland is seen most impressively in the cow, for the pressure in the udder cistern can be raised 10–15 mm Hg by a single injection of the hormone.

Uterine Contraction

Effects of oxytocin on uterine smooth muscle vary according to species, phase of estrus or menstrual cycle, and stage of pregnancy. Generally, estrogen sensitizes the myometrium to stimulation by oxytocin, and progesterone makes it more resistant to such stimulation. Attempts to demonstrate a physiologic role for oxytocin in the initiation of labor, or even during delivery, have been unsuccessful. The concentration of oxytocin in *fetal* blood is very high at the time of labor (see next section).

Cellular Mechanism of Action

High affinity binding sites for ^3H oxytocin have been found in plasma membrane-enriched fractions of rat uterus and mammary gland (see Soloff et al.). The affinity of these receptors for analogues of oxytocin generally correspond to their rank-ordered biologic potency.

The oxytocin receptor concentration in uterine smooth muscle increases in pregnant women and reaches a maximum early in labor. Receptors also increase in the endometrium and reach a maximum at parturition. Oxytocin stimulates the production of prostaglandins in the endometrium but not in smooth muscle. Oxytocin may participate in the onset of labor directly by stimulating smooth muscle contraction and indirectly by causing the endometrium to produce prostaglandins that are powerful smooth muscle stimulants and can act in a paracrine manner. Thus, the onset of labor may represent collaboration between oxytocin and locally produced prostaglandins. Since the fetus announces when it is prepared to be born, it has been suggested (Fuchs et al.) that one component of its announcement may be the oxytocin that causes the endometrium to synthesize prostaglandins. That prostaglandins play an important role in the onset of labor is indicated by the fact that PG synthesis inhibitors delay the onset of labor in women.

During stimulation of mammary myoepithelial cells to contract (the cellular basis for milk let-down) oxytocin causes phosphorylation of myosin. Oxytocin stimulation of these cells causes an increase in cyclic AMP, but myosin phosphorylation is not affected by cAMP protein kinase. Both myosin phosphorylation and contraction are blocked by agents that block Ca^{2+}

influx into the cells. Therefore, Ca^{2+}-calmodulin is the major messenger system in this response (Olins and Bremel).

Clinical Uses

No oxytocin deficiency state has been described. However, the peptide has been used to stimulate uterine contractions during and after labor.

BIBLIOGRAPHY

Bartter FC: The syndrome of inappropriate secretion of antidiuretic hormone (SIADH). *DM* 1973; 1.

Baylis P: Posterior pituitary function in health and disease. *Clin Endocrinol Metab* 1983;12:747.

Cobb WE, Spare S, Reichlin S: Neurogenic diabetes insipidus: Management with DDAVP (1-Desamino-8-D arginine vasopressin). *Ann Intern Med* 1978; 88:183.

Cross BA, Leng G (eds): *The Neurohypophysis: Structure, Function, and Control: Progress in Brain Research*, vol 60. New York, Elsevier North-Holland, Inc, 1983.

DeWied D: Central actions of neurohypophysial hormones, in Cross BA, Leng G (eds): *The Neurohypophysis: Structure, Function, and Control: Progress in Brain Research*, vol 60. New York, Elsevier North-Holland, Inc, 1983, pp 155–167.

Dousa TP: Cyclic nucleotides in the cellular actions of neurohypophysial hormones. *Fed Proc* 1977; 36:1867.

Fitzsimons JT: The physiological basis of thirst. *Kidney Int* 1976; 10:3.

Fuchs A-R, Fuchs F, Husslein P, et al: Oxytocin receptors and human parturition: A dual role for oxytocin in the initiation of labor. *Science* 1982; 215:1396.

Gainer H, Sarne Y, Brownstein MJ: Neurophysin biosynthesis: Conversion of a putative precursor during axonal transport. *Science* 1977; 195:1354.

Handler JS, Orloff J: Antidiuretic hormone. *Ann Rev Physiol* 1981; 43:611.

Hays RM: Alteration of luminal membrane structure by antidiuretic hormone. *Am J Physiol* 1983; 245 (*Cell Physiol* 14):C289.

Jard S, Butlen D, Cantau B, et al: The mechanism of action of antidiuretic hormone. *Adv Nephrol* 1984; 13:163.

Kachadorian WA, Wade JB, Di Scala VA: Vasopressin: Induced structural change in toad bladder luminal membrane. *Science* 1975; 190:67.

Kirk CJ, Creba JA, Hawkins PT, et al: Is vasopressin-stimulated inositol lipid breakdown intrinsic to the mechanism of Ca^{2+} mobilization at V_1 vasopressin receptors? in Cross BA, Leng G (eds): *The Neurohypophysis: Structure, Function, and Control: Progress in Brain Research*, vol 60. New York, Elsevier North-Holland, Inc, 1983, pp 405–411.

Litosch I, Lin S-H, Fain JN: Rapid changes in hepatocyte phosphoinositides induced by vasopressin. *J Biol Chem* 1983; 258:13727.

McNeill JR: Role of vasopressin in the control of arterial pressure. *Can J Physiol Pharmacol* 1983; 61:1226.

Moses AM, Miller M: Osmotic threshold for vasopressin release as determined by saline infusion and by dehydration. *Neuroendocrinology* 1971; 7:219.

Moses AM, Miller M, Streeten DHP: Pathophysiologic and

pharmacologic alterations in the release and actions of ADH. *Metabolism* 1976; 25:697.

Olins GM, Bremel RD: Oxytocin-stimulated myosin phosphorylation in mammary myoepithelial cells: Roles of calcium ions and cyclic nucleotides. *Endocrinology* 1984; 114:1617.

Perks AM: Developmental and evolutionary aspects of the neurohypophysis. *Am Zool* 1973; 17:833.

Reaven E, Maffly R, Taylor A: Evidence for the involvement of microtubules in the action of vasopressin in toad urinary bladder. *J Membr Biol* 1978; 40:251.

Robertson GL: Diseases of the posterior pituitary, in Felig P, Baxter JD, Broadus AE, et al (eds): *Endocrinology and Metabolism*. New York, McGraw-Hill Book Co, 1981, pp 251–280.

Robertson GL: Vasopressin, in Ingbar SH (ed): *Contemporary Endocrinology*, vol 2. New York, Plenum Publishing Corp, 1985, pp 403–450.

Sawyer WH: Evolution of active neurohypophysial principles among the vertebrates. *Am Zool* 1977; 17:727.

Schlondorff D, Levine SL, Salisbury J: Interaction of cAMP and calcium-calmodulin in the action of vasopressin. *Adv Nephrol* 1984; 13:319.

Share L (ed): Vasopressin and cardiovascular regulation (symposium). *Fed Proc* 1984; 43:78–106.

Soloff MS, Schroeder BT, Chakrabarty J, et al: Characterization of oxytocin receptors in the uterus and mammary gland. *Fed Proc* 1977; 36:1861.

Thomas AP, Alexander J, Williamson JR: Relationship between inositol polyphosphate production and the increase of cytosolic free Ca^{2+} induced by vasopressin in isolated hepatocytes. *J Biol Chem* 1984; 259:5574.

Verbalis JG, Robinson AG: Neurophysin and vasopressin: Newer concepts in secretion and regulation, in Imura H (ed): *The Pituitary Gland*. New York, Raven Press, 1985, pp 307–339.

Williamson JR, Cooper RH, Joseph SK, et al: Inositol triphosphate and diacylglycerol as intracellular second messengers in liver. *Am J Physiol* 1985; 248 (*Cell Physiol* 17):C203.

7

The Pineal Gland

	Some Landmarks in Pineal Chronology	
Date		**Investigator(s)**
300 B.C.	Pineal said to control flow of memory	Herophilus
17th century	Pineal the seat of the soul	Descartes
18th century	Pineal associated with madness	Many
1899	Pineal tumors in children associated with precocious puberty	Ogle; Heubner
1941	Exposure of rats to light caused estrus cycle disturbances	Fiske
1954	Pinealocyte tumors cause decreased gonadal function; pineal-destroying tumors = premature puberty	Kitay

Discovery of Melatonin and Its Synthesis

Beginning with the elucidation of the structure of melatonin in 1959 by Lerner and associates, information about the pineal progressed rapidly at both the biochemical and physiologic levels. Weissbach and Axelrod worked out the biosynthetic pathway for melatonin from its precursor amino acid tryptophan and demonstrated the presence of the necessary enzymes in the pineal (Fig 7–1). In parallel studies in the same laboratory, Wurtman et al. demonstrated that environmental light depresses pineal function, including the rate of melatonin synthesis. A neural pathway from the retina → retino-hypothalamic tract → sympathetic ganglia → pineal had been discovered by Kappers.

Assay of Melatonin

Progress in this field was aided by the development of extremely sensitive bioassays for melatonin, which are based on the lightening effect on previously darkened amphibian skin. The availability of the pure compound for standard curve construction was a great advantage. Radioimmunoassays for melatonin are now the most commonly used methods.

Storage and Secretion

Unlike glands that contain prepacked hormone poised for secretion on signal, the pineal appears to alter its melatonin secretory rate in response to changes in the *rate of synthesis* of the hormone. In this it resembles steroid hormone-producing glands, which tend to store very little finished hormone, but rather hormone precursor instead. In the case of the pineal, the availability of the hormone precursor tryptophan does not appear to be limiting.

Signals for Melatonin Synthesis and Release

The proximate stimulus for increasing synthesis and release is norepinephrine. Figure 7–2 is a summary of factors influencing the size of the catecholamine pool that acts on the pineal cell. The major factor is light, or the absence of light: the former *inhibits* norepinephrine production and, in the dark, norepinephrine release at sympathetic nerve endings near the pinealcyte is increased. Information about environmental light is transmitted from the retina to the CNS and thence to the superior cervical ganglion and adrenal medulla by way of preganglionic fibers. Postganglionic neurons arising in the superior cervical

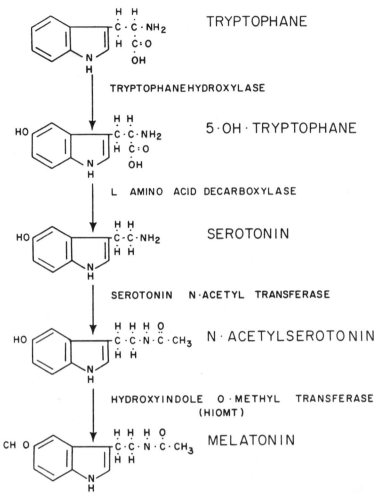

FIG 7–1.
Biosynthesis of melatonin.

ganglion may be traced directly to the pineal cells.

Melatonin synthesis and release in rats also may be stimulated by immobilization stress and hypoglycemia. Other factors, e.g., periodicity of feeding and availability of dietary tryptophan, may affect rate of melatonin secretion. In rats and other species, light-dark cycles entrain rhythmic secretion rates, with high rates in the dark and low rates in the light. In man about 70% of the daily melatonin secretion occurs at night, between 11 P.M. and 7 A.M.

One of the most striking effects of melatonin is the inhibition of gonadotropin secretion, suggested by the earliest work and demonstrated in more recent studies. A characteristic feature of one endocrine stress response (to be discussed more fully in Chapter 11) is that, whereas the secretion of some hormones in-creases as a result of stress (adrenal glucocorticoid, aldosterone, vasopressin, growth hormone), there is evidence of a *decrease* in insulin secretion and gonad-otropin secretion. The mechanism of the latter is not known, but since melatonin secretion is stimulated by stress, it may be involved in stress-related decreases in gonadotropin secretion.

Microregulation of Melatonin Synthesis

Norepinephrine interacts with the β and α adren-ergic receptors on the plasma membrane of the pin-ealocyte with several results (Fig 7–3). *Adenylate cyclase* is stimulated via the β receptor and the G_s protein, and cyclic AMP synthesis is increased. *Poly-phosphatidyl inositol* turnover is stimulated (α recep-

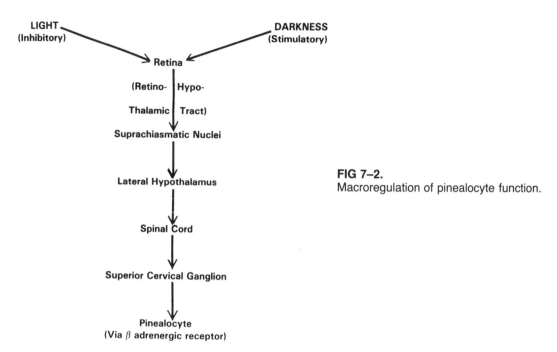

FIG 7–2.
Macroregulation of pinealocyte function.

tor) and IP$_3$ and diacylglycerol are released. *Arachidonic acid release* from membrane phospholipids occurs and prostaglandin E accumulation has been documented, though other arachidonic acid metabolites may also appear. All of these messengers collaboratively cause the phosphorylation of proteins that elicit a selective increase in the synthesis of messenger RNAs for the rate-limiting enzyme of melatonin synthesis, S. N acetyltransferase, and for HIOMT (see Fig 7–1). Since the supply of precursor, tryptophan, is not limiting, the newly synthesized enzymes are responsible for the increased synthesis and release of melatonin.

Pineal cells show the phenomenon of down regulation. Kebabian et al. have used the β blocker, [³H] alprenolol, as an indicator of norepinephrine receptor number. They have demonstrated an *increased* binding in the pineals of animals kept in continuous light (i.e., when norepinephrine release is inhibited) and *decreased* binding in pineals stimulated by β agonist drugs.

Fate of Secreted Melatonin

Melatonin has a short half-life in blood. It is extracted by both hepatic inactivation and urinary excretion. The accumulated urinary excretion generally is regarded as indicative of secretory rate. In fact, studies of urinary melatonin secretion make it possible to do noninvasive experiments in human subjects.

Biologic Effects of Melatonin

The major known effect is that of *gonadotropin secretion inhibition*. This is believed to be due to inhibition at two loci: (1) the constellations of cells that control the function of those peptidergic neurons that secrete LHRH into hypophyseal portal blood, and (2) a direct action on the pituitary gland. Since effects on gonadotropin output are demonstrable following intraventricular administration of melatonin, the melatonin secreted in response to catecholamine may reach gonadotropin control centers by way of the CSF. That this is not the only mechanism for inhibition of gonadotropin secretion is suggested by the fact that the response of the pituitary to LHRH stimulation is inhibited by melatonin.

In addition to inhibition of gonadotropin function, injection of melatonin has been observed to decrease thyroid hormone, adrenal hormone, and growth hormone production as well. All of these functions are increased, and mitotic activity of the pituitary is stimulated, following pinealectomy in young animals. The biologic significance of these observations is not known.

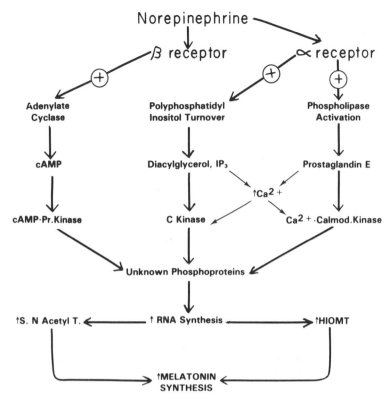

FIG 7–3.
Microregulation of melatonin synthesis in the pinealocyte.

Applications in Humans

The amplitude of light-induced changes in melatonin production, particularly in relation to gonadal activity, are much greater in seasonal breeders and nocturnal rodents than in humans. Disturbances in the circadian rhythm of melatonin secretion are demonstrable in people, however, as a component of *jet lag,* particularly when as many as seven time zones are crossed. These observations are difficult to interpret because they involve sleep deprivation in addition to altered lighting pattern.

That the pineal is involved in modulating gonadal function in people is suggested by the fact that there is a sharp decrease in serum melatonin levels in boys at the time of the onset of puberty. It is possible that melatonin decrease is an important component of the signal complex that triggers the beginning of puberty. In women, the highest levels of melatonin are seen at the time of menstruation and the lowest at the time of ovulation. These times, of course, correspond reciprocally to estrogen levels (see Chapter 9).

The pineal tumor story appears to be much the way Kitay summarized it in 1954 (see chronology above).

Pineal tumors can *decrease* gonadal function by secreting melatonin or by compression or destruction of nerve cells or tracts that are important in the maintenance of LHRH secretion. They, or other tumors in the vicinity, may *increase* gonadal function by destroying pineal cells. Since germ cell tumors may occur in the region of the pineal (especially in Japan), some pineal tumors overproduce chorionic gonadotropin. Pineal tumors of all types constitute between 0.4% and 1% of all intracranial neoplasms.

Finally, we must leave open the possibility that the 18th-century physicians who associated the pineal with behavioral abnormalities may not have been completely wrong. Injection of melatonin in humans induces mild euphoria, and sleep.

BIBLIOGRAPHY
Binkley SA: Circadian rhythms of pineal function in rats. *Endocr Rev* 1983; 4:255.
Cardinali DP: Melatonin: A mammalian pineal hormone. *Endocr Rev* 1981; 2:327.
Fèvre-Montange M, Van Cauter E, Refetoff S, et al: Effects of "jet lag" on hormonal patterns. II. Adaptation of melatonin circadian periodicity. *J Clin Endocrinol Metab* 1981; 52:642.

Kebabian JW, Zatz M, Romero JA: Rapid changes in rat pineal β adrenergic receptor: Alterations in ^{3}H alprenol binding and adenylate cyclase. *Proc Natl Acad Sci USA* 1975; 72:3735.

Kolata G: Puberty mystery solved. *Science* 1984; 223:272.

Martin JE, Klein DC: Melatonin inhibition of the neonatal pituitary response to luteinizing hormone releasing factor. *Science* 1976; 191:301.

Preslock JP: The pineal gland: Basic implications and clinical correlations. *Endocr Rev* 1984; 5:282.

Reiter RJ: The pineal and its hormones in the control of reproduction in mammals. *Endocr Rev* 1980; 1:109.

Reiter RJ (ed): *The Pineal Gland*. New York, Raven Press, 1984.

Relkin R (ed): *The Pineal Gland*. New York, Elsevier North-Holland, Inc, 1983.

Sugden D, Vanacek JV, Klein DC, et al: Activation of protein kinase C potentiates isoprenaline-induced cyclic AMP accumulation in rat pinealocytes. *Nature* 1985; 314:359.

Tamarkin L, Baird CJ, Almeida OFX: Melatonin: A coordinating signal for reproduction? *Science* 1985; 227:714.

PART **IV**

Reproductive Endocrinology

8

The Male

Date	Some Landmarks in the History of Andrology	Investigator(s)
2000 B.C. et seq.	Castration as punishment for adultery and other sexual offenses	Code of Hammurabi
?	Prepuberal castration for social purposes: slaves, stewards, harem attendants, male soprano singers, etc.	Greek authors Chinese, Indian, North African authors
400 B.C.	Testicular anatomy described	Aristotle
400 B.C.	Denial of necessity of testes for fertility	Aristotle
17th century	Castration of human war captives by cannibals to increase weight and tenderness of flesh	Caribbean, NE Brazil natives
1667	Spermatozoa (''animalcules'') seen in seminal fluid	v. Leuwenhoek
1668	Studies on testicular anatomy	De Graaf
1840	Spermatozoa developed in tubules, not preformed ''animalcules''	v. Koelliker
1849	First demonstration of an endocrine role for any gland: prevention of atrophy of cock's comb by transplanting testis to abdominal site	Berthold
1878	Proscription of castration for church singing (last castrato died in 1922)	Pope Leo XIII
1889	Report of dramatic increase in vigor and libido after self-injection of extracts of animal testes (later retracted).	Brown-Sequard

(Adapted from Bremner WJ, in Burger H, de Kretser D (eds): *The Testis*. New York, Raven Press, 1981.)

Reproductive Endocrinology: Population Homeostasis

The reader is no doubt aware of the major theme of *regulatory* biology in *individual* people and animals. The concept of homeostasis is built on the idea that some quantity—that of blood glucose, serum calcium, blood pressure, blood volume, or other entity—is regulated within a range of "normal" values. When the equilibrium level is disturbed, monitor cells respond by setting in motion forces that tend to correct the disturbance. These forces generally act in ways that appear to us to be teleonomically adapted to survival of the individual. Regulations of this type occur in single, more or less free-living organisms who are clearly at a disadvantage when the regulatory mechanisms are compromised.

Reproductive biology, of which endocrinology is an important part, represents a qualitatively different, and more complex, kind of homeostasis, since reproductive biology no longer involves only individual people or animals. Sexual reproduction goes far beyond the individual, since the smallest unit we can examine is what can be called the *reproductive unit,* which consists of female, male and offspring (Fig 8–1). The biology of sexual reproduction differs from that of the individual because *regulations occur in one member of the reproductive unit that are complementary to functions in one or more of the other members of the triangle.* For example, gametogenesis occurs in the male and in the female. Although the processes in the two sexes show certain similarities, they are also very different. However, they are complementary since the maturation of gametes, the anatomical arrangements for their rendezvous, and the mechanisms involved in the nidation, growth and development of the fertilized ovum all represent collaborative contributions of all three parties to the transaction.

Reproductive endocrinology deals with nothing less than the perpetuation of the species, with the homeostatic regulation of populations. The preoccupation of human individuals and populations with sexual reproduction is clearly evident in much of the world's history, art and literature, not to mention its economics, politics and theology. Large numbers of people reproduce while others devote considerable effort to preventing reproduction. Contemplation of the biology of reproduction provides a basis for the study of infertility on the one hand and "birth control" on the other.

Fertilization

The recent achievement by Steptoe and Edwards of in vitro fertilization of the human ovum reminds us

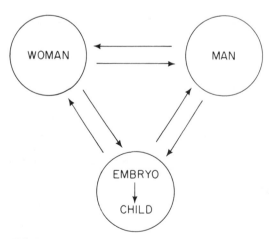

FIG 8–1.
The reproductive unit.

that all of reproductive biology is ultimately concerned with fertilization of the ovum by a competent spermatozoon. Gametogenesis in the two sexes, the growth and maintenance of the secondary sex characteristics, the complex social and behavioral activities associated with reproduction all converge at the instant that the sperm fertilizes the egg and renders it impermeable to the entry of other spermatozoa.

Although the sperm cell is not a hormone, the stimulus-response character of the events of fertilization is very similar to the response of a sensitive cell to a hormone. The species specificity of fertilization is based on a molecular "receptor" built into the vitelline membrane of the ovum, which reacts only with a species-specific protein (called "bindin") on the surface of its homologous spermatozoon. Lennarz and colleagues (see Schmell et al.) have isolated a single glycoprotein (from sea urchin egg membranes) which, when added in vitro to a suspension of spermatozoa and an ovum, successfully competes for spermatozoa with the ovum and thereby prevents fertilization. The attachment of the spermatozoon entrains the series of events that, together, constitute fertilization.

The "turning on" of the ovum by the spermatozoon is a prototype of one form of stimulation, i.e., *stimulation by releasing inhibition.* The unfertilized ovum can be imagined as poised to begin its developmental program but inhibited from doing so by the presence of a complement of hypothetical inhibitors. When the sperm interacts with the membrane of the ovum, profound alterations in membrane permeability occur, which result in marked changes in intracellular fluid and electrolyte composition and pH. The hypothetical inhibitors are unable to function in the new environment and the ovum is then released to begin development. In some ova the process can be initiated by mechanically damaging the ovum membrane or by acutely changing intracellular calcium concentration with the calcium ionophore, A23187.

The consequences of the sperm bindin-receptor interaction have been studied extensively by scanning electron microscopy and by bioelectric methods as well as biochemically. The earliest perceptible change is a minor influx of sodium ions, which occurs within the first two seconds and is perceptible as an action potential. The membrane modification indicated by this action potential is believed to be associated with the early block to polyspermy. Within 8 seconds calcium ions are liberated from intracellular storage depots and, by 20 seconds, the cortical reaction begins, first at the sperm attachment point and then propagated radially over the whole surface of the cell. Thousands of cortical granules, about 1μ in diameter, fuse with the plasma membrane and discharge their contents between the plasma membrane and the vitelline layer. The discharged granule components are a complex mixture of enzymes, structural proteins used to construct the occlusive fertilization membrane, and other unknown materials. One enzyme actually alters the configuration of the sperm receptor on the vitelline membrane so that supernumerary sperm are no longer able to remain attached. Thus, the discharge of cortical granules generates the second block to polyspermy and triggers formation of the fertilization membrane, which is completed within a minute of sperm attachment.

The major ion fluxes that are initiated by the sperm-receptor interaction are a calcium influx, which peaks at about 80 seconds and a large sodium influx, associated with a striking alkalinization of the intracellular environment, which achieves its maximum at about 150 seconds. Whether the ovum is stimulated to develop by a sperm, a needle prick or a calcium ionophore, similar changes are seen. For an extraordinary account of a multidisciplinary approach to a fundamental problem in biology the reader is referred to the essay by Epel.

Reproductive Function in the Male

The testis is a compound organ composed of two main populations of cells: (1) Leydig cells, which synthesize and secrete the principal circulating androgen testosterone, and (2) the cells of the seminiferous tubules, or the germinal epithelium, in which gametogenesis occurs. Leydig cells are stimulated to synthesize and release testosterone by pituitary LH (luteinizing hormone), which in the male is sometimes referred to as ICSH (interstitial cell-stimulating hormone). The stimulatory effect of LH on the Leydig cell is duplicated by chorionic gonadotropin (CG). Neuroendocrine control of reproduction is outlined diagrammatically in Figure 8–2.

Gametogenesis, or spermatogenesis, is controlled by testosterone and pituitary FSH. Since high local concentrations of testosterone at the periphery of the seminiferous tubules are required to sustain spermatogenesis, testosterone secreted by adjacent Leydig cells may be said to perform a paracrine function in this case. The duct system through which newly formed spermatozoa must pass to reach the ejacula-

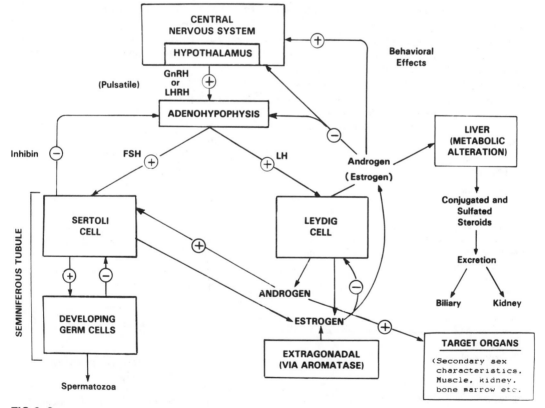

FIG 8–2.
Diagrammatic outline of neuroendocrine control of reproduction in the male ($\oplus$ = stimulation; $\ominus$ = inhibition).

tory duct is also dependent on high concentrations of androgen.

The main functions of androgens are summarized in Table 8–1.

Sex Chromosomes

Sex determination is a genetically directed phenomenon and the result that is determined is the *sex genotype,* or *genetic sex*. The results of the developmental process are referred to as the *sex phenotype*. In most cases the sex genotype and sex phenotype are congruent, but there are many conditions in which there is an apparent discrepancy between the two.

Both oogonia and spermatogonia contain 46 chromosomes: the former's complement can be designated as 44 XX, that of the latter 44 XY. At the stage of oogenesis between the primary and secondary oocyte, halving of the chromosome number occurs, so that each secondary oocyte (and therefore each ovum) receives 22 X. At the analogous stage in the development of the spermatozoon, two kinds of secondary spermatocytes are formed, 22 X and 22 Y. Genetic maleness or genetic femaleness is therefore determined by the chance that an ovum is fertilized by an X- or Y-bearing sperm: XX = female; XY = male.

In 1949 Barr and Bartram discovered that the somatic tissues of females carry a visible chromatin mass, which is believed to be due to the apposition of certain regions of the XX pair. It is therefore possible to determine sex genotype by examining smears of buccal mucous membrane for Barr bodies. More recently, techniques for detecting the presence of the Y chromosome by fluorescence microscopy have also been used extensively. Growth of human cells and direct examination of chromosomes (karyotype determination) have added to our knowledge of genetic abnormalities. The availability of the technique of amniocentesis, which permits examination of cells obtained from amniotic fluid aspirated in the 14th to 16th week of pregnancy, has made possible the detection of chromosomal abnormalities of the fetus (and, incidentally, diagnosis of the sex of the fetus).

Several diseases have been shown to be associated with chromosomal abnormalities. Down's syndrome (mongolism) in both males and females is characterized by the presence of an extra autosomal chromosome and therefore a total chromosome number of 47 instead of 46. Klinefelter's syndrome (apparent male with small testes and feminine stigmata) is often, but not invariably, accompanied by an XXY chromatin pattern and a positive Barr test. (Rare individuals are found with as many as five X chromosomes but, as long as there is a Y, the testis develops.) Patients with Turner's syndrome (small stature, amenorrhea, undeveloped secondary sex characteristics) are often, but not always, found to have only one X chromosome and a total number of 45.

The XYY combination occurs once in 1,000 male births, and nearly all such individuals are phenotypically normal. There have been reports that people with this chromosomal configuration are statistically more likely to occur in "mental-penal institution" settings, but it has been estimated that no more than 1% of XYY individuals are confined, which means that 99% are not. XYY individuals tend to be very tall and have a higher incidence of severe acne than XY counterparts.

The "super female" cluster of chromosomes (XXX) occurs once in 1,600 female births, and most individuals are normal in appearance. There is some evidence that offspring of these individuals have a higher incidence of chromosomal abnormalities than do XX women.

A small sample of chromosomal abnormalities is presented in Table 8–2. For a profound review of this subject, the interested reader is referred to the essay by Grumbach and Van Wyk.

TABLE 8–1.

Main Functions of Androgens

Differentiation
  Genital apparatus and tracts
  Central nervous system
Growth and maintenance of secondary sex characteristics
  External genitalia
  Accessory glands
  Voice timbre
  Skin
  Others
Anabolic and general metabolic effects
  Skeletal growth
  Skeletal muscle growth
  Renotropic effects
  Subcutaneous fat distribution
Gametogenesis (in FSH-primed tubules)
Processing of immature spermatozoa for fertilization
Behavioral effects

Functions of Androgens in Differentiation

Developmental Biology of Reproductive Structures

In mammals, the primordial gonad is programmed to develop a female reproductive tract in the absence of a Y chromosome (Fig 8–3). When the Y chromo-

TABLE 8–2.

Chromosomal Abnormalities in Man*

CLINICAL STATE	BARR CHROMATIN BODIES	SEX CHROMOSOMES	NO. OF AUTOSOMAL CHROMOSOMES	TOTAL NO. OF CHROMOSOMES
Normal female	1	XX	44	46
Normal male	0	XY	44	46
Superfemale	2	XXX	44	47
Klinefelter's†	1	XXY	44	47
Turner's†	0	X	44	45
Female, mongolism	1	XX	45	47
Male, mongolism	0	XY	45	47

*Barr ML: *Science* 1959; 130:679.
†See text for qualification.

some is present, however, the indifferent gonad begins to develop in the human male fetus at about six weeks. Between 6 and 16 weeks, male sexual differentiation occurs.

Organization of the testis occurs through the agency of a remarkable surface glycoprotein identifiable immunologically as histocompatibility Y (H-Y) antigen, which is either directly or indirectly elicited by a gene on the Y chromosome. This protein, studied by Ohno and by Wachtel, is the first cell surface

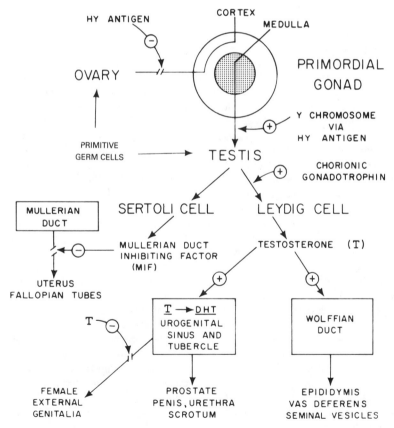

FIG 8–3.

Differentiation of male and female reproductive systems. *DHT* = dihydrotestosterone. (For references to original data upon which this diagrammatic summary is based, see Wilson JD: *Ann Rev Physiol* 1978; 40:279, and Ohno S: *JAMA* 1978; 239:217.)

protein to which a specific organogenesis function has been assigned, and thus represents a landmark in the history of developmental biology. If the cells of a very early testis are dispersed by trypsinization and stripped of H-Y antigen by an anti-H-Y antibody, they aggregate into a follicular structure that is typically ovarian. If they are treated with control serum (i.e., if the surface H-Y is allowed to persist), they self-assemble into a tubular (more appropriately, cord-like, for there is as yet no lumen) structure that is the precursor of seminiferous tubules.

When the original aggregation into primitive tubules occurs, germ cells, which have completed their long, pseudopodal journey from the yolk sac to the urogenital ridge, are entrapped by the aggregating pre-Sertoli and pre-Leydig cells. Thus, all of the cellular elements necessary for the further development of the seminiferous tubule are already in place in the very early embryo. The identity of the chemotactic signals that direct the migration of the germ cells precisely to the place where they can be incorporated into the nascent tubule is unknown, but the phenomenon has its analogue in the migration of leukocytes to the site of inflammation.

At the time of organization of the primitive testis, the fetal pituitary is not yet producing LH. However, embryos of both sexes are exposed to CG (chorionic gonadotropin) of placental origin. Receptors on the newly developed Leydig cell are already capable of recognizing and binding CG.

The Sertoli cell produces a protein substance known as müllerian inhibiting factor (MIF), which actively induces the regression of the müllerian duct. This is a protein with a molecular weight of 30,000 daltons. Rare male individuals have been described with a persistence of müllerian duct structures in the presence of a normal male reproductive system, and they are presumed to have had a genetic defect, which resulted in either a missing or inadequately functioning MIF.

The Leydig cell is stimulated by CG to produce testosterone, which is either directly or indirectly responsible for organizing the development of the other structures of the male tract. Testosterone itself has been found by Wilson et al. (see review) to stimulate the wolffian duct development system. This duct is the precursor of the epididymis, vas deferens and seminal vesicles. However, the structures derived from the urogenital sinus and tubercle—prostate, penis, outer two-thirds of urethra, and the scrotum— require conversion of testosterone to dihydrotestosterone (see p. 110) for their development.

Disturbances in development of the reproductive tract may be seen either as a result of inborn errors of metabolism or because an androgenic steroid is given to a pregnant woman during the crucial time when development of the tract occurs. Female infants with genetic disorders of adrenal steroid production (see Chapter 11) may be born with ambiguous external genitalia, as were female infants whose mothers were treated with androgenically active progestins during pregnancy.

One of the most interesting examples of disordered development in boys was described in a kindred of people in the Dominican Republic by Imperato-McGinley, Peterson, and colleagues. These investigators described a high incidence of boys who had a prepuberal deficiency of the enzyme 5α reductase, which catalyzes the conversion of testosterone to dihydrotestosterone. These genetic boys showed a typical female phenotype and feminine external genitalia, though wolffian duct-derived structures were normal since they had normal levels of testosterone. At the time of puberty, 5α reductase was induced and they became phenotypically male individuals.

ROLE OF ANDROGENS IN DIFFERENTIATION OF THE CNS

There is an analogy between the developing generative tract and the developing brain, as in both cases the female pattern of development occurs in the absence of androgen. When androgen is present, however, the male pattern is induced. When we talk about a female and male pattern of development in the brain, we mean *those structures in the brain that are associated with the control of pituitary gonadotropin secretion and sexual behavior.*

In 1936, Pfeiffer transplanted the gonads of newborn male rats into newborn females and demonstrated that, when the animals matured, they did not show estrus cycles, although they did have persistent vaginal cornification indicative of high estrogen output. In 1954, Barraclough and colleagues discovered that administration of a single injection of androgen to a neonatal female rat during a ''time window'' between day two and day five resulted in the development of sterile adult rats with polyfollicular ovaries that contained no corpora lutea. These ovaries were perfectly capable of making corpora lutea if transplanted to normally cycling female animals, so the original effect of the testosterone was not on the ovary.

The androgen effect is now believed to occur in parts of the brain that are associated with cyclic control of LHRH release and behavior. Before the characteristic features of the biologic clock in the preoptic region of the hypothalamus become fixed, androgen can imprint the clock in such a way as to prevent it from performing its cyclic function.

We now have actual morphologic evidence that generally supports the idea of the plasticity of the neonatal hypothalamus. Raisman and Field have shown that in normal female rats there is a larger number of a certain population of (nonamygdaloid) synapses on dendritic spines in the preoptic area than in male rats. Moreover, they have demonstrated that treatment of the neonatal female rat with androgen results in male morphology, whereas castration of the male within 12 hours of birth results in the development of a female neuronal pattern. Thus we now have endocrinologic, behavioral and morphologic evidence to support the view that androgens are involved in the differentiation of the brain.

The discovery that large amounts of estrogen in the newborn male can duplicate the masculinizing effects of androgens on "gonadostat" development was difficult to explain until Ryan and colleagues described the aromatization of testosterone (i.e., the formation of estrogen from testosterone) in the hypothalamus. It now seems that certain functions of testosterone in the CNS, especially those related to behavior and differentiation of gonadostat function, are accomplished not by testosterone itself but by estrogen synthesized from testosterone in specific neurons. Dihydrotestosterone (DHT) (see below), a steroid that is not susceptible to aromatization, cannot duplicate the effects of testosterone or estrogen in gonadostat development experiments such as those described above or in correction of disturbances in sexual behavior caused by castration. Embryos of both sexes are protected from high maternal levels of estrogen by α *fetoprotein,* which binds estrogen avidly.

All of these experiments were done in the rat, a species that is relatively more immature at birth than are primates, including the human. We do not know whether they have relevance for man. However, Goy and Phoenix have described behavior modification in female monkeys treated with androgen prenatally.

The concept that the functioning of hypothalamic "hormonostats" can be modified in neonatal life has been extended to the thyroid and the adrenal glands.

Chemistry and Metabolism of Androgens and Related Compounds

The main hormonal product of the Leydig cell is testosterone (Fig 8–4), which is synthesized at the rate of about 7 mg/day in man. Cholesterol ester, the major precursor for testosterone biosynthesis, is stored in lipid droplets in the Leydig cell. The general features of the testosterone synthetic pathway are shown in Figure 8–5. (A more detailed presentation of steroid hormone biosynthesis will be given in Chapter 11.) The testis also makes and secretes a very small amount of 5α dihydrotestosterone, but its source is the Sertoli cell.

The stimulus for testosterone synthesis is pituitary LH, or ICSH or, in the developing male fetus, CG. These hormones work by way of the cAMP mechanism. The LH, or CG, receptor on the plasma membrane of the Leydig cell binds the hormone with such high affinity that it can be used in a useful radioligand assay. LH and CG demonstrate the phenomenon of spare receptors, since maximal testosterone production can be achieved when only a small percentage of the available binding sites are occupied. Steroidogenesis also occurs when it is impossible to measure an increase in cAMP concentration. If one measures intracellular availability of cAMP binding sites, it is clear that doses of LH that effectively stimulate steroidogenesis also activate cAMP-dependent protein kinase (see Dufau et al.).

The effects of activation of the kinase have been worked out in connection with the entirely analogous stimulation of adrenal glucocorticoid stimulation by ACTH, a subject that will be discussed more fully in Chapter 11. As in the case of other steroid hormone-producing cells, the Leydig cell stores primarily hormone precursor in the form of cholesterol ester, and the finished hormone is promptly secreted. In addition to testosterone, the testis also makes and secretes small amounts of estrogen.

The Sertoli cell, stimulated by FSH, is also capable of making estrogen from androgen by the aromatase reaction. Estrogen production within the testis inhibits androgen production either in an autocrine (Leydig cell) or paracrine (Sertoli cell → Leydig cell) manner. Estrogen that originates in the testis may also participate in the feedback inhibition of gonadotropin production.

Only a small fraction of circulating estrogen in human males is actually secreted by the testis. The major part represents a metabolic product of circulating androgens from the testis and the adrenal. The ability to aromatize steroids to estrogen has been discovered in many nongonadal tissues including adipose tissue.

Like all other lipid-soluble hormones, testosterone is transported in the blood by a specialized transport protein synthesized in the liver, known as steroid hormone-binding globulin (SHBG, sometimes designated as TeBG; testosterone, estrogen-binding globulin). This is the same protein that carries estrogen and, as in the case of estrogen, carrier-bound steroid is biologically inactive. The combined affinity of testosterone for SHBG and albumin is such that less than 3%

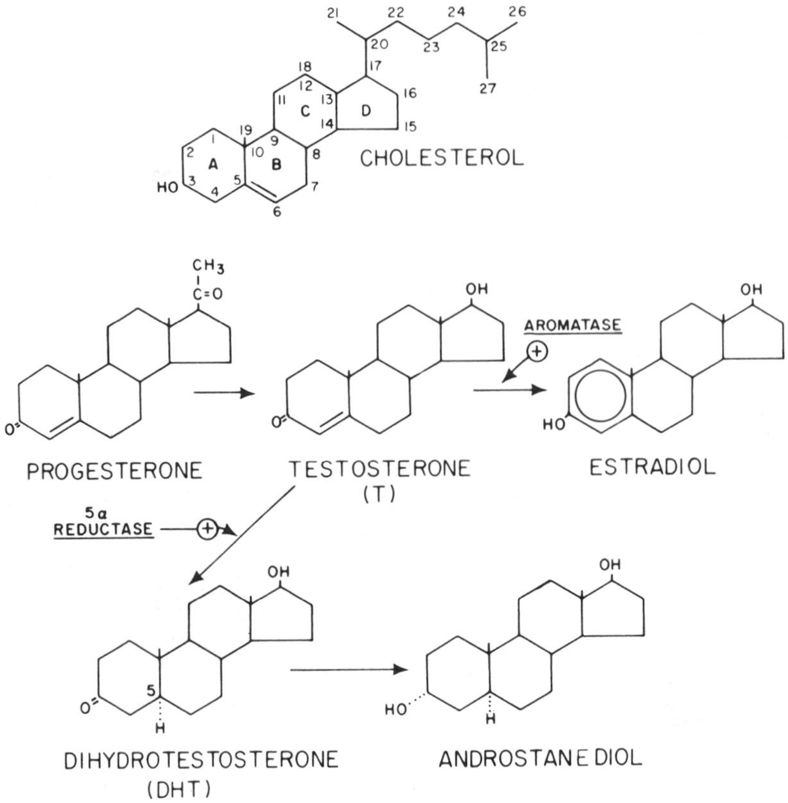

FIG 8–4.
Relationship of testosterone to other steroids. (In the human, the predominant pathway proceeds via pregnenolone, as shown on the left side of Figure 8–5.)

of the total testosterone in the blood is in the free, or biologically active, form. Regulation of SHBG concentration in the blood is of some practical significance, since there may be either an increase in total carrier protein (e.g., by estrogens) or a decrease (by androgens). In either case, measurement of total hormone concentration may not accurately reflect the concentration of free hormone.

Androgens can be measured by exquisitely sensitive bioassays, by chemical analytical methods, and by various kinds of radioligand assays, particularly by radioimmunoassay. Since there is about a 20% fluctuation in serum testosterone, with the highest blood levels occurring in the morning, and since androgen secretion in response to pulsatile gonadotropin secretion is episodic, there is some renewal of interest in urinary excretion of metabolic products of testosterone over measured time periods, a sort of integrated steroid secretion record.

Testosterone undergoes metabolic alteration to compounds of less androgenicity, or none, primarily in the liver, and these compounds are excreted in the urine as 17-ketosteroids (17-ks). Figure 8–6 summarizes the source of 17-ks and emphasizes the fact that only 30% of excreted 17-ks are of testicular origin. This does not mean, however, that women, who generally excrete about 70% of the ketosteroids excreted by men are necessarily 7/10 as androgenized as men. The major steroid contributed by the adrenals is dehydroepiandrosterone, a very weak androgen. The plasma testosterone concentration, a better index of biologically active androgen, is 0.73μg/100 ml in men and 0.037μg/100 ml in women.

SYNTHETIC MODIFICATIONS OF TESTOSTERONE

Testosterone is readily inactivated by the liver and is therefore of limited value for replacement of deficiencies when administered orally. Prototypes of many testosterone and progesterone analogues developed for specific purposes are shown in Figure 8–7. Esters of testosterone, such as the propionate illus-

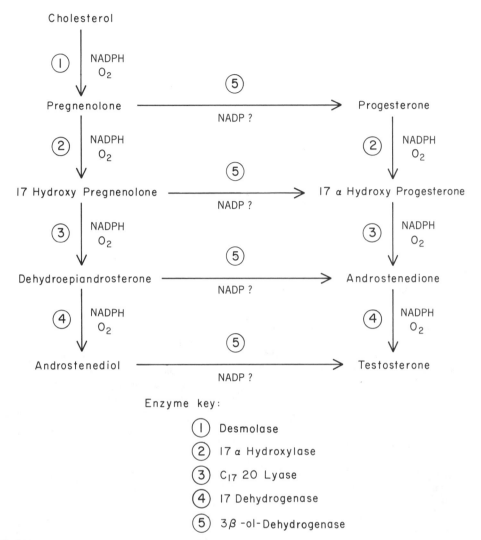

Enzyme key:

① Desmolase

② 17 α Hydroxylase

③ C₁₇ 20 Lyase

④ 17 Dehydrogenase

⑤ 3β -ol-Dehydrogenase

FIG 8–5.
Metabolic pathways for conversion of cholesterol to testosterone. *NADP* = nicotinamide adenine dinucleotide phosphate; *NADPH* = reduced *NADP*.

trated, are absorbed from the injection site more slowly and therefore have a more sustained biologic effect than does the native hormone. This type of compound, however, must still be injected or given in the form of subcutaneously implanted pellets. The 17-methyl ester of testosterone resists inactivation and may be given by mouth. It has the disadvantage occasionally of causing biliary tract stasis and jaundice. Injectable testosterone esters are preferred for replacement therapy.

Anabolic steroids will be discussed in connection with androgen effects.

Antiandrogens, of which two examples are shown, are compounds capable of binding to the androgen receptor, thereby denying it to environmental androgen. However, although they bind, the antiandrogens are incapable of initiating a biologic response. Such compounds are very useful in experimental circumstances when involvement of androgens in a physiologic process is in doubt. They were, in fact, used in this way in elucidating the role of androgens in differentiation of the reproductive tract of the male fetus. If a process is blocked by antiandrogens, one can infer that androgens are involved in it. This is analogous to the blocking of hormone effects by inhibitors of protein and DNA synthesis.

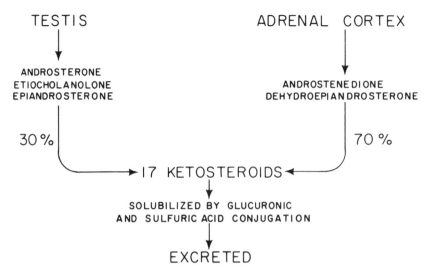

FIG 8–6.
Source of 17 ketosteroids. (Percents shown are those of total 17 Ks.)

Testosterone: Hormone and Prohormone?

The discovery by Wilson that injected tritiated testosterone was primarily recoverable from the nuclei as *dihydrotestosterone* initiated a long series of studies, which indicate that, in androgen-dependent tissues, testosterone exerts its effect in large part by way of its 5α reduction product, DHT (see Fig 8–4). In the normal human male, very little DHT circulates: it is formed from circulating testosterone in responsive cells. When tested for its androgenic potency (increase of prostate or seminal vesicle weight) in castrated male rats, DHT has about twice the potency of testosterone. It also shows a higher affinity for SHBG than does the parent steroid. We have already mentioned its role in the development of the male generative tract. This is an example of target tissue activation of a hormone. In another case, that of vitamin

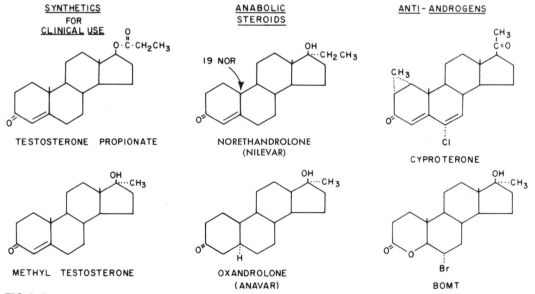

FIG 8–7.
Synthetic androgens and antiandrogens.

D, the precursor, cholecalciferol, is progressively activated by the liver and kidney to 1,25 dihydroxycholecalciferol, which then acts on the intestine, bone and kidney tubule.

Another metabolic route for testosterone is aromatization to *estrogen* (see Fig 8–4). This is an important reaction, particularly in cells in the CNS involved in hormonal control of sexual behavior and in differentiation of these cells.

There is no evidence for action of any metabolite of testosterone on skeletal muscle and bone. As we have seen, testosterone itself is responsible for the differentiation of several structures in the male genitourinary tract (see Fig 8–3). After they are fully differentiated, testosterone stimulates them via dihydrotestosterone.

In several species, 5β derivatives of testosterone have a highly specialized function: stimulation of RBC development.

Therefore, the total biologic effect of testosterone can be achieved, not only by testosterone but also by a family of testosterone-derived metabolites. A summary of this concept is presented in Figure 8–8.

Testicular Function at Different Ages

INFANCY

The concentration of testosterone in peripheral blood of the male neonate is higher than that of the female. However, by the end of one week it is virtually undetectable in both sexes. From age 1 month to 4–7 months in normal male infants, there is a substantial *increase* in circulating testosterone to about one-half the level seen in adult males. LH levels are also high at this time. By 6–7 months, both LH and testosterone levels fall to insignificant concentrations and do not rise again until puberty. This is known as the infantile testosterone surge (ITS), and its biologic significance is not known. It is possible that some important imprinting experience occurs during this period.

PUBERTY

From age 6–10, there is a slight but significant increase in both FSH and LH, with the FSH rise anticipating that of LH. There is a small increase in mean testis size without a change in plasma testosterone level. The "set" of the gonadostat is such that it is exquisitely sensitive to feedback inhibition, even by the very small concentrations of steroid circulating in the prepuberal boy.

At age 10–17, FSH rises at a slow rate and reaches adult levels by age 15. LH rises at a more rapid rate and reaches the adult mean by age 17. In both sexes there are extraordinary sleep-related bursts of gonadotropin output, the levels returning to progressively higher daytime levels until, at the end of puberty, gonadotropin concentrations, though still episodic, are fairly steady over the sleep-wake cycle at the adult level. These sleep-related episodes of gonadotropin release are reminiscent of the secretory patterns of other pituitary hormones that fluctuate in characteristic diurnal rhythms. The difference is that sleep-re-

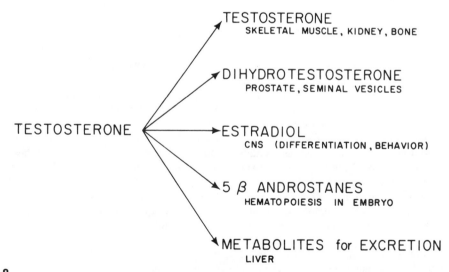

FIG 8–8.
Testosterone and its transformation products. Effects of testosterone on muscle, kidney, and bone may be indirect.

lated GH, ACTH, and PRL (prolactin) secretions persist through adult life, but large nocturnal bursts of gonadotropin secretion do not continue beyond the completion of puberty.

The mechanism for increased gonadotropin secretion at puberty is not understood. The usual explanation is related to a resetting of the gonadostat in the brain so that it becomes less sensitive to feedback inhibition and therefore more capable of sustaining a high output of LHRH in the presence of adult levels of circulating gonadal steroids. The increase in LHRH at puberty is accompanied by both increased sensitivity of gonadotrophes to LHRH and increased sensitivity of the Leydig cells to LH.

Feedback inhibition of gonadotropin secretion occurs at the levels of both the hypothalamus and the pituitary. Inhibition is accomplished by testosterone (via conversion to estradiol in the brain), by estradiol of testicular origin, and by dihydrotestosterone. Dihydrotestosterone decreases the frequency and estradiol decreases the amplitude of GnRH pulses.

LH receptors are up-regulated in the immature testis and down-regulated in the mature testis. On the other hand, estradiol decreases the steroidogenic response to LH in the mature testis but fails to do so in the immature one. Thus, the Leydig cell, like the Sertoli cell, has its own life cycle.

In both sexes, an increase in adrenal androgen secretion occurs about two years before the reactivation of the pituitary-gonad axis. The significance of this event for the onset of puberty is unknown. A summary of the sequence of events at the onset of male puberty is given in Table 8–3.

PITUITARY-GONAD FUNCTION IN AGING MEN

The events surrounding menopause in the female and occasional reports of new paternity in nonagenarian males led to the misconception that gonadal function in males does not deteriorate in the elderly. More recent studies (e.g., Baker et al.) by many observers have indicated that there is a gradual decline in testicular function, which begins some time after age 40 in many men. The changes are less striking than are those seen in women, and variability of both rate and extent of change among individuals is large.

A composite picture constructed from many reports reveals that plasma concentration of total and free testosterone and DHT declines as plasma FSH and LH slowly rise. The carrier protein, SHBG, increases, sometimes resulting in a higher free estrogen to testosterone ratio than that found in younger men. There is an increased FSH response to LHRF, which may indicate a deficiency of inhibin. There may be a slight

TABLE 8–3.

Sequence of Events at Onset of Male Puberty*

1. Decrease in melatonin production by pineal gland.
2. Decreased feedback sensitivity of gonadostat.
3. Increased GnRH secretion: increased amplitude of pulses during deep sleep.
4. Increased pituitary cell sensitivity to GnRH.
5. Increased LH:FSH ratio in response to GnRH.
6. Increased Leydig cell sensitivity to LH: increased testosterone synthesis.
7. Cessation of division, activation of Sertoli cells.
8. Sequential development of testes, pubic hair, penis, deepening of voice timbre, growth spurt.
9. Stimulation of spermatogonial division and production of mature spermatozoa.

*Adapted from Grumbach MM: *Excerpta Med* 1983; 598:3.

decrease in testis size and there is a gradual decline in libido. Although these observations do not warrant the adjective climacteric, they suggest that the male gonad, like the ovary, is susceptible to aging.

Prolactin in the Male

Circulating PRL concentrations in the male are only slightly lower than those in the female. Androgen deficiency results in a decrease in plasma PRL, and androgen replacement restores PRL levels to normal.

By itself, PRL has little apparent effect on the male reproductive apparatus. However, PRL receptors are present on the plasma membrane of Leydig cells, and PRL significantly potentiates the effect of LH on steroidogenesis in Leydig cells. In a strain of dwarf mice that produce little PRL because they lack pituitary acidophils, administration of pure PRL stimulates the production of motile sperm and substantially increases fertility.

Prolactin also has a significant effect on structures of the male reproductive tract, notably the prostate and seminal vesicles. It is believed to act by increasing the molecular population of androgen receptors in those tissues, thus improving the responsiveness of the tissues to androgen.

Hyperprolactinemia, on the other hand, is associated with testicular atrophy and *decreased* circulating testosterone levels in male rats. In men with PRL-producing tumors, an impressive behavioral effect of PRL is observed: these men are impotent in spite of normal circulating levels of testosterone. Removal or suppression of the tumor's secretion with bromocryptine results in restoration of potency. In this connection, PRL has striking behavioral effects in animals, mainly manifested as mothering and nest-building behavior. The implication is that PRL produced by pituitary tumors can reach loci in the brain that are associated with patterns of sex-related behavior.

Androgen Deprivation and Replacement

The physiologic effects of androgen can be appreciated by examining the effects of androgen deprivation, or by observing changes that occur during the transition from boyhood to manhood. Androgens, in addition to their participation in embryogenesis, have prominent effects on *primary* and *secondary sex characteristics;* on the *skeleton, skeletal muscle,* and *fluid balance;* and in the sphere of *behavior.* In all cases a distinction should be made between prepuberal and postpuberal castration, since in the former, both the physiologic and behavioral marks of maleness fail to develop. Postpuberal castration, on the other hand, does not necessarily cause regression of already established androgen-dependent tissue. Behavioral changes will be discussed below.

The primary *sex structures* are the gonads themselves, their associated glands and duct system—in summary, the production and delivery system for male germ cells. All of these components are absolutely dependent on androgen for their growth, development and maintenance. This dependence can be seen best in bioassays for androgen in which the weight of the empty seminal vesicles or ventral prostate can be used as a very precise indicator of the amount of androgenic stimulus that the structure has received. On histologic examination after castration the columnar epithelial cell lining of the seminal vesicle shows a striking shrinking in height and a loss of normal basophilic granulation and cell organelles in the cytoplasm. The nucleolus disappears from the nucleus and there is a generalized loss of much of the enzyme activity associated with the tissue. On androgen replacement the nucleolus becomes very prominent, cell organelles and basophilia reappear and the height of the columnar cells reflects the dose of androgen. The activity of cell-specific enzymes returns to normal. The external genitalia, similarly androgen dependent, fail to develop after prepuberal castration or androgen deficiency but may remain within normal limits following postpuberal castration.

The *secondary sex characteristics* are often far more colorful in some animal species than in man, as Charles Darwin noted more than a century ago. Structures such as deer antlers, rooster head dressing, peacock feather displays, sexual skin of primates, male odor of goats and the distinctive songs of birds are all examples of visual, olfactory, tactile and auditory mechanisms for communication between males and females. It is unnecessary here to belabor the point that, in the case of the human species, communication between male and female is far more complex than are the most colorful courtship rituals in animals. It can involve infinitely graded nuances from a facial expression to Shakespeare's poetry, and it may be profoundly affected by social custom and prevailing cultural patterns.

Androgen deficiency produces marked changes in the texture and distribution of *body hair.* The prepuberal castrate fails to develop facial, axillary or pubic hair and the head hair may remain soft and silky. Postpuberal castration causes slowed growth of the beard and regression and thinning of body hair. Hair distribution and texture is determined largely by inheritance. Certain races of men of undoubted virility and proved procreative capacity lack beards and have minimal body hair. In these cases, since there is obviously no lack of androgen, we must assume that there is a genetically determined, selective failure of hair follicles to respond to androgen. Facial, axillary and pubic hair in females is also androgen dependent.

Common bitemporal baldness is a genetically determined condition as well, but it does not develop in eunuchoid males. Some such individuals who have been hereditarily predisposed to baldness begin to manifest it only after treatment with replacement doses of androgen. This is an instance of the requirement of androgen for *hair loss.* The mechanism of this effect of androgen is unknown.

Androgens have a stimulating effect on *sebaceous glands,* which is evident from the fact that oiliness of the skin appears at puberty and on treatment with androgen. The disease *acne vulgaris,* multiple infections of the sebaceous glands, is not seen in castrate or eunuchoid males or in prepuberal children. It is extremely common in adolescents of both sexes and it may appear in patients who are treated with androgens or with proandrogens such as cortisol. Not uncommonly, acne is seen in menopausal women, who may experience an uneven diminution of androgen and estrogen secretion, with a transitory preponderance of androgen.

Skin pigmentation is affected by availability of androgen. The skin of castrates and eunuchoids is soft, pale yellow and very finely wrinkled, particularly at the corners of the eyes. It does not tan readily on exposure to sunlight, but the ability to tan appears on treatment with androgen.

The *timbre of the voice* is a well-recognized secondary sex characteristic. Androgen administration to the eunuchoid male or to the female results in lowering of the pitch of the voice and in some degree of hoarseness.

The *general metabolic effects* of androgen deficiency and replacement are difficult to separate from those on secondary sex characteristics. For example, the eunuchoid male often shows a typically feminine distribution of subcutaneous fat, particularly in the region of the hips and lower abdomen. Conversely, the virilized female who suffers from diffuse adrenal hyperplasia fails to show this typically feminine distribution of subcutaneous fat. Although there is some doubt that feminine fat distribution of the eunuchoid male is invariably influenced by androgen, there is no doubt whatever that typically feminine fat padding appears in female patients whose adrenal virilism is successfully treated with replacement doses of cortisol (see Chapter 11).

The effects of androgen on *skeletal growth* are complex. Prepuberally androgen-deficient boys are often tall, suggesting failure of epiphyseal closure and overgrowth of long bones. However, the adolescent growth spurt in males is due in part to androgens, which act by stimulating growth hormone synthesis and secretion by the pituitary. Skeletal growth is controlled by a complex array of nutritional, genetic, and hormonal factors, of which androgen availability or excess is one; premature closure of the epiphyses and short stature can result from excessive androgenization prepuberally.

The aggregate *skeletal muscle mass* of castrate and eunuchoid men is smaller than that of normal men, and an increase in muscle strength has occurred on treatment with androgen. As the sculptors of antiquity noted, the muscle markings of the male figure are prominent, whereas those of the feminine figure tend to be obscured by subcutaneous fat. Treatment with androgen, or with inappropriate androgen in the female, accentuates visible muscle contours.

A common denominator of skin, skeletal and muscle effects of androgens may be a *general protein anabolic effect* of these compounds. In many balance experiments, it has been found that androgens cause nitrogen, potassium, and phosphorus retention and an increase in total skeletal muscle mass. The magnitude of such effects is greater on treating castrate or eunuchoid men with androgen than it is when normal males are given androgen.

The discovery of the anabolic effects of androgen stimulated a search for synthetic analogues of androgen that would have a maximum amount of anabolic activity and minimum androgenicity. Some promising compounds have been developed in which the anabolic-androgenic ratio has been markedly altered. For example, certain steroids in the 19-nor series (i.e.,

lacking the methyl group in the 19 position; see Fig 8–7) have an anabolic:androgenic ratio of 20:1 compared with 1:1 for testosterone. Although the 19-nor compounds are less androgenic than testosterone, none has so far failed to exhibit androgenic activity in clinical trials.

There has been no convincing, well-controlled experiment that has demonstrated an enhancing effect of anabolic agents on athletic performance beyond that which can be achieved by training alone. Moreover, there are substantial risks involved in the use of these agents for such purposes. Since they are taken orally, they may cause various kinds of liver damage, including (rarely) liver tumors. The abuse of these substances is widespread in athletes of both sexes, including adolescents. Most medical authorities we respect condemn this practice.

Cellular Mechanism of Action of Androgens

Most work on the cellular mechanism of action of androgens has been done on rat prostate or seminal vesicle and therefore may not be relevant to other tissues in which 5α-DHT is probably *not* testosterone's active intracellular deputy steroid (see Fig 8–8). Although the findings have generally been in harmony with the all-purpose steroid hormone action model presented in Chapter 2, there is still no certainty that all of the stimulatory effects of androgens on prostate or seminal vesicle cells are explicable on the basis of increased gene transcription. Investigators of estrogen's action were fortunate in having available a model system (chick oviduct) in which synthesis of very large amounts of specific proteins (ovalbumin and others) was stimulated by estrogen. No such distinctive marker characterizes androgen's effect on target cells.

What androgen does to a prostate cell can be inferred from Liao's succinct description of what happens in a prostate cell immediately following castration or after androgen deprivation. Nuclear DHT is half gone in a few hours and virtually completely undetectable within 24 hours. Rate of RNA synthesis is half that of control cells by about 18 hours and persists at about 20% of the normal rate for four days and beyond. Both the nuclear RNA polymerase proteins and the DHT-receptor protein persist near control levels for 48 hours, but between the third and fourth days they have decreased to 50% of the control value.

Treatment of the deficient cell with testosterone results in a reversal of these changes. The earliest observable *nuclear* change is DHT accumulation. Increased RNA synthesis occurs in 1 hour. Repletion of polymerase proteins begins soon afterward, and finally restitution of receptor is accomplished. These effects are compatible with the basic steroid hormone action already developed. However, there are suggestions (by Liao) that the hormone may have important effects on initiator transfer RNA-binding activity of prostate cytosol proteins. The latter effect is evident only 10 minutes after androgen administration and it is not eliminated by inhibitors of protein and RNA synthesis. The antiandrogens inhibit this non-nuclear effect.

These interesting findings suggest that when we understand more about steroid hormone action, we will probably discover that stimulation of transcription is part of a coordinated cellular response that involves extranuclear events as well as transcriptional ones.

Genetics and the Pituitary-Testis Axis

Like other endocrine systems, the pituitary-testis axis is involved in a great variety of inborn errors of metabolism. Although some of these may concern the trophic complex in the brain and pituitary, these have not yet been clearly identified. Mutations have been described in (1) the enzymes responsible for steroid hormone biosynthesis and in (2) the response of target organs to stimulation by androgens.

Each of the enzymes listed in Figure 8–5 has been found to be deficient in patients with steroidogenesis defects. Since some of these also participate in synthesis of adrenocortical steroids, the same biochemical deficiency may appear in both glands. A discussion of genetic defects in steroidogenesis will be deferred until Chapter 11.

In addition to the 5α reductase deficiency syndrome (described above to illustrate mechanisms of development of the male generative tract), some related conditions, collectively classified as *testicular feminization syndromes,* have been described both in human beings and in experimental animal models. Although these abnormalities were originally believed to represent a single defect, we now believe them to be expressions of a number of different inborn errors, not unlike those described in Chapters 2 and 3 in connection with response failures to other steroid or peptide hormones. Thus, in some cases, the response failure is attributable either to a *deficiency of a normal receptor* or to the presence of a *receptor with a low affinity for the hormone*. In others, although adequate receptor is present, the *hormone-receptor complex is unable to initiate a biologic response*. The consequences of a 5α reductase deficiency, particularly on development, already have been discussed. These disorders may be either total or partial.

In the complete form in the human being (sometimes called male pseudohermaphroditism), inheritance is X linked and the disorder may be found in several members of the same family, almost always reared as females, although their genotype is XY and they have testes but no internal female generative tract structures. Their external genitalia are unambiguously female, but they lack pubic and axillary hair. Their serum testosterone levels are either normal or supernormal, and they are usually unresponsive to either exogenous testosterone or DHT. They often develop breasts at puberty, presumably because the inhibitory effect of testosterone on the breast anlagen, which is exerted at puberty in normal males, is missing.

An excellent discussion of disorders of sexual development is given by Jaffe.

Spermatogenesis

PARTICIPATING CELLS AND HORMONAL CONTROL

In both male and female, meiosis (halving of the diploid chromosome number) occurs prior to the complete differentiation of spermatozoon and ovum. Meiosis and subsequent pairing of male and female chromosomes at the time of fertilization have the effect of giving each nascent individual a fresh start. Bernstein has suggested in an interesting essay called "Why Babies Are Young" that close pairing of two sets of chromosomes may allow the chromosomes to assume a configuration that establishes especially favorable conditions for excision and repair of DNA. According to the cumulative DNA damage hypothesis of aging, the pristine DNA of the fertilized ovum must be as error-free as it will ever be.

The overall process of gametogenesis in the male is called spermatogenesis. The process of *spermiogenesis* begins with the spermatid stage (22 X or 22 Y); the process is characterized not only by the absence of cell division but, except for its early stages, by an absence of RNA synthesis as well. The many striking morphologic and biochemical changes that occur in developing spermatids are evidently accomplished by the turning on and off of the translation of prepackaged, long-lived mRNAs in a sequential program.

The complementary process of *oogenesis* occurs in the female. The mathematics of gametogenesis in the two sexes is an interesting lesson in statistical probability. In the human female 800,000 primitive germ cells are present in the embryonic ovary, but in a reproductive life of about 35–40 years, only 350–400 of these will mature into competent ova. In contrast, in the male, assuming a duration of sexual maturity of 60 years, the order of magnitude of germ cell production might be 30,000,000 per day! The discrepancy in production rate must be related to the fact that the ovulated ovum is escorted to the site of fertilization in the fallopian tube. Of the 2–300,000,000 or so spermatozoa in an average ejaculate, only 100 may reach the fallopian tube. The apparent redundancy of male gamete production is simply an expression of the odds that a spermatozoon will reach an ovum when an ejaculate is deposited in the female generative tract.

Our insight into the process of spermatogenesis has been enormously enriched by investigators, most notably Clermont and Fawcett, who have used a battery of morphologic approaches. Clermont used mainly histologic and autoradiologic methods at the level of the light microscope, whereas Fawcett has illuminated this difficult field with the electron microscope. It is beyond our competence to present a detailed morphologic account of spermatogenesis. The student who is not familiar with the work of Clermont and of Fawcett is urged to review their elegant studies.

The main lesson of these advances has been emphasized mainly by Fawcett, i.e., that the isolation and study of individual cellular elements of the seminiferous tubule does not begin to suggest the extraordinarily complex exchange of information that occurs among them and with the interstitial cells of Leydig. Although we do not yet understand all of the subtle cross-talk that goes on among these cells, their architectural arrangements are evidently part of the overall control mechanisms that operate to initiate and sustain sperm production. There are five main categories of cell involved in spermatogenesis and sperm transport and maturation: (1) Leydig cell, (2) myoepithelial cell, (3) Sertoli cell, (4) developing germ cells and

(5) epithelial cells of the efferent duct system. Each member of this federation has direct or indirect effects on the function of others. Cells of the various types communicate with each other either by secreting chemical messengers or by cell–cell interaction. We know very little about the mechanisms of cell–cell interaction, but we have already seen an example of it in the induction of tubular organization in the embryonic testis by the H-Y antigen. We suspect that it may occur by way of surface glycoproteins. The organization and cooperation of these cells result in a whole that is clearly greater than the sum of its parts.

In Figure 8–9, an attempt is made to summarize a vast amount of experimental data. Although this cryptic depiction is obviously an oversimplification, it describes many well-documented features of spermatogenesis. A cartoon of the relationships of Sertoli cells to developing germ cells is shown in Figure 8–10.

The *interstitial cell of Leydig* has a complicated life history of its own within the life cycle of the individual. It is large and active in the late embryo, in early neonatal life and during the infantile testosterone surge. It then becomes quiescent until puberty, when it is stimulated by LH to produce testosterone from stored cholesterol. It has LH receptors but no FSH receptors. However, it is now known that FSH treatment of an immature animal increases the number of LH receptors on the Leydig cell plasma membrane and increases the sensitivity of the Leydig cell to LH stimulation. This is probably an indirect effect of FSH (via Sertoli cell?), but the mechanism is unknown.

The high concentration of testosterone produced at the base of the seminiferous tubules is essential for spermatogenesis. If gonadotropin secretion is suppressed by exogenous testosterone, the Leydig cells atrophy and spermatogenesis ceases in spite of the fact that the exogenous testosterone is sufficient to maintain secondary sex characteristics and libido. (*High*

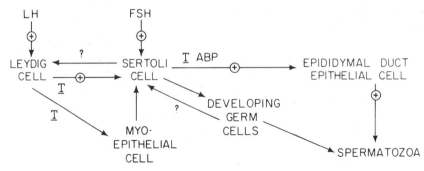

FIG 8–9.
Hormonal control of spermatogenesis and sperm maturation. *ABP* = androgen-binding protein. (With help from I. Fritz.)

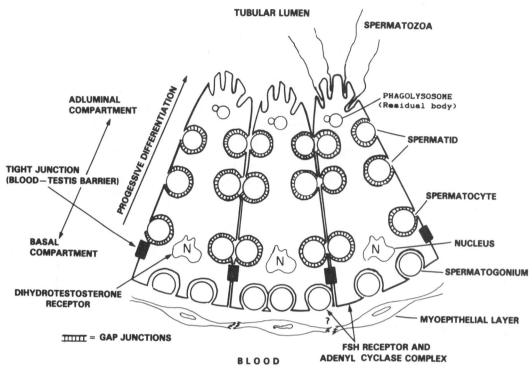

FIG 8–10.
Relationship of Sertoli cells with developing germ cells.

doses of testosterone can *maintain* established spermatogenesis without FSH.) As we have seen, LH stimulation involves the cAMP response system, not necessarily by measurably increasing cAMP concentration.

The *Sertoli cell*, like the ovarian *granulosa cell*, is of mesenchymal origin. Each of these remarkable cells has a life cycle of its own within the embryonic, immature, and mature phases of the life cycle of the individual. There are many similarities between the two cells (among them, FSH responsiveness, steroid hormone responsiveness, aromatase activity stimulated by FSH, inhibin or folliculostatin synthesis, etc.), but there are also significant differences (see Fritz). They are united in our imagination because each, in its own way, has the main function of maintaining a highly specialized microenvironment in which its germ cells can develop.

The changing roles of the Sertoli cell begin with the formation of the primitive testis, when pre-Sertoli cells, which recognize each other by their surface display of H-Y antigen, assemble to form the spermatic cords. In the *embryo*, the Sertoli cell synthesizes and secretes müllerian inhibiting factor or hormone, a paracrine signal. The fact that the hormone works by local diffusion is underscored by the observation that,

in individuals in whom a testis develops on only one side, there is persistence of the müllerian duct on the contralateral side.

In the *immature* animal or person, Sertoli cells proliferate and have the capacity to synthesize estradiol from testosterone via the aromatase reaction. FSH increases cyclic AMP only in immature rats. The failure of the Sertoli cell in the adult to respond to FSH with an increase in cyclic AMP is due neither to an increase in phosphodiesterase nor to a decrease in FSH receptors. The suggestion has been made that the cyclic AMP response does not occur in an environment of developing germ cells.

In adults there is no Sertoli cell proliferation but a new set of capabilities is acquired:

1. Androgen-binding protein synthesis in response either to FSH or testosterone (the androgen-binding protein is immunologically related to, but not identical with, TeBG: see below);

2. The ability to secrete a potassium and bicarbonate-rich fluid into the lumen;

3. Inhibin synthesis and secretion;

4. Synthesis of *Seminiferous Growth Factor* (SGF), which is different from all other known growth factors (Bellvé);

5. The capacity to phagocytose residual bodies, the debris of spermatogenesis; and

6. The establishment and maintenance of the blood:testis barrier which consists of tight junctions between adjacent Sertoli cells.

The lumina of the seminiferous tubules and the duct system that must be traversed by the spermatozoon on its way to the ejaculatory duct are operationally outside the body in the same sense that the contents of the gastrointestinal and urinary tracts are outside the body. The effects of sealing off the adluminal compartment by Sertoli-Sertoli tight junctions are to maintain a potassium-bicarbonate-rich microenvironment within the tubule that has little resemblance to a sodium-rich ultrafiltrate of plasma, and to protect the developing germ cells from potentially toxic materials in blood. But, in addition to sealing off the intratubular environment, the barrier also prevents egress of the contents of the tubule back into the blood. For spermatozoa carry surface antigens that are classified as ''not-self'' by the individual who carries them. When the barrier becomes permeable, as in men who have undergone vasectomy for the purpose of contraception, antisperm antibodies are commonly produced (see Lepow).

The Sertoli cell is unusual in the fact that it is a target cell (i.e., it contains specific receptors) for both a glycoprotein hormone, FSH, and a steroid, testosterone. Both of these hormones are essential for spermatogenesis but they need not be present at the same time for spermatogenesis to be sustained. If FSH is removed by hypophysectomy, spermatogenesis can be sustained by large doses of testosterone if testosterone is given immediately. If the testis is permitted to regress after hypophysectomy, FSH is required to reinstitute spermatogenesis. Evidently, FSH priming is essential in order to make the Sertoli cell responsive to androgen. Two of the most prominent effects of FSH priming in the regressed testis are (1) stimulation of the formation of tight junctions and (2) inhibition of spermatogonium degeneration, a process that occurs continuously in the basal compartment (Means).

Whether spermatogonia, which exist in the basal compartment on the blood side of the blood-testis barrier, respond directly to FSH is uncertain. Steinberger, Orth, and their colleagues have described FSH binding to spermatogonia. Moreover, gap junctions, which occur between developing germ cells and Sertoli cells in the adluminal compartment, do not occur between Sertoli cells and spermatogonia in the basal compartment. Means' finding that FSH causes an increase in spermatogonia number by decreasing their rate of disappearance certainly suggests the possibility

that FSH may have a direct effect on the most primitive germ cells.

When a clone of spermatogonia is selected for spermatocyte development instead of oblivion, the primitive gametes are ushered from the basal compartment into the adluminal compartment by an amazing process: two adjacent Sertoli cells obligingly dissolve the tight junction that blocks the entry of the spermatogonium into the adluminal zone and immediately re-form another tight junction under it. The molecular mechanisms involved in this maneuver are unknown, but the Sertoli cell is known to synthesize and secrete at least two proteolytic enzymes that may participate in the dissolution of the original tight junction barrier.

Once within the luminal compartment, clones of cells, connected by intercellular bridges, synchronously follow their developmental program, always in the embrace of Sertoli cell processes. When the completed spermatozoa are released, the Sertoli cell functions as a phagocytic scavenger of residual bodies, materials left over after the individual gametes are released into the lumen.

Some features of Sertoli cell structure are suggested in Figure 8–10. One of the effects of FSH on the Sertoli cell is to stimulate the production of a special protein known as ABP (androgen-binding protein). This is a carrier protein that binds testosterone and DHT with high affinity and whose synthesis and secretion are also stimulated by testosterone. (Although ABP may be similar to SHBG found in the plasma, it is distinguished from that protein both immunologically and with respect to its steroid hormone-binding profile.) Thus, the Sertoli cell responds to FSH (or to cAMP or to cholera toxin) by making ABP and responds to testosterone, presumably by the prototypical steroid hormone mechanism, by making the same protein. Simultaneous stimulation by both hormones results in more ABP production than stimulation by either alone. The presence of ABP in the intraluminal fluid insures a high concentration of androgen in that fluid, about that of testicular venous blood. Although the role of this androgen is not entirely clear, it is presumed to be required for maintenance of highly specialized endothelial cells that line the duct system, especially those in the epididymis (see below).

Although the importance of FSH- and androgen-stimulated Sertoli cells for spermatogenesis is well recognized, there is a possibility that the presence of developing germ cells may influence the function of the Sertoli cell. In Sertoli cell-only testes, which may be produced either by subjecting testes to the relatively high temperature of the abdominal cavity or by destruction of gametes by radiation (see below), the circulating levels of FSH are high. This has been attributed to a lack of the FSH secretion inhibitor *inhibin*. Since the source of inhibin is said to be the Sertoli cell, we can only conclude that, when germ cells are properly developing in the tubule, the Sertoli cells secrete inhibin, which regulates FSH secretion. When germ cells are missing, there is a failure of inhibin production and FSH secretion is unrestrained.

The *myoepithelial cell* (see Fig 8–10) has relationships with both the Leydig cell and Sertoli cell. It is absolutely dependent on androgen for its differentiation and maintenance, and its anatomical juxtaposition to the Leydig cell insures a high local concentration of androgen. The suspicion that it may be functionally related to the Sertoli cell is based on the observation (see Fritz) that Sertoli cells grown in tissue culture survive for a relatively short time. However, if they are plated on an underlying layer of myoepithelial cells, they grow very well for a long time. Fibroblasts or other mammalian cells cannot substitute for myoepithelial cells in this circumstance.

EFFECTS OF PHYSICAL AGENTS AND DRUGS ON SPERMATOGENESIS (Figure 8–11)

Heat

The close approximation of the major artery and vein supplying the testis results in a countercurrent transfer of heat from artery to vein. This causes the temperature of the contents of the scrotal sac to be lower than intra-abdominal temperature. If the testis of an experimental animal is imprisoned in the abdominal cavity by a ligature, or if a human testis fails to descend into the scrotum, the condition of cryptorchidism exists. In this circumstance, most of the germinal elements in the tubule disappear, leaving only surviving Sertoli cells. These cells are now known to be functionally damaged by exposure to intra-abdominal temperature.

The vulnerability of developing germ cells at intra-abdominal temperature is due to the fact that spermatocytes and spermatids have lysosomes that are much more labile at 37 C than are those of either

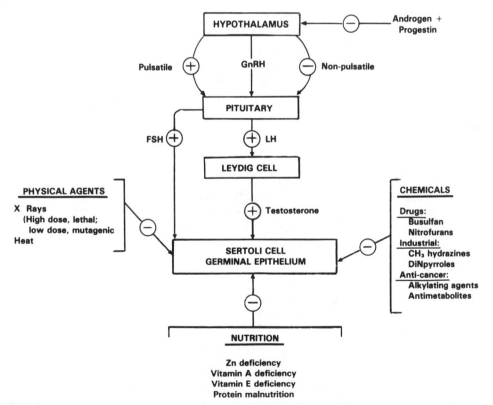

FIG 8–11.
Summary of effects of physical agents, chemicals, and certain nutritional deficiencies on gametogenesis in the male.

Sertoli cells or liver cells. The release of lysosomal enzymes is the apparent cause of the regression of germinal elements.

X-irradiation

X-irradiation has two different but mechanistically related effects on male germ cells. At high doses, radiation can kill spermatogonia by generating free radicals in cells. These highly reactive species can interact with the genetic material and with other macromolecules and destroy cells, particularly rapidly dividing ones. The testis shares vulnerability to radiation damage with other rapidly proliferating cells such as intestinal epithelial cells and bone marrow stem cells.

In lower doses, radiation can cause mutations by a similar mechanism. This is of some practical importance in the field of diagnostic radiology. Lead shielding of gonads to prevent their exposure to x-ray is routinely done.

Drugs and Toxins

Many drugs and toxins have been shown to have a deleterious effect on spermatogenesis, and many of these have been examined for their potential usefulness as male contraceptives. In general they have proved highly toxic and, in some cases (nitrogen mustard), mutagenic. Busulphans and methylhydrazines generally inhibit at the spermatogonium replication phase of the process, i.e., before reduction division. Dinitropyrroles inhibit early spermatid development. The antimetabolite, 6-azauracil, and the nitrofurans inhibit indiscriminately over the whole cycle. The antiandrogens inhibit both at the early spermatogonium stage and at reduction division, but such compounds are of no use as male contraceptives, since they decrease libido and interfere with maintenance of secondary sex characteristics.

The most promising chemical approach to male contraception has been the use of testosterone-progestogen combinations, which inhibit gonadotropin secretion and thus result in Leydig cell atrophy while supplying adequate replacement concentrations of testosterone. This method has not had widespread trial.

The second most extensively used method of contraception in the male (after the condom) is vasectomy, which involves segmental removal of a small portion of the vas deferens. Although this method effectively eliminates spermatozoa from the ejaculate after 90–120 days, it was regarded as practically irreversible. However, recent reports suggest that reestablishment of continuity of the vas by microsurgery is feasible in many individuals.

Intraductile Sperm Maturation and Capacitation

The newly released spermatozoon is nonmotile, incapable of fertilization and generally immature. Its development continues as it travels via the tubuli recti to the rete testis → efferent ducts → epididymal ducts → vas deferens → ejaculatory duct. The immature, immotile germ cells are carried through the duct system largely by the contractile energy generated by *myoepithelial cells* that embrace the tubules. These are noninnervated, androgen-dependent smooth muscle cells, which have an inherent rhythmicity. Although they are stimulatable by oxytocin, little information is available on the subject of their physiologic control mechanisms. Some of the epithelial cells lining the duct system are ciliated and probably participate in propulsion of duct contents.

The most striking changes—morphologic, physiologic and biochemical—are seen when spermatozoa entering the epididymal duct system are compared with those leaving it. The cells linking this duct system perform both secretory and absorptive functions and are utterly androgen dependent. The androgen concentration of rete testis fluid is about 15 times that of peripheral venous blood, or about the same as spermatic vein blood. Thus, the duct system, largely through the agency of ABP, is exposed to very high androgen concentrations.

The processing of spermatozoa that occurs during transit through the epididymal duct system has been studied most successfully in the bull (see Hoskins et al.). When the proximal caput (nearest the testis) is sampled, spermatozoa are nonmotile. By the time they have reached the cauda (at the vas deferens end), they are capable of *linear mobility*. One stage toward the development of linear mobility is a sort of aimless, circular swimming movement. Associated morphologic changes in the sperm may be seen by both light and electron microscopy. Linear, or forward mobility, is essential for the successful completion of spermatozoon function in the female generative tract.

Forward mobility is associated with at least two conditions: (1) an increase in cAMP content of spermatozoa and (2) the presence of a specific protein (partially purified), which has been called forward mobility protein (FMP). The ingenious assay for FMP is based on the fact that a time exposure of a moving sperm produces a linear streak on Polaroid film reminiscent of the physicist's photographs of subatomic particles. FMPs are glycoproteins, which may exist in different states of aggregation, and are found throughout the duct system. If nonmotile spermatozoa are treated with active FMP when cAMP concentration of the sperm is low, no stimulation of forward motility occurs. The glycoprotein is believed to act by attaching to the membrane of the sperm in an unspecified location. Although changes in cAMP during transit of the epididymal duct system have been well documented, the mechanism by which the change is accomplished is presently unknown.

SPERM CAPACITATION

In 1951, Austin and Chang discovered that spermatozoa acquired the capacity to fertilize ova only after a minimum period of residence in the female tract. The event or events that had to occur during this time in order to transform the spermatozoa from incompetent to competent were called "capacitation." The process was studied intensively in rats, mice, hamsters, and rabbits over a period of decades, mostly with epididymal sperm, but until recently, there was disagreement about whether or not the phenomenon occurs in humans. Now, however, there is universal acceptance of the fact that it does.

The acrosome is a highly specialized lysosomal sac that is interposed under the plasma membrane between the forward tip of the spermatozoon and its nucleus. It contains a variety of enzymes capable of degrading macromolecules, and it is essential for these enzymes to be released in the vicinity of the ovum before sperm-ovum fusion, and therefore fertilization can occur. The escape of the contents of the acrosomal sac and the exposure of the posterior acrosomal membrane is called the *acrosomal reaction*.

Capacitation consists of at least two components: (1) preparation of the spermatozoon for the acrosomal reaction and (2) increased flagellar activity (hyperactivity). The second of these has, so far, been observed only in laboratory animals.

Until recently, it was difficult to devise appropriate assay methods for the study of capacitation in human sperm, but the discovery of the fact that hamster eggs stripped of their *zona pellucida* were able to incorporate heterologous spermatozoa made the development of such an assay possible.

Although the molecular details of the process of capacitation are not yet known in detail, it is interesting to contemplate current ideas of investigators in this field and see how closely these ideas resemble those we have previously discussed as mechanisms of action of hormones on their sensitive cells. In the first place, seminal fluid contains something that *inhibits* the ability of previously capacitated sperm to fertilize ova, so the first step in capacitation is the removal of such inhibitory materials. Although surface alterations in the spermatozoa must be important, intrinsic plasma membrane proteins as well as phospholipids are modified during the capacitation process. The net result of these dimly understood membrane modifications is an increased intracellular Ca^{2+} concentration. This is essential for the fusion and fragmentation of the anterior plasma membrane and the outer acrosomal membrane. It is this event that permits the release of acrosomal enzymes and exposes the inner acrosomal membrane at the anterior end of the spermatozoon. The Ca^{2+} influx is also responsible for putting the sperm's flagellar motor into high gear. Cyclic AMP may also play a role in the acrosomal reaction, since many features of the reaction can be induced by cAMP analogues and by phosphodiesterase inhibitors.

The conclusion is inescapable that nature has invented a comparatively small number of strategies for disseminating information intracellularly and that these are integrated into the responses of many different kinds of cells in distinctive ways. Ca^{2+} is no less essential for the acrosomal reaction and flagellar stimulation than it is for secretory processes and muscle contraction.

Androgens and Sexual Behavior

The earliest recorded observation linking a product of the testis to behavior was made in castrated chickens in 1949 by Berthold who observed a lack of sexual interest in hens and a renewal of such interest in castrated cockerels treated with intra-abdominal implants of single testes. The subject of androgens and behavior has been studied extensively, mostly in experimental animals.

In some species (e.g., the rat), sexual behavior is stereotyped and quantifiable. When prepuberal rats (or other species) are castrated, sexual behavior does not appear. When adult male rats are castrated, mating behavior is lost in a predictable sequence: (1) ejaculatory behavior, (2) intromission, (3) finally, mounting behavior. There is a variable time lag in every species studied: it may vary from weeks to months and even (in the human) years. In other words, the gradual loss of sexual behavior following castration occurs long after testosterone has disappeared from the blood. In other experiments it has been shown that adrenal androgens make no important contribution to the sustaining of sexual behavior after castration in the male.

Sexual behavior may be restored by treating the castrate with androgen, but higher doses of testosterone are required for restoration of sexual behavior than are required for restoration of prostate or seminal vesicle weight. This has been interpreted as a loss of sensitivity by the CNS target tissue involved in re-initiating sexual behavior. On the other hand, the blood levels of testosterone necessary to *maintain* normal sexual behavior after castration are much less than those found in normal male animals of the same age. Thus, from a behavioral point of view, a considerable safety factor is built into the normal level of circulating testosterone. In this connection, studies in men have revealed no consistent relationships between circulating testosterone levels and sexual activity, as evaluated by questionnaire techniques.

Although there is evidence that testosterone facilitates spinal reflexes associated with copulation, the major site of action of testosterone on behavior is in the anterior hypothalamic preoptic area (AHPO). This statement is based on experiments in which crystalline testosterone implants were made in various parts of the hypothalamus in castrate rats and the behavioral effects noted. Although some behavior restoration was achieved with posterior hypothalamic implants (near the mamillary body), the most consistent results were obtained with AHPO implants. Testosterone implants elsewhere in the brain do not restore normal sexual behavior, and the results are *not* due to systemic absorption of androgen, since blood levels following negative intracerebral implants were higher than those after hypothalamic implants.

It is now generally agreed that testosterone repairs behavioral deficits by conversion to estradiol in the involved neurons. Estrogens or DHT alone are ineffective in restoring normal sexual behavior in castrates but the combination of estrogen plus DHT is as effective as testosterone alone.

Results of a study of several hundred men legally castrated in Norway generally conform to those of work on rats. The most striking difference was the extreme variability of the lag period in the loss of libido and potency following the operation. In some men, the loss occurred very soon, whereas other individuals continued to have sexual intercourse for years.

The relationship between androgen, or androgen deficiency, and male homosexuality is under continuing discussion. There are two general theories concerning the origin of homosexuality: (1) temporary androgen deficiency during sexual differentiation and development of the brain may result in homosexual orientation; and (2) sexual preference is determined postnatally by psychosocial learning and experience. This is the old nature-nurture argument, and each side has its articulate proponents. There need not be an either-or decision in favor of either side. Human sexual behavior, including object preference, is so complex that it would be an oversimplification to attribute it to any single determinant.

Arguments in support of a contributory endocrine factor in the origin of male homosexuality have been marshalled by Dörner and his colleagues. On the basis of plasma FSH, LH, and testosterone levels, he has observed statistically significant (but always overlapping) differences among three groups: heterosexuals, noneffeminized homosexuals, and effeminized homosexuals. The inference is that variable degrees of androgen deficiency during the critical time window of brain differentiation may produce different degrees of changed behavior, but this is obviously an impossible theory to prove retrospectively. One of the most interesting findings (shared by Gladue et al.) is the difference in response of serum LH to injected estrogen in effeminized male homosexuals as compared with that in heterosexual males. In the female, injected estradiol first depresses and then positively feeds back to result in a higher-than-baseline level of LH. In the heterosexual male, LH stays well below the baseline throughout the period of observation. Positive feedback responses to injected estradiol were observed in effeminized homosexual males, who showed final LH concentrations intermediate between those of females and male heterosexuals.

There can be little doubt that nurture, as well as nature, has an effect on sexual orientation (see Erhardt, for example). Environmental, social, and cultural experiences obviously contribute importantly to sexual behavior of heterosexual people of both sexes, and there is no reason to doubt that they do so in homosexual individuals as well. In most nature-nurture controversies in the past (the etiology of obesity is a good example), protagonists on both sides turned out to be partly right.

There are suggestions that behavioral or situational events may work in the opposite direction, i.e., they may stimulate or inhibit GnRH release and thus alter the level of circulating testosterone. There is one often-cited study (Anon., see Bibliography) in which an increased rate of beard growth was observed by a man in *anticipation* of sexual activity. Similarly, in studies in monkeys a young male subjected to punishment by a dominant male was shown to have a striking decrease in serum testosterone. The level returned to normal when he was put into a cage with females. Decrease in gonadotropin output in psychologically stressed monkeys has been well described by Mason. Generally these effects have been more extensively studied in females than in males.

The student who wishes to learn more about this interesting subject is referred to the writings of Beach and Davidson (also see Bermant and Davidson), and the Goy-McEwen monograph.

BIBLIOGRAPHY

Anonymous: Effects of sexual activity on beard growth in man. *Nature* 1970; 226:869.

Arbatti MJ, Seidah NE, Rochemont J, et al: β_2 inhibin contains the active core of human seminal plasma β inhibin: Synthesis and bioactivity. *FEBS Lett* 1985; 181:57.

Baker HWG, Bremner WJ, Burger HG, et al: Testicular control of follicle-stimulating hormone secretion. *Recent Prog Horm Res* 1976; 32:429.

Baker HWG, Burger HG, de Kretser DM, et al: Changes in the pituitary-testicular system with age. *Clin Endocrinol* 1976; 5:349.

Bardin CW, Bullock LP, Sherins RJ, et al: Androgen metabolism and mechanism of action in male pseudohermaphroditism: A study of testicular feminization. *Recent Prog Horm Res* 1973; 29:65.

Bardin CW: Pituitary-testicular axis, in Yen SSC, Jaffe RB (eds): *Reproductive Endocrinology.* Philadelphia, WB Saunders Co, 1978.

Bartke A: Prolactin and the physiological regulation of the mammalian testis, in Troen P, Nankin H (eds): *The Testis in Normal and Infertile Men.* New York, Raven Press, 1977.

Beach FA: Behavioral Endocrinology: An emerging discipline. *Am Sci* 1975; 63:178.

Bellvé AR, Feig LA: Cell proliferation in the mammalian testis: Biology of the seminiferous growth factor (SGF). *Recent Prog Horm Res* 1984; 40:531.

Bermant G, Davidson JM: *Biological Bases of Sexual Behavior.* New York, Harper & Row, 1974.

Bernstein C: Why are babies young? Meiosis may prevent aging of the germ line. *Perspect Biol Med* 1979; 22:539.

Burger H, de Kretser D (eds): *The Testis.* New York, Raven Press, 1981.

Catt KJ, Dufau ML (eds): Hormone action and testicular function (Symposium, 107 papers). *Ann NY Acad Sci* 1985.

Channing CP, Gordon WL, Liu W-K, et al: Physiology and biochemistry of ovarian inhibin. *Proc Soc Exp Biol Med* 1985; 178:339.

Cheng CY, Frick J, Gunsalus GL, et al: Human testicular binding protein shares immunodeterminants with serum testosterone estradiol-binding globulin. *Endocrinology* 1984; 114:1395.

Clermont Y: Kinetics of spermatogenesis in mammals: Seminiferous epithelium cycle and spermatogonial renewal. *Physiol Rev* 1972; 52:198.

Decker GL, Joseph DB, Lennarz WJ: A study of factors involved in induction of the acrosomal reaction in sperm of the sea urchin. *Arbacia Punctulata. Dev Biol* 1976; 53:115.

de Kretser DM, Burger HG, Hudson B (eds): *The Pituitary and Testis.* New York, Springer-Verlag New York, 1983.

Donohoe PK, Hutson JM, Fallat ME, et al: Mechanism of action of müllerian inhibiting substance. *Ann Rev Physiol* 1984; 46:53.

Dörner G, Rohde W, Stahl F, et al: A neuroendocrine predisposition for homosexuality in men. *Arch Sex Behav* 1975; 4:1.

Dufau ML, Tsuruhara T, Horner KA, et al: Intermediate role of adenosine $3':5'$ cyclic monophosphate and protein kinase during gonadotropin-induced steroidogenesis in testicular interstitial cells. *Proc Natl Acad Sci USA* 1977; 74:3419.

Edwards RG: Current status of human conception in vitro. *Proc R Soc Lond (Biol)* 1985; 233:417.

Epel D: The program of fertilization. *Sci Am* 1977; 237:128.

Erhardt AA: Prenatal androgenization and human psychosexual behavior, in Money J, Musaph H (eds): *Handbook of Sexology.* Amsterdam, Excerpta Medica, 1977.

Ewing LL, Robaire B: Endogenous antispermatogenic agents: Prospects for male contraception. *Ann Rev Pharmacol Toxicol* 1978; 18:167.

Ewing LL, Zirkin B: Leydig cell structure and function. *Recent Prog Horm Res* 1983; 39:599.

Fawcett DW: The cell biology of gametogenesis in the male. *Perspect Biol Med* 1979; 22:556.

Forest MG: Role of androgens in fetal and puberal development. *Horm Res* 1983; 18:69.

Franchimont P, Verstraelen-Proyard J, Hazee-Hagelstein MT, et al: Inhibin: From concept to reality. *Vitam Horm* 1979; 37:243.

Fritz IB, Rommerts FG, Louis BG, et al: Regulation by FSH and dibutyryl cyclic AMP of the formation of androgen-binding protein in Sertoli cell-enriched cultures. *J Reprod Fertil* 1976; 46:17.

Fritz IB: Sites of action of androgen and follicle-stimulating hormone on cells of the seminiferous tubule, in Litwack G (ed): *Biochemical Actions of Hormones,* vol 5. New York, Academic Press, 1978, pp 249–281.

Fritz IB: Comparison of granulosa and Sertoli cells at various stages of maturation: Similarities and differences. *Adv Exp Med Biol* 1982; 147:357.

Gerald PS: Sex chromosome disorders. *N Engl J Med* 1976; 294:706.

Glabe CG, Vaquier VC: Egg surface glycoprotein receptor for sea urchin sperm bindin. *Proc Natl Acad Sci USA* 1978; 75:881.

Gladue BA, Green R, Hellman RE: Neuroendocrine response to estrogen and sexual orientation. *Science* 1984; 225:1496.

Goy RW, Phoenix CH: The effects of testosterone propionate administered before birth on the development of behavior in genetic female rhesus monkeys, in Sawyer CH, Gorski RA (eds): *Steroid Hormones and Brain Function.* Berkeley, University of California Press, 1971, pp 192–202.

Goy RW, McEwen BS (eds): *Sexual Differentiation of the Brain.* Cambridge, Massachusetts, The MIT Press, 1980.

Griffin JE, Wilson JD: The testes, in Wilson JD, Foster DW (eds): *Williams Textbook of Endocrinology,* ed 7. Philadelphia, WB Saunders Co, 1985.

Grumbach MW, Conte FA: Disorders of sex differentiation, in Williams RH (ed): *Textbook of Endocrinology,* ed 6. Philadelphia, WB Saunders Co, 1981, pp 422–505.

Grumbach MM: Control of onset of puberty. *Excerpta Med ICS* 1983; 598:3.

Hoskins DD, Brandt H, Acott TS: Initiation of sperm motility in the mammalian epididymis. *Fed Proc* 1978; 37:2534.

Huhtaniemi IT, Warren DW, Catt KJ: Functional maturation of the rat testis Leydig cell. *Ann NY Acad Sci* 1984; 438:283.

Lepow IH, Crozier R (eds): *Vasectomy: Immunologic and pathophysiologic effects in animals and man.* New York, Academic Press, 1979.

Liao S, Chang C, Salzman AG: Androgen-receptor interaction—an overview, in Eriksson H, Gustafsson J-A (eds):

Steroid Hormone Receptors: Structure and Function (Nobel Symposium No 57). New York, Elsevier North-Holland, Inc, 1983, pp 407–418.

Lipsett MB: Physiology and pathology of the Leydig cell. *N Engl J Med* 1980; 303:682.

Mainwaring WIP: The mechanism of action of androgens. *Monogr Endocrinol* 1976; 10:1.

Mann T, Lutwak-Mann C: *Male Reproductive Function and Semen.* New York, Springer-Verlag New York, 1981.

Ohno S: The role of H-Y antigen in primary sex determination. *JAMA* 1978; 239:217.

Ojeda SR, Andrews WW, Advis JP, et al: Recent advances in the endocrinology of puberty. *Endocr Rev* 1980; 1:228.

Orth WD, Christensen AK: Autoradiographic localization of specifically bound ^{125}I-labelled follicle-stimulating hormone on spermatogonia of the rat testis. *Endocrinology* 1978; 103:1944.

Orth JM: The role of follicle-stimulating hormone in controlling Sertoli cell proliferation in testes of fetal rats. *Endocrinology* 1984; 115:1248.

Parker MW, Johanson AJ, Rogol AD, et al: Effect of testosterone on somatomedin C concentrations in pubertal boys. *J Clin Endocrinol Metab* 1984; 58:87.

Parvinen M: Regulation of the seminiferous epithelium. *Endocr Rev* 1982; 3:404.

Peterson RE, Imperato-McGinley J, Gautier T, et al: Male pseudohermaphroditism due to steroid reductase deficiency. *Am J Med* 1977; 62:170.

Plant TM, Dubey AK: Evidence from the rhesus monkey (Macacca mulatta) for the view that negative feedback control of luteinizing hormone secretion by the testis is mediated by deceleration of hypothalamic gonadotropin-releasing hormone pulse frequency. *Endocrinology* 1984; 115:2145.

Raisman G, Field PM: Sexual dimorphism in the neuropil of the preoptic area of the rat and its dependence on neonatal androgen. *Brain Res* 1973; 54:1.

Roy AK, Chatterjee B, Demyan WF: Hormone and age-dependent regulation of $_{2\mu}$-globulin gene expression. *Recent Prog Horm Res* 1983; 29:425.

Ryan AJ: Anabolic steroids are fool's gold. *Fed Proc* 1981; 40:2682.

Schmell E, Earles BJ, Breaux C, et al: Identification of a sperm receptor on the surface of the eggs of the sea urchin *Arbacia punctuluata. J Cell Biol* 1977; 72:35.

Schrag SD, Dixon RL: Occupational exposures associated with male reproductive dysfunction. *Ann Rev Pharmacol Toxicol* 1985; 25:567.

Snyder PJ: Clinical uses of androgens. *Ann Rev Med* 1984; 35:207.

Steinhardt RA, Epel D: Fertilization of sea urchin eggs by a calcium ionophore. *Proc Natl Acad Sci USA* 1974; 71:1915.

Troen P, Nankin H (eds): *The Testis in Normal and Infertile Men.* New York, Raven Press, 1977.

Vermeulen A: Androgen secretion after age 50 in both sexes. *Horm Res* 1983; 18:37.

Wachtel SS: H-Y antigen and the genetics of sex determination. *Science* 1977; 198:797.

Wilson JD: Sexual differentiation. *Ann Rev Physiol* 1978; 40:279.

Wolf DP, Quigley MM (eds): *Human in Vitro Fertilization and Embryo Transfer.* New York, Plenum Publishing Corp, 1984.

9

The Female

DATE		INVESTIGATOR(S)
1672	Ovarian follicles, corpus luteum	de Graaf
1896	First experimental demonstration of ovarian activity	Knauer
1896	Origin of corpus luteum described	Sobotta
1897	Relationship between corpus luteum and pregnancy suggested	Beard
1900	Prevention of uterine atrophy and loss of sexual function by ovarian grafts in castrate animals	Knauer
1903	Interruption of early pregnancy by corpus luteum removal in rabbits	Fraenkel
1905	Concept of endocrine function of placenta introduced	Halban
1910	First demonstration of endocrine activity of corpus luteum	Ancel and Bouin
1912	Gonadal atrophy posthypophysectomy	Aschner
1927	Chorionic gonadotropin in urine of pregnant women	Ascheim, Zondek
1928	Prolactin discovered	Stricker and Grüter
1919–1930	Isolation of crystalline estrogen by three independent groups	Doisy; Butenandt; Marrian
1918–1930	Purification and bioassay of luteal extracts; prevention of abortion after ovariectomy in early pregnancy in rabbits	Corner and Allen
1932	Structure of estrone and estriol	Marrian; Butenandt
	Structure of progesterone	Butenandt
1932	Feedback control of pituitary gonadotropin output suggested	Moore and Price
1932	Participation of CNS in feedback control of gonadotropins suggested	Hohlweg, Junkmann
1935	Isolation of estradiol 17β	Doisy et al.
1936	Discovery of synthetic estrogens (stilbenes)	Dodds

Like the testis, the ovary is a compound organ with a dual function: production and release of ova and production of certain hormones, steroids and polypeptides, which have important regulatory roles in the growth, development, and maintenance of the structures necessary for the continuation of the species. Among these are the reproductive organs themselves, including both the gravid and nongravid uterus; the secondary sex characteristics; and the mammary glands. Figure 9–1 is intended to convey some idea of the complexity of the interrelationships of the neural, endocrine and end-organ tissues concerned

with reproductive function in the female. It is suggested that the reader examine the diagram, mainly to get a panoramic view of the structures and substances that will be discussed in this chapter; read the chapter and return to the diagram to see how the individual components in this communications system fit the larger pattern.

The following subjects will be discussed (the numbers correspond to those circled in Fig 9–1):

1. Chemistry, biosynthesis, and metabolism of estrogens and progestins

2. Gonadotrophic hormones

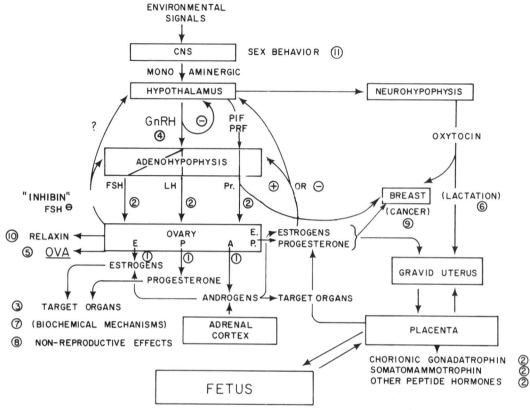

FIG 9–1.
Overview of reproductive endocrinology in the female.

3. Effects of estrogens and progestins on reproductive tissues

4. Role of the CNS in the hypophyseal-ovarian relationship

5. Oogenesis and the hormonal control of ovulation and the menstrual cycle

6. Hormonal regulations in pregnancy and lactation

7. Cellular mechanism of action of reproductive hormones.

8. Nonreproductive effects of ovarian steroids

9. Steroid hormones and breast cancer

10. Relaxin

11. Sex behavior

Chemistry, Biosynthesis, and Metabolism of Estrogens and Progestins

The estrogen produced and secreted by the ovary of many species, including the human, is estradiol 17β. This compound is in equilibrium with estrone, which can be converted by the liver and placenta to estriol, the principal estrogen secreted by the placenta. The structural relationships of these compounds are shown in Figure 9–2. All of them have estrogenic effects, estradiol 17β being the most active. Estriol is synthesized in the placenta from a precursor steroid (dehydroepiandrosterone), which is provided by the adrenal gland of the fetus. Although the ovaries of some species make female sex hormones that are not precisely the same as these, all naturally occurring estrogens have an unsaturated A ring, a phenolic hydroxy group at position 3, and a methyl group at 13. Synthetic congeners of the naturally occurring estrogens have been prepared, and one of these will be discussed in the section on nonreproductive functions of estrogens.

Estrogens are comparatively inactive when taken by mouth, mainly because they are inactivated in the liver, where they are conjugated with glucuronic or sulfuric acids or otherwise modified. The discovery that certain nonsteroidal compounds, especially stilbene derivatives, were able to produce all of the physiologic effects of naturally occurring estrogens,

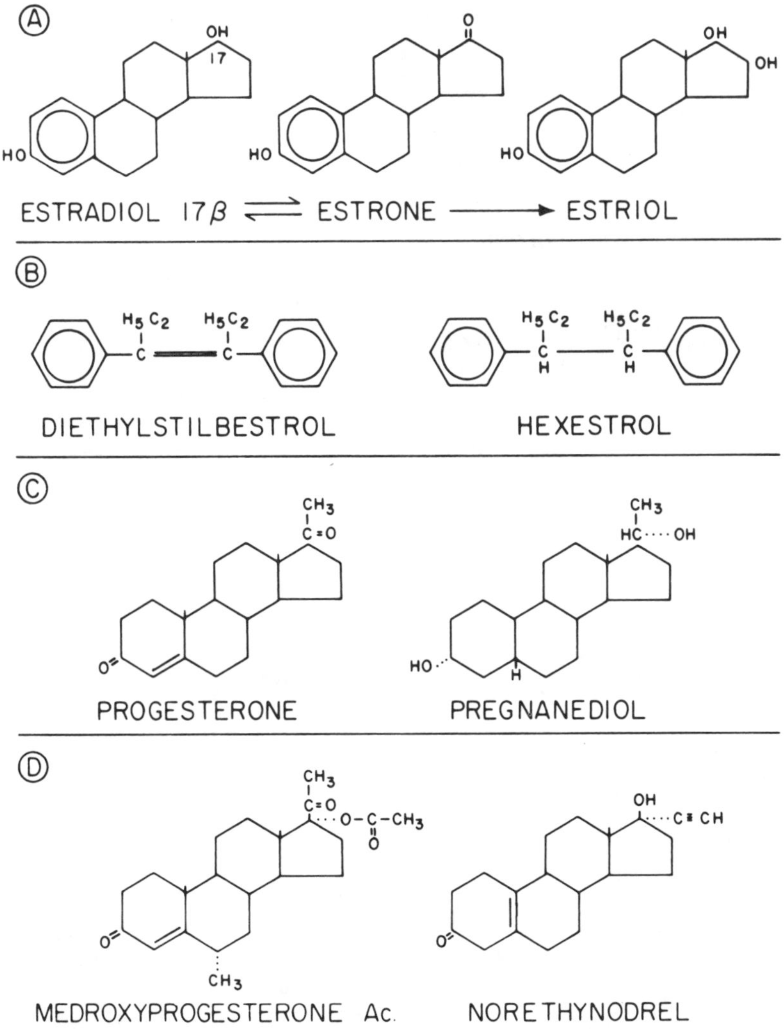

FIG 9–2.
A–D, estrogens, synthetic estrogens, progesterone, synthetic progestins.

even when given by the oral route, proved to be of great therapeutic importance. Two of the most widely used synthetic estrogens are diethylstilbestrol and hexestrol, shown in Figure 9–2.

The naturally occurring hormone of the corpus luteum is progesterone, shown in Figure 9–2 with its excretion product, pregnanediol. Progesterone is important not only because of its role in maintenance of pregnancy but also because it is an intermediate in the biosynthesis of adrenal, testicular, and gonadal steroids from cholesterol. Figure 9–3 is a schematic representation of some of the intermediates in the synthesis of estradiol 17β and progesterone. It is designed to suggest that steroid synthesis in the preovulatory

ovary proceeds by way of the Δ^5 pathway and involves aromatizing androgens (supplied by the thecal cells) to estrogens by the granulosa cells. In the corpus luteum, the full complement of enzymes necessary to produce progesterone and estrogens is present and these are the major steroids secreted.

The synthetic route from androgen to estradiol 17β is the main route of estrogen formation in the ovary. We do know that ovarian slices incubated with ^{14}C-labeled testosterone make labeled estradiol 17β. The corpus luteum cell evidently differentiates further by producing progesterone as a secretory product while retaining the ability to produce estrogen. It is emphasized that the various steroid-producing cells may re-

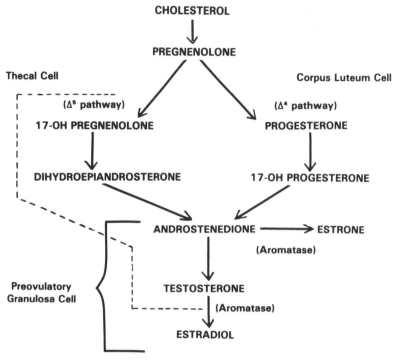

FIG 9–3.
Patterns of steroidogenesis in the thecal cell, corpus luteum cell, and preovulatory granulosa cell. See text for discussion.

tain some capacity to make hormonal products in addition to the main ones. For example, estrogen is made by Leydig cells, androgens are produced in adrenocortical cells and in the ovary. In this connection it is interesting to recall that mutants of ovarian or testicular cells that undergo metaplasia and form tumors may specialize in making estrogens or androgens, whether they developed in a testis or an ovary.

As in the case of androgens, the naturally occurring estrogens and progestins are metabolized too rapidly in the liver to be useful as replacement therapy for deficiencies. A few examples of synthetic substances with estrogenic and progestational activity are shown in Figure 9–2. Technically, diethylstilbestrol and hexestrol are not steroids, but if one inspects three-dimensional models of these compounds, it is easy to imagine how they would fit into the estrogen receptor pocket. Like androgens, estrogens have their synthetic antagonists such as tamoxifen, which is widely used in the treatment of breast cancer (see below).

The *biosynthesis* of estrogens and progesterone, in its broad outlines, resembles that of other steroid hormones such as testosterone and the adrenal cortical hormones. In all steroid hormone-producing cells,

readily available hormone precursor is stored in the form of cholesterol ester droplets. The earliest phases of steroidogenesis are identical in all such cells: (1) cholesterol ester hydrolysis; (2) cholesterol side chain cleavage; and (3) pregnenolone synthesis. Together, these three reactions are the rate-limiting reactions of steroid hormone biosynthesis, and they are the major site of the acute effect of trophic hormones: LH, ACTH, and angiotensin II. When these hormones are active over a longer time scale, they are capable of inducing other enzymes that catalyze reactions distal to side chain cleavage.

The fate of pregnenolone in different cell types (ovary, corpus luteum, Leydig cell, adrenal cell) depends on the distinctive array of steroidogenic enzymes that is expressed in each of the cells. The flow of substrate through the biosynthetic pathway is punctuated by a series of hydroxylation reactions, each of which is catalyzed by a specific cytochrome P450 complex. Whether the secreted steroid is estradiol, progesterone, aldosterone, or cortisol ultimately depends on the particular collection of P450 enzymes a cell "decided" to transcribe when it differentiated.

In the case of the ovary, the sequence following

pregnenolone is shown in Figure 9–3. As we have seen, the synthesis of estradiol in the preovulatory phase of the menstrual cycle involves collaboration between two different cell types, one of which (the thecal cell) exports testosterone which its granulosa cell neighbor imports and aromatizes to estradiol.

Cells of the corpus luteum, while still capable of synthesizing estradiol, secrete large amounts of progesterone. This could be due to so rapid a progesterone production rate that the capacity of the enzymatic machinery to metabolize it is overwhelmed.

The naturally occurring steroids are rendered water soluble when they are conjugated in the liver with glucuronic or sulfuric acid. The conjugated steroids are excreted in the urine and are themselves biologically inactive.

Gonadotropic Hormones

LH, FSH, hCG

As we saw in Chapter 5, pituitary LH, FSH, TSH, and hCG (human chorionic gonadotropin) are composed of two noncovalently linked subunits, α and β. LH, TSH, and hCG share an α subunit (MW 14,000) of identical structure; hormone specificity of each is determined by its distinctive β subunit. The α subunit of FSH differs from that of the others. Carbohydrate groups are linked to the polypeptides of both subunits. The molecular weight of LH is about 28,000, that of FSH, about 33,000.

One aspect of the structure of LH, FSH, and hCG concerns the sialic acid residues that occur at the ends of carbohydrate chains attached to the hormones. If these amino sugars are removed by treatment with the enzyme neuraminidase, the half-life of the hormones is greatly reduced. The liver recognizes and binds the desialylated forms of the peptides and catabolizes them. Sialic acid evidently functions as protection from hepatic inactivation.

The cells of origin of the glycoprotein hormones, the gonadotropes, appear to be exceptions to the statement that each pituitary hormone is secreted by its own private cell type. In the rat both immunocytochemical and electron microscopic analysis has revealed *both* LH and FSH in the same cell, though other cells can be found that contain one or the other hormone. The finding of both gonadotropins in the same cell makes it easier to account for the concurrent appearance of FSH with LH at the midcycle surge, but it makes accounting for dissociation of FSH from LH secretion more difficult.

All of the pituitary hormones are stored in granules that are characteristic for each. There is some evidence that there is a readily releasable pool, possibly granules poised at the plasma membrane for discharge, and a second, more slowly mobilizable one. Release from both pools is stimulated by the appropriate releasing factor and/or by removal of a tonic inhibition. Release from the first pool does not require protein synthesis, but release from the second does. Stimulus-secretion coupling is brought about by an inositol phosphate turnover-mediated modification of calcium concentration in the secretory cell (Naor et al.).

The gonadotropins apparently circulate in their monomeric form and are assayable either by a radioligand receptor assay (dispersed Leydig cells) or by radioimmunoassay. The latter has been refined by the use of antibodies specifically directed to the respective β subunits of the hormones. This has made it possible to distinguish between such closely related molecules as LH and hCG.

Circulating levels of gonadotropins are low in the prepuberal female. Studies of gonadotropin reserve by measuring responses of circulating gonadotropins to LHRH administration show that infant boys have more LH reserve and infant girls more FSH reserve. In both sexes prepuberal increase in FSH anticipates the rise in LH. Also in both sexes, the time of puberty is marked by sleep-related pulsatile swings in circulating gonadotropin levels. At the end of puberty, pulsatile fluctuations at the adult level, no longer sleep-related, are seen. At menopause or after castration, circulating gonadotropins, particularly FSH, are greatly elevated, though still pulsatile.

The liver and kidneys collaborate to remove gonadotropins from the circulation. The half-life of LH is 12–45 minutes, that of PRL 12 minutes. Chorionic gonadotropin resists removal from the circulation and has a half-life of several hours. The role of sialic acid in the removal process has already been mentioned. Although only 10% of synthesized LH is excreted in the urine, urinary excretion is a good index of integrated pituitary secretory activity.

FSH is important in both sexes for its action on somatic cells (granulosa cell, Sertoli cell) which control the microenvironment in which their respective germ cells develop and mature. Estrogen stimulates the replication of granulosa cells primed with FSH and synergizes with FSH to increase the induction in them of the aromatase enzyme that converts testosterone to estradiol. In addition, estrogen also collaborates with FSH in the induction of receptors for both LH and FSH. FSH receptors are present only on granulosa cells, but LH receptors occur on thecal, interstitial, luteal, and (variably) on granulosa cells as well. As granulosa cells acquire LH receptors, they lose some FSH receptors and the capacity to respond to FSH.

The granulosa cell, like the Sertoli cell, responds to FSH via a cyclic AMP-mediated mechanism that involves phosphorylation of key proteins by cAMP-dependent protein kinase, but none of these has been identified. Whether or not other messenger systems described in Chapter 3 are involved in the granulosa cell response to FSH is not yet known. An important action of LH is its stimulation of steroid hormone production by an ACTH-like mechanism. It shows the well-known phenomenon of spare receptors and, though biologic effects on stimulation of steroid hormone synthesis may be seen without measurable changes in cAMP concentration, protein kinase activity ratio measurements suggest that protein kinase activation and protein phosphorylation are involved in the action of the hormone.

A second essential function of LH is in ovulation. It stimulates the synthesis of progesterone and prostaglandins, both of which participate in the process (see below).

NEUROTRANSMITTERS AND GnRH RELEASE

Although there is no reason to doubt that GnRH peptidergic neurons are controlled by a system of monoaminergic neurons, it is difficult to present a coherent scheme by which the control is accomplished. Serotonin, dopamine, and norepinephrine have all been implicated in the control of GnRH discharge, but advocates for acetylcholine and gamma amino butyric acid argue for their participation as well. Fuxe et al. have shown that dopamine and GnRH-containing neurons cluster in the same lateral external layer of the median eminence. If one contemplates data obtained in rats and in human beings, one is dismayed to discover that at times dopamine inhibits gonadotropin release, whereas at others it stimulates it. In human beings infusion of dopamine (or L-Dopa or bromocryptine, given orally) causes a significant decrease in circulating levels of LH as well as of prolactin. A tentative scheme, suggested by Yen, is as follows: norepinephrine and dopamine have reciprocal effects on GnRH; norepinephrine stimulates and dopamine inhibits. If dopamine is continuously infused in human beings, circulating gonadotropin concentrations decrease. When infusion is stopped, there is a large overshoot above the original baseline.

The relation among estrogens, GnRH and catecholamines involves a newly discovered class of compounds known as *catecholestrogens*. Fishman and Norton described the formation of catecholestrogens by brain tissue, which can hydroxylate estrogens at the 2 position of the A ring (Fig 9–4). Paul and Axelrod reported that catecholestrogen concentrations in pituitary and hypothalamus are more than 10 times as high as those of unaltered estrogens. Interestingly these catecholestrogens are devoid of estrogenic activity by the usual bioassay methods. However, their structural similarity to catecholamines in the brain is so close that they are metabolized by the same enzymes. Whether these compounds participate in feedback regulation of gonadotropin release is not known, but it is easy to imagine ways in which they could function in a *positive* feedback mechanism. For example, if the catecholestrogens competitively inhibited the enzyme COMT (see Fig 9–4), the stimulatory effect of norepinephrine on GnRH release would be amplified. Or if they functioned as antiestrogens, they could block out feedback inhibitory effects of estrogens and facilitate GnRH release. Although we cannot now give any definitive description of the role of catecholestrogens in regulation of gonadotropin secretion, their occurrence in the hypothalamus in high concentration and their distinctive molecular features make them difficult to ignore.

PROLACTIN AND SOMATOMAMMOTROPHIN

Until 1970 the existence of a specific lactogenic hormone in the human being was questioned by investigators who suggested that lactogenic function was a property of hGH (human growth hormone). However, with the purification of PRL and development of a highly discriminating radioimmunoassay, the tempo of research on this hormone was accelerated.

Prolactin (MW 20,000) is *synthesized* as a prohormone (MW 40,000) by lactotrophes of the anterior pituitary. The number of PRL-producing cells increases sharply during pregnancy, probably as a result of estrogen stimulation of growth and replication. When the entire *amino acid sequence* for sheep and pig PRL and the partial sequence of the hGH were established, it became obvious that PRL, hGH and hPL (human placental lactogen) shared many homologous amino acids, suggesting an evolutionary relationship among these hormones.

The most striking feature of *prolactin control* is the inhibitory effect of dopamine on PRL secretion. Since dopamine injected directly into the hypophyseal portal circulation decreases circulating PRL levels, some authorities believe that the catecholamine is itself the long-sought PIF (prolactin inhibitory factor). Sero-

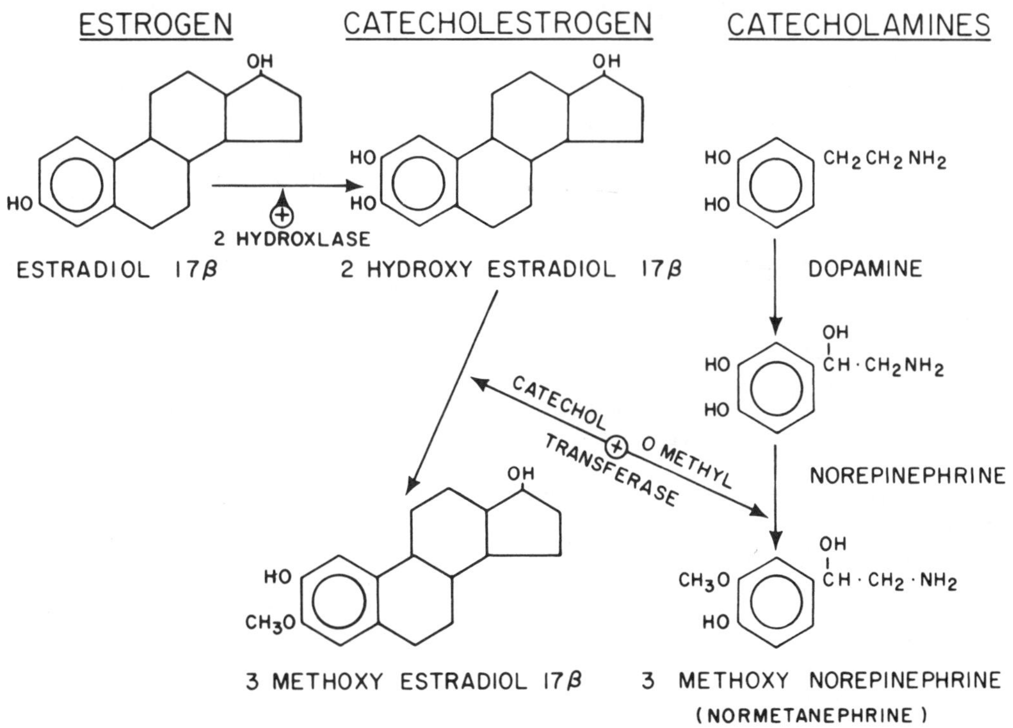

FIG 9–4.
Catecholestrogens and their relation to catecholamines.

tonin *increases* PRL secretion by an unknown mechanism. Serotonin is probably involved in sleep-related increases in serum PRL levels. TRH stimulates the release of PRL practically as well as it stimulates TSH release, but TRH is not generally believed to be "the" physiologic PRF because TSH and PRL secretion rates are readily dissociable from one another.

Plasma prolactin levels in human females are 8–10 ng/ml and, in males, almost as high: 5–8 ng/ml. The physiologic role of PRL, if any, in the male has not been established, though it has been implicated in spermatogenesis (see Chapter 8). Newborn infants of both sexes have circulating levels of PRL (100–500 ng/ml) that exceed the highest levels seen in pregnancy and in maximally stimulated nursing mothers. Adult levels are achieved after 2–3 months. The reason for this high neonatal level is completely unknown.

Like most peptide hormones, PRL has a short half-life when it is injected: 15–20 minutes. Like other pituitary hormones, PRL is released episodically, with a spiking frequency of 30–90 minutes. As has been mentioned, it also shows diurnal fluctuations in plasma concentrations, the highest levels seen 6–8 hours after the onset of sleep.

The major *physiologic function* of PRL is stimulation of milk secretion. It is appropriate, therefore, that the physiologic stimulus for PRL secretion is suckling. This is a typical neuroendocrine reflex: the afferent component is neural (nipple to CNS) and the efferent component is endocrine (prolactin secretion). This is an excellent example of the biology of a reproductive unit as opposed to the biology of an individual. If we trace the origin of the information involved in the nursing of an infant by its mother, the following signals are entrained by the empty gastrointestinal tract of the infant: (1) hunger signal(s) in baby; (2) crying; (3) anticipatory oxytocin response in mother; milk let-down; (4) breast made available to infant; (5) suckling; (6) afferent signals from nipple for prolactin to stimulate milk secretion and oxytocin to insure continued milk let-down; (7) integration of signals in hypothalamus; release of correct mix of pituitary releasing and release-inhibiting signals; (8) pituitary secretion of the two hormones; (9) satiety in baby, termination of suckling; and (10) readjustment of hormone secretory rates.

The maximum rise in serum PRL evoked by nursing (to 200–400 ng/ml) occurs about 30 minutes after stimulation begins. By 3–4 months post partum, in spite of continued nursing, little increase in plasma PRL occurs. However, a continuing supply of PRL is necessary to sustain nursing, since hypophysectomy (in animals) or pharmacologic inhibition of PRL secretion by a dopamine agonist (bromocryptine, in human beings) effectively stops milk secretion under any circumstances. The oxytocin response, however, continues unchanged even in long-term lactation.

Prolactin release may inhibit LHRH release and may therefore account in part for the anovulatory cycles associated with breast feeding. Although physiological concentrations of PRL are required for normal ovarian follicular development and function, amounts associated with lactation have a direct antiovulatory effect in the ovary. Thus, large-scale introduction of bottle feeding as a replacement for breast feeding could have the effect of increasing the birth rate in countries in which artificial methods of contraception are not in wide use.

In addition to circumstances mentioned in which PRL levels increase (estrogen, pregnancy, nursing, sleep), PRL secretion is stimulated by stress (e.g., hypoglycemia). Its role in the stress response, if there is one, has yet to be described.

These fundamental studies already have resulted in impressive clinical advances. For example, Frantz and colleagues have found that 70% of all pituitary tumors are associated with increases in serum PRL levels. Thus, radioimmunoassay for PRL may be very helpful as a diagnostic aid. Another example: gynecomastia, or breast development in the male, occurs not uncommonly, sometimes as a side effect of therapy with dopamine-blocking agents (e.g., phenothiazines). It also may occur spontaneously. In the latter case, a dopamine-mimetic drug (e.g., the ergot derivative bromocryptine) may be used with some success. Also, women with infertility associated with hyperprolactinemia are successfully treated with appropriate doses of bromocryptine. Radioimmunoassay for PRL is now in routine use for monitoring efficacy of treatment.

The *cellular mechanism of action* of PRL is not well understood. Sensitive cells bind the hormone with high affinity—so high, in fact, that a binding protein and radioligand assay for PRL has been used. The hormone has an insulin-like action on breast tissue, in which it stimulates glucose uptake and lipogenesis. Prolactin stimulates synthesis of milk proteins (casein, α lactalbumin) by increasing synthesis of their mRNAs. Synthesis of lactose by lactose synthetase requires galactosyl transferase and α lactalbumin, and is therefore secondarily stimulated by increased α lactalbumin synthesis.

Finally, in many species, prolactin appears to have distinctive behavioral effects, which caused it to be dubbed the "mother love hormone." The location of the CNS structures involved in this effect and the route by which this 20,000-dalton protein reaches them are not immediately obvious. The role of PRL in the male is discussed in Chapter 8.

Another placental hormone, hPL, or *somatomammotrophin,* is secreted by the trophoblast in very large amounts. As we have seen, hPL is closely related in structure to both GH (growth hormone) and PRL. It shares with GH the ability to produce some degree of peripheral insulin resistance. Since the fetus requires large amounts of carbohydrate, diversion of glucose from the peripheral tissues of the mother to the fetus may be regarded as a teleonomically useful tactic. By the same token, hPL may be largely responsible for the mild glucose intolerance that is commonly seen in pregnant women.

Effects of Estrogens and Progestins on Tissues

ESTROGENS

Embryonic

Although differentiation of the female reproductive tract and organs seems to be determined largely by the absence of androgen, estrogen (from either the fetus or mother) appears to be essential for the full development of the uterus and vagina in some species. If androgens, progesterone, or synthetic progestins are given to the mother at the critical time at which sex differentiation is occurring, masculinization of the external genitalia of the female fetus may occur.

Prepuberal

Throughout childhood estrogen is secreted at levels too low to cause development of the reproductive tissues. Like the immature testis, the immature ovary can be stimulated to a high level of activity by exogenous gonadotropin; therefore, persistence of the prepuberal state does not signify any lack of competence of the ovaries to respond to gonadotropic stimulation, but rather a lack of such stimulation. The pituitary of the prepuberal animal, male or female, can readily assume adult responsibility if it is transplanted to the sella turcica of the hypophysectomized adult.

This suggests that lack of maturation or its presence is determined not by the ovary or pituitary but by the state of suprahypophyseal tissues, i.e., the brain. The small amount of estrogen secreted by the ovaries of the prepuberal female is still sufficient to inhibit output of gonadotropins at the level of the CNS. At puberty there is a crucial change in sensitivity of these tissues, so that they require very much more estrogen to signal inhibition of gonadotropins. Gonadotropin is called for up to the new set of the "gonadostat" and sexual maturation occurs.

Puberty

An increase in adrenal androgens (adrenarche) normally precedes the onset of puberty (menarche in females) by about two years. The physiological significance of this event is unknown. That it is not essential is suggested by the fact that puberty proceeds normally even in the presence of adrenal cortical insufficiency.

Puberty is initiated by an increased output of gonadotropins by the pituitary acting on instructions from the hypothalamus. This may occur as the result of the removal of an inhibitory influence on GnRH release. The best candidate for such an inhibitory influence is *melatonin*, which decreases with waning pineal secretory activity (Chapter 7) at the beginning of sexual maturation in both sexes. Whether the marked decrease in sensitivity of the GnRH feedback mechanism that occurs at this time is entirely due to melatonin withdrawal is not known. In any case, this change in the "set" of the gonadostat must occur as increasing amounts of steroids are secreted by the ovary at puberty. Increasing supplies of both estrogens and androgens secreted by the ovaries in response to the new levels of gonadotropins result in accelerated growth of the uterus, vagina, accessory sex glands, external genitalia, pelvis, breasts, and pubic and axillary hair. (Hair growth, the occurrence of acne, and some deepening of the voice timbre all signify that androgen participates in the process of sexual maturation in the female.) This growth is specific, i.e., it occurs at rates far more rapid than those at which somatic growth is occurring at the same time. The process begins at the age of 9 or 10, and the first menstrual period may appear at age 12 or may be delayed until age 16. Some of the wide variation in time of onset may be genetically determined. Whenever the menarche occurs, it may take several months before the establishment of typical, regular, adult ovulatory menstrual cycles (see below).

The average age at which the first menstrual period occurs in the United States is between 12 and 13 years. The age of onset of puberty has declined steadily since the last century until about two decades ago when it stabilized. Better nutrition is believed to be the main reason for earlier incidence of menarche. For reasons unexplained, a certain proportion of adipose tissue to total body weight is essential for the onset of puberty. Strenuous exercise delays the appearance of the first menstrual period. The combination of exercise and food restriction that is often seen in ballet dancers may have striking effects on the maturation of the hypothalamic-pituitary-gonad axis.

Nonpregnant Adult

During the (approximately) 35-year period of fertility in the adult woman, estrogen production fluctuates in a cyclic way, which will be described in greater detail in a later section. In general, estrogen functions as a growth hormone for those tissues that are either immediately or secondarily related to the reproductive process.

There are some observations that suggest that estrogen may have local effects in the *ovary* that are quite analogous to those described for testosterone in the testis, and that they may be similarly exerted by local diffusion. An important effect of estrogen is to stimulate the production of progesterone receptors in granulosa cells, uterus, mammary gland, and other tissues. In both immature and hypophysectomized rats, priming with rather high doses of estrogen enhanced the ovarian response to gonadotropin. The synergistic effect of FSH and LH on the ovary may be visualized as a synergism between FSH- and LH-stimulated estrogen produced in the gland. Just as spermatogenesis may be stimulated in the hypophysectomized male rat by large doses of testosterone, estrogen may stimulate follicular growth in the hypophysectomized female. Estrogen pellets implanted in rabbits maintain the corpora lutea beyond their normal span in both intact and hypophysectomized animals.

In the *uterus*, estrogen stimulates growth of the glandular epithelium of the endometrium. The earliest detectable effect is hyperemia and transudation of water and salt into the tissues of the uterus. Estrogen also is a growth hormone for the smooth muscle of the uterus, and (possibly indirectly) for the uterine vascular system.

The epithelium of the *vagina* is so sensitive to the action of estrogen that examination of vaginal smears is used as a bioassay of the effect of the hormone. The vaginal epithelium of the castrate or immature female consists of only two or three layers of low cuboidal cells. At the height of estrus, there are about 10 layers of cells, and those near the surface are squamous and cornified. These large flat cells with small nuclei appear in the vaginal smears of women under estrogen stimulation, and examination of such smears is important in analyzing a menstrual cycle or in gauging the effect of estrogen replacement therapy.

Estrogen effects on the *mammary gland* are seen best during pregnancy, since the glandular elements of this structure are under the combined influence of estrogen and progesterone. Growth of the ductile components is stimulated by the former, whereas that of the glands themselves is stimulated by the latter. Growth of the mammary glands and duct development are seen in the nonpregnant animal given large doses of estrogen.

Ovarian Function in Peri- and Postmenopause

The average life expectancy of a female in the United States is 75 years. If one subtracts the premenarche and postmenopause years from the total, only half of the mean life span is associated with cyclic ovarian function and reproductive competence. Even beginning with age 15 through 35, there is a progressive shortening of mean menstrual cycle length with increasing age. The shortening is entirely associated with the follicular phase of the cycle; the luteal phase normally remains fairly constant.

At about age 45 there is an even further shortening of the follicular phase, and an increase in FSH (but not LH) may occur at the midcycle gonadotropin surge. This may be related to a decline in inhibin secretion by the aging ovary in which atresia of follicles, begun in the female embryo, continues throughout reproductive life. Menstrual irregularity of variable length (owing to irregularly occurrring anovulatory cycles), accompanied by more or less severe symptoms of the menopause, may appear. Estradiol secretion by the ovary progressively decreases, and finally estradiol serum levels decline to very low levels: < 20 pg/ml (normal mean for young women, 120 pg/ml). The perimenopausal woman, however, is not entirely devoid of estrogen because adrenal (and ovarian) androstenedione can be converted to estrone by muscle and adipose tissue. In fact, obese women may have persistence of high levels of circulating estrogen since their aromatization capacity in adipose tissue is large. Estrone does not bind well to SHBG (steroid hormone-binding globulin) and thus circulates largely as the free or active form. In competitive tests for estradiol-receptor binding, estrone is about 15%–25% as potent as is estradiol. The younger postmenopausal woman may derive circulating estrogen from ovarian testosterone and androstenedione, which the ovary may continue to secrete when it no longer makes much estrogen. For some reason, more apparent peripheral aromatization of androgens occurs in both men and women who have disease of the liver. This may be due to failure of the liver to abstract the inactivated estrone.

Many of the symptoms associated with the menopause are attributable to estrogen deficiency and can be relieved by small doses of estrogen. One of the most prominent of these is vascular instability leading to "hot flushes (or flashes)" and night sweats, which are due to episodic vasodilation in the face and upper extremities and are experienced to some degree by more than half of menopausal women. Atrophic changes in the epithelium of the vagina and in the accessory sex glands are associated with a variety of complaints and are also amenable to amelioration by estrogen replacement therapy. Another serious health problem in postmenopausal women is *osteoporosis*, which predisposes to pathological bone fractures (i.e., fractures that occur with minimal trauma). Although the causes of this condition are complex, there is now general agreement that decreasing estrogen availability is a major contributory factor in its development, and that replacement doses of estrogen can delay the onset and retard the progress of the disease.

The relationship of other menopause-related events to estrogen deficiency is less clear. A wide spectrum of emotional and psychological problems may occur at the time of the menopause which happens to be, for many women, a time for complex new adaptations. Obviously, it would be simplistic to suggest that estrogen deficiency is the underlying cause of such difficulties, though it may contribute to them. Genetic and experiential predisposition are probably the major determinants of many of these problems, and each individual who seeks help must be assisted in ways appropriate for her.

The question of estrogen replacement in postmenopausal women is controversial, for the benefit to be derived from such therapy must be weighed against the risk of inducing endometrial cancer. The addition of progestin during the last 7–10 days of cyclic estrogen replacement therapy may decrease the endometrial cancer risk. Many thoughtful physicians believe that the prospect of developing clinically significant osteoporosis represents a greater risk than that involved in estrogen-progestin replacement therapy, especially in women with one or more of the following demonstrated risk factors for osteoporosis: slight stature, heavy smoking, early menopause, and positive family history.

PROGESTERONE

In the mature, nonpregnant individual, small amounts of progesterone are synthesized in the ovarian follicle *before* ovulation, and are involved in the process of ovulation (see below). Much larger amounts are secreted by the corpus luteum which, in the human, is composed mainly of ex-granulosa cells that have developed LH receptors and are enzymatically equipped to synthesize and secrete estrogen as well as progesterone.

Progesterone probably has effects on the mammary gland of the nonpregnant individual, but these are not prominent or clearly described. There is little doubt that the compound plays a part in development of the secretory apparatus of the mammary gland during pregnancy. With estrogen, progestins participate in modulating the activity of hypothalamic regions that control the secretion of gonadotropins. Progesterone derivatives are important components of contraceptive pills (see below).

ANDROGEN IN THE FEMALE

The normal human female, like females of most species, synthesizes and secretes testosterone and testosterone precursors, though at a much lower level than the male (testosterone 250 µg/day versus 7,000 µg/day). The mean total androstenedione secretion/day varies between 1.4–1.6 mg/day; 1.2 mg from the adrenal and 0.2–0.4 mg from the ovary. Adrenal steroids have far less androgenic potency than testosterone. Androgens in females maintain sexual drive and are necessary for stimulation of growth of pubic and axillary hair.

Androgen production in normal women covers a very wide range. At the higher levels of testosterone production, various manifestations of virilism may be manifest, from moderate increases in body and facial hair through menstrual irregularities, acne, clitorimegaly and muscle hypertrophy and bitemporal balding. The degree of virilism/hirsutism correlates very well with testosterone production rate. In some populations of women (e.g., in the Mediterranean area), facial and abundant body hair are seen so frequently that they are not a source of concern. In other geographic areas, hirsutism is perceived as a distressing stigma. The interested reader is referred to the review by Kirchner et al.

Role of CNS in Hypophysial-Ovarian Relationship

Either ovarian hyperfunction or hypofunction may be seen in patients with destructive lesions of the CNS, particularly those at the base of the brain. That emotional disturbances can cause profound irregular-

ities of the menstrual cycle and that they can impair fertility in women are commonplace knowledge. The realization that the hypophyseal-portal system of blood vessels represents a route of information transfer from the hypothalamus to the adenohypophysis, and the increasingly wide application of stereotactic exploration of the brain by neuroendocrinologists, have begun to suggest a physiologic basis for some of the older studies.

Many kinds of evidence in addition to that obtained in the clinic suggest that gonadotropin output is controlled by messages that reach the pituitary gonadotrophes from the brain, and the locus of the feedback action of estrogens may well be in the CNS. In ferrets, for example, exposure to light induces a condition known as "constant estrus," which is believed to be due to an increased output of FSH induced by photic stimulation. This, of course, is very similar to the introduction of off-season gametogenesis in seasonally breeding males by exposing them to light. There now seem to be excellent data in support of the view that in some species certain special odors, by their presence of absence, can have a dramatic effect on gonadotropin output. In these cases, sensory afferents send information to the CNS, which then sends a humoral message to the pituitary by way of the portal system of blood vessels. The light effect, at least, has been prevented by stalk section and placement of a mechanical barrier to regeneration of the portal vessels across the section.

The structure of GnRH, or LHRH, is shown in Figure 5–1. Materials purified from ovine and porcine hypothalami have the same amino acid sequence, and synthetically prepared GnRH is biologically indistinguishable from the naturally occurring peptide. The participation of GnRH in the LH-FSH ovulatory surge is indicated by the fact that the surge can be prevented by antibodies to GnRH. Many GnRH analogues have been synthesized and tested by Schally and coworkers. They have found that certain molecular variants of natural GnRH are much more biologically active than is the native hormone. They have also described analogues that function as competitive inhibitors of GnRH.

As we have seen in our discussion of the male, the gonadotrope responds to GnRH not only because it is equipped with a specific plasma membrane receptor and appropriate transducing and effector systems but also because it can sense the pulse frequency and amplitude of GnRH secretion by the hypothalamus or administration via a programmed pump. As in the male, continuous, nonpulsatile presence of GnRH desensitizes the gonadotrope to stimulation and effectively shuts off gonadotropin secretion. Pulsatile injection of GnRH in an amplitude-frequency mode that simulates hypothalamic secretion can restore gonadal function in hypogonadal females as well as males as long as their pituitaries are competent to respond to the releasing hormone.

So far, only one releasing factor for gonadotropins has been discovered, although some students of the problem believe that separate FSH- and LH-releasing factors may exist. At present, it is difficult to explain the fact that FSH and LH circulate in different concentration ratios in various circumstances. The recent discovery that both gonadotropins can be found in single anterior pituitary cells by immunofluorescent examination is no great help in resolving the problem. In general, two ideas have been suggested to account for shifting ratios of FSH to LH secretion in response to a single peptide-releasing factor: (1) the frequency pattern of GnRH secretion may affect the FSL/LH ratio because a *decrease* in frequency favors FSH accumulation over LH accumulation since FSH has a longer half-life than LH. Conversely, an *increased* frequency would favor an increased LH/FSH ratio since there would be less time for clearance of LH from the circulation. (2) a selective feedback inhibitor (e.g., inhibin) could alter FSH secretion independently of that of LH. In either case, it is likely that a differential response to GnRH by the pituicyte may be achieved by alterations in that cell's secretory activity.

Ovulation, as we have seen, does not occur in the hypophysectomized animal and is brought about by the release of pituitary LH (and FSH?) in the intact animal. The event can be triggered in the hypophysectomized animal and in some hypophysectomized women by administration of hypophyseal gonadotropins in proper proportion. Ovulation is therefore used in many experiments as an indicator of LH release.

In animals that normally ovulate only in response to coitus or to mechanical stimulation of the vagina (rabbit, cat), ovulation can be produced in the animal in estrus by electric stimulation of very precisely demarcated regions of the hypothalamus. Ovulation does not occur in such species if the hypophysis is removed immediately following vaginal stimulation, but it does if the operation is delayed for as short a time as one hour after stimulation. The compound neuroendocrine reflex in rabbits is blocked by certain drugs (i.e., atropine, morphine, pentobarbital), which act in the CNS. In drug-blockaded animals, electric stimulation of the hypothalamus near the pituitary still produces ovulation. Similar experiments on electrically induced ovulation may be performed in drug-blockaded animals that normally ovulate sponta-neously. Electrolytic lesions of the same regions in which stimulation is effective produce a block in ovulation in reflex ovulators.

In many experiments, pituitary glands have been grafted into a hypophysectomized animal at a site remote from the brain, i.e., the anterior chamber of the eye or beneath the renal capsule. The tissue becomes revascularized in its new site and recovers a certain amount of its original capacity to secrete trophic hormones, but LH and FSH are not secreted in sufficient amounts to support normal gonadal function. If such a transplanted gland is retransplanted in the sella turcica, where it can be shown to be revascularized by the hypophyseal vessels, perfectly normal gonadal function is observed to occur in animals in which portal revascularization is most successful.

There is evidence that the brain is involved in feedback inhibition of gonadotropin secretion by estrogens and androgens. Flerko and colleagues have discovered that lesions in the hypothalamic paraventricular nuclei prevent the gonadal atrophy that occurs on steroid hormone administration. When they autotransplanted tiny pieces of ovarian tissue to this region of the brain, they demonstrated suppression of gonadotropin secretion, presumably by the estrogen secreted by the graft.

Recent studies suggest that the *negative* feedback effect of estrogen results from the stimulation of the secretion of an endogenous opioid peptide, beta endorphin, which inhibits GnRH secretion by modulating catecholamine release (Ferin). The *positive* feedback of estrogen that causes the ovulatory LH surge, in addition to its major direct effect on the pituitary, is also achieved by way of increasing GnRH secretion (amplitude and frequency), but the neuronal circuitry involved in estrogen's ability to increase GnRH is unknown.

All the experiments mentioned above were concerned with FSH and/or LH release. The data for prolactin also suggest a role for the hypothalamus in the stimulation of prolactin secretion (see above). When the hypophysis is transplanted to a site remote from the sella, all evidence suggests an *increase* in PRL output rather than a decrease. This could be explained if signals of hypothalamic origin constantly inhibit PRL output, and transplantation constitutes a form of release from this inhibition.

Pituitary glands incubated without hypothalamic tissue produce more prolactin in vitro than in the presence of such tissue.

Infusion of dopamine directly into the pituitary portal circulation, or direct addition of dopamine to anterior pituitary glands in vitro decreases PRL secretion. Therefore, dopamine has been proposed as the physiologic PIF, but at least one peptide with PIF activity has been described recently (see Chapter 5).

TRH is a positive signal for PRL release, but whether or not it plays a physiological role is not clear. There is some evidence that there may be an additional PRL-RH that has not yet been isolated and characterized. The suckling stimulus probably generates CNS signals for the release of serotonin, vasoactive intestinal peptide (VIP), and possibly other stimulatory hypothalamic mediators.

Oogenesis

Gametogenesis in the female contrasts sharply with the complementary process in the male. During differentiation of the ovary, primary germ cells differentiate into oogonia and primary oocytes. This results in a total germ cell population of 6–7,000,000 germ cells in the human fetus at five months. From this point, there is a progressive decrease in the number of germ cells; of the original high of 7,000,000, only 400 or so are destined to be ovulated during the reproductive life of the woman. Some are enveloped by granulosa cells, but many others aggregate into clusters and disappear by the process of atresia. Since the surviving oocytes are arrested in the prophase of the first meiotic division and do not undergo final division until the ovum is fertilized, some arrested oocytes that are destined to ovulate eventually may persist for up to 50 years. Meiosis arrest is probably brought about by one or more *meiosis inhibiting factors* produced in the ovary but not yet chemically identified. Meiosis arrest over many decades may account for the observation that there is a progressive increase in chromosomal abnormalities, including the one associated with Down's syndrome, with increasing maternal age.

The statistical probabilities built into the sperm-ovum rendezvous (one ovum versus *at least* 60 million sperm per ejaculate) require that many trillions of spermatozoa be produced during the reproductive life of the male which has been observed to extend into the 10th decade of life. In contrast to the cessation of germ cell division which occurs in the five-month-old human female fetus, spermatogonia continue to divide during the reproductive years of a man's life. While an ovulated ovum may be as old as 50 years, all sperm mature in about 74 *days*.

FERTILIZATION AND IMPLANTATION

After ovulation occurs (see below for description of mechanism), the ovum is trapped by the fimbria of the fallopian tube and is carried by ciliary action to the ampullary-isthmic junction where fertilization occurs. The cellular cumulus, which surrounds the newly ovulated ovum, may carry important hormonal information for the epithelial cells lining the fallopian tube.

The fertilized ovum remains in the tube for about four days. It enters the uterus in the morula-blastocyst stage, when it contains up to 50 cells. The time of residence within the tube is critical for the success of subsequent implantation in the endometrium. A "correct" estrogen-progesterone ratio is required for the process to proceed normally for coordination of endometrial and fertilized ovum development. The theory of the "morning-after pill," which consists of a massively large amount of stilbestrol, or a somewhat smaller dose of estrogen combined with progestin, is based on a disruption of the coordinated processes of tubal transport, retention, discharge of the developing morula into the uterine cavity and nidation of the structure in the endometrium.

Hormonal Control of Ovulation and the Menstrual Cycle

The menstrual cycle in primates, like the estrus cycle in other mammals, represents an extraordinarily complex relationship in time and in function among a number of anatomically distant structures. Since the cycle can be modified by fertilization of an ovum and successful implantation, it involves not only many structures in a single individual but also the male and female members of a reproductive unit. The cycle is at once a periodic preparation of the endometrium for implantation of an embryo; maturation of an ovum and ovulation; changes in activity of the trophic structures in the brain and pituitary that control the gonadotropin mix; and changes in secondary sex characteristics associated with the procreative act. Much of the coordination of these events is achieved by precisely timed fluctuations in the production and secretion rates of a number of hormones. In recent years, largely due to the application of radioimmunoassay for both peptide and steroid hormones, it has been possible to give a reasonably good phenomenologic description of changes in circulating hormone levels and how they correlate with endometrial morphology, ovarian follicle maturation, ovulation, corpus luteum formation and menstruation.

It is widely assumed that gonadotropin secretion is regulated by two discrete "centers" in the hypothalamus: (1) a "tonic" center, which controls more or less continuous release of gonadotropins, and (2) a "cyclic" center, which is associated with the periodic release of very large amounts of LH and FSH at mid-cycle. Most of the work on which this concept is based was done in the rat. There is no compelling evidence to support the idea that precisely the same arrangement exists in primates. Not the least important dividend produced by the recent revolution in radioimmunoassay technology has been a series of elegant studies in women by Van de Wiele, Speroff, and others and in subhuman primates by E. Knobil and his associates.

The cycle can be described most conveniently in two phases: pre- and postovulatory. The *preovulatory phase* is characterized by ovarian follicular growth and maturation and by a gradual increase in thickness of the endometrium. The *postovulatory phase* is often referred to as the luteal phase, for it is dominated by the growth, development and involution of the corpus luteum. During this period, when the estrogen-primed uterus is under the influence of progesterone, the endometrial glands become tortuous, glycogen deposition occurs and the uterus is anatomically and biochemically prepared to receive the conceptus. Coincident structural and functional alterations occur in the vagina. At about the time of ovulation vaginal smears show a sharp increase in the number of large, acidophilic squamous cells with small, dark-stained nuclei. The character of cervical mucus at this time is watery and offers least resistance to penetration by spermatozoa. Later, during the luteal phase, cervical mucus becomes scanty and more viscous. These changes in the character of the cervical secretions may be important in the mechanism of action of certain antifertility compounds.

Although we can describe hormonal fluctuations in association with ovarian and endometrial events, it is difficult to establish cause-and-effect relationships among these events. Therefore, some investigators have introduced the technique of assessing the contribution of a particular hormone by neutralizing its effect by means of a specific antibody and then watching for the consequences of this selective neutralization on later developments. This type of analysis has been conducted successfully with anti-FSH, anti-LH and antiestrogen antibodies, and the essential contribution of FSH, LH and estrogens at each phase of the cycle has been confirmed. For example, anti-FSH prevents early follicular growth; anti-LH prevents ovulation; and antiestrogen, just before midcycle, prevents the ovulatory surge of gonadotropins.

EVENTS OF THE MENSTRUAL CYCLE

The hormonal control of the menstrual cycle in women is illustrated in Figure 9–5. The events can be described as follows (numbers here refer to the circled numbers in Fig 9–5):

1. As the corpus luteum involutes, there is a precipitous fall in circulating levels of both estrogen and progesterone.

2. In consequence, there is a small but constant increase in circulating FSH concentration, which may persist through the 4–5 days of menstrual bleeding.

3. The rising FSH concentration stimulates several follicles to begin to develop. After a few days, one of these begins to mature rapidly, while the others begin to involute. This occurs while FSH is diminishing and LH may be very low and perhaps slowly rising. It may be due in part to the fact that the "chosen" follicle secretes estrogen, which increases its sensitivity to gonadotropin stimulation, whereas that of the "rejected" follicles may diminish. The atretic follicles may continue to make steroids, which may have some as yet unknown physiologic importance. Some investigators believe them to be a source of androgen, which would give them some significance in maintenance of libido.

4. The maturing follicle produces increasing amounts of estrogen. If the rising estrogen concentration is neutralized with antiestrogen antibody, the midcycle gonadotropin surge does not occur. Therefore, the rising estrogen concentration just before the surge is believed to be the proximate stimulus for the sharp peak in both LH and FSH that occurs just before ovulation.

5. Progesterone synthesis by granulosa cells is stimulated by the rise in LH that occurs just before the midcycle LH surge. Progesterone contributes to the positive feedback signal that elicits the LH surge. In addition, progesterone participates in the process of ovulation in a paracrine manner, for the hormone is essential for the synthesis of enzymes that are responsible for locally thinning the follicular wall through which the ovum and its cumulus will be extruded.

6. During the immediate postovulatory period (when there is a transitory drop in circulating steroids), the ruptured follicle becomes filled with luteal cells, which are yellow and lipid-laden. As these cells proliferate into the cavity, new blood vessels form. The enzymatic "emphasis" in these cells is such that they produce large and increasing amounts of progesterone, as well as estrogen, under the influence of LH working via the adenyl cyclase mechanism. Stimulation of steroidogenesis occurs mainly at the desmolase step, as it does in all steroid-producing cells that are regulated by way of cyclic AMP.

7. The high circulating levels of estrogen and progesterone inhibit the release of gonadotropins by the pituitary, mainly at the hypothalamic locus.

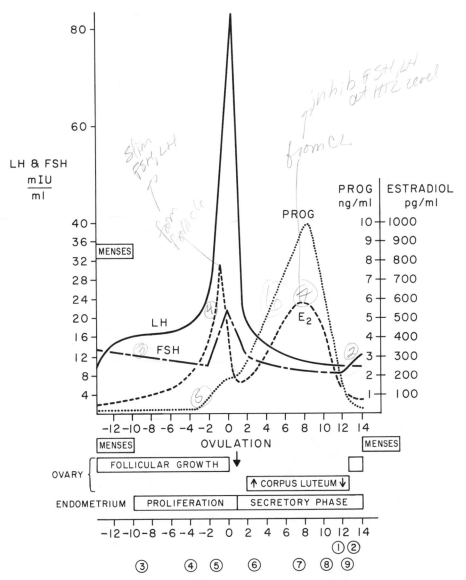

FIG 9–5.
Circulating hormone levels during ovarian and endometrial events in the human menstrual cycle.

(From Speroff L, Van de Wiele RL: *Am J Obstet Gynecol* 1971; 109:234. Used by permission.)

8. In some species, a luteolytic substance produced by the uterus is responsible for involution of the corpus luteum. In primates there is no evidence that such a substance exists, since the corpus luteum degenerates even if the uterus is removed. The primate corpus luteum may be programmed to degenerate at a fixed time without the necessity of external signals. It has been suggested that the prostaglandins, particularly $PGF_2\alpha$, may be involved in luteolysis.

9. When the corpus luteum degenerates, there is a sharp decrease in circulating estrogen and progester-

one levels. As this occurs, there is a selective increase in serum FSH concentration, which initiates a new wave of follicle maturation. At the same time, the secretory endometrium, now suffering from withdrawal of its steroid stimulants, undergoes hemorrhagic and degenerative changes, which culminate in the bleeding and discharge that constitute the menstrual flow.

The details of this process have been observed directly in endometrial transplants placed in the anterior chamber of the eyes of experimental animals and inspected through the transparent cornea with a microscope. At the time of sloughing, there is marked constriction of the arterioles and a slowing of circulation, with extravasation and pooling of blood in the stromal layer. The submucosal blood pools coalesce, and the superficial layers of endometrium, leukocytes and mucus are shed as menstrual discharge. The blood of this discharge does not clot readily, and it may vary in amount from 20 to 200 ml for a single period. The flow lasts 3–7 days in 95% of women. In 30–40 years of active reproductive life, a woman menstruates 300–500 times. At 100 ml per period, 400 periods could account for a cumulative loss of 40 liters of blood—a figure that helps to explain why some women tend to have a mild to moderate degree of chronic iron deficiency anemia.

AN OVARIAN FOLLICULAR VIEW OF THE MENSTRUAL CYCLE

At the level of organization of the intact woman, one can describe the menstrual cycle in terms of fluctuating circulating hormone concentrations and morphologic changes in the endometrium. This kind of phenomenologic description understates the importance of events in the cycle that are occurring in the *ovarian follicle*. In fact, one can defend the point of view that the ovarian follicular program is the major director of the cycle; i.e., the events in the intact woman represent responses to a sequence of initiatives taken by the developing follicle. The mitotic and biosynthetic activity of granulosa (G) cells (analogous to Sertoli cells in the testis) and steroid-producing thecal cells (Leydig-like cells) correlates better with changing gonadotropin and steroid concentration patterns in *follicular antral fluid* than it does with those in the general circulation (McNatty).

The G cell undergoes a series of changes as the follicular phase leads to ovulation and the corpus luteum is organized thereafter. During the early follicular phase, the analogy to the Sertoli cell is close, since the G cell is FSH dependent for the initial phases of follicular development, which occur in an environment in which steroid hormone concentrations are far higher than they are in the circulating blood. At this stage the G cell has FSH receptors but few LH receptors, and it proliferates rapidly. It does not have the ultrastructure of a steroid-producing cell, but it rapidly acquires the capacity to aromatize androgens to estrogen. Early in follicular development, production of estrogen is achieved by a collaboration between the thecal cell, which makes primarily androgen from cholesterol, and the G cell, which uses the androgen as an estrogen precursor. The estrogen

so produced synergizes with FSH to promote further replication of G cells, an increase in FSH and estrogen receptors, induction of aromatase enzyme (among others), and an increase in LH receptors. One of the follicles is selected early in the cycle to become the dominant follicle that contains the germ cell that will be ovulated eventually. (Although there are many theories about the mechanism of the selection process, none is generally accepted.) The designated follicle continues to produce large amounts of estrogen in spite of the *decrease* in *circulating* FSH resulting from a combination of the negative feedback effects of estrogen and inhibin.

During the latter part of the follicular phase, the base of the follicle shows proliferation of an extensive capillary circulation. Thus, it becomes possible for the very large amounts of estrogen produced in the follicle to gain access to the general circulation. Concurrently, more and more LH receptor capacity develops both in thecal and G cells in preparation for ovulation and the luteal phase of the cycle.

In midfollicular phase, when the G cell is under FSH dominance and thecal cells are still producing mainly androstenedione and a smaller amount of estradiol, an inhibin-like protein (Channing et al.) is produced. The source of this selective inhibitor of FSH secretion is believed to be the G cell itself, and the locus of inhibition by inhibin is probably the pituitary gonadotrope. Deficiency of this material may be the basis for the appearance of very high circulating levels of FSH in the postmenopausal woman. The granulosa cell produces a number of other peptides, including one that resembles GnRH, but their functions are not completely understood.

As the follicular stage progresses to *late* follicular, there is extensive aromatization of androstenedione to estrogen, which now becomes the dominant steroid and is secreted in sufficient amounts to increase its level in the blood. This has the effect of establishing the positive feedback demand that elicits the midcycle LH surge.

Very late, i.e., just before ovulation, LH stimulates the G cell to produce *progesterone*, which is now the principal antral fluid steroid. At the same time LH inhibits G cell mitosis, probably by a mechanism involving cAMP. Ovulation occurs (see below) by a mechanism that importantly involves progesterone.

After ovulation has occurred, both the remaining G cells and thecal cells are transformed into full-fledged steroid hormone-secreting cells. Under the electron microscope, luteal cells resemble adrenocortical cells, with their prominent lipid droplets filled with cholesterol ester and their mitochondria specialized for steroid hormone hydroxylation reactions. Their most important steroid product is progesterone, though they produce more estrogen than was required to initiate the LH surge (this estrogen may be important for implantation). Gonadotropin secretion, however, is finally inhibited by the progesterone-estrogen combination if conception does not occur.

The corpus luteum cell produces prostaglandin $F_2\alpha$ in response to LH, and the LH effect on the corpus luteum cell is enhanced by prolactin.

The microenvironment provided by the antral fluid of the ovarian follicle is just as special as that surrounding the developing male germ cells in the seminiferous tubule. The oocyte in the early-developing follicle increases in size, but its growth is arrested in the first meiotic division. It is interesting that growth of the arrested oocyte may occur even when no gonadotropins are available to the follicle, i.e., when enough antigonadotrophic serum is given to retard follicular development.

If a mammalian oocyte is removed from a follicle and placed in a suitable medium in vitro, it will resume nuclear maturation. From this it was concluded that follicular fluid contains an oocyte maturation inhibitor (OMI), which has been partially purified (MW 2,000). This inhibitor is made by the G cell, is not species specific (follicular fluid from species A will inhibit maturation of ova from species B) and does not appear related to steroidogenesis in the ovary.

When we described the Sertoli cell, we pointed out that the cell had a complex life cycle, beginning with the production of MIF (müllerian inhibitory factor) in the embryo and proceeding through an FSH sensitivity change to the acquisition of testosterone sensitivity. The G cell in the developing follicle telescopes its life cycle in time. First, it develops aromatase activity in response to FSH. Then, as FSH receptors diminish, it acquires LH receptors. As it does so, it expresses enzymes required for steroidogenesis from cholesterol. Finally, those G cells that remain in the ruptured follicle are transformed into large, lipid-laden, progesterone-secreting cells. There is some evidence for a requirement for hormones in addition to estradiol (insulin, thyroxine, cortisol) when LH receptors are induced in G cells.

The events involved in the *rupture of the follicular wall at ovulation* have been studied extensively. Initially there is a swelling of the follicle associated with fluid accumulation within. (Contrary to older teachings, the hydrostatic pressure within the follicle is *not* increased: the ovum is not discharged from the surface of the follicle as if it were being shot from a gun.) There are coordinate changes in blood flow (hyperemia and increased capillary permeability in the thecal layer) and in the intercellular matrix within the follicle (a general "loosening" and separation of intercellular bridges). The increased progesterone concentration is accompanied by increased synthesis of prostaglandin $F_2\alpha$ and an increase in free proteolytic enzyme activity of the follicular fluid. Both progesterone synthesis and prostaglandin synthesis are necessary for rupture of the follicle, since that phenomenon does not occur if either progesterone synthesis is inhibited by a steroid hormone synthesis inhibitor, (cyanoketone) or if prostaglandin synthesis is inhibited (by indomethacin). However, prostaglandin synthesis is not required for stimulation of progesterone synthesis by LH, which occurs by a mechanism such as that for LH stimulation of androgen synthesis in the Leydig cell and that for ACTH stimulation of cortisol synthesis in the adrenal cell.

Follicle rupture is difficult to demonstrate in very late follicles by in vitro addition of LH. When it occurs in situ, it is probably the result of a combination of hormonal, circulatory and possibly neurogenic factors.

INDICATORS OF SUCCESSFUL OVULATION

There are a number of ways of distinguishing ovulatory cycles from anovulatory ones. Following hormone levels in the blood by frequent serial estimations is one way, but the following techniques are far less technically demanding:

1. Basal body temperature taken in the morning immediately on awakening varies between 36.3 C and 36.8 C during the preovulatory phase of the cycle and increases by 0.3–0.5 C at the time of ovulation. It continues at the higher level throughout the latter half of the cycle and falls to the initial level at the time of menstruation. The temperature elevation is related to production of progesterone. This simple observation reveals not only whether a cycle is ovulatory or anovulatory but also the approximate time of ovulation—a useful datum for women with a history of infertility. Probability of conception is greatly enhanced by concentrating sexual activity at the time of ovulation.

2. An increase of urinary gonadotropins occurs in conjunction with the midcycle surge.

3. An increase in urinary estrogen excretion can be observed just before ovulation.

4. Vaginal smear reveals typical large, flat squamous cells in the immediate preovulatory period.

5. A rise in pregnanediol excretion (a reflection of increased progesterone secretion) occurs 3–4 days after ovulation.

6. Cervical mucus is examined for viscosity.

CONTROL OF FERTILITY AND INFERTILITY

When overpopulation threatens animal populations, fertility control may be imposed on them by environmental forces (e.g., food scarcity) or by the phenomena of "crowd stress," which presumably work by interfering with the normal functioning of the hypothalamic cells, which secrete gonadotropin-releasing factors. Men and women who wish to control their fertility have resorted to a wide variety of mechanical, surgical, and chemical methods of preventing conception, implantation or maturation of a fetus.

The introduction of chemical methods of fertility control by Pincus, Chang and Rock has had important repercussions on population growth and has contributed to changing social mores. Commonly used steroid contraceptives consist of synthetic estrogens (ethinyl estradiol or mestranol) in combination with progestogens derived from 19-nortestosterone. They may be given concurrently, and they have been used in many combinations and at widely varying dose levels. The oral contraceptives currently approved for use in selected individuals contain much less estrogen and progestin than did those prescribed earlier. Evidence is accumulating that they have fewer serious side effects than older forms although all undesirable complications have not been eliminated. Women at risk for developing thromboembolic disease, coronary heart disease, or other side effects (for example, heavy smokers or women over 30) are urged to use alternative methods of fertility control to lessen the occurrence of dangerous side effects. In fact, recent reports suggest that there may be beneficial effects of the "pill," among them a decreased incidence of anemia and a diminished risk of endometrial cancer.

It is difficult to describe their mechanisms of action with precision, since the same compound may exert an antifertility effect at two different doses by different mechanisms. The agents may interfere with fertility by perturbing function at the following loci: (1) the hypothalamic-pituitary gonadotropin-secreting apparatus, (2) the ovary, (3) the fallopian tubes, (4) sperm transport to the site of fertilization (capacitation, (5) endometrium and (6) cervical secretory glands.

Estrogens may interfere with follicular development by inhibiting FSH release, and estrogens and progestins may eliminate the ovulatory surge of gonadotropins, presumably by acting at the hypothalamic level and, possibly, by acting directly on the pituitary as well. Some may have direct effects on the ovary, inhibiting steroidogenesis. Low-dose "pills" may suppress fertility, even when they permit ovulation, by rendering the endometrium unsuitable for nidation, by altering transit time of the ovum through the fallopian tube or by causing a thickening of cervical mucus, thereby rendering it comparatively impermeable to penetration by sperm. All of these effects are readily reversible on discontinuation of the contraceptive pill.

Mechanical devices for preventing fertilization, such as the condom and the diaphragm, are statistically less effective than steroid contraceptives, but they do not involve the risk of certain undesirable side effects, such as an increased susceptibility to thromboembolic diseases, which has been observed in a small percentage of women on "the pill." Since the total number of women who use chemical contraception is very large (many millions), a small percentage may represent a large absolute number. Current research with low-dose steroid contraceptives and with progestogens alone may reveal a diminished risk of thromboembolic complications, since these complications are generally related to estrogen dose. However, reports of increased incidence of pelvic inflammatory disease that can cause infertility in women using IUDs have tempered enthusiasm for this form of contraception, especially in women who plan to become pregnant at a later time.

The mechanism of action of the IUD in preventing fertilization is still not entirely known, but it is believed to work by setting up a sterile inflammatory process in the endometrium. The leukocytic infiltration and breakdown of leukocytes, with the release of a high local concentration of lysosomal enzymes, impairs the ability of the endometrium to accommodate the fertilized ovum. The presence of the device may stimulate tubal motility so that the transit time of the fertilized ovum through the tube is unfavorable for implantation. Access of spermatozoa to the usual site of fertilization is unimpaired.

Shortly after 1900, von Grafenberg introduced metal devices for insertion into the uterine cavity as contraceptives (intrauterine devices, or IUDs). Early experience with these devices was unsatisfactory and they were abandoned for almost 50 years. Experience with various plastic IUDs has been more favorable; they have been found to be about 96% effective. However, a recent wave of lawsuits by injured users of one type of IUD has sharply inhibited the use of these devices in the United States.

On the other side of the coin, other strategies have been used successfully in the *management of infertility*. Gonadotropin mixtures have been used successfully in some women, many of whom were induced to superovulate and, therefore, give birth to multiple babies. The tendency to multiple births is now under somewhat better control due to improved dosage and treatment schedules and the development of noninvasive techniques for detecting the number of preovulatory follicles present. A drug called *clomiphene* (Fig 9–6) has also proved to be effective in inducing ovulation in women with a history of infertility. This drug requires the presence of a functioning hypothalamo-hypophysial unit, for it works by cancelling out influences that impede the release of GnRH by hypothalamic neurones.

In one of the most dramatically prompt applications of new physiologic knowledge to clinical practice ever seen, Knobil's description of the pulsatile release of GnRH in the monkey was quickly followed by the pulsatile administration of GnRH (via a programmable pump) to anovulatory women who had demonstrated the ability to respond to GnRH with an increase in circulating gonadotropin levels. A number of women have had successful pregnancies as a result of this treatment. We predict that, in properly selected individuals, it will continue to be effective in the future.

Until recently, ovulating women with damaged fallopian tubes were hopelessly infertile. Now, following the pioneering studies of Steptoe and Edwards, many such women have been able to experience successful pregnancies as a result of *in vitro fertilization and embryo transfer*. The many successful programs in this field are based on the enormous amount of detailed information that has accumulated during the last two or three decades about the basic biology of human reproduction, much of which was inspired by studies on animal models. The birth of a baby who began as an encounter between a sperm and an ovum in a petri dish is the result of our ability to measure hormone concentrations in blood and antral fluid, to assess oocyte maturation, to apply pharmacologic methods to induce ovulation, to regulate the number of preovulatory follicles and the time of ovulation, and to monitor follicle development. The biology of these processes is complex enough, but when one adds the human, ethical, and legal dimensions of the enterprise, not to mention the logistic challenge of co-ordinating a large number of professional people with complementary skills into an effective team, progress has been phenomenal (see Wolf and Quigley; also G.S. Jones).

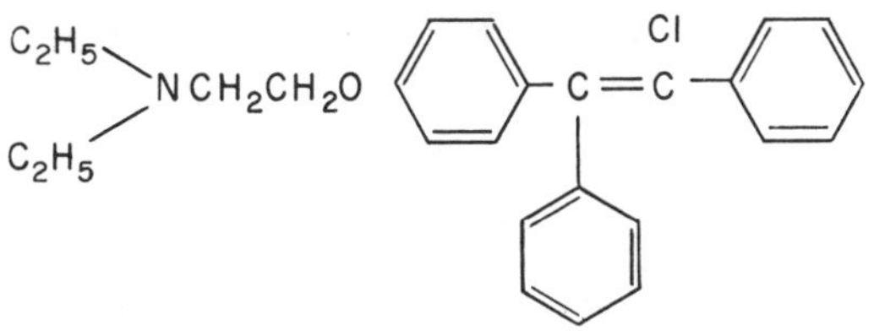

Hormonal Regulations in Pregnancy and Lactation

The participation of the hormones in pregnancy begins before fertilization and implantation of the fertilized ovum, for all of the uterine changes of the menstrual cycle may be regarded as preparation for these events. If fertilization does not occur and there is a decrease in the production of estrogen and progesterone by the corpus luteum, endometrial shedding and bleeding appear, as we have seen. If fertilization and endometrial implantation of the fertilized ovum do occur, there is no drop in production of sex steroids by the corpus luteum, and both estrogen and progesterone continue to exert their effects on the pregnant uterus.

In some species, estrogen and progesterone are produced by the corpus luteum, which remains critically functional throughout pregnancy. In other species, including the human, the corpus luteum provides these steroids during early pregnancy, but later the placenta takes over the job of producing them. Though the corpus luteum persists because it is stimulated by a gonadotropin made by the placenta (chorionic gonadotropin, CG, or hCG), it is not essential for the successful continuation of the pregnancy after about the third month of gestation.

The persistence of the functioning corpus luteum in very early pregnancy, and hence the prevention of menstrual bleeding, is due to the fact that the chorionic tissue begins to produce hCG at least as early as two weeks after ovulation. Thus, the corpus luteum is sustained, although the pituitary trophic influences that normally stop stimulating it at this time are removed. The appearance of chorionic gonadotropin in the urine is the basis for many tests for pregnancy, the first of which was the famous Aschheim-Zondek, or A-Z test. All of these tests are based on the fact that hCG has essentially the same biologic effect as pituitary LH, and therefore is capable of stimulating the ovaries or the testicular Leydig cells to produce their respective steroid hormones in sexually immature animals of many species. Older bioassay pregnancy tests have been replaced by immunologic methods.

As the placenta grows and differentiates, it begins to make more and more estrogen and progesterone, and as the output of these steroids mounts, that of hCG diminishes. The most obvious changes that occur in pregnancy are the great growth of the uterus to

FIG 9–6.
Clomiphene.

accommodate its growing contents, and the growth of the mammary glands, as if in anticipation of their use following parturition. Both estrogen and progesterone participate in the continuing growth and further differentiation of both of these structures. Estrogen, which functions as a specific growth hormone for uterine smooth muscle cells, stimulates the growth of the uterine muscle mass, and thus contributes to the contractile force that will ultimately be needed to expel the fetus at the time of delivery. Progesterone, by its inhibiting effect on uterine smooth muscle, prevents the establishment of effective, coordinated uterine muscle contractions and insures that feeble, ineffectual, fibrillatory contractions persist until the appropriate signals for the expulsion of the fetus are given.

Progesterone, in partnership with estrogen, helps to prepare the mammary glands for lactation by stimulating the formation of new glandular elements. Estrogen and progesterone prevent lactation during pregnancy by blocking the secretory action of prolactin on the mammary gland.

The *placenta* is practically a whole endocrine system in one tissue package. From the rich variety of its hormonal products, it appears to combine the biochemical capability of the pituitary, the ovaries and the corpus luteum. The placenta produces hCG, estrogens (particularly estriol in the human) as well as progesterone. In addition, it produces somatomammotrophin (placental lactogen), placental corticotrophin and placental thyrotrophin. Hypothalamic-releasing factors are also present in the placenta.

The fetus and placenta are so closely associated functionally that they are often referred to as the *fetal-placental unit*. As an example of a biochemical collaboration between the components of the reproductive unit, one can cite the synthesis of estriol by the placenta. The precursor of placental estriol is dehydroepiandrosterone, which is synthesized in large quantities by the fetal adrenal. In fact, maternal estriol excretion may be used as an index of fetal viability. The contributions of mother, placenta, and fetus to the synthesis of estriol are shown in Figure 9–7.

There is indirect evidence that steroids produced by the placenta act locally within the uterus. The birth of twins at different times from the two horns of a bicornuate uterus suggests the possibility of a local ac-

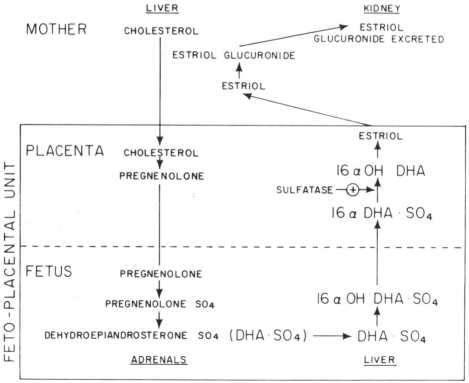

FIG 9–7.
Contributions of mother, fetus, and placenta to synthesis of estriol.

tion of progesterone. Also, Csapo has measured the membrane potential of the endometrium and has found that it is higher at the placental implantation sites than between such sites. The potential of the interplacental sites can be raised to the level of that of the placental sites by local application of progesterone.

The mechanisms involved in *parturition* are not clearly understood, and the stimulus that initiates the train of events that we call labor has not been identified. The mechanisms in all species may not be precisely the same. For example, *progesterone withdrawal* may explain onset of labor in the rabbit, but there is no convincing evidence that a fall in blood progesterone level must occur before the onset of labor in women. *Oxytocin stimulation* could be a component of a complex of labor initiation signals.

One of the most intriguing hypotheses concerning the onset of labor is the *fetal cortisol surge hypothesis* advanced by Liggins, mainly on the basis of observations in pregnant sheep. In imaginative studies, Liggins found that hypophysectomy, adrenalectomy, or blocking the hypophysial-portal circulation of the fetus resulted in prolonged pregnancy. Infusion of cortisol or ACTH into the fetus with intact adrenals brought about premature labor in the pregnant ewe. Although significant reasons exist for not extrapolating the sheep data to the human in toto, it is interesting that as early as 1933 Malpas described prolonged gestation in human pregnancy with an anencephalic (brainless) fetus, and even suggested that a fetal defect in the brain-pituitary-adrenal axis could have been the basis for the delayed labor. (This was 50 years before the chemical characterization of CRF!) One of the appealing features of the cortisol surge hypothesis is the fact that cortisol plays an important role in the final preparation of the lung for extrauterine life (Chapter 11).

The formation of *prostaglandins* by the amnion occurs just before parturition, and there is circumstantial evidence that these compounds, particularly PGF_2 and PGE, may initiate uterine contractions. As mentioned in Chapter 4, the administration of aspirin or other prostaglandin synthesis inhibitors to either women or animals near delivery prolongs gestation. A substance has been found in fetal urine near term that stimulates the production of prostaglandins by amnion cells in monolayer culture.

Synthesizing all of this information into a tidy statement is difficult. The most important concept is that the fetus announces when it is ready to be born. The cortisol surge occurs *within* the fetus and may cause the urinary excretion of a phospholipase-activating substance. This may accumulate in the am-

niotic fluid in sufficiently high concentration to induce synthesis of prostaglandins which then activate the myometrium. Progesterone withdrawal makes its contribution by increasing the number of low resistance junctions between adjacent myometrial cells, thus making coordinated contractions possible. Oxytocin is undoubtedly involved as well, since it has been demonstrated that myometrial cells have an increased number of oxytocin receptors at parturition. Interested readers should consult reports by MacDonald and colleagues (see M.L. Casey et al.).

Other hormones, notably thyroxine and cortisol, circulate in greater than normal amounts during pregnancy and their concentration in the blood progressively increases up to the time of parturition. In both cases, the specific hormone-carrying globulins appear to be synthesized rapidly in the pregnant woman as a result of estrogen action, and they accumulate in the blood. The increased blood levels appear to be set by the fact that more carrier protein accumulates in the blood. In the case of the thyroid hormone, we know that the level of activity of the thyroid gland itself is high because the uptake of tracer doses of ^{131}I by the gland is elevated. This has been attributed to the production of TSH by the placenta. The concentration of free thyroid hormone is the same as in the nonpregnant woman, but free cortisol is slightly elevated because of a decreased rate of removal. Whether or not these events are physiologically important in the maintenance and completion of pregnancy is not known.

In the latter part of pregnancy, urinary excretion of aldosterone is markedly elevated (Venning and Beck). This may be a compensatory response to the salt-losing effect of progesterone. A summary of the hormonal excretion pattern in pregnancy is given in Figure 9–8.

As we have already seen, some of the events associated with parturition may function as important signals for the initiation of *lactation*. Most prominent among these are progesterone and estrogen withdrawal, and the subsequent release of prolactin from inhibition. Prolactin participates in the growth and milk secretory activity of the mammary gland, but the initiation of milk flow, or let-down, is accomplished by way of a neuroendocrine reflex that is initiated by the tactile sensation from the nipple induced by the infant's sucking. The afferent nerves from the nipple carry the message to the CNS, where a connection is made with the preoptic nucleus and a "request" for the posterior pituitary hormone, oxytocin, is made. This octapeptide hormone is then released from the neurohypophysis and travels by way of the bloodstream to the mammary gland where it facilitates the

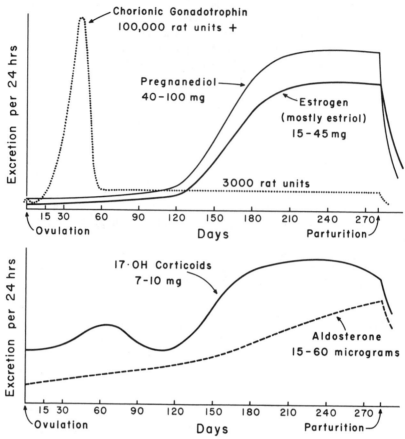

FIG 9–8.
Urinary excretion of hormones in pregnancy. (From Venning EH, Beck JC, in Lloyd CW [ed]: *Endocrinology of Reproduction.* New York, Academic Press, 1959, and also from Houssay BA [ed]: *Human Physiology.* New York, McGraw-Hill Book Co, 1955. Used by permission.)

flow of milk by acting on the myoepithelial cells in the mammary gland (see Chapter 6). As mentioned earlier, oxytocin can also be released in *anticipation* of nursing.

Lactation markedly increases spontaneous food intake in both women and experimental animals. In fact, Kennedy has shown that the lactating rat eats as much spontaneously as the nonlactating animal does if its medial hypothalamic satiety "centers" are destroyed by electrolytic lesions (see Chapter 16). It is almost as if something about the process of lactation resulted in the production of a transitory functional (i.e., reversible) hypothalamic "lesion" of the type that causes obesity in the nonlactating animal. The mechanism of the effect of lactation on spontaneous food intake is not known, but it could somehow be related to the same afferent stimuli that arise in the nipple and that trigger the release of oxytocin. We know of another circumstance in biology in which a

neural signal produces transitory overeating–light-induced premigratory hyperphagia in birds. A possible alternative explanation states that the lactating mammary gland abstracts so much glucose (and other metabolites) from the body pool that the "appestat" is reset at a higher level, in much the way it must be reset as a result of exercise or cold exposure.

The importance of food and water intake in preparation for lactation is suggested by experiments on hypophysectomized rats, in which it was possible to prepare mammary glands for lactation by giving a combination of estrogen, progesterone, growth hormone and prolactin. When insulin was given, however, only estrogen and progesterone were required. This suggests that the pituitary hormones may have functioned by increasing food intake. An adequate supply of food and water is also necessary for the maintenance of lactation at optimal levels.

Insulin and prolactin may have very similar effects

on the mammary gland, since, as we have seen, PRL markedly accelerates the rate of glucose utilization and secondarily stimulates various synthetic processes in the mammary gland, such as lipogenesis from carbohydrate. The mammary gland cell must synthesize fat and protein for secretion in milk, and it appears to combine the metabolic characteristics of an adipose tissue cell, which synthesizes fat for storage, and (for example) an exocrine pancreatic cell, which synthesizes large amounts of protein enzyme precursors.

In addition to an adequate food and water intake, the continuation of lactation, once established, appears to require many hormones. Hypophysectomy prevents lactation, and the thyroid hormone, adrenal hormones and hypophyseal growth hormone all have been implicated in the process.

The return of menstruation and ovulation after parturition is delayed in nursing mothers. The antifertility effects of lactation are associated with high levels of prolactin that fall progressively as the infant's suckling decreases in response to supplementary feeding and weaning. In many nursing mothers, however, the conditions for ovulation may return during lactation, and pregnancy may occur even while lactation continues. In this circumstance, at least, a rising production rate of estrogen and progesterone is not sufficient to prevent the continuation of established lactation.

Cellular Mechanisms of Action of Reproductive Hormones

ESTROGENS

The broad outlines of the mechanism of action of estrogen on sensitive cells were given in the discussion of steroid hormone action in Chapter 2. In fact, much of the work that supports this model was done by students of estrogen action. Some readers may want to review Chapter 2 in relation to information presented in this chapter.

PROGESTERONE

Progesterone appears to have an inhibitory effect on uterine muscle; for example, progesterone treatment renders the myometrium comparatively unresponsive to the stimulatory effect of oxytocin in the rabbit (but *not* in the human!). A similar refractoriness to oxytocin stimulation can be produced by changing the fluid bathing the uterine muscle strips to a high-potassium, low-sodium buffer. Progesterone treatment does, in fact, result in a decrease in potassium and an increase in sodium in the myometrium. The quieting effect of progesterone on uterine contractility may be achieved by a change in the differential permeability of the membranes of smooth muscle cells to sodium and potassium. Progesterone also decreases the number of low resistance pathways (nexuses) among smooth muscle cells (see Ichikawa and Bortoff). As we have seen, this calming effect of progesterone on the uterus may have some importance in the initiation of labor in some species, for the progesterone influence on the uterine muscle may have to be withdrawn before powerful rhythmic contractions can occur.

GONADOTROPINS

Although the mechanism of action of the *gonadotropins* is by no means as well understood as is that of ACTH, recent work has begun to illuminate this problem. Bovine corpus luteum slices increase their production of progesterone when pituitary LH preparations or hCG are added in vitro. These hormones stimulate steroidogenesis in target cells by activating adenyl cyclase. The cAMP thus generated then activates protein kinase, which stimulates steroidogenesis primarily at the cholesterol → pregnenolone step. All of the molecular details of the process are not known, but they are believed to be analogous to those involved in the action of ACTH on adrenal cells (see Chapter 11).

An interesting in vitro effect of prolactin on slices of rat mammary gland of the pregnant rat has been described by McLean, who found that the hormone caused increased glucose utilization, especially for fat formation, and that substrate traffic via the direct oxidative pathway was markedly stimulated.

As noted above, prolactin stimulates synthesis of milk proteins (casein, α lactalbumin) and of lactose, milk sugar. Synthesis of lactose is accomplished by the enzyme lactose synthase, which requires participation of galactosyl transferase and α lactalbumin. Synthesis of casein and α lactalbumin evidently requires new synthesis of the mRNAs for the two proteins. The mechanism by which the protein hormone elicits the selective synthesis of specific mRNAs is presently unknown.

Nonreproductive Effects of Ovarian Steroids

BONE METABOLISM

Estrogen deficiency that occurs prior to completion of puberty may cause a failure of epiphyseal

Girls with this condition may show a retarded bone age on x-ray and may grow abnormally tall. Estrogen treatment accelerates epiphyseal closure in this circumstance. But just as in the case of androgen, severe deficiency of estrogen during the immediate prepuberal growth phase may cause stunting of growth.

The possible role of estrogen deficiency in the development of osteoporosis in postmenopausal women has already been mentioned. The mechanism by which estrogens inhibit bone resorption is not presently understood. Many investigators have searched in vain for estrogen receptors on bone cells; estrogen effects on the bone mineral balance, therefore, are thought to be indirect. Among possible indirect effects of estrogen on bone are the following: (1) stimulation or potentiation of calcitonin release, and, therefore, inhibition of bone resorption; (2) a small compensatory increase in parathyroid hormone release in response to (1); (3) stimulation by parathyroid hormone of the activation of vitamin D in the kidney with the result that (4) intestinal absorption of calcium is increased. The biology of mineral balance in bone will be discussed in detail in Chapter 17.

OTHER EFFECTS

Other nonreproductive effects of estrogens include those on nitrogen retention and on water and electrolyte balance. Estrogens have been reported to have some general protein anabolic effect, but less than that of androgens. Both estrogens and androgens show some activity in anti-inflammatory assays, such as inhibition of the development of paw edema in the rat following the administration of an irritating substance. They also show a minor degree of salt-retaining activity, but less than either the adrenal steroids or androgens. In mice, local application of estrogen to the skin produces cutaneous edema, which reminds us that they are frequently dispensed as a constituent of cosmetics. This kind of self-medication with a powerful drug is not generally encouraged by physicians because some of the material may be absorbed percutaneously and may produce undesirable systemic effects.

In experimental animals, large doses of estrogen may produce cancer of estrogen-sensitive tissues such as the uterus. This may be explained on the basis of the marked stimulation of mitotic activity and cell division that occurs when the hormone is given. This is readily visible in the endometrial gland cells, for example. If such stimulation is intense and prolonged and many cells divide, the statistical probability of the

occurrence of a somatic mutation in the direction of the cancer cell type is greatly increased. There has been a recent report of a high incidence of vaginal cancer among daughters of mothers who were treated with stilbestrol during their pregnancies.

The administration of progesterone to men or women results in salt loss. This effect is more pronounced in treated addisonian patients deficient in adrenocortical hormones. Therefore, the salt loss is believed to be due to an antialdosterone effect of progesterone, which means that (to reverse the usual designation) progesterone is a sort of naturally occurring spirolactone (see Chapter 11).

HEPATIC PROTEIN SYNTHESIS

Estrogens have important effects on the synthesis of specific proteins by the liver. Among such proteins are the following:

1. Hormone carrier proteins (for adrenal glucocorticoid, thyroid, and sex steroid hormones)
2. Clotting factors (II, VII, IX, X)
3. Angiotensinogen (renin substrate)
4. Very low-density lipoproteins (VLDL)
5. High-density lipoproteins (HDL)

This effect of estrogens may complicate diagnosis (as in the case of the hormone carrier proteins) and predispose to thromboembolic disease (clotting factors) or to elevation in blood pressure (angiotensinogen). The effect on HDL may be related to the observation that premenopausal women are less likely than men of similar age to have myocardial infarction (MI). High levels of circulating HDL are associated with decreased risk of MI. (See Chapter 15.)

Hormones and Breast Cancer

Premenopausal breast cancer is often treated by means of some form of estrogen withdrawal or denial, since cancer cells often retain the capacity to respond to hormones that acted upon their cells of origin. This is most often accomplished by surgical removal of the ovaries. If a relapse occurs, tamoxifen, an antiestrogen that prevents the stimulatory effect of estrogen on growth, is commonly used. Progesterone receptors are induced by estrogen; therefore, when tumors are positive for both estrogen and progesterone receptors (indicating that the estrogen receptors are functional), about two-thirds of the patients show remissions. In general, patients with tumors that lack estrogen receptors are unlikely to benefit from estrogen deprivation. Overall, only about 50% of estrogen receptor-positive cancers respond to ovariectomy. This may be due to the fact that the presence of estrogen receptors does not necessarily indicate that they are functional, i.e., that they articulate with a growth-promoting effector system.

Individual cancer cells, whether estrogen-dependent or -independent, synthesize and secrete a variety of identifiable growth factors (somatomedin-like, epidermal growth factor, etc.) when they are grown in culture. Estrogen-dependent cells synthesize these substances (which may act in an autocrine manner on their cells of origin or paracrinely on neighboring cells) in response to the hormone. Estrogen-independent cells apparently can make them without stimulation. The biological behavior of an individual tumor may depend ultimately on the quality and/or quantity of the growth factors it is either induced to synthesize or that it can synthesize autonomously. Study of the relationships among cancer cells, hormones, and growth factors is likely to be among the most exciting areas of research in the near future (Lipman).

Another possible reason for the failure of ovariectomy to cause remission in cancer patients is the variable capacity of women to synthesize estrogen in extraovarian sites, particularly in adipose tissue. The ability of aromatase to transform androgen precursor to estrogen is clearly limited by the supply of androgen. Formerly, hypophysectomy or adrenalectomy was used to eliminate the adrenal as a source of androgen. Currently, a ''medical adrenalectomy'' is achieved by administering the drug *aminoglutethimide,* which inhibits both cholesterol side chain cleavage (important in adrenal androgen synthesis) and (more significantly) the aromatase reaction by interfering with the action of the specific cytochrome P450 enzyme that catalyzes it. To avoid compensatory overstimulation of the adrenals due to the inhibition of cortisol synthesis by aminoglutethimide, cortisol is given to suppress ACTH secretion.

It is obviously inappropriate here to discuss the detailed management of breast cancer, which involves surgery, radiotherapy, and chemotherapy as well as manipulation of the endocrine environment of the tumor. The main points, not only about breast cancer but also about endometrial cancer and cancer of the prostate, are (1) these cancers retain some of the hormone responsiveness of their cells of origin, and this can be exploited in their management; and (2) the more it becomes possible to categorize these cancers with respect to their estrogen, androgen, progesterone, prolactin and growth hormone binding and to correlate hormone-binding characteristics with the results of therapy, the more likely it will be that patient selection for alternative procedures will be done confidently and with a high probability of success.

Relaxin

In 1926, Hisaw discovered that aqueous extracts of sow ovary contained a substance that caused relaxation of the pelvic ligaments of the guinea pig and widening of the symphysis pubis. From this modest beginning, we have witnessed over the past six decades (1) the chemical characterization, synthesis, and cDNA cloning of *relaxins* in several species, including the human; (2) the development of an interesting and important chapter in molecular evolution; and (3) the possibility that a new strategy may be developed in the future that will decrease the need for cesarean section in some women.

Before relaxin was purified, characterized, and synthesized, it was established that it had effects not only on the symphysis pubis (relaxation) but also a softening effect on the cervix of the uterus and a relaxing effect on uterine smooth muscle. Together, two of these effects (widening of the symphysis pubis and cervical softening) appear teleonomically to facilitate the passage of the fetus through the birth canal. Inhibition of uterine contraction would not help the process of parturition very much, so we must assume that this effect of relaxin is overridden by powerful stimulants of uterine muscle contraction we have mentioned.

When the amino acid sequences of human, porcine, and rat relaxin were deduced from the corresponding nucleotide sequences of cloned, complementary DNA, the relaxin molecules were found to resemble insulin and insulin-like growth factor I, or somatomedin C (Chapters 5 and 14). All of these hormones consist of A and B chains bound together by two disulfide bonds which, like the third intra A chain S-S bond, are invariant among them. Although only six amino acids in the A chain (out of 21–29) and eight in the B chain (out of 30–33) are identical in all three hormones, hypothetical three-dimensional models of relaxin and IGF I suggest that these hormones assume tertiary structures similar to that of insulin's, which was determined by x-ray diffraction analysis of Zn-insulin crystals (Chapter 14). All of these hormones are transcribed from their respective genes with a connecting peptide (CP) of varying length between the beginning of the A chain and the end of the B chain, and the CPs are excised from the molecules by surgically precise proteolytic enzymes before they are secreted. The CP excising enzymes for insulin and relaxin differ (trypsin-like versus chymotrypsin-like) but the appropriate one seems to have coevolved with its proper substrate. The placement of S-S bonds, the similarities in biosynthesis and posttranslational processing, the amino acid homologies, and the postulated similarities in three-dimensional shape all argue for the fact that the genes responsible for these three proteins all evolved from a common ancestral gene.

The source of relaxin has long been known to be the corpus luteum, but a beautiful new technique, hybridization histochemistry, has been applied to this problem. In suitably prepared sections of tissue, a high specific activity ^{32}P-labeled cDNA probe for relaxin hybridizes only with its complementary messenger RNA. Cells that contain the message and are therefore actively transcribing the gene can be differentiated from those that do not because they bind the radioactive probe. With this method, high levels of relaxin mRNA were identified in corpora lutea and not in other tissues. Thus, CL cells, which we have been accustomed to think of as steroid hormone-producing factories, also synthesize and secrete a protein hormone.

The *mechanism of action* of relaxin has been studied most intensively in uterine smooth muscle, which is simulated to contract by a Ca^{2+} Calmodulin-mediated phosphorylation of myosin kinase. This, in turn, phosphorylates a specific protein that is associated with the contractile protein, myosin. The myometrium is stimulated to contract by many agonists, including acetyl choline, oxytocin, angiotensin, and prostaglandins, all of which raise the cytosolic Ca^{2+} concentration. Relaxation is caused by two agents, primarily β adrenergic agonists and relaxin. Both of these activate adenylate cyclase and cause an increase in cyclic AMP.

The way in which relaxin and catecholamines cause relaxation of smooth muscle is worth examining as a particularly elegant example of the power of protein phosphorylation in metabolic control mechanisms (see Adelstein). The two kinases, cyclic AMP-dependent and Ca^{2+} Calmodulin-dependent, phosphorylate myosin kinase in different patterns, though they share one phosphorylation site. Cyclic AMP-dependent protein kinase phosphorylates in an additional site, but the double phosphorylation does not activate the enzyme in spite of the fact that one of the sites is the same one used by the activating kinase. However, the double phosphorylation renders the enzyme refractory to activation by Ca^{2+} Calmodulin, and the muscle relaxes because of the removal of its tonic stimulation.

Relaxin also increases cyclic AMP in the chondrocytes of the symphysis pubis, which consists largely of proteoglycans and collagen. When relaxin stimulates chondrocytes, they either secrete depolymerizing enzymes or activators of proteoglycanase or procollagenase, resulting in the breakdown of the major molecules that hold the symphysis pubis together. It is interesting that relaxin, readily demonstrable in fol-licular fluid and ovarian (thecal) cells before ovulation, has been implicated in the process of ovulation, which is brought about by the local production at the site of follicle rupture of depolymerizing enzymes similar to those described above.

Relaxin, found in seminal fluid, may play a role in sperm activation or in modulating some aspect of the physiology of the female generative tract. However, such suggestions, as well as others concerned with possible effects of relaxin in the nonpregnant female, are still speculative. There have been interesting pilot studies in which porcine relaxin has been applied topically to the uterine cervix of women in labor with some labor-shortening effect. Since the human gene has been cloned, it is likely that the human hormone will be made available by recombinant DNA technology and that these studies will be repeated.

Sexual Behavior

Each species has encoded in its DNA elaborate blueprints for the construction of certain kinds of sexual behavioral patterns. In many species, mating behavior may be observed in the decorticate animal but not in the spinally transected animal. Therefore, the neural integrative circuits for sexual behavior in these species lie below the cortex and above the spinal cord. These circuits must be extraordinarily complicated. We may think of them as preprogrammed computers into which information is fed in the form of visual, tactile, olfactory and auditory stimuli, which elicit a response that involves the many widely scattered muscles and nerves involved in mating behavior. There are skeletal muscle reflexes associated with posture and movement and there is a widespread involvement of the autonomic nervous system, particularly those parts of it that are concerned with cardiopulmonary reflexes and those associated with the act of copulation.

Both sexes are believed to possess the central nervous integrative circuitry that is essential for the mediation of both masculine and feminine sex behavior. It is easier to demonstrate this ambivalence in the female than in the male, for one can frequently observe male copulatory thrusting movements in an untreated spayed female dog. In many species, the androgen-treated female may show typical male mounting behavior and assume dominance over females—and even over males. An androgen-treated hen quickly climbs to the top of the barnyard peck order.

The effects of castration on sexual behavior vary from species to species. In man, as has been indicated, prepuberal castration abolishes sexual behavior, whereas postpuberal orchiectomy may only diminish it. In woman, oophorectomy does not eliminate sex interest and activity or interfere with any major aspect of female sexual behavior, but adrenalectomy does. Full sexual activity can be restored to the prepuberally castrate male animal by androgen treatment, and the same is true of female animals treated with estrogen if they belong to a species in which sexual activity is abolished by estrogen deprivation.

Certain regions of the hypothalamus have been identified that are deeply involved in the central integration of sexual behavior. Lesions in the posterior hypothalamus in both male and female rats abolish such behavior, and these lesions are not in the same place as are those that interfere with the production and release of hypophysial gonadotropins.

It had been assumed that the central structures associated with mediating and integrating sexual behavior are under the influence of the sex steroids. There was, however, no direct proof of a local effect of a sex steroid in the brain until Harris performed the ingenious experiment of inserting an ester of a synthetic estrogen (stilbestrol) into that part of a spayed cat's hypothalamus that had previously been associated with sexual behavior. The stilbestrol ester's solubility characteristics were such that it could diffuse for short distances locally, but not enough of it entered the bloodstream to affect the reproductive organs. By this maneuver, a cat that had greeted potential mates with hostile, vicious, spitting, back-arching behavior was transformed into one that readily assumed the female copulatory posture when confronted with a male. Implantation of similar amounts of estrogen into the cerebellum, preoptic region, caudate nucleus, thalamus or amygdaloid nucleus did not elicit normal sexual behavior in similar experiments. Hypothalamic lesions prevent sexual behavior in animals, even in the presence of adequate estrogen.

Although the neural machinery for sexual behavior may be subcortical, there is abundant evidence that cortical influences play heavily upon it, especially in man, certain primates, and the guinea pig. Young has demonstrated that guinea pigs reared in solitary confinement have an impairment of sexual activity compared with those raised in litters. This immediately brings to mind the experiments of Harlow, who raised baby monkeys with artificial cloth-and-wire mothers and discovered that adult males so raised, when confronted with female monkeys, were completely disinterested in them. Successfully bred female monkeys with the same history showed not just an absence of affection for their young but actual hostility toward them. These experiments vividly illustrate the role of learning and conditioning in the modulation and modification of instinctive patterns of behavior.

In man, a moral, social and cultural environmental mosaic of influences has produced a complex cortical overlay on the basic central integrative structures for sexual behavior. That "problems of living" in the sphere of sexual behavior can occur in the absence of any readily detectable disorder of the endocrine or nervous system is beyond doubt. It is equally true that emotional difficulties can work either through the behavioral brain mechanisms or through those brain mechanisms involved in maintaining the integrity of the endocrine system to produce functional changes in the physiologic machinery concerned with reproduction. It is also true that behavioral disorders may be secondary to disease of the endocrine glands.

Our comments on the origins of homosexuality in the male (Chapter 8) apply to the female as well.

BIBLIOGRAPHY

Abe H, Engler D, Molitch ME, et al: Vasoactive intestinal polypeptide is a physiological mediator of prolactin release in the rat. *Endocrinology* 1985; 116:1383.

Adelstein RS, Pato MD, Conti MA: The role of phosphorylation in regulating contractile proteins. *Adv Cyclic Nucleotide Protein Phosphorylation Res* 1981; 14:361.

Barraclough CA, Wise PM, Selmanoff MK: A role for catecholamines in the regulation of gonadotropin secretion. *Recent Prog Horm Res* 1984; 40:487.

Beyer C (ed): *Endocrine Control of Sexual Behavior*. New York, Raven Press, 1979.

Bryant-Greenwood CD: Relaxin as a new hormone. *Endocr Rev* 1982; 3:62.

Bugnon C, Bloch B, Fellman D: Cytoimmunologic study of the ontogenesis of the gonadotropic hypothalamopituitary axis in the human fetus. *J Steroid Biochem* 1977; 8:565.

Casey ML, Winkel CA, Porter JC, et al: Endocrine regulation of the initiation and maintenance of parturition in women. *Clin Perinatol* 1983; 10:709.

Channing CP, Tsafriri A: Mechanism of action of the luteinizing hormone and follicle-stimulating hormone on the ovary in vitro. *Metabolism* 1977; 26:413.

Channing CP, Gordon WL, Liu W-K, et al: Physiology and biochemistry of ovarian inhibin. *Proc Soc Exp Biol Med* 1985; 178:339.

Davidson JM, Levine S: Endocrine regulation of behavior. *Ann Rev Physiol* 1977; 34:475.

Dickson RB, McManaway ME, Lippman ME: Estrogen-induced factors of breast cancer cells partially replace estrogen to promote tumor growth. *Science* 1986; 232:1540.

Espey LL: Ovarian proteolytic enzymes and ovulation. *Biol Reprod* 1974; 10:216.

Ferin MF, Van Vugt D, Wardlaw S: The hypothalamic control of the menstrual cycle and the role of endogenous opioid peptides. *Recent Prog Horm Res* 1984; 40:441.

Fishman J: Aromatic hydroxylation of estrogens. *Ann Rev Physiol* 1983; 45:61.

Gibbons JM, Mitnick M, Chieffo V: *In vitro* synthesis of TSH- and LH-releasing factors by human placenta. *Am J Obstet Gynecol* 1975; 121:127.

Gray LA, Christopherson WM, Hoover RN: Estrogens and endometrial carcinoma. *Obstet Gynecol* 1977; 49:385.

Grumbach MM: Control of the onset of puberty. *Excerpta Med ICS* 1983; 598:3.

Hsu CJ, McCormack SM, Sanborn BM: The effect of relaxin on cyclic adenosine 3′, 5′-monophosphate concentrations in rat myometrial cells in culture. *Endocrinology* 1985; 116:2029.

Hsueh AJW, Adashi EY, Jones PBC, et al: Hormonal regulation of the differentiation of cultured ovarian granulosa cells. *Endocr Rev* 1984; 5:76.

Ichikawa S, Bortoff A: Tissue resistance of the progesterone-dominated rabbit myometrium. *AM J Physiol* 1970; 219:1763.

Jones GS: Update on *in vitro* fertilization. *Endocr Rev* 1984; 5:52.

Jordan VC: Biochemical pharmacology of antiestrogen action. *Pharmacol Rev* 1984; 36:245.

Jost A, Picon I: Hormonal control of fetal development and metabolism. *Adv Metab Disord* 1970; 4:123.

Kemp BE, Niall HD: Relaxin. *Vitam Horm* 1984; 41:79.

Kirchner MA, Zucker IR, Jespersen D: Ovarian and adrenal vein studies in women with idiopathic hirsutism, in James VHT, Serio J, Giusti G (eds): *Endocrine Function of the Human Ovary*. New York, Academic Press, 1976, pp 443–455.

Kumar R, Cohen WR, Silva P, et al: Elevated 1,25-dihydroxyvitamin D plasma levels in normal human pregnancy and lactation. *J Clin Invest* 1979; 63:342.

Leake RD, Waters CB, Rubin RT, et al: Oxytocin and prolactin responses in long-term breast feeding. *Obstet Gynecol* 1983; 62:565.

Leblanc H, Lachelin GCL, Abu-Fadil S, et al: Effects of dopamine infusion on pituitary hormone secretion in humans. *J Clin Endocrinol Metab* 1976; 43:668.

LeMaire WT, March JM: Inter-relations between prostaglandins, cyclic AMP, and steroids in ovulation. *J Reprod Fertil* 1975; 22(suppl):53.

Leong DA, Frawley LS, Neill JD: Neuroendocrine control of prolactin secretion. *Ann Rev Physiol* 1983; 45:109.

Liggins GC: Initiation of parturition. *Br Med Bull* 1979; 35:145.

Longscope C, Pratt JH, Schneider SH, et al: Aromatization of androgens by muscle and adipose tissue in vivo. *J Clin Endocrinol* 1978; 46:146.

McNatty KP: Cyclic changes in antral fluid hormone concentrations in humans, in Ross GT, Lipsett MB (eds): *Clinics in Endocrinology and Metabolism*, vol 7. Philadelphia, WB Saunders Co, 1978, pp 577–600.

McNatty KP, Lun S, Fannin J, et al: The recruitment of an ovarian follicle for ovulation. *Excerpta Med ICS* 1983; 598:73.

McNeilly AS, Robinson ICAF, Houston MJ, et al: Release of oxytocin and prolactin in response to suckling. *Br Med J* 1983; 286:257.

Naor Z, Molcho J, Hermon J, et al: Phospholipid turnover and GnRH action in the pituitary and gonads. *Excerpta Med ICS* 1984; 56:245.

Nicol CS (ed): Prolactin symposium. *Fed Proc* 1980; 39:2561–2598.

Odell WD: Physiology of the reproductive system in women, in DeGroot LJ (ed): *Textbook of Endocrine Physiology*. New York, Grune & Stratton, 1978.

Page EW, Villee CA, Villee DB: *Human Reproduction: Essentials of Reproductive and Perinatal Medicine,* ed 3. Philadelphia, WB Saunders Co, 1981.

Rondell P: Role of steroids in the process of ovulation. *Biol Reprod* 1974; 10:199.

Salhanick HA: Basic studies on aminoglutethimide. *Cancer Res* 1982; 42:3315S.

Serra GB: The ovary, in Martini L (ed): *Comprehensive Endocrinology Series*. New York, Raven Press, 1983.

Speroff L, Van de Wiele RL: Regulation of the human menstrual cycle. *Am J Obstet Gynecol* 1971; 109:234.

Talo A, Csapo AI: Conduction of electrical activity in late pregnant and parturient rabbit uteri. *Physiol Chem Phys* 1970; 2:489.

Tepperman HM, Beydoun SN, Abdul-Karim RW: Drugs affecting myometrial contractility in pregnancy. *Clin Obstet Gynecol* 1977; 20:423.

Wolf DP, Quigley MM (eds): *Human In Vitro Fertilization and Embryo Transfer*. New York, Plenum Publishing Corp, 1984.

Yen SCC, Jaffe RB (eds): *Reproductive Endocrinology: Physiology, Pathophysiology, and Clinical Management*. Philadelphia, WB Saunders Co, 1978.

Zuckerman S, Baker TG: The development of the ovary and the process of oogenesis, in Zuckerman S, Weir BJ (eds): *The Ovary*, vol 1. New York, Academic Press, 1977, pp 41–76.

The Thyroid

10

The Thyroid

Physicians have been interested in the thyroid gland from the beginning of recorded medical history. The accompanying chronology points to a long tradition of cooperation between clinician and laboratory worker in the study of thyroidology. The main reason for the modern physician's preoccupation with the thyroid is the existence of certain diseases, which are grouped as hypothyroid and hyperthyroid states. With increasing knowledge of the facts of thyroid physiology and biochemistery, more and more refined diagnostic and therapeutic methods have been, and are being, applied to this group of disorders.

The purpose of this chapter is not so much to discuss diseases of the thyroid gland as to describe, insofar as this is possible, some of what is known about the iodine cycle and its relation to thyroid physiology in animals and man. Each animal is part of a continuum with its environment with respect to such factors as food and water supply, oxygen and temperature. He or she is also dependent on his or her environment for certain trace substances, such as iodide. A knowledge of the way in which iodide is used by the body for synthesis of thyroid hormones and the role of these hormones in the vital economy of the body is the basis of modern management of thyroid disease.

Nutritional Requirement for Iodide

Although dried seaweed and sea sponge had been fed to patients with goiter by Egyptian physicians in antiquity, a clear relationship between iodine lack and goiter was established only in this century by Marine.

He showed convincingly the high incidence of endemic goiter in an inland population and demonstrated that the disease could be prevented by the administration of as little as 2 gm of potassium iodide twice yearly. The amounts of iodine involved in goiter prevention are small: only about 100–700 μg of iodide is ingested daily. When the amount of iodide available to the thyroid is markedly lowered, there is a sort of "work hypertrophy" of the gland, which may take the form of diffuse hypertrophy and hyperplasia. Whenever cell division is stimulated, there is the statistical possibility of an increased rate of somatic mutation; therefore, it is not surprising to see adenomatous growth in some iodine-deficient glands.

Most patients with endemic goiter compensate successfully for the lack of iodine intake and are able to maintain normal levels of thyroid hormone output. Some, however, become hypothyroid, and in these instances the disease probably represents the result of the interplay between an unfavorable environment and an inborn predisposition. When endemic goiter was much more prevalent than it is now, it was not unusual for iodine-deficient goitrous mothers to give birth to cretinous babies. One of the most effective methods of preventing goiter in endemic areas is the addition of iodide to table salt.

A quantitative accounting for the iodine economy in the human being is given in Figure 10–1. In this diagram, the areas of the bars are drawn to scale so that one can quickly see the relationship among the intrathyroidal iodine pool, ingested iodide, excreted iodide, and circulating organic and inorganic iodine. It is apparent that, in terms of daily requirement, a large store of hormone is maintained in the follicles of the thyroid. The system is a remarkably parsimonious one, since at low intakes the thyroid adapts by increasing its ability to take up I⁻. This is due to enhanced iodide transporting capacity, but, since iodide transported into the thyroid cell is quickly oxidized and incorporated into organic molecules ("organified"), it is effectively "trapped." The fecal loss in most animals is extremely small owing to the efficient enterohepatic retrieval of conjugated thyroid hormones secreted in bile. In humans, there is very little enterohepatic circulation of thyroid hormones.

The structures of some biologically important iodinated compounds are given in Figure 10–2.

Hypothalamic-Pituitary Control of TSH Secretion

The general outline of the control of TSH (Fig 10–3) secretion conforms with the model presented in Chapter 5. As we have seen, peptidergic neurons in the preoptic area of the hypothalamus synthesize and release TRH into the pituitary portal system. Measurements of circulating TSH over 24-hour sleep-wake cycles show that TRH, like other releasing factors, is secreted episodically day and night, but that a peak in TSH occurs just before the onset of sleep. The level declines through the night thereafter, sug-

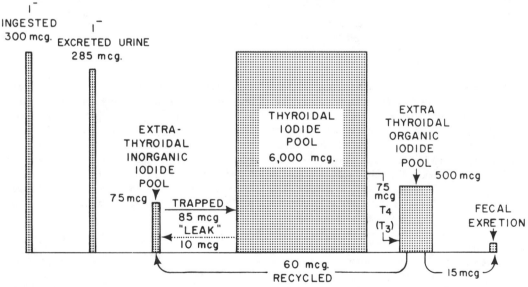

FIG 10–1.
Iodide balance in the human.

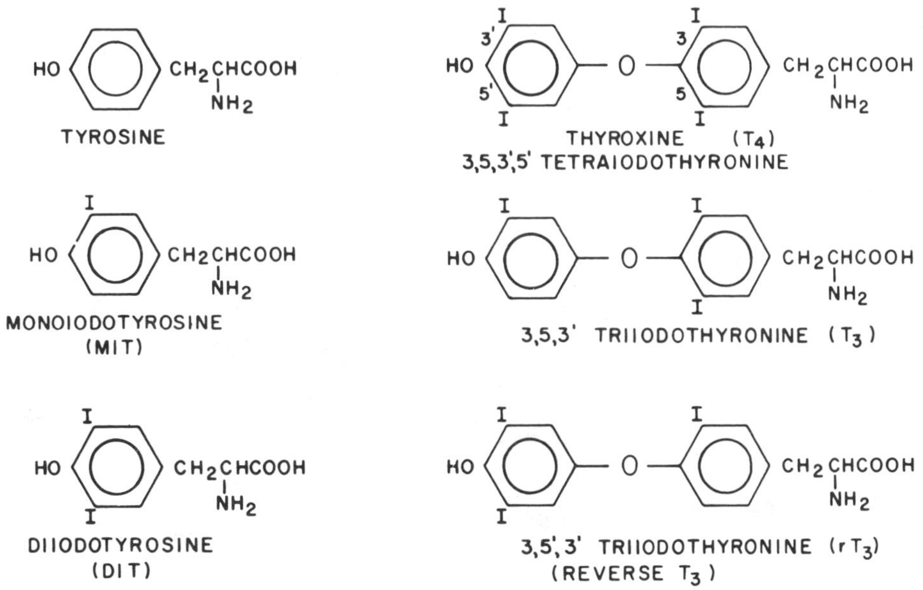

FIG 10–2.
Tyrosine and some of its iodinated derivatives.

gesting that an inhibitory influence on TRH secretion is generated during sleep.

In addition to *sleep-related* fluctuations in TRH, there is evidence to suggest participation of the TRH-TSH system in *stress responses* and in *adaptation to cold temperature*. In nonspecific stress (e.g., trauma, anesthesia), TRH secretion is inhibited and is thus in the category of gonadotropins. Thyroid function has long been associated with adaptation to cold temperature; indeed, the temperature-regulating center of the hypothalamus is near the area occupied by TRH-producing neurons. Increased production of thyroid hormone participates in the adaptive nonshivering thermogenesis that occurs in animals, but an increase in TSH in response to cold exposure in humans has been demonstrated only in infants and in young children during surgical hypothermia. The adaptation of adult humans to cold temperatures involves mainly the wearing of clothing and controlling the temperature of the environment.

Although the identity of "the" thyrotrophin release-*inhibiting* factor is not known with certainty, there is some evidence that *somatostatin* may perform this physiologic function. Arimura and Schally have found that passively immunizing rats with antisomatostatin antiserum resulted in both an elevation of basal TSH levels and an enhanced TSH response to TRH infusion. This suggests that somatostatin may exert a tonic control on TRH release. In addition, inhibition of TSH release by *dopamine* and increased

release of TSH following administration of a dopamine-blocking drug (metoclopramide) indicate a physiologic role for dopamine in TSH release inhibition. As in the case of prolactin release inhibition, dopamine probably acts directly on the pituitary cell.

The major inhibitory influence on TSH secretion is an increase in the level of circulating thyroid hormone, by which, after a lag period during which protein synthesis must occur, the thyrotrophe in the pituitary is rendered resistant to the stimulatory action of TRH. This is now believed to be the major site of feedback inhibition by thyroid hormone, but binding sites for triiodothyronine (T_3) have been found in the hypothalamus, and a regulatory role of thyroid hormones on TRH cannot be ruled out.

Other hormones also modulate the response of the pituitary to TRH. *Estrogen* sensitizes the thyrotrophe to TRH and exaggerates its TSH secretory response. *Glucocorticoids* and *growth hormone* inhibit the thyrotrophe response to TRH.

The *monoaminergic neural control* of TRH-secreting neurons has not been as clearly worked out as it has for other peptidergic neurons, but it is probable that the three known suprahypothalamic influences on TRH secretion—sleep, cold temperature and nonspecific stress—use different brain circuits, which employ different neurotransmitters. Norepinephrine, acting via α receptors, is probably the most important transmitter involved in stimulating TRH release.

TRH, as we saw in Chapter 5, is a powerful stim-

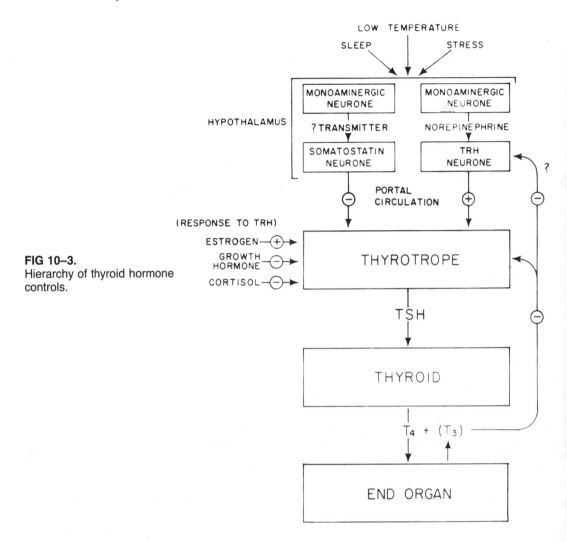

FIG 10–3.
Hierarchy of thyroid hormone controls.

ulator of prolactin secretion as well as that of TSH. In fact, it has been used to stimulate milk secretion in mothers with inadequate lactation response to suckling. It is improbable that TRH is "the" PRL-releasing factor, since TSH and PRL secretion are readily dissociable.

The discovery of TRH, the first hypothalamic peptide to be purified, identified and synthesized, was a major event in biology. The development of extremely sensitive methods of detecting the tripeptide led to the remarkable finding that, though the concentration of TRH in the hypothalamus is very high, more than 80% of the TRH in brain is extrahypothalamic. The pineal gland contains large amounts of TRH. That the extrahypothalamic TRH originates where it is found is suggested by the fact that it persists all over the brain when the hypothalamic neurons that produce it are destroyed. Although the function

of TRH outside the hypothalamus is unknown, the tripeptide has been reported to have both behavioral and electrophysiologic effects on the nervous system (see Reichlin).

The cellular mechanism of action of TRH on the thyrotrope involves binding to a specific receptor and TSH secretion stimulation by an increase in cytosolic Ca^{2+} concentration. It is likely that stimulated polyphosphatidyl inositol turnover supplies the significant second messengers in the response since increased diacylglycerol concentrations have been reported in a pituitary cell line (GH_3) following TRH stimulation (Martin and Kowalchyk). It is not yet certain that thyrotropes respond to the hormone as GH_3 cells do (Woeber and Braverman). Stimulation of TSH secretion initially does not require protein synthesis, but continued TRH stimulation ultimately results in enhanced TSH synthesis by an unknown mechanism.

Thyroid-Stimulating Hormone

Thyrotrophin (TSH) is a glycoprotein with a molecular weight of about 29,000. As we have seen, it shares a subunit with pituitary LH and with hCG. TSH may have a *developmental effect* on the thyroid follicular cell even before the appearance of thyroid follicles, for Lissitzky et al. have shown that thyroid cells in vitro, dispersed by treatment with proteolytic enzymes, reassemble into recognizable follicles when TSH is added to the medium. The reassembly occurs only after several hours, and it is prevented by inhibitors of RNA and protein synthesis. The inference is strong that TSH elicits synthesis of one or more membrane components that are important for cell-cell recognition.

The developed follicular cell is dependent on continuing stimulation by TSH for its normal function. Although the thyroid cell of a TSH-deprived animal can still concentrate iodide to a small extent, hormone synthesis and secretion are greatly depressed. TSH stimulation arouses the cell in two phases: (1) a series of events occur that do not require RNA synthesis; and (2) later, cell growth, mitotic activity and cell division occur. The thyroid cell can be stimulated to produce and secrete inappropriately large amounts of thyroid hormone either by TSH or by a variety of TSH-like globulins that have the characteristics of antibodies.

The *TSH receptor* has been studied extensively (see Kohn et al. for a recent review). One distinctive feature of the receptor is its apparently compound nature; it consists of two separate domains, one, a glycoprotein, and the other, a ganglioside (i.e., a sialic acid containing glycolipid). The TSH molecule must interact with both of these in order to initiate a complete biological response.

The glycoprotein part of the receptor consists of a tetramer with a molecular weight of about 160–180 K. It bears a family resemblance to the insulin receptor (to be discussed in detail in Chapter 14) and the IgG molecule, which consists of pairs of heavy and light chains linked by S-S bonds. The IgG molecule acts as a lymphocyte receptor. Many observers have commented on the possible evolutionary significance of similarities in receptor chemical morphology.

It is remarkable that the ganglioside with the greatest ability to inhibit TSH binding to thyroid membranes could not be detected in brain (i.e., it is tissue specific). Reinsertion of the specific ganglioside into ganglioside-deficient membranes corrected the inability of these membranes to bind TSH and to produce cyclic AMP in response to the hormone.

The TSH receptor complex, as a consequence of TSH binding, initiates complex biological responses to at least four intracellular messengers: cyclic AMP, inositol triphosphate, diacylglycerol, and Ca^{2+} Calmodulin (Fig 10–4). The activation of adenylate cyclase in thyroid membranes by TSH was discovered early, but since the discovery of the stimulatory and inhibitory G proteins, G_s and G_i, the problem has been reexamined. In experiments in which TSH was given alternatively with either cholera toxin (a G_s protein activator) or pertussis toxin (a G_i protein inhibitor), the conclusion was reached that most of the adenylate cyclase activation resulting from TSH was due to inhibition of G_i. In any case, cyclic AMP accumulates in thyroid cells following TSH stimulation. Many of the biological effects of such stimulation, including the complex morphological ones to be described below, can be duplicated by dibutyryl cyclic AMP. Until recently, all of these effects were attributed to the phosphorylation of an unknown number of unidentified proteins by cyclic AMP-dependent protein kinase.

When a new discovery is made, old observations are quickly reexamined in its light. Thus, when the phosphatidyl inositol-inositol triphosphate-diacylglycerol-C kinase story unfolded, it was found that this messenger system is responsive to TSH, particularly in the dog thyroid. Since it was known that the full biological response of the thyroid cell to TSH stimulation requires Ca^{2+}, it was already apparent that Ca^{2+} Calmodulin was a likely mediator and/or modulator of the intracellular events set in motion by TSH. Thus, as in so many other systems, we can conceive of the TSH-receptor interaction as the first step in a complex chain of events that leads, by phosphorylation, to alterations in the activity state of multiple, strategically placed proteins—in membranes, microtubules, microfilaments, enzyme systems, and ribosomes. Some of these are substrates for cyclic AMP-dependent protein kinase; others, for C kinase; still others, for Ca^{2+} Calmodulin-activated kinase; perhaps others may be affected by Ca^{2+} directly. The identification of protein kinase substrates and elucidation of their individual roles in the total TSH response will require much future work.

Attempts have been made to analyze the effects of a large battery of monoclonal antibodies raised to the TSH receptor. Some of these proved to be stimulatory, i.e., they mimicked the effect of TSH. Others were inhibitory, i.e., they blocked the stimulatory effect of TSH. A third group, called "mixed," stimulated both TSH-like growth stimulating activity in thyroid cells as well as adenylate cyclase-activating activity, but in comparison with TSH, they were much more powerfully growth stimulating than cy-

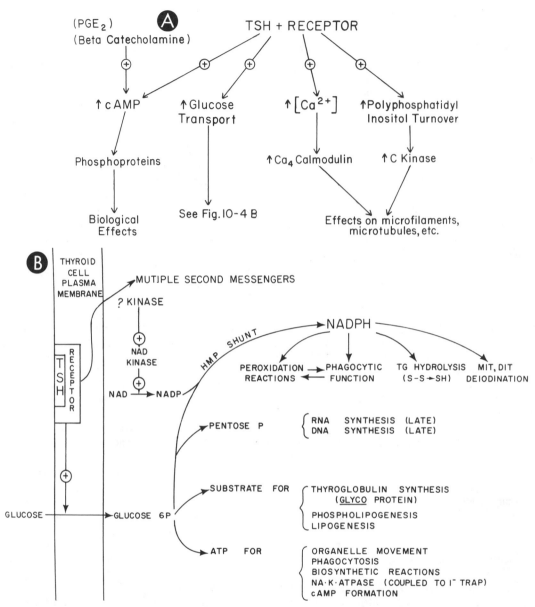

FIG 10–4.
A, a summary of multiple intracellular second messengers elicited by TSH interaction with its receptor. **B,** some of the consequences of stimulation of glucose transport by TSH and activation of NAD kinase by one of the many second messengers generated by TSH-receptor interaction. By "steering" glucose metabolism over the hexose monophosphate (HMP) shunt, NADP stimulates the production of NADPH, which is distinctively required for many thyroid cell functions. (*NADP* = nicotinamide adenine dinucleotide phosphate; *NADPH* = reduced NADP.)

clase stimulating. This suggests that different agonists can bind to the same receptor but entrain different transducing responses. This has some significance for the TSH-mimetic immunoglobulins (to be discussed below) for it has become apparent that many different kinds of antithyroid autoantibodies may be generated in people.

The *morphologic changes* in the thyroid follicular cell following TSH stimulation are impressive (Fig 10–5). The thyroid cell is highly polarized: it displays

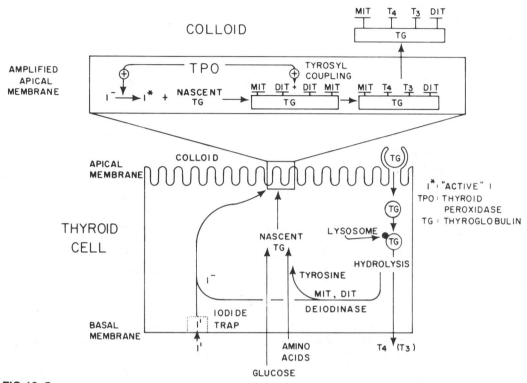

FIG 10–5.

Intrathyroidal iodide cycle. *MIT* = monoiodotyrosine; *DIT* = diiodotyrosine; T_4 = thyroxine; T_3 = triiodothyronine; *TRAP* = I^- transporter.

many microvilli (and thus a very large surface area) at its apical end, which is adjacent to the colloid store of the follicle. Its basal surface communicates with the circulation and presumably carries the receptor-cyclic AMP generating complex. Within a few minutes after exposure to TSH, colloid droplets appear at the apical ends of cells near the colloid surface. Microvillous processes "bite" small droplets of colloid from the large community store.

Concurrently, electron-dense organelles identifiable as lysosomes begin to migrate from the basal end of the cell toward the apical end. There, fusion of lysosomes and colloid droplets occurs and the phagolysosome so formed migrates to the basal end of the cell, becoming progressively smaller as it moves. Thyroglobulin (TG) hydrolysis occurs within the phagolysosome and the products of hydrolysis diffuse into the cell water. The hormones, largely T_4 and a small amount of T_3 under ordinary circumstances, diffuse out of the cell and into the general circulation. Monoiodotyrosine (MIT) and diiodotyrosine (DIT), also products of TG hydrolysis, are deiodinated by an intrathyroidal deshalogenase enzyme, which functions as a scavenger of iodide and tyrosine, which are then

recycled. All of these striking morphologic changes are seen not only after TSH administration but also after treatment with db cAMP.

Microtubular and microfilamentous processes must participate in some of these events, most probably in colloid ingestion and in organelle translocation. The effect of either TSH or cAMP on the overall morphologic response is blocked either by colchicine, a microtubule toxin, or by cytochalasin B, which interferes with microfilament function.

TSH affects all phases of *iodine metabolism*. The earliest effect is that just described: a stimulation of TG hydrolysis and hormone release. Within several hours a membrane change ocurs as a result of synthesis of new RNA and protein. As a result, I^- *efflux* is first stimulated, but later I^- *uptake* is increased. There is an early stimulation of the organification of iodine and increase in the capacity of the I^- pump, or trap. All components of the intracellular iodine cycle operate at a higher level, and concurrently the rate of synthesis of thyroglobulin is accelerated.

TSH effects on *carbohydrate metabolism* are striking, and it is interesting to attempt to understand how these effects are related to those on iodine metabolism and to other parts of the overall TSH response (see Fig 10–4,B). The early stimulation of glucose utilization and oxygen consumption does not require protein synthesis. Glucose influx is increased, possibly by a mechanism that depends on the TSH-receptor transaction but does not require cAMP. There is an increase in NAD kinase activity, which has the effect of increasing NADP. Although the percent of glucose believed to traverse the hexose-monophosphate (HMP) (pentose phosphate) shunt is small, the large influx of glucose has the effect of generating NADPH, the cofactor that is required for so many reactions involved in iodine metabolism in the thyroid cell. Moreover, pentose produced by the direct oxidative pathway may be important in RNA and DNA metabolism. Glucose is also required for synthesis of thyroglobulin and other proteins, as well as for lipid synthesis. Energy generated by glucose oxidation by the Emden-Meyerhof pathway and oxidative metabolism may be used by the newly activated cell for a variety of purposes, a few of which are listed in Figure 10–4,B.

The effects of TSH on *phospholipid* metabolism are striking and complex. We assume that the stimulation of phospholipid synthesis, which occurs after a brief initial period of phospholipid breakdown, is somehow required for the extensive membrane-remodeling processes suggested by our description of the morphologic effects of TSH. Curiously, however, this is one aspect of TSH function that has not yet been convincingly duplicated by cAMP. The stimulation of polyphosphatidyl turnover by TSH has been mentioned.

TSH has stimulatory effects on *protein* synthesis that may involve accelerated amino acid transport, increased ATP (and GTP) availability, as well as effects at the translational and transcriptional levels. RNA and DNA synthesis, as measured by the rate of incorporation of radioactively labeled precursors, is increased by TSH.

In summary, the coordinated set of events that results from the interaction of TSH with its plasma membrane receptor includes changes in membrane permeability, increased influx of substrates, cAMP formation, polyphosphatidyl inositol turnover, increased cytosolic Ca^{2+} concentration, and phosphorylation of an unknown number of protein kinase substrate proteins. The highly specialized thyroid cell responds to TSH by increasing proteolysis of stored thyroglobulin, increasing the rate of discharge of T_4 and T_3 and increasing the trapping and organification of iodide. As the stimulus continues to be applied, cell hypertrophy and, eventually, cell replication occur.

TSH-MIMETIC IMMUNOGLOBULINS

In Graves' disease, TSH is essentially absent from the circulation and, unlike the normal response, thyroid function is not suppressible by T_3. The cause of Graves' disease is not known, but most observers believe it to be in the category of autoimmune diseases.

In the 1960s, there was considerable interest in the possibility that a substance known as long-acting thyroid stimulator (LATS) was the force behind the inappropriate overproduction of thyroid hormone in Graves' disease. LATS was found to be an immunoglobulin of the IgG class, and it generally duplicated the thyroid-stimulating effect of TSH by a cAMP mechanism. Subsequently it was shown to displace TSH from its receptor on thyroid cell membranes. Initial enthusiasm waned when careful study of many patients revealed no convincing correlation between either the presence and absence of hyperthyroidism or the titers of LATS and severity of the disease when LATS was demonstrable.

However, out of the work on LATS, a new family of globulins, HTSI (human thyroid stimulatory immunoglobulins), has been found that resembles both TSH and LATS in its stimulatory effect on the thyroid. HTSI appears to be present in most patients with Graves' disease. The duration of their stimulatory effect is slightly longer than that of TSH (peak at 30 minutes versus 7 minutes for TSH), it is much shorter than that of LATS, whose stimulatory effect persists for hours. HTSI displaces both TSH and LATS from thyroid membrane receptors, which suggests that all of these substances, hormone and immunoglobulins alike, share some configuration that not only binds to the receptor but activates adenylate cyclase as well. There are many different kinds of autoantibodies to thyroid antigens. In addition to stimulatory ones mentioned above, there are also destructive ones that may cause inflammatory devastation of the thyroid gland (Hashimoto's disease). TSH-blocking antibodies have also been described.

Intrathyroidal Iodine Cycle

THE IODIDE CONCENTRATING MECHANISM

The iodide trap is sometimes called the iodide pump, or concentrating mechanism (see Fig 10–5). The blood flow of the thyroid gland is so great and the avidity of the thyroid cell for I^- so great that the gland, in spite of its comparatively small size, is able to sequester 20%–40% of an administered dose of radioactive iodine. Most of what is not retained by the thyroid appears in the urine; together, thyroid trapping and urinary excretion account for over 90% of a test dose. Small amounts may be secreted in gastric juice, salivary glands, and sweat.

The iodide pump shows all the characteristics of an active transport system, since I^- is concentrated to the extent of 30–40 times the serum concentration against both an electric and chemical gradient and since the transport process is inhibited by ions of similar size and shape (perchlorate and thiocyanate). Energy expenditure is required for the successful operation of the I^- concentrating mechanism. The system is saturable and is autoinhibited by large excesses of I^-. The observation that cardiac glycosides (e.g., oubain) inhibit the action of the trap led to the hypothesis that NA^+K^+ ATPase activity is coupled with the I^- trapping function of the thyroid cell.

The most important single factor responsible for the level of operation of the trap is the amount of trophic stimulation that the gland receives. The hypophysectomized animal or the hypopituitary patient shows very low thyroid I^- trapping ability. Treatment with TSH may increase trapping ability to supernormal levels. In hyperthyroidism, trapping of I^- is much higher than normal; it must therefore be assumed that globulins that mimic TSH also can maintain the trapping mechanism at a high level. In general, radioactive iodine uptake parallels thyroid status: it is low in hypothyroidism and high in hyperthyroidism. However, the antecedent iodine intake history of the subject must be taken into account in interpreting uptake results, since iodine deficiency results in extremely high uptakes, and intake of iodine (iodine-containing medications and white bread processed with iodate) may cause spurious low values. The radioactive iodine uptake test, although still useful in diagnosis, has been overshadowed by recent developments in the field of hormone measurements in blood. Diagnostic use of radioiodine uptake requires administration of only a few *microcuries* of a seven-day half-life isotope. The substitution of technetium for I^- reduces the radiation dose even more.

Certain ions are inhibitors of the iodide transport system, notably SCN^-, ClO_4^-, NO_3^-, and BF_4^-. Perchlorate (ClO_4^-) is used in the diagnosis of one of the inborn errors of thyroid metabolism, a defect in organification (others will be mentioned later). When a tracer dose of radioactive iodide is administered, the normal gland retains the radioactivity at five hours, even if perchlorate is given two to three hours after the radioactive iodide. If an organification defect is present, perchlorate administration causes the discharge of a large amount of iodide from the gland (previously accumulated but neither oxidized nor incorporated into thyronines) with a striking decrease in radioactivity measured over the gland five hours after the tracer dose of radioactive iodide.

The trapping function of the thyroid is exploited for the radiologic ablation of the thyroid in Graves' disease. Radioactive iodine (^{125}I or ^{131}I) emits both gamma and beta radiation. The former makes possible monitoring radiation externally over the gland. The latter is nonpenetrating but is very destructive at short range, intracellularly. When radioactive iodine is given in millicurie doses, the iodine trap concentrates the material in thyroid cells and local radiation destroys them. This is often the preferred method of treating a patient with a hyperactive gland.

The penetrating character of gamma radiation has transformed the art of diagnosis of nodular disease of the thyroid. It is possible, by external scanning of the thyroid after it has been permitted to trap a test dose of radioactive iodide, to localize nodules and to characterize them with respect to their ability, or lack of ability, to concentrate I^-. This information is crucial in constructing appropriate management strategies.

"ORGANIFICATION" OF IODINE

Thyroglobulin is synthesized in the rough endoplasmic reticulum whence it progresses to the Golgi for posttranslational modification, which consists mainly of the acquisition of complex carbohydrate side chains. Thyroglobulin consists of two polypeptide chains with an aggregate of about 5,000 amino acids. Its molecular weight is about 670,000 and it contains 10% carbohydrate. It is remarkable that 115 tyrosyl residues constitute 3% of the weight of the molecule. Of these, only about 10%, on the surface of the globular protein, are eventually iodinated. Surprisingly, only about 1–3 thyronine molecules (T_4, T_3) are produced when the entire protein is hydrolyzed. Most authorities now believe that organification (i.e., iodination of tyrosyl residues) occurs on tyrosyl residues that are already incorporated in TG.

Here, I^- supplied by the iodide transporter; thyroid peroxidase (TPO), a membrane-bound hemoprotein; H_2O_2 generated in an unknown manner, but involving NADPH cytochrome C reductase; and nascent thyroglobulin (TG) all assemble so fast and so effectively that organification in this region of the cell (at or near the apical membrane) occurs almost instantaneously when radioactive iodide enters the cell at the basal membrane. TPO catalyzes the oxidation of I^- to a reactive species of iodine (free radical?) which then iodinates a small number of accessible surface tyrosyl groups in the nascent TG. TG is a prohormone in the sense that its three-dimensional configuration, determined by its amino acid and carbohydrate composition, aligns a very few iodinated tyrosyl groups with near neighbors so that TPO-catalyzed coupling can occur. Fully iodinated TG, containing MIT, DIT, T_4, and a small amount of T_3, is secreted into the colloid so fast that autoradiographic studies often show the earliest grains in the colloid adjacent to the villous border only minutes after the administration of radioactive iodide. In hyperthyroidism and in iodine deficiency, there is an increase in the ratio of T_3 to T_4 in TG, and, therefore, an increase in T_3 secretion when the TG is hydrolyzed. Since T_3 is more active biologically than T_4, this shift in the T_3:T_4 ratio has the effect of making hyperthyroidism more severe in the first case, or maximizing the biological effectiveness of iodide when it is in short supply in the second.

COLLOID RESORPTION AND HORMONE SECRETION

When a secretory stimulus is perceived by the thyroid cell (see section on TSH above), the apical membrane villi surround and ingest small droplets of colloid, which are thus transported across the apical membrane. The last TG to be iodinated is the first to be endocytosed for secretion. Lysosomal proteolysis of droplet contents hydrolyzes TG to its constituent amino acids and carbohydrates. Two of the products of hydrolysis, T_4 and T_3, are secreted into the circulation; however, MIT and DIT are promptly deiodinated, and the resulting I^- and tyrosine are retained for recycling. T_4 and T_3 are resistant to the action of the intrathyroidal scavenger deshalogenase. Since 80% of iodotyrosines in TG are MIT and DIT, this enzyme is important for the conservation of iodide.

A small amount of radioimmunoassayable thyroglobulin normally gains access to the circulation. In inflammatory disease of the thyroid, much larger amounts of TG are found in the blood.

The intrathyroidal iodine cycle is an excellent example of a microhomeostatic regulatory mechanism that functions within a larger system. The thyroid cell is able to integrate a very large number of environmental messages—e.g., iodine availability, substrate availability, presence of TSH or TSH-like stimulators—into a coherent, coordinated, continuing level of hormone biosynthesis, storage, and secretion.

Circulating Thyroid Hormone

When the TG protease frees T_4 and T_3 from their storage depot in the follicular colloid, they traverse the cell and enter the bloodstream. There they are selectively bound by one of several carrier proteins, which have been exhaustively studied. By far the largest amount of hormone in the blood is in the form of T_4, but small amounts of T_3 also are detectable. In thyrotoxicosis or acute infections of the thyroid, larger amounts of T_3 may appear. The nature of the thyroxine-binding proteins has been determined by chemical fractionation of the serum proteins and by ingenious combinations of paper electrophoresis with localization by means of ^{131}I labels on the specific compounds under study. It has been found that most of the protein-bound iodine (PBI) migrates with a mobility between that of α_1 and α_2 globulin (thyroxine-binding globulin [TBG]). A smaller portion examined under certain precise conditions of buffering and pH migrates with a prealbumin fraction (thyroxine-binding prealbumin [TBPA]), while up to 10% is bound to albumin.

There is no evidence that protein-bound thyroxine or T_3 can enter cells, so we must presume that the hormone-protein complex dissociates at the tissue sites where the hormone exerts its effect. These may be either in the peripheral tissues (to be discussed below) or in those structures in the nervous system and the hypophysis that participate in the feedback regulation of TSH output regulation.

Measurements of free and bound thyroid hormones and estimation of their binding affinities for carrier proteins have led to a reconsideration of the comparative importance of T_4 and T_3 in metabolic control. Sixty percent of circulating T_4 is bound to thyroxine-binding globulin (TBG), 30% to prealbumin (TBPA) and 10% to albumin. T_3 binds only loosely to TBPA, and it binds to TBG only to the extent of 3% of T_4. Thus, although the thyroid gland may produce 10 times as much T_4 as T_3, the protein-binding characteristics of the two hormones may result in free T_3 plasma concentrations of up to 50% of free T_4. In hyperthyroidism and in iodine deficiency the ratio of T_3 to T_4 may be even higher. Since the calorigenic effect of T_3 is greater than that of T_4, circulating T_3 contributes very substantially to the aggregate metabolic effect of the two hormones.

THYROID FUNCTION TESTS

Historically, estimation of the basal metabolic rate (BMR) was used to assess thyroid function, but this has been superseded by many tests of a more specific kind—tests that have become progressively more specific and discriminating. The proliferation of tests has been due in part to the fact that iodide-containing medications, especially those contained in x-ray contrast media, interfere with certain tests. Furthermore, fluctuations in the levels of circulating binding proteins have stimulated a search for reliable methods of estimating free thyroxine and T_3.

While it is unrealistic to expect a beginning student to develop a working knowledge of thyroid function tests, it is important to make the point that this armamentarium of tests enables the physician to make very precise judgments about the functional status of individual components of the hypothalamo-pituitary-thyroid system. All of these tests are grounded in basic chemical, physical, biochemical, and physiologic studies. An outline of thyroid function tests is given in Table 10–1. Together they constitute an extraordinary advance in the application of new biologic information to the analysis of human disease.

EFFECTS OF THYROID HORMONE

Table 10–2 is a summary of some of the effects of thyroid hormone deficiency and excess that have been noted by observers working at virtually every wavelength of the biologic spectrum. The purpose of this discussion is to examine these effects in an effort to discover the extent to which observations made at different levels of organization may either complement one another or confound the searcher after unity.

Gross effects of thyroid hormone lack and surfeit are obvious. In general, the earlier the hormone deficiency appears, the more far-reaching the effects on the CNS. If the deficiency in the cretin goes untreated for too long, irreversible damage may be done to the brain.

Although some of the CNS effects of thyroid hormone deficiency may be regarded as a developmental failure, it is clearly not completely so, for if the deficiency occurs in a previously healthy adult, the same kind of mental sluggishness, torpor, and somnolence appears as one sees in a cretinous child, and the clearing away of the mental fog on treatment with replacement doses of thyroid hormone can be nothing less than astonishing. The thyrotoxic patient—restless, anxious, emotionally unstable—not infrequently finds his or her way to the internist by way of the psychi-

TABLE 10–1.
Summary of Some Thyroid Function Tests (Normal Ranges in Parentheses)*

General tests
  BMR (− 10% to + 10%)
  Deep tendon reflex. Delayed relaxation in hypothyroidism
  Serum cholesterol (approx. 170–230)
Special tests
  Circulating antithyroid antibodies. In Hashimoto's disease and in Graves' disease
  Thyroid biopsy. In neoplasia, thyroiditis
Radioactive iodine uptake
  2 hr (2–10% of dose)
  6 hr (4–20%)
  24 hr (6–33%). Poor test for hypothyroidism
  Scan: localization of sites and intensity of radioactivity in thyroid or elsewhere
Plasma hormone measurements
  PBI (4–8 mg/100 ml: include MIT, DIT. Useful for screening only)
  T_4 by column chromatography (2.9–6.4 μg %). Measures total circulating T_4 without interference of iodine-containing compounds
  T_4 by competitive binding protein (3–7 μg %). A radioligand assay based on human TBG saturated with radioactive T_4. May be done in presence of contaminating iodine
  Free T_4 (about 3 ng/100 ml). Accurate even when TBG levels are abnormal
  Free T_4 index (indirect estimate of free T_4). From total T_4 and partition of protein-bound and resin-bound hormone, it is possible to estimate free T_4
  Total T_3 by radioimmunoassay or gas-liquid chromatography (100–200 ng/100 ml, 1.5 ng/100 ml free). May be used when other standard plasma measurements are normal, i.e., in T_3 thyrotoxicosis
  Reverse T_3 and other metabolites of T_4
Suppression and stimulation tests
  T_3 suppression (RAIU suppresses to < 50% of initial value on 75 μg T_3/day; RAIU in hyperthyroidism not suppressible)
  TSH stimulation (RAIU p̄ TSH). Differentiates primary from secondary hypothyroidism
  Plasma TSH by radioimmunoassay (3.9 ± 2 μU/ml). Elevated in hypothyroidism
  TRF stimulation test: TSH response to TRH. Differentiates between hypothalamic and pituitary hypothyroidism

*Modified from Theodore Dalakos.

TABLE 10–2.

Effects of Thyroid Deficiency and Excess Observed at Different Levels of Organization

LEVEL OF ORGANIZATION	HYPOTHYROID	HYPERTHYROID
Behavior	Mental retardation	Often quick mentally
	Mentally and physically sluggish	Restless, irritable, anxious, hyperkinetic
	Somnolent	Wakeful
	Sensitive to cold	Sensitive to heat
Whole individual	Deficient growth	Negative nitrogen balance
	Low BMR	High BMR
	Hypercholesterolemia	Hypocholesterolemia
	Myxedema	Exophthalmos
Organ systems	$\downarrow$ Cardiac Output	$\uparrow$ Cardiac output
Cardiovascular	$\uparrow$ BP ($\uparrow$ peripheral resistance)	$\uparrow$ Systolic BP, pulse pressure ($\uparrow$ ejection force)
	Weak heart beat	Tachycardia, palpitations
	$\uparrow$ Circulation Time (i.e., sluggish circulation)	$\downarrow$ Circulation time (i.e., rapid circulation)
Gastrointestinal	Hypophagia	Hyperphagia
	Constipation	Frequent bowel movements
	Low glucose absorption rate	High glucose absorption rate
Muscle	Weakness	Weakness
	Hypotonia	Fibrillary twitchings, tremors
Immune mechanism	Infection susceptible	Infection susceptible (? related to excess protein catabolism)
Tissues	$\downarrow$ QO_2 of liver, kidney muscle, etc. in vitro	$\uparrow$ QO_2 of same tissues
	Normal QO_2 of brain, testis, retina, etc.	Normal QO_2 of brain and same tissues
	Decreased sensitivity of some tissues to epinephrine	Potentiation of epinephrine effects by thyronines
Organelle	Increased no. of mitochondria per cell.	Increased no. of mitochondria per cell.
	$\downarrow$ Plasma membrane β receptors	$\uparrow$ Plasma membrane β receptors
Organelle component		Mitochondrial swelling (action on mitochondrial membrane?)
Enzymes	$\downarrow$ Oxidative enzymes/mitochondrial mass	$\uparrow$ Oxidative enzymes in chronically treated animals
	$\downarrow$ $Na^+K^+ATPase$, NADPH malic enzyme, α GPDH, etc.	$\uparrow$ $Na^+K^+ATPase$, etc.

atrist. These symptoms, too, subside dramatically with successful treatment.

The hypothyroid patient prefers the hot weather and complains bitterly about the cold; the hyperthyroid individual is just the reverse. One of the most striking features of hypothyroidism is impaired heat production. On the other hand, the hyperthyroid individual is inappropriately "adapted" to the cold even at warm temperatures. In effect, he or she is unable to turn off his or her cold-adapting machinery; hence, his or her misery at ambient air temperatures that seem only mildly warm to euthyroid individuals.

Thyroid hormone deficiency or excess can cause profound changes in behavior. For example, it is sometimes difficult to differentiate between anxiety and hyperthyroidism.

Among important observations made in the nonbehavioral sphere of the whole person, those on growth are of great interest. Thyroxine is a growth hormone in replacement doses, for growth failure occurs in hypothyroid infants and children, and rapid growth spurts regularly follow the treatment of such patients with adequate amounts of thyroid hormone. A surplus of the hormone, on the other hand, produces excessive protein catabolism with tissue wasting in severe cases. The patient with Graves' disease literally burns up his own substance.

In 1895, the great pioneer Magnus-Levy discovered that hypothyroid patients were hypometabolic and hyperthyroid patients had high basal metabolic rates. These changes are still most striking, although their specificity is not great, as the BMR can be high or low for many reasons other than thyroid dysfunction.

Disturbances in lipid metabolism have been associated with altered states of thyroid function for many years. In hypothyroidism there may be lipemia, hypercholesterolemia and a fatty infiltration of the liver, whereas in hyperthyroidism there is characteristically a decrease in serum cholesterol. Recent studies with ^{14}C-labeled metabolites have revealed that the rate of cholesterol catabolism by the liver may be responsible for the comparative plasma levels. For in hyperthyroidism, in spite of accelerated cholesterol synthesis rates from acetate by liver slices, there is an even greater acceleration of the destruction of cholesterol by the liver, thus contributing to low circulating levels. Another factor that may influence serum cholesterol in the hyperthyroid individual is that, even when such people overeat, they may be underfed with respect to their total caloric requirement. Whereas the serum cholesterol in adults is so variable that it is not very useful diagnostically in investigating thyroid status, an elevated level in small children may be very helpful in alerting the physician to the possibility of hypothyroidism.

There is no major organ system that is uninfluenced by either the absence or excess of thyroid hormone. The behavioral aspects of thyroid physiology represent expressions of hormone effect on the CNS and the neuromuscular apparatus. Just as impressive, dependence on thyroid hormone and disturbances due to its presence in excess are seen in many other systems.

In the *cardiovascular system* the cardiac output tends to be proportional to the metabolic rate, being low in hypothyroidism and high in thyrotoxicosis. The same generalization can be made about changes in blood volume and in systolic blood pressure. One of the most distinctive findings in hyperthyroidism is a moderate elevation in systolic blood pressure with little change in diastolic, or a marked increase in pulse pressure. This is often associated with vigorous, brisk and rapid contractions of the heart, which are in contrast with the weak heart beat (which often produces low voltage deflections in the ECG) of hypothyroidism. The arm-to-lung or arm-to-tongue circulation time is prolonged in hypothyroidism and shortened in hyperthyroidism.

Although the regulation of food intake and food intake behavior are not regarded primarily as local *gastrointestinal tract functions,* altered thyroid status is accompanied by striking differences in the quantity of food ingested. Hypofunction of the thyroid is usually associated with decreased food intake, whereas thyrotoxic patients often eat voraciously without becoming obese. The mechanisms by which these attempted adjustments of intake to caloric need are made are not known, but some of the implications of these findings for current theories of food intake regulation are discussed in Chapter 16.

A prominent gastrointestinal tract function that is often markedly influenced by thyroid dysfunction is motility. The cretin or adult hypothyroid often suffers from constipation, whereas frequent bowel movements may be a prominent complaint of the hyperthyroid patient. The mechanism of these effects is not known. They may be due in part to modifications of the CNS and in part to alterations in the sensitivity of the gastrointestinal smooth muscle cells to their customary neurohumoral transmitter substances.

The rate of intestinal absorption of glucose parallels the basal metabolic rate and the general level of thyroid activity. Hypothyroidism is associated with slow absorption rates and hyperthyroidism with rapid ones. Since the rate of hepatic and peripheral removal of absorbed glucose also parallels the level of metabolic activity, the oral glucose tolerance curve of a hypothyroid and a hyperthyroid patient may look much the same.

The effects of thyroid hormone lack or excess on *muscle* are extremely complex. Weakness, or the consciousness of diminished muscle strength, is one of the commonest complaints heard by physicians, but the pathophysiology of weakness is not commonly discussed. It is convenient to think of weakness as a derivative of three potential contributory factors: (1) the central perception or awareness of weakness, (2) a cardiopulmonary-circulatory component and (3) the state of the muscle as a contractile machine. The central perception of weakness must be at least as complicated as the perception of hunger, satiety, thirst or similar sensations, and although thyroid hormone availability or lack may have effects on the perception of the sensation of fatigue, we cannot describe these at present. The cardiopulmonary-circulatory contribution to fatigue in hyperthyroidism must be considerable, for the reserves of the heart and lungs in this condition are inadequate to deal with the increased oxygen and fuel requirements even of moderate exercise. In the severely hyperthyroid person, the tissue demands may be so outrageously high that even a tachycardia, a high-pulse pressure, and a markedly diminished circulation time fail to keep up with them. Moreover, extremely hypermetabolic individuals are susceptible to vitamin deficiencies, so that a sort of beriberi heart syndrome may develop and lead eventually to cardiac failure. If hyperthyroidism occurs in a middle-aged or elderly person and the peremptory demands of a racing metabolic motor are made on a heart that is supplied by narrowed, atherosclerotic vessels, cardiac decompensation may occur.

Both hypothyroidism and hyperthyroidism are characterized by disturbances in the muscle tissue itself. In hypothyroidism, a generalized hypotonia and sluggishness is a characteristic finding. In children and growing animals, the failure of growth is just as apparent in muscle as in other tissues. In hyperthyroidism, there is a negative nitrogen balance, and the presence of creatinuria and a low concentration of creatinine and phosphocreatine in the muscle of hyperthyroid animals suggests that there is a very rapid catabolism of muscle protein. Thus, the weakness of hyperthyroidism is the complicated sum of circulatory failure, local muscle factors and, possibly, heightened perception of fatigue centrally. In addition to these, the fibrillary twitching and tremors seen in a patient with severe hyperthyroidism represent a relentless bombardment of the muscles by nerve impulses, so that in a sense such an individual is always exercising, and any muscle work that he does is superimposed on an existing load.

This constant muscular activity of the hyperthyroid animal or man may not be obvious to inspection but is clearly evident in electromyograms. Since the muscle mass constitutes 50% of the body weight and since muscle has the widest range of oxygen requirement of any tissue, muscular activity must contribute substantially to the elevated basal metabolic rate seen in hyperthyroidism even under the conditions of the test, although, as we shall see, other tissues removed from hyperthyroid animals show a high rate of oxygen consumption when studied in vitro.

Hypothyroid patients and animals are said to have an increased susceptibility to infectious disease. This may be related to defective function of the immune mechanism and to the subnormal phagocytic capacity of leukocytes described in this condition. Hyperthyroid individuals, too, are hypersusceptible to infections, but the mechanism of this susceptibility is not clearly understood. Possibly the general debility resulting from prolonged negative nitrogen balance may account for most of it.

Many studies have been made on the in vitro metabolism of surviving tissues obtained from animals with altered thyroid function. Certain tissues, particularly liver and kidney, accurately reflect the thyroid status of the donor animal, since they show high oxygen consumption if they are obtained from a hyperthyroid animal and a low consumption if they are taken from a hypothyroid animal. These effects are not seen immediately: a week or more of treatment of the donor animal is required before the tissue effects are seen. The events that occur during the latent period will be discussed below.

Just as impressive as the high "tissue BMR" of the tissues of hyperthyroid animals is that certain other tissues—particularly such tissues as brain, testis, and retina—do not show decreased or increased rates of oxygen consumption when they are obtained from animals with thyroid hormone lack or excess. Since altered thyroid hormone availability has unmistakable effects on the function of the brain in situ, our inability to detect an obvious metabolic aberration (though admittedly a gross one) is an arresting finding. We are left with the conclusion that thyroid hormone effects on the brain can occur without a change in oxygen consumption, which leaves plenty of other possibilities to explore.

Cellular Mechanisms of Action of Thyroid Hormone

The thyroid hormones do not fit comfortably into the conventional model of steroid hormone action or that of amine or peptide hormone action. They differ significantly from other amines and peptides in their lipid solubility, in which feature they resemble steroid hormones. Thus there is no reason to suppose that the plasma membrane lipid bilayer effectively excludes thyroid hormones from the cell interior.

A distinction should be made between the role of thyroid hormone in the process of *differentiation*, which is seen most strikingly in the metamorphosis of amphibia, in the neonatal development of the central nervous system in the human infant, and its role in *maintenance of function in fully differentiated cells*. In mammals, including man, calorigenesis is deficient in hypothyroid states and supernormal in hyperthyroid states. Calorigenesis is an *indicator* of the maintenance function referred to above. (Encircled numbers refer to those in Figure 10–6.)

① PERIPHERAL DEIODINATION OF T_4 and T_3

Peripheral tissues, particularly pituitary, liver, and kidney, contain a deiodinase enzyme complex, coupled to an NADPH-generating system, that converts T_4 to T_3. When radioactively labeled T_4 is administered, less than 15% of it appears in the nucleus of thyroid hormone-sensitive cells. Most of the labeled hormone bound in the nucleus is T_3. Deiodination of T_4 to T_3 in the pituitary is essential for the expression of the chronic decrease in sensitivity of the pituitary to TRH stimulation that occurs after T_4 administration.

However, T_4 does bind to the thyroid hormone nuclear receptor (to be described), though with less affinity than T_3, and therefore may have nuclear effects. There is at least one circumstance in which T_4 is *the* biologically active form of the hormone; i.e., in the premetamorphic tadpole. In fact, in that animal the

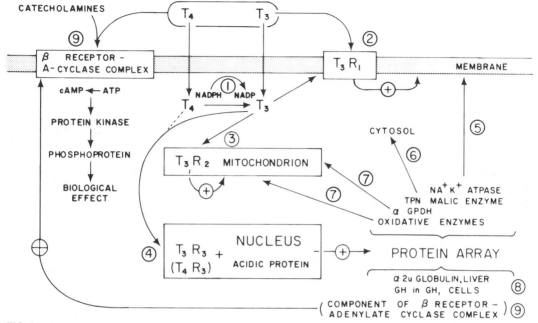

FIG 10–6.
Cellular mechanisms of action of thyroid hormones. TPN = NADP.

deiodinase responsible for T_3 synthesis does not appear until after the process of differentiation has been initiated by T_4. Whether there is a stage in mammalian embryonic development when analogous events occur is unknown.

The development of specific radioimmunoassays for T_4, T_3, reverse T_3 (rT_3), and their deiodinated products has permitted a detailed analysis of the peripheral breakdown of thyroid hormones. The general scheme is shown in Figure 10–7.

Practically all of the circulating T_4 is of thyroid origin. However, most of the circulating T_3 is derived from peripheral deiodination of T_4. T_3 derived from T_4 may be retained by the cells bound to its receptors, but some diffuses back into the general circulation. As we have already mentioned, in two circumstances,

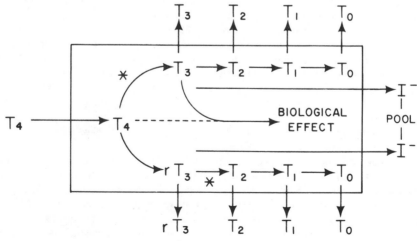

FIG 10–7.
Serial peripheral deiodinations of thyroxine (T_4). (See text for explanation of *.)

hyperthyroidism and iodine deficiency, a larger proportion of T_3 may be secreted by the thyroid because of the relative preponderance of MIT to DIT in those conditions.

There are two different deiodinating enzymes in T_4-sensitive tissues: the outer ring deiodinase catalyzes the formation of T_3 and the inner ring deiodinase catalyzes that of rT_3 (see Fig 10–7). Reverse T_3 is either noncalorigenic or feebly antagonistic to T_3, and therefore inhibitory to the peripheral actions of thyroid hormones.

Outer ring deiodination (T_3 formation) is inhibited in a variety of circumstances that may exist even in the presence of a normally functioning hypothalamic-pituitary-thyroid axis. Among these are the following: severe illness or trauma; fasting or carbohydrate deprivation; after glucocorticoid treatment; following iodinated drugs (example: x-ray contrast agents); in the human fetus; following treatment with a catecholamine β blocker; during propylthiouracil treatment (except in pituitary); in severe liver or kidney disease.

In contrast, in obesity there is a tendency to *enhanced* conversion of T_4 to T_3.

As a result of these findings, the inhibition or accentuation of T_4 outer ring deiodination has been considered adaptively significant. One of the consequences of starvation (undernutrition is a prominent feature of many illnesses) is a decrease in basal metabolic rate. A decreased rate of T_3 formation, therefore, would be a teleonomically useful energy conservation tactic. Conversely, an increased rate of T_3 formation in obesity would have the effect of limiting the further development of the obesity by stimulating the oxidation of excess substrates (see Chapter 16). Thus, control mechanisms operating at the site of T_4 to T_3 conversion have important implications for energy balance in the whole individual.

When T_4 deiodination to T_3 is blocked, more T_4 is available for inner ring deiodination, and more rT_3 may be formed. The further deiodination of rT_3 may be impaired (asterisks [*] in Fig 10–7) and rT_3 may rise. Although the fall in T_3 and the rise in rT_3 are not precisely reciprocally related, they tend to change in opposite directions.

There is no universally accepted mechanism for the $T_3 \rightarrow rT_3$ shift in starvation and other circumstances. We favor the idea that, since the outer ring deiodinase requires NADPH, availability of that cofactor may determine the rate of the reaction. Since NADPH is generated by glucose oxidation via the pentose phosphate shunt pathway, glucose availability may be an important determinant of the level of T_4 to T_3 deiodination. This hypothesis is consistent with a decrease in T_3 formation in starvation and an increase as a consequence of overeating.

② Plasma Membrane Effects

While most of the emphasis in elucidating the mechanism of thyroid hormone action has been on nuclear events, undeniable T_3 effects on plasma membrane function have been described (Goldfine et al.). High affinity binding sites on the plasma membranes of thyroid hormone-sensitive cells have been reported, but they are probably not identical with the much more extensively studied nuclear receptors. The major effect seen following T_3 administration was a stimulation of amino acid transport; the response was rapid and did not require either RNA or protein synthesis.

③ Mitochondrial Effects

The association between thyroid hormone action and mitochondria has been a long and complicated one. Morphological and biochemical effects of thyroid hormones on mitochondria are so prominent in hyper- and hypothyroidism that hyperthyroidism has been called a "disease of mitochondria." At one time, the calorigenic effect of T_3 was ascribed to uncoupling of oxidative phosphorylation, but this view has been generally abandoned. Receptors for T_3 have been described in mitochondria (Sterling et al., 1984), and a variety of morphological changes in mitochondria have been seen after T_3 administration, including striking swelling of the organelles. Curiously, there is an increase in total mitochondrial mass in thyroid hormone-sensitive cells in both hypo- and hyperthyroidism, but the concentration of oxidative enzymes per unit of mitochondrial mass is low in the former and, despite the increase in total mitochondrial mass, high in the latter.

For some time it has been recognized that transport of ADP into mitochondria is decreased in hypothyroidism and increased in hyperthyroidism. In this connection, it is interesting that even in severe hyperthyroidism, cells are able to sustain comparatively normal ATP concentrations in spite of the fact that ATP is obviously being hydrolyzed at a rapid rate (Sestoft). Also, Sterling has observed a correlation between mitochondrial production of ATP from labelled ADP and thyroid status (an immediate effect that could not possibly involve gene transcription) even with concentrations of T_3 as low as 10^{-9} M. All of these observations should be reviewed in light of Beck and Sterling's recent (1985) finding that T_3 binds to partially purified adenine nucleotide translocase (AdNT), the ADP inward transporter that exerts at least partial control over the rate of mitochondrial oxidative phosphorylation. (It has been long recognized that this process is stimulated by ADP.) If it can be demonstrated that there is a connection between T_3 binding and activation of AdNT, one interesting facet of thyroid hormone action will be illuminated.

Long-term effects of thyroid hormones on mitochondrial function will be discussed under (7) below.

(4) THE NUCLEUS

Oppenheimer and others have described high-affinity receptors for T_3 in the nuclei of a variety of thyroid hormone-sensitive cells. In general, the rank order of binding of thyroid hormone analogues in these cells parallels the thyroid hormone biologic potency of the compounds. As we remarked above, following the administration of a pulse of radioactively labelled T_4, about 85% of the label appears in the nucleus as T_3 and less than 15% is recoverable there as T_4. These binding sites generally conform to accepted criteria for hormone receptors, but some skepticism has been expressed about their biologic significance (Tata). It is odd, for example, that most of the T_3 receptors are associated with "occluded" segments of the genome; i.e., with genes that are never expressed. While the nuclear receptors, which appear to be integral chromatin constituents, bind T_3 with higher affinity than T_4, they do bind T_4 at physiological concentrations.

The nuclear localization of these receptors raises the question of how the iodothyronines, which are lipid-soluble, get into the cell and gain access to high-affinity binding sites in the nucleus and mitochondria. It is possible that the plasma membrane binding sites, discussed above, may play a role in transporting the hormones into the cell. Cytosolic proteins that bind the hormones with lower affinity than do those in the cell's organelles have been described, and these may function as intracellular molecular ferryboats.

Older studies (by Cohen and by Frieden) on the initiation of metamorphosis in amphibia and the classical analysis of thyroid hormone effects on the nucleus by Tata strongly support the view that thyroid hormone action (like that of steroids) involves stimulation of the transcription of specific genes and the induction of a distinctive battery of proteins for each cell. (The box that is bound by hormone binding on one side and increased mRNA synthesis on the other is no less black for thyroid hormones than it is for steroids.) Figure 10–8 is a summary of Tata's findings in rat liver following the injection of a single dose of T_3. The time scale of these responses is longer than that seen with steroid hormones, although in both cases, immediate, extranuclear events precede the nuclear ones. Also in both cases, a small number of nuclear effects can be seen long before most of the nuclear excitement occurs. Indeed, in the case of T_3, stimulation of the transcription of a specific mRNA (identified only as its translated protein product, a spot in a two-dimensional chromatogram) was observed as early as 20 minutes after administration of the hormone (Narayan). This is reminiscent of the induction of a single protein (IP) by estrogen long before other proteins appear. However, the increase in

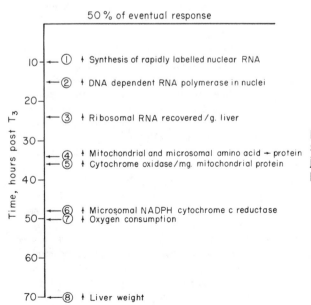

FIG 10–8.
Sequence of events following a single injection of triiodothyronine (T_3) into a hypothyroid rat.

oxygen consumption after T_3 (transcription-dependent) does not reach its half-maximal response until 50 hours after the administration of the hormone. As in the case of steroid hormones, only a limited number of mRNAs are elicited by T_3. Some of these, and how they are related to the manifestations of thyroid function in the whole animal or person, will now be discussed.

⑤ SODIUM-POTASSIUM ATPASE

(Reviewed by Guernsey and Edelman in Oppenheimer and Samuels.)

Edelman and his colleagues were impressed by their estimates of the fraction of resting metabolism contributed by the osmotic work associated with maintenance of high intracellular $[K^+]$ and high extracellular $[Na^+]$. The maintenance of this uneven distribution of ions across the plasma membranes of cells is the work of the sodium pump, Na^+-K^+ATPase, which is powered by a continuing supply of ATP. After finding that the Na^+-K^+ATPase activity in kidney and muscle was low in hypothyroidism and high in hyperthyroidism, they proceeded to demonstrate, in a series of elegant studies, that the rate of incorporation of labelled amino acids into both subunits of the enzyme was greatest in hyperthyroidism, intermediate in untreated controls, and least in hypothyroid animals. Although there has not yet been a demonstration that the rate of mRNA synthesis for this enzyme is increased by T_3, studies with an inhibitor of RNA synthesis suggest that this is so, particularly since the extent of occupation of nuclear T_3 receptors can be correlated with the increase in Na^+-K^+ATPase elicited by the hormone.

While the action of the hormone on the sodium pump may account for some of the increased oxygen consumption caused by T_3 (increased number of pump units→increased ATP utilization→increased ADP→stimulation of oxidative phosphorylation), it now appears unlikely that it accounts for the major part of the increased thermogenesis brought about by the iodothyronines. Various estimates of the metabolic cost of osmotic work vary widely: from 15%–80% of the basal oxygen consumption. Sestoft is impressed by the large energy cost of cardiac work in hyperthyroidism. We are inclined to agree with others that, in hyperthyroidism, the concurrent stimulation of opposing metabolic processes, for example, lipogenesis (see next section) and lipolysis, is extremely inefficient and costly in terms of ATP utilization since energy used in synthesis is wasted by rapid catabolism. Such futile cycling could contribute substantially to the increased heat production of hyperthyroidism. Increased oxidative deamination brought about by increased protein catabolism could make an additional contribution.

⑥, ⑧ TPN MALIC ENZYME, α2u GLOBULIN, GROWTH HORMONE

Unfortunately, investigators of thyroid hormone action did not have an oviduct-ovalbumin model and were, therefore, forced to study hormone-induced proteins that represented only small fractions of the total amount of protein synthesized by certain cells. In spite of this handicap, they have been able to establish that the thyroid hormones, like the steroids, stimulate transcription of specific genes, notably those coding for NADP malic enzyme (a cytosolic enzyme important as a NADPH generator for the process of lipogenesis) and α2u globulin (a protein excreted in large quantities in the urine of rodents) in liver and growth hormone in cultured GH_1 cells. All of the techniques of modern molecular biology pioneered by investigators of steroid hormone action have been applied successfully to T_3, including the titration of mRNA by cDNA (Magnuson). There are many reviews on this subject (notably those of Towle, Roy, Goodridge, and Mariash and Oppenheimer) in the Oppenheimer-Samuels monograph.

As we shall see in more detail in Chapter 14, NADP malic enzyme is one of a number of lipogenic enzymes that increase when carbohydrate is ingested. Others include acetyl CoA carboxylase and fatty acid synthetase, which are also induced to a lesser extent by thyroid hormone as well as by insulin. Insulin is believed to affect gene transcription of lipogenic enzymes not directly but by increasing the amounts of glucose that enter lipogenic cells (liver, adipocyte). (Whether an insulin-generated "second messenger" is involved in these actions of insulin is an open question. If the signal for new enzyme synthesis is some metabolite or other molecule derived from accelerated glucose oxidation, its identity is not known.) In any case, insulin and T_3 act synergistically to cause the synthesis of more NADP malic enzyme mRNA. It is not even known whether insulin supplies a positive inductive signal for new enzyme synthesis or whether it removes an inhibitory influence. In either case, the partnership between T_3 and insulin is only one of a number of similar collaborative arrangements in which T_3 participates.

The induction of new GH mRNA by T_3 is markedly potentiated by the simultaneous presence of adrenal glucocorticoids. Similarly, α2u globulin induction, intensively studied by Feigelson and Roy and their coworkers, is a complex process that involves no less than *four* hormones: T_3, testosterone, glucocorticoids, and growth hormone. T_3 joins with other hormones in switching on other genes: those for glutamine synthase (GH and glucocorticoids); for hepatic δ aminolevulinic acid (ALA) synthase (insulin, glucocorticoids); and for α lactalbumin in mammary gland explants.

We cannot give a molecular explanation for the way in which various hormones, carbohydrate metabolites (?), and cofactors (?) cooperatively affect chromatin to open up gene sites for transcription. Indeed, each hormone combination may have its distinctive mechanism. In a general way, we can imagine that the unraveling of chromatin by one hormone may make the "open" DNA more accessible to another transcription signal. Until we learn more about the details of the turning on and off of gene sites for transcription (processes that may involve phosphorylation and dephosphorylation of control proteins, and probably other reversible covalent modifications such as acetylation-deacetylation and methylation-demethylation as well), we cannot give better than a vague description of the basis for these multiple hormone effects on gene expression, effects that are probably more pertinent to "real life" than are the single hormone models we discuss so frequently.

⑦ ⑧ Mitochondrial α Glycerophosphate Dehydrogenase: Enzymes of Oxidative Phosphorylation and Others

Under ③ above we discussed acute effects of T_3 on mitochondrial function, rapid events which require neither protein synthesis nor gene transcription. It has long been known that the activity of oxidative enzymes (succinic dehydrogenase, cytochrome oxidase) is low in hypothyroidism and high in hyperthyroid states. More recently it has been discovered that T_3 strikingly and selectively induces a manyfold increase in mitochondrial α glycerophosphate dehydrogenase (α GPDH in Fig 10–6). Since over 90% of mitochondrial proteins are encoded by nuclear genes, effects on these enzymes are achieved by the interaction of T_3 with nuclear receptors (R_3 in Fig 10–6). Thus, the long-range effects of T_3 on the mitochondrion are in the same category as are those on Na^+-K^+ATPase, NADP malic enzyme, α2μ globulin and growth hormone; i.e., an increased rate of transcription of specific mRNAs. They are part of a massive, coordinated reorganization of the metabolic machinery throughout the cell brought about by T_3: acute membrane effects (amino acid transport, adenine nucleotide translo-

case), chronic membrane transport effects (Na^+-K^+ATPase); cytosolic changes (lipogenic enzymes), mitochondrial alterations, and, finally, modifications of the cell that make it more responsive to β catecholamines (next section).

⑨ Thyroid Hormones and Catecholamines

Many of the signs and symptoms of hyperthyroidism suggest overactivity of the sympathetic division of the autonomic nervous system. Prominent among these are those seen in the cardiovascular system: palpitations, tachycardia, cardiac arrhythmias, dilatation and hypertrophy of the heart, increased contractility of the heart and increased cardiac output, a widening of the pulse pressure (systolic minus diastolic blood pressure) and heart failure. In addition to these, tremor and muscle weakness, restlessness and anxiety and diarrhea may involve autonomic nervous system malfunction. Older studies had shown that drugs that interfere with the function of the sympathetic nervous system (reserpine and guanethidine) often caused an amelioration of the constellation of symptoms enumerated above but did not affect indicators of the presence of hyperthyroidism, e.g., increased oxygen consumption and increased levels of circulating thyroid hormone. These drugs, however, had some undesirable side effects and have been replaced by the β blocker propranolol and related drugs. This compound is now an important adjunct in the management of symptoms in hyperthyroid patients.

Although much effort has been expended on the problem of thyroid-catecholamine interrelations, there is no satisfactory single explanation for the fact that many manifestations of thyroid hormone excess are controllable by the β blocker propranolol. *Circulating* catecholamine levels, in fact, are decreased in hyperthyroidism. Therefore, the apparent hyperadrenergic state associated with hyperthyroidism must be related to events at the sympathetic nerve endings, to the responses of catecholamine-sensitive cells, or both.

Williams et al. have described an increased number of β receptor-binding sites on cardiac muscle cells induced by thyroid hormone administrations. The authors are cautious about attributing the increase to a selective synthesis of β receptors induced by thyroid hormone, since the decrease in circulating catecholamines may have "up-regulated" the β receptor population. However, the possibility exists that thyroid hormone-induced DNA transcription may include the transcription of components of the catecholamine-adenylate cyclase complex. This need not involve only the receptor: the coupling mechanism or the phospholipid environment of the complex could be affected by the action of the hormone.

Another interesting possibility is suggested by Dratman, who calls attention to the fact that both the catecholamines and the thyroid hormones are tyrosine analogues and, as such, may be modifiable by the same enzymes (Fig 10–9). According to this hypothesis, the norepinephrine and epinephrine analogues of the thyroid hormones could function as pseudocatecholamines by way of the β receptor. Dratman has demonstrated not only that thyroxine can serve as a substrate for tyrosine hydroxylase, but also that the thyroxine label can be concentrated in adrenergic nerve endings (synaptosomes).

Propranolol therefore may exert its effect by blocking the catecholamine receptor to either naturally occurring catecholamine or a spurious, thyroxine-derived transmitter. The block could involve either a "normal" receptor-cyclase complex or a hyperresponsive one. In addition to these possibilities, there is another propranolol effect that could contribute to the evident amelioration of the catecholamine-related symptoms of hyperthyroidism, i.e., propranolol decreases the peripheral conversion of T_4 to T_3. Since T_3 is biologically more active than T_4 and since $T_4 \rightarrow T_3$ conversion is accelerated in hyperthyroid tissues, a decrease in T_3 synthesis could contribute to the beneficial effect. Thus, it seems likely that there will be multiple answers to the old question: How are catecholamines related to the symptoms ameliorated by propranolol?

Pharmacology of Pituitary-Thyroid System and Hyperfunctional Thyroid States

It is possible to describe the effects of drugs on the component parts of the iodine cycle. Some of these agents have been used to decrease the production or effect of thyroid hormones in hyperthyroid patients, and others are important because they may confound diagnosis.

IODINE

Iodine was the first truly effective antithyroid drug to be used in preparation of hyperthyroid patients for surgery. The antithyroid effect of large doses of iodine (known as the Wolff-Chaikoff effect) is expressed as a resistance of the thyroid to stimulation by TSH (or, presumably, TSH-like globulins). Although there are many hypotheses to explain this effect, no single explanation is satisfactory. In normal people and animals, the effect is transient; the thyroid is evidently able to adapt to the new level of I^- in the environment. In hyperthyroid glands, however, the effect is more sustained, and preoperative preparation of patients for thyroid surgery includes the use of inhibitory amounts of iodide and other antithyroid drugs.

DRUGS THAT INTERFERE WITH THYROID HORMONE SYNTHESIS

These include I^- trap blockers, perchlorate, and thiocyanate (mentioned above), and blockers of hormone synthesis such as propylthiouracil and methimazole. The trap blockers function as competitive inhibitors of I^- transport. Although they are not used therapeutically, they are of some importance in the field of nuclear medicine.

Structures of the thiourylene group of antithyroid drugs are shown in Figure 10–10, which shows their shared features. Their effects are complex: they interfere with the TPO (thyroid peroxidase)-mediated re-

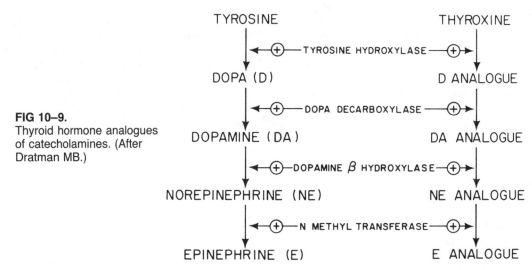

FIG 10–9.
Thyroid hormone analogues of catecholamines. (After Dratman MB.)

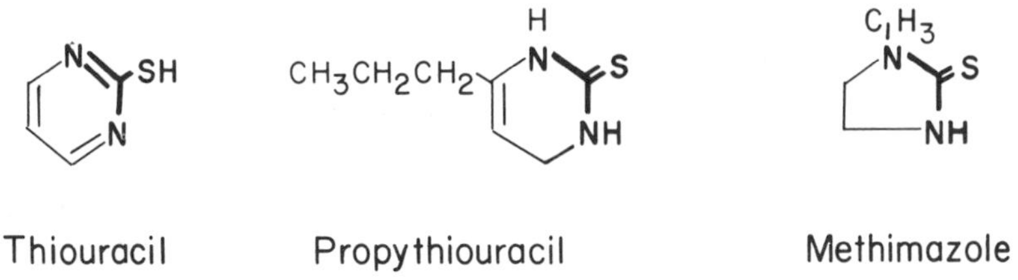

Thiouracil   Propythiouracil   Methimazole

FIG 10–10.
Some commonly used antithyroid drugs.

actions (see Fig 10–5); namely, oxidation of I^- and tyrosyl coupling. They may inhibit intrathyroidal deiodinase. Also, propylthiouracil has recently been found to inhibit peripheral deiodination of T_4, except in the pituitary.

Antiadrenergic drugs such as propranolol (see preceding section), are directed not against the underlying disease of hyperthyroidism but against its symptoms. This adjunctive treatment may ameliorate many of the catecholamine-mediated symptoms and signs of thyroid hormone excess, but abnormally high circulating levels of thyroid hormone persist. The thiourea-derived drugs take effect only after weeks of treatment, whereas propranolol's effect is rapid. Thus the ability to ameliorate symptoms rapidly is often desirable and may be lifesaving.

DRUGS THAT AFFECT THYROXINE-BINDING GLOBULIN (TBG)

These drugs are important because they may introduce artifacts into the interpretation of diagnostic laboratory data. Salicylates and diphenylhydantoin, an anticonvulsive agent, displace circulating T_4 from TBG and may thus indicate a low circulating level of T_4 in a euthyroid individual. In this circumstance, there is no change in total TBG.

In other instances, the *rate of synthesis of TBG by the liver* may be either stimulated or inhibited by an agent, thus yielding high or low values for serum T_4, again in clinically euthyroid people. Estrogens, contraceptive pills and pregnancy all *increase* TBG concentration in plasma, whereas androgens and pharmacologic doses of glucocorticoids *decrease* TBG. In none of these cases is there a remarkable change in the circulating level of *free* T_4, a quantity that clearly correlates better with thyroid function status than with total circulating hormone.

Iodine-containing x-ray contrast media and other iodine-containing drugs no longer interfere with accurate serum hormone estimations by modern methods, but they may confuse interpretation of radioactive iodine uptake studies.

Screening for Congenital Hypothyroidism

Congenital hypothyroidism is the most commonly occurring preventable cause of mental retardation. However, if it is untreated for as short a time as three months, the probability that treatment will be associated with an IQ of more than 85–90 falls very sharply. For example, in one study, 14 of 19 hypothyroid children treated before age 3 months achieved an IQ of 90, whereas less than 30% of children in whom treatment was delayed until after the third month attained a similar level. To see the problem in perspective, it has been estimated that less than one third of congenitally hypothyroid infants less than 3 months old are diagnosed on purely clinical grounds.

The development of highly potent anti-TSH serums has made possible the development of a radioimmunoassay for TSH, which can be done on a spot of blood on a piece of filter paper. Extensive screening experience with this and other tests of thyroid status (such as serum T_4) has revealed that it is possible to detect hypothyroidism in the newborn infant with a high degree of accuracy (Klein and Fisher).

Inborn Errors of Pituitary-Thyroid System

The study of human mutants has provided confirmatory evidence for the general outline of pituitary-thyroid function that has been developed largely as a result of experiments on animals. In addition to congenital absence of the thyroid gland, which may be a developmental defect, individuals with greater or lesser degrees of clinical hypothyroidism have been found with a large variety of biochemical deficiencies. These can be classified as (1) intrathyroidal and (2) extrathyroidal biochemical lesions (Table 10–3).

Most individuals with one of these genetic abnormalities would present with symptoms, signs, and laboratory evidence of hypothyroidism. With the exception of three categories of extrathyroidal errors (transport, deiodination, response failure to T_4/T_3) (see Table 10–3), these individuals would be likely to respond to appropriate thyroid hormone replacement.

TABLE 10–3.

Intrathyroidal and Extrathyroidal Biochemical Lesions*

Intrathyroidal errors
  Decreased responsiveness to TSH (receptor?)
  Transport defect or iodide leak
  Diminished thyroid peroxidase (TPO) function
    Decreased $I^-\rightarrow I^+$
    Decreased coupling
  Decreased H_2O_2 generation
  Thyroglobulin abnormality
    Imperfect protein synthesis
    Disordered secretion into follicle
    Poor resorption, resistance to protease
  Failure of "scavenger" intrathyroidal deiodinase
    function, loss of MIT and DIT in urine
Extrathyroidal hereditary errors
  Diminished or ineffective TSH
  Transport abnormalities
  Defective peripheral deiodination, $T_4\rightarrow T_3$
  Failure of usually sensitive tissues to respond to T_4 and/
    or T_3
  Excessive loss of T_4, T_3 because of too rapid metabolism
    and excretion

*Adapted from DeGroot LJ, Niepomniszcze H: *Metabolism* 1977; 26:665.

Although some of these "experiments of nature" are extremely rare, others, e.g., organification and coupling defect (reminiscent of the loci of action of antithyroid drugs), are no longer considered uncommon. Together they constitute human counterparts of (1) mutant cells grown in tissue culture, which show abnormal responses to catecholamines and glucocorticoids (see Chapter 3), and (2) people with defects in steroid hormone synthesis (see Chapter 11).

BIBLIOGRAPHY

Arimura A, Schally AV: Increase in basal and TRH-stimulated secretion of TSH by passive immunization with antiserum to somatostatin in rats. *Endocrinology* 1976; 98:1069.

Beck JC, Sterling K: The role of adenine nucleotide transferase (AdNT) in the early hormonal stimulation of mitochondrial oxidative phosphorylation by the thyroid hormone triiodothyronine (T_3). *Endocr Soc* (abstract) 1985; 1118.

Burman KD, Baker JR: Immune mechanisms in Graves' disease. *Endocr Rev* 1985; 6:183.

Cavalieri RR, Rapoport B: Impaired peripheral conversion of thyroxine to triiodothyronine. *Ann Rev Med* 1977; 28:57.

Chopra IJ, Hershman JM, Pardridge EM, et al: Thyroid function in nonthyroidal illnesses. *Ann Intern Med* 1983; 98:946.

Cohen PP: Biochemical differentiation during amphibian metamorphosis. *Science* 1970; 168:533.

Cooper DS: Antithyroid drugs. *N Engl J Med* 1984; 311:1353.

Danforth E Jr, Burger A: The role of thyroid hormones in the control of energy expenditure. *Clin Endocrinol Metab* 1984; 13:581.

Davies TF: Diseases of the TSH receptor. *Clin Endocrinol Metab* 1983; 12:79.

DeGroot LJ, Niepomniszcze H: Biosynthesis of thyroid hormone: Basic and clinical aspects. *Metabolism* 1977; 26:665.

DeGroot LJ, Larsen PR, Refetoff S, et al: *The Thyroid and Its Diseases.* New York, John Wiley & Sons, 1984.

DeVisscher M (ed): The thyroid gland, in Martini L (ed): *Comprehensive Endocrinology Series.* New York, Raven Press, 1980.

Dratman MB: On the mechanism of action of thyroxine, and amino acid analogue of tyrosine. *J Theor Biol* 1974; 46:255.

Dratman MB, Crutchfield FL, Axelrod J: Localization of triiodothyronine in nerve ending fractions of rat brain. *Proc Natl Acad Sci USA* 1976; 73:941.

Edelman IS, Ismail-Beigi F: Thyroid thermogenesis and active sodium transport. *Recent Prog Horm Res* 1974; 30:235.

Goldfine ID, Simons CG, Ingbar SH: Stimulation of uptake of aminoisobutyric acid in rat thymocytes by L-triiodothyronine: A comparison with insulin and dibutyryl cyclic AMP. *Endocrinology* 1975; 96:802.

Greenspan FS, Forsham PH (eds): *Basic and Clinical Endocrinology.* Los Altos, California, Lange Medical Publications, 1983.

Hamada S, Fukase M: Demonstration and some properties of cytosol binding proteins for thyroxine and triiodothyronine in human liver. *J Clin Endocrinol Metab* 1976; 42:302.

Ingbar SH, Braverman LE (eds): *The Thyroid.* Philadelphia, Harper & Row, 1984.

Jackson IMD: Thyrotropin-releasing hormone. *N Engl J Med* 1982; 306:145.

Klein AH, Fisher DA: Thyroid function in the neonatal period, in Kelley VC (ed): *Practice of Pediatrics.* New York, Harper & Row, 1977.

Klein I, Level GS: New perspectives on thyroid hormone, catecholamines, and the heart. *Am J Med* 1984; 76:167.

Kohn LD, Aloij SM, Tombaccini D, et al: The thyrotropin receptor, in Litwack G (ed): *Biochemical Actions of Hormones,* vol 14. Orlando, Florida, Academic Press, 1985.

Kurtz DT, Feigelson P: Multihormonal control of the messenger RNA for hepatic protein globulin, in Litwack G (ed): *Biochemical Actions of Hormones,* vol 5. New York, Academic Press, 1978, p 433.

Larsen PR: Thyroid-pituitary interaction: Feedback regulation of thyrotropin secretion by thyroid hormones. *N Engl J Med* 1982; 306:23.

Larsen PR, Silva JE, Kaplan MM: Relationship between circulating and intracellular thyroid hormones: Physiological and clinical implications. *Endocr Rev* 1981; 87.

Lever EG, Medeiros-Neto GA, DeGroot LJ: Inherited disorders of thyroid metabolism. *Endocr Rev* 1983; 4:213.

Levey GS: The adrenergic nervous system in hyperthyroidism: Therapeutic role of beta adrenergic blocking drugs. *Pharmacol Ther* 1976; 1:431.

Lissitzky S, Fayet G, Verrier B: Thyroid stimulating hormone binding to cultured cells. *FEBS Lett* 1973; 29:20.

Lo CS, Edelman IS: Effect of triiodothyronine on the synthesis and degradation of renal cortical (Na$^+$ + K$^+$)-adenosine triphosphatase. *J Biol Chem* 1976; 251:7834.

Magnuson MA, Nikodem VM: Molecular cloning of a cDNA sequence for rat liver enzyme. *J Biol Chem* 1983; 258:12712.

Malbon CC, Moreno FJ, Cabelli RJ: Fat cell adenylate cyclase and β adrenergic receptors in altered thyroid states. *J Biol Chem* 1978; 253:671.

Martin TFJ, Kowalchyk JA: Evidence for the role of calcium and diacylglycerol as dual second messengers in thyrotropin-releasing hormone action: Involvement of diacylglycerol. *Endocrinology* 1984; 115:1517.

Narayan P, Liaw CW, Towle HC: Rapid induction of a specific nuclear mRNA precursor by thyroid hormone. *Proc Natl Acad Sci USA* 1984; 81:4687.

Nunez J: Effects of thyroid hormones during brain differentiation. *Mol Cell Endocrinol* 1984; 37:125.

Nunez J, Pommier J: Formation of thyroid hormones. Vitam Horm 1982; 39:175.

Oppenheimer JH: Thyroid hormone action at the nuclear level. *Ann Intern Med* 1985; 102:374.

Oppenheimer JH, Samuels HH (eds): *Molecular Basis of Thyroid Hormone Action.* New York, Academic Press, 1983.

Petrick P, Weintraub BD: Inappropriate secretion of TSH, in Krieger D, Bardin W (eds): *Current Therapy in Endocrinology and Metabolism.* Philadelphia, BC Decker, 1985.

Pliam WB, Goldfine ID: High affinity thyroid hormone binding sites on purified rat liver plasma membranes. *Biochem Biophys Res Commun* 1977; 79:166.

Portnay GI, McClendon FD, Bush JE, et al: The effect of physiological doses of thyroxine on carrier-mediated ADP uptake by liver mitochondria from thyroid-ectomized rats. *Biochem Biophys Res Commun* 1973; 55:17.

Scanlon F, Chan V, Heath M, et al: Dopaminergic control of thyrotropin α subunit, thyrotropin β subunit and prolactin in euthyroidism and hypothyroidism: Dissociated responses to dopamine receptor blockade with metoclopramide in hypothyroid subjects. *J Clin Endocrinol Metab* 1981; 53:360.

Segal J, Gordon A, Gross J: Evidence that L-triiodothyronine (T$_3$) exerts its biological action not only through its effects on nuclear activity, in Robbins J, Braverman LE (eds): *Thyroid Research.* New York, Elsevier North-Holland, Inc, 1976, p 331.

Sestoft L: Metabolic aspects of the calorigenic effect of thyroid hormone in mammals. *Clin Endocrinol* 1980; 13:489.

Shapiro LE, Samuels HH, Yaffe BM: Thyroid and glucocorticoid hormones synergistically control growth hormone mRNA in cultured GH$_1$ cells. *Proc Natl Acad Sci USA* 1978; 65:45.

Shiroozu A, Taurog A, Engler H, et al: Mechanism of action of thioureylene antithyroid drugs in the rat: Possible inactivation of thyroid peroxidase by propylthiouracil. *Endocrinology* 1983; 113:362.

Sterling K: Thyroid hormone action at the cell level. *N Engl J Med* 1979; 300:117.

Sterling K, Campbell GA, Taliadouros GS, et al: Mitochondrial binding of triiodothyronine (T$_3$). *Cell Tiss Res* 1984; 236:321.

Tata JR: How specific are nuclear receptors for thyroid hormones? *Nature* 1975; 257:18.

Williams LT, Lefkowitz RJ, Watanabe AM, et al: Thyroid hormone regulation of adrenergic receptor number. *J Biol Chem* 1977; 252:2787.

Woeber KA, Braverman LE: The thyroid. *Contemp Endocrinol* 1985; 2:87.

PART VI

The Adrenals

11

ACTH and Adrenal Glucocorticoids

The physician's interest in adrenal cortical physiology covers a wide spectrum of disorders. Adrenal insufficiency (Addison's disease) and adrenal hyperfunction (Cushing's disease) are not very common, but with increasingly accurate diagnostic methods in the face of our population explosion, they can no longer be considered rare. In addition, there are certain well-recognized inborn errors of metabolism of the adrenal cell that manifest themselves as a group of syndromes called congenital adrenal hyperplasia. Like the cells of other endocrine glands, adrenal cells sometimes undergo metaplasia and form tumors, which may cause a number of different clinical disturbances, depending on the predominant hormonal product of the tumor cell. One tumor cell type produces an excess of the salt-retaining hormone aldosterone, which is discussed below. Others may produce an excess of androgenic steroids, or estrogenic steroids with manifestations appropriate to internal "overdoses" of these substances.

In addition, the adrenals are believed to play an important role in adaptation to many kinds of "stresses," such as trauma (accidental or surgical), severe infectious disease, severe intoxication, and other similar challenges. The mechanism of the participation of adrenal hormones in these complex events is not known and the role of many other hormonal, neural, and nutritional influences in them is just beginning to be appreciated, but current and future studies of these phenomena must involve an understanding of the hypophyseal-adrenal cortical machinery.

Since 1949, adrenal cortical hormones, and various modifications of the naturally occurring materials that have been made by the organic chemist, have been used for their anti-inflammatory effect in the treatment of many diseases. The ability of these substances to suppress inflammation is one of their most fascinating attributes, and the importance of this effect in the management of patients with rheumatoid arthritis, disseminated lupus erythematosus and various allergic states is well recognized though not well understood. The successful use of these compounds in the fields of dermatology and ophthalmology alone would have justified the work that went into discovering and producing them.

There are important effects of adrenocortical insufficiency and excess on mood and even on adjustment to reality. Patients with Addison's disease are often depressed or anxious, and these symptoms are ameliorated by proper hormonal replacement therapy. The use of pharmacologic doses of adrenal steroids in the long-term management of patients with arthritis or other diseases may result in euphoria or even overt psychosis in certain individuals who are presumably predisposed to such a condition. In some instances the CNS effects can be correlated with changes in the character of the electroencephalogram. Thus, there is scarcely a medical field of interest in which a knowledge of the adrenal cortex is without pertinence.

Structures of glucocorticoids and mineralocorticoids are given in Figure 11–1.

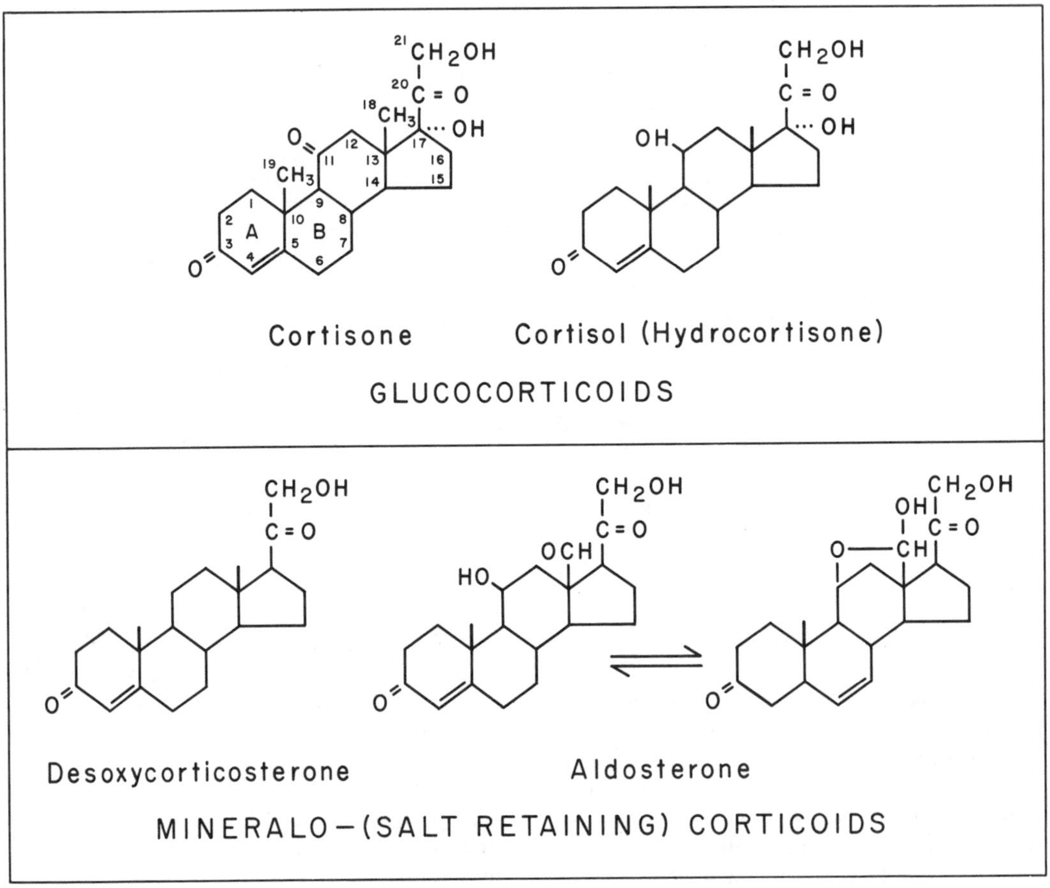

FIG 11–1.
Adrenal glucocorticoids and mineralocorticoids.

Effects of Adrenalectomy

Adrenal ablation in animals or man causes a far-reaching metabolic disturbance that has repercussions in virtually every area of physiology. The untreated condition is characterized by *weakness* and *easy fatigability;* by *hypotension;* by a variety of *gastrointestinal disturbances* including anorexia, nausea, vomiting, abdominal pain, and diarrhea; by various ill-defined *emotional* difficulties including anxiety and depression; and (in man) by increased *pigmentation* of the skin. There may be a striking intolerance to fasting, and there is certainly decreased ability to withstand trauma, infections, hemorrhage, or other similar insults. In man, the untreated deficiency may lead to a condition known as "adrenal crisis," which is characterized by prostration and peripheral circulatory failure. There are certain analogies between the diseases diabetes mellitus and adrenal insufficiency in man: both are due to a hormone deficit; both require careful, long-term week-to-week management; both kinds of patients may be made worse by a sudden, unexpected event, such as an injury or an infection; and both may lead to a kind of collapse that can be described only as a medical emergency (adrenal crisis and diabetic acidosis).

It is traditional to separate the sequelae of adrenal ablation into two general physiologic compartments: (1) associated with the metabolism of carbohydrate and protein, and with the capacity to withstand stresses of many types; and (2) with water and electrolyte metabolism and the ability to reabsorb sodium from the glomerular filtrate, and thus conserve this ion when it is available only in limited amounts. Although this compartmentalization is sometimes useful, it may also be misleading, for a primary effect on electrolyte and water excretion may lead to a severe circulatory disturbance, which in turn may have a devastating effect on carbohydrate and protein metabolism. For example, the sequence of events following adrenalectomy may be as follows: Loss of aldosterone → sodium loss in urine → dehydration → peripheral circulatory failure → tissue hypoxia → protein catabolism. The integrity of metabolic processes in cells depends in part on their blood supply and a serious hemodynamic derangement may result in a profound metabolic disturbance.

One of the most constant characteristics of the adrenalectomized animal or the patient with adrenal insufficiency is the inability to excrete a large water load and the susceptibility to water intoxication. This defect persists even when the salt-wasting tendency has been corrected hormonally or compensated for by an increased salt intake. It is corrected not by the typical salt water adrenal steroids such as desoxycorticosterone but by steroids of the cortisol type, which are active in organic metabolism.

The two general areas of activity of adrenal hormones—salt conservation and organic metabolism—may be affected differentially or unequally in both animals and man. Aldosterone, which is the main salt-retaining hormone of the adrenal cortex, is synthesized in the glomerulosa layer of cortical cells, whereas cortisol (in man) and corticosterone (in the rat), which are the principal glucocorticoids of adrenal vein blood, are made primarily in the fasciculata layer. When tuberculosis was a prominent cause of bilateral adrenal destruction, far more pronounced defects in salt conservation were seen than are observed in idiopathic adrenal insufficiency, which may sometimes express itself as an almost pure glucocorticoid deficiency. The hypophysectomized animal shows many of the organic metabolic defects of the adrenalectomized animal, but it does not die of adrenal insufficiency because the glomerulosa appears to be able to secrete a sufficient amount of aldosterone to fill its limited needs. The trophic control of secretion from the different zones of the adrenal will be discussed in Chapter 12.

The *electrolyte-water* defect of adrenal insufficiency is far more complex than a simple renal incontinence for sodium. The most prominent feature of the defect is an inability to reabsorb sodium and chloride from the tubular urine rapidly enough to prevent a net sodium loss from the body under conditions of normal or reduced sodium intake. This effect is accompanied by potassium retention and rising concentrations of this ion in the extracellular fluid. The increase in serum potassium is due to a combination of the animal's inability to excrete it and an accompanying discharge of potassium from the intracellular into the extracellular fluid compartment of the body. This may be partly the result of an effect of adrenal cortical hormone deficiency on cell membranes generally and partly the tissue hypoxia that develops as a result of the hemodynamic disturbance of the untreated deficiency state. As the dehydration becomes more severe due to the loss of progressively more sodium, the ensuing hypotension and diminished renal blood flow contribute to an accumulation of phosphate and nonprotein nitrogen in the blood as well as potassium. Associated with this sequence of events there may be gastrointestinal disturbances, such as vomiting and diarrhea. These accentuate the salt and fluid loss and may tend to telescope the events described above within a shorter time just as they tend to accelerate the development of diabetic acidosis.

Although the renal aspects of salt conservation

have been studied most extensively, effects of adrenalectomy and salt-water adrenal hormone treatment on salt escape from the body by other routes are also striking. Desoxycorticosterone, a powerful salt-retaining hormone, not only can promote the reabsorption of sodium by the renal tubule but also can diminish the sodium concentration of sweat, saliva, and intestinal secretions. The effect on sweat adds a new dimension to our thoughts about the adrenal cortex and evolutionary survival value, for heat exposure is a powerful stimulus to aldosterone secretion and we may assume that the additional aldosterone secreted functions to diminish the sodium concentration of sweat, as desoxycorticosterone has been shown to do. Thus, the salt-retaining activity of the adrenal hormones is of adaptive value, not only when there is less salt available in the environment for ingestion but also when a hot environment leads to increased salt loss through sweating.

The adrenals are essential to life because their salt-retaining function is a vital one. The lives of hypoadrenal animals and patients may be prolonged by feeding them large amounts of sodium chloride. A salt-maintained adrenalectomized animal, or a similar animal maintained with just a salt-water hormone such as desoxycorticosterone, lives a precarious life because it lacks those hormones that function primarily in the sphere of organic metabolism.

The *organic metabolic defects* of adrenal insufficiency are extremely complicated, and it is impossible to give a tidy or appealing summary of them at this time. Some of the metabolic effects of adrenalectomy that have been described are due to glucocorticoid hormone deficiency, others to hemodynamic effects of salt loss on metabolism, and still others to the fact that adrenalectomized animals do not eat well and have an abnormally low rate of total metabolism.

Adrenalectomized animals show a rapid fall in blood glucose and tissue glycogen levels on fasting. Patients with Addison's disease often show a typical reactive hypoglycemia, or overshoot, during the performance of a glucose tolerance test, suggesting that the intact individual uses his adrenal steroids as a sort of brake on the falling blood glucose concentration (see Chapter 14). In fact, insulin sensitivity is a prominent feature of adrenal insufficiency. Pancreatic diabetes is ameliorated by adrenalectomy partly because the insulin lack is compensated by the absence of adrenal hormones. Many experiments suggest that the fasting adrenalectomized animal is unable to adapt to carbohydrate deprivation by drawing upon its muscle protein and lymphoid tissue stores for the process of gluconeogenesis. Although there is much experimental evidence to support the view that peripheral tissue protein, particularly that of muscle and lymphoid tissue, is not readily available for gluconeogenesis in the adrenally deprived animal, other evidence suggests that the liver cell in such an animal may not be able to convert amino acids to glycogen at a normal rate.

In addition to the effects described, the adrenal glucocorticoids often appear to play a "permissive" role in metabolism. This simply means that many cells that are responsive to a variety of humoral and neural influences perform well only when they are exposed to a certain baseline concentration of adrenocortical steroids. For example, the adrenalectomized animal does not respond to trauma or hemorrhage with an increased nitrogen excretion as the normal intact animal does. Comparatively small doses of a cortisone-like compound "permit" this response to occur.

Glucocorticoids are involved in both the synthesis and actions of catecholamines. The induction by glucocorticoids of the methyl transferase enzyme, PNMT, which is responsible for synthesizing epinephrine from its precursor, norepinephrine (see Fig 13–2), occurs in the adrenomedullary cell. Glucocorticoids "permit" the calorigenic, lipolytic, pressor, and bronchodilator effects of catecholamines to occur. That is, in the absence of glucocorticoids (as in the adrenalectomized animal), these catecholamine actions are either absent or incompletely expressed. In some tissues, glucocorticoids increase the number and hormone affinity of β adrenergic receptors. The detailed mechanism by which they do this is not yet known.

It now seems that the hepatic effect of glucocorticoids on gluconeogenesis, like the effect of these substances on peripheral protein mobilization, is basically a permissive one. Exton and Park (1967) have described a failure of the isolated perfused liver of the adrenalectomized rat to respond to a gluconeogenic stimulus such as glucagon, epinephrine or $3',5'$ cyclic adenylic acid. Pretreatment of such an animal with glucocorticoids results in restoration of the normal gluconeogenic response to these agents. Partial restoration of the response can even be achieved by perfusing the hormone-deficient liver with an adrenal glucocorticoid (dexamethasone) in vitro. Adrenal insufficiency does not result in a diminished production of $3',5'$ cyclic AMP in response to the gluconeogenic stimulus. It apparently interferes with the capacity of a component of the gluconeogenic machinery to respond to the cyclic nucleotide.

In human adrenal insufficiency, pigmentation of the skin is a prominent finding. The possible role of the high hypophyseal corticotrophin output that is characteristic of this condition in the mechanism of the hyperpigmentation will be discussed.

The behavioral and emotional disturbances seen in Addison's disease and the fact that these may be accompanied by abnormal electroencephalographic tracings has already been referred to. These changes can be reversed by the administration of glucocorticoids.

Design of Hypothalamo-Pituitary-Adrenocortical System

The fasciculata zone of cells in the adrenal cortex is trophically controlled by hypophyseal corticotrophin (ACTH), which stimulates them to produce steroids, such as cortisol, which are concerned especially with organic metabolism. The aldosterone-producing cells in the glomerulosa zone are controlled separately by other trophic substances, which may require permissive concentrations of ACTH in order to raise secretory activity to high levels (see Chapter 12). It has been suggested that adrenal androgens arise predominantly in the cells of the reticularis, or juxtamedullary, portion of the cortex. The glomerulosa cells have a degree of freedom from ACTH direction, for the glomerulosa zone does not become depleted of lipid on ACTH stimulation as does the fasciculata, and it can be shown to vary in width with salt deprivation and repletion even in the hypophysectomized animal. Thus, there are at least two feedback systems that regulate the activity of the adrenal cortex: one that involves principally ACTH and cortisol, and the other, aldosterone and its own trophic substances. In the case of the former, the level of output of cortisol in adrenal vein blood is almost entirely determined by the intensity of the ACTH stimulus. The cortisol produced then feeds back on the trophic tissues and "instructs" them to decrease ACTH release. The rate of ACTH production at which the shut-off signal is perceived and acted upon apparently can be reset at higher or lower levels in a manner that is not now understood. The regulation of aldosterone secretion will be considered in Chapter 12.

The adrenal androgens and their regulation have been discussed in Chapter 9. They play an important role in the steroid hormone economy of the pregnant woman and the fetal-placental unit. They also serve as precursors for estrogen synthesis in both males and females.

If we use Figure 11–2 as a diagrammatic outline of the entire neurohypophyseal-adrenocortical end-organ system, we will be able to see how each of the following subdivisions of the discussion fits into the larger picture.

Adrenocortical Cell: Hormone Biosynthesis

The marked variations in activity that occur in adrenocortical cells are due to varying amounts of chemical stimuli that are brought to them in the bloodstream. Of these stimuli, ACTH has been most studied. In the absence of ACTH, the adrenal cortex narrows, the glands become small and production of glucocorticoids falls to negligible levels. Aldosterone production decreases somewhat but remains sufficiently high to prevent serious salt loss.

Unlike the islets of Langerhans, the hypophysis, and the thyroid, adrenocortical cells do not store large quantities of hormone. The glands are extremely vascular and the cells appear to secrete hormone into the blood as soon as it is made. In order to extract milligram quantities of cortisol or aldosterone from adrenal glands, it is necessary to process very large amounts of material. Many steroids (25–30) have been extracted from adrenal tissue and identified, but most of these are believed to be metabolic intermediates in synthesis of the few final hormonal products. With the perfection of a variety of analytic methods, it is now possible to detect and quantify steroids that appear in adrenal vein blood on ACTH stimulation. The main glucocorticoid in man and the dog is cortisol (hydrocortisone, Kendall's compound F); in the rat it is corticosterone.

As a result of the application of a large number of methods (e.g., histochemical, analytical chemical, radioactive tracer studies, paper chromatography, adrenal perfusion, study of urinary excretion products), it is now possible to reconstruct a plausible account of hormone biosynthesis in the adrenal cell. Although the adrenal cell does not store much finished hormone, it does contain very large amounts of what is presumed to be hormone precursor, esterified cholesterol.

Figure 11–3 illustrates a typical postulated reaction sequence for the synthesis of adrenal steroids. The importance of this scheme transcends the fasciculata cells of the adrenal cortex, as similar events doubtless take place in all steroid hormone-producing cells, whether the final product is cortisol, aldosterone, estrogen, androgen, or progesterone. All of the structures that produce these materials (adrenals, ovarian cells, testicular cells) are embryologically derived from the primitive urogenital ridge and eventually differentiate to specialize in the production of one or more steroid hormones. Whether the final product turns out to be one steroid or another depends on the enzyme profile of the hormone-producing cell.

A striking feature of steroid hormone biosynthesis

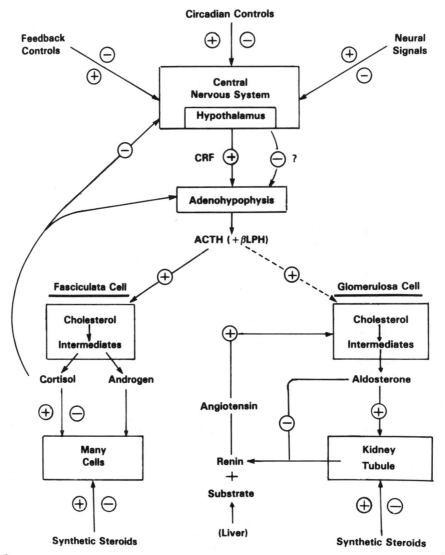

FIG 11–2.
Neuroendocrine control of the adrenal cortex.

is sequential hydroxylation (emphasized in Figure 11–3 by OH). The side chain cleavage (SCC) reaction consists of a preliminary hydroxylation of carbons 20 and 22 of cholesterol followed by cleavage of the molecule to pregnenolone and isocaproaldehyde. Depending on the product, hydroxylations of the steroid nucleus may occur at carbons 17, 21, 11, and 18. The general molecular mechanism is the same in each case: NADPH, molecular oxygen, and a cytochrome P450 oxygen donor system are required. These components interact as shown in Figure 11–4. *While a P450 enzyme performs the same function in all hydroxylations, it is specific for each substrate.* Thus, the side chain cleavage cytochrome P450 is desig-

nated as $P450_{SCC}$, while the others are known respectively as $P450_{17\alpha}$, $P450_{11\beta}$, $P450_{C21}$, and $P450_{C18}$. Since each of these is the product of a different gene, the steroid hormone-producing capability is determined, in an adrenal cell or a Leydig cell or a corpus luteum cell, at the time of differentiation, when the cell is committed to transcribe a certain battery of P450 enzymes in a particular ratio.

INBORN ERRORS OF ADRENAL HORMONE SYNTHESIS

One practical yield from basic studies on steroid transformations in the adrenal gland has been the rec-

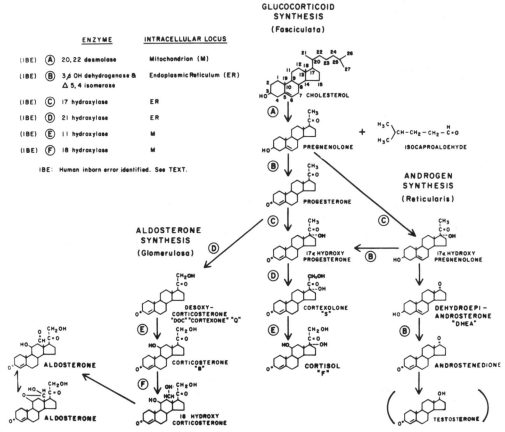

FIG 11–3.
Summary of steroidogenesis in the adrenal cortex.

ognition of many different types of inborn errors in patients. The enzymatic loci of some of these errors are indicated in Figure 11–3.

The general principles involved in clinical manifestations of an inborn error are worth examining. When an enzymatic defect exists—it may be a deficiency of enzyme protein or a defective enzyme protein—the product of the reaction is not made in sufficient quantities. The precursor tends to accumulate. Thus, for example, in type I adrenal hyperplasia, the block is at the 21-hydroxylation reaction, which catalyzes the transformation of 17-OH progesterone to compound

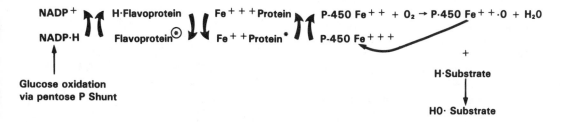

FIG 11–4.
Mechanism of steroid hydroxylation in mitochondria. (In endoplasmic reticulum, electrons are passed directly from flavoprotein to P-450.)

S. Metabolites below the block decrease, and those proximal to the block accumulate. The resulting failure of cortisol production results in low circulating cortisol, which in turn elicits CRF (corticotrophin-releasing factor) from the median eminence gland. Intense CRF stimulation causes a high level of circulating ACTH, which stimulates steroidogenesis at a site above the genetic block. This has the effect of generating large amounts of adrenal androgens (see Fig 11–3), which are manifest as virilization in the female or precocious puberty in the male. The locus of the block can be inferred from the nature of the excreted steroids (in this case, predominantly pregnanediol) as well as by the absence of water and sodium retention.

If there is a deficiency of 11-hydroxylase (type II), compound S cannot be converted to cortisol. Again, cortisol deficiency elicits overproduction of ACTH, with consequent increase in adrenal androgen output. However, the accumulation of S is reflected in the secretion of large amounts of desoxycorticosterone, a powerfully salt-retaining steroid. Thus, the hallmark of type II disease is salt retention and hypertension in the presence of virilization and cortisol deficiency. The predominating urinary steroid in this instance is tetrahydro S.

In both of these circumstances, the failure of feedback inhibition of ACTH production because of the cortisol deficiency causes overproduction of ACTH and, hence, the accumulation of large amounts of steroids whose production is not impaired by the genetic defect. Thus, by replacing the cortisol deficiency, ACTH secretion is inhibited and excessive production of androgens is stopped. In the case of 11-hydroxylase deficiency, overproduction of 11-desoxycorticosterone (DOC) is also interrupted. Since the hypertension in this group is associated with overproduction of 11-desoxycortisol and DOC, this abnormality is also corrected.

Female fetuses exposed to androgen as a result of an inborn error of metabolism in the adrenal show virilization of the external genitalia at birth, though there is persistence of the müllerian duct-derived structures because of the absence of testes, the source of müllerian inhibiting factor (see Chapter 8). This condition can be corrected by inhibiting ACTH production with replacement (not anti-inflammatory) doses of a glucocorticoid.

The development of radioimmunoassays for individual steroid intermediates in the biosynthetic pathway for adrenal hormones has made possible the *prenatal diagnosis* of the locus of certain inborn errors of the adrenal. For example, elevated levels of 17OH progesterone and δ^4 steroids in amniotic fluid indicate a 21-hydroxylase deficiency in the fetus, while increased levels of tetrahydrodeoxycortisol are associated with 11-hydroxylase deficiency. Histocompatibility (HLA) genotyping of amniotic cells is also useful as a predictor of 21-hydroxylase deficiency if the HLA genotype is identical with that of an affected sibling (see New).

The same genetic error need not be expressed to the same extent in two different types of steroid hormone-producing cells. For example, in four distinct inborn errors, 21-, 11β-, 17β-hydroxylase and 3-hydroxysteroid dehydrogenase deficiencies, fasciculata cells (cortisol) and glomerulosa cells (aldosterone) may show different degrees of enzymatic defects. In spite of their anatomical juxtaposition, fasciculata and glomerulosa cells are, functionally, elements of two distinct glands in which the locus of genes for the same enzymes, as well as their control mechanisms, may have been arranged differently at the time of differentiation. (For a contemporary view of inborn errors of the adrenals, see reviews by New and colleagues.)

EFFECTS OF DRUGS ON STEROIDOGENESIS

Several drugs and toxins inhibit steroid hormone production by the adrenal cortex. These are potentially useful when excessive amounts of hormone are being produced and, in one instance, as a diagnostic agent to test the competency of the feedback regulatory aspect of the pituitary-adrenal system.

Mitotane

Mitotane or DDD (Fig 11–4) is closely related to the DDT family of chlorinated hydrocarbon insecticides. During the course of routine toxicity tests, the compound was found to have a highly selective destructive effect on normal adrenocortical cells, and later the same effect was seen in neoplastic cells of adrenocortical origin. Although its mechanism of action is not known, the compound has been used as a palliative chemotherapeutic agent in management of inoperable adrenocortical carcinoma. Although therapeutic doses cause anorexia, nausea, and somnolence in many treated individuals, treatment is continued. In this case, potential benefits outweigh the risk of unpleasant side effects.

Aminoglutethimide

Aminoglutethimide (α ethyl-p-aminophenol-glutarimide) inhibits at the first reaction of steroid hormone biosynthesis, i.e., at the cholesterol side chain cleavage step. This decreases or stops all steroid hormone synthesis.

Metyrapone

Metyrapone is a rather selective inhibitor of 11β-hydroxylase. Steroid synthesis stops at 11-desoxycortisol, or cortexolone (Fig 11–5). This metabolite accumulates, but since it has no feedback inhibitory effect on ACTH production, ACTH is greatly overproduced and stimulates the synthesis of large amounts of steroid intermediate compounds above the pharmacologic blockade. It is possible to assess the ability of the ACTH trophic complex to respond to acute deprivation of the target organ hormone by measuring either the urinary excretion of 17-hydroxysteroids or by radioimmunoassay for ACTH. The test was used extensively to evaluate hypothalamic-pituitary function with respect to ACTH.

Corticotrophin-Releasing Factor

See discussion on page 64, Chapter 5.

Corticotrop(h)in, ACTH

The structure of human ACTH is shown in Figure 11–6. Hofmann and his colleagues first synthesized de novo a 23 amino acid peptide (1–23) with all of the ACTH activity of the naturally occurring material. Then they succeeded in synthesizing the entire 39 amino acid peptide, beginning with individual amino acids.

The relationship between and among ACTH, α MSH, β LPH, and the opiate-like peptides was discussed in Chapter 5. A high molecular weight glycoprotein precursor molecule is synthesized in one type of pituitary basophil. ACTH and β LPH are among the cleavage products of this glycoprotein. Both ACTH and β LPH have now been identified in clusters of neurons in the brain in locations distant from the pituitary and hypothalamus. There is some uncertainty about the origin of these extrahypothalamic peptides, and this uncertainty has been compounded by Bergland and Page's demonstration of pituitary-to-brain blood flow in the hypophyseal portal system. However, the persistence of ACTH in extrahypothalamic locations in the brain after hypophysectomy in the rat favors local origin.

The entire human pituitary contains about 50 units, or 250 μg, of ACTH. The daily secretion rate is 1–5 units (5–25 μg), but many times this amount may be secreted in stressful circumstances (e.g., surgical trauma).

The development of radioimmunoassay and radioreceptor assay methods for ACTH made it possible to sample blood levels very frequently by means of indwelling catheters. Like all other pituitary hormones, ACTH is secreted in a pulsatile manner with a pulse frequency of about 7–9 per three-hour period. These small pulses are superimposed on a characteristic diurnal fluctuation, which has a much greater amplitude. In normal individuals the lowest ACTH levels are found late in the day and near the beginning of the sleep period. The highest levels usually occur at about 6–8 A.M., upon awakening. The morning surge characteristically begins toward the end of the sleep period. A knowledge of the normal diurnal pattern is important diagnostically because in conditions in which ACTH secretion is autonomous (as in Cushing's disease due to an ACTH-producing pituitary tumor, or ectopic ACTH production by a neoplasm), high concentrations of ACTH may be found late in the day or at the beginning of sleep; i.e., there is a disruption of the normal diurnal pattern.

ACTH has a biologic half-life in the circulation of 15–25 minutes. Although the affinity of the adrenal cell ACTH receptor for the hormone is very high, only a very small fraction of the 5–25 μg of ACTH secreted daily by the pituitary is fixed by the adrenals. Since the adrenals respond to this by secreting 20–50 mg of cortisol daily and since the anatomical position of the pituitary vis-à-vis the hypothalamus is so favorable, this represents an extraordinary amplification of the neural and humoral signals that elicited the secretion of CRF in the hypothalamus. By this system, information can be integrated, decoded and acted upon by CRF neurons rapidly and efficiently, since the cortisol secretion elicited can be disseminated throughout the general circulation. If we follow ACTH and cortisol in the blood simultaneously, the target organ hormone concentration can be seen to follow closely that of the trophic one.

It is instructive to compare levels of circulating ACTH in a variety of circumstances, as shown in Table 11–1.

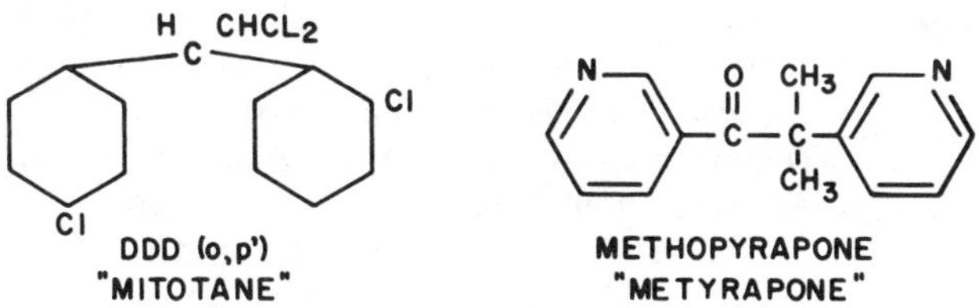

FIG 11–5.
Inhibitors of steroidogenesis.

1   10

H₂NSer-Tyr-Met-Glu-His-Phe-Arg-Trp-Gly-Lys-
13   18   20

Lys-Pro-Val-Gly Lys-Lys-Arg-*Arg-Pro-Val-*
30

Lys-Val-Tyr-Pro-Asn-Gly-Ala-Glu-Asp-Glu-
39

Ser-Ala-Glu-Ala-Phe-Pro-Leu-Glu-Phe·COOH

FIG 11–6.
Amino acid sequence of human ACTH. Amino acids 1–13 *(bold)* are αMSH; those for corticotropin-like intermediate lobe peptide (CLIP) are 18–39 *(italics)*. (Based on data of Lerner and Buettner-Janusch *(J Biol Chem* 1961; 236:2970.)

CELLULAR MECHANISM OF ACTION OF ACTH

The *ACTH receptor* has all the characteristics of a stereospecific, high affinity, saturable plasma membrane receptor. It shows the phenomenon of spare receptors, since a maximal steroidogenic response can be obtained with only 5% occupancy of available receptors. In fact, steroidogenesis can be measurably increased when it is not possible to detect an increase in the concentration of cAMP in the adrenal tissue or dispersed cell preparation. On the other hand, adenylate cyclase *is* activated by ACTH, and steroidogenesis *can* be stimulated by cAMP in the absence of ACTH. The lack of correlation between measurable hormone synthesis and cAMP concentration, like that which has been observed in the Leydig cell stimulated by LH, is due to increased binding of cAMP to the regulatory subunit of cAMP-dependent protein kinase when no significant increase in tissue cAMP concentration can be measured.

Calcium is necessary for ACTH stimulation of steroidogenesis in adrenal cells. According to Cheitlin et al., its primary effect is to facilitate the association of the hormone with its receptor, although there is evidence to suggest that the calcium ion may also be involved in the action of cAMP on steroidogenesis. (Indeed, calcium may mimic certain actions of ACTH in the absence of cAMP.)

ACTH effects on the adrenal fasciculata cell can be divided into three general categories on the basis of the time required for the response: (1) acute, i.e., within minutes, and not involving transcription of new messenger RNAs; (2) subacute, i.e., those dependent on the transcription of mRNAs for specific enzymes involved in steroidogenesis (hours); (3) chronic growth effects—hypertrophy and hyperplasia of the gland (hours to days).

1. Acute Effects of ACTH (Fig 11–7,A)

Historically, the discovery that cAMP is involved in the action of ACTH was the first extension of the cAMP second messenger idea beyond Sutherland's famous glycogenolysis experiments (Haynes and Berthet). Indeed, it was possible to stimulate steroidogenesis in adrenal cells with the cAMP analogue, dibutyryl cAMP. Since neither ACTH nor dbcAMP could stimulate steroid hormone synthesis in the presence of an inhibitor of translation (cycloheximide), it was postulated by Garren and his associates that one of the effects of cAMP was to stimulate the translation of a short half-life protein ("labile protein") from a readily available, long half-life mRNA. The existence of "labile protein" has been proved, but the precise role of cAMP-dependent protein kinase in either stimulating its translation or activating it is still a matter of conjecture. That the translation process itself may be affected by cAMP is suggested by the phosphorylation of a ribosomal protein of unknown function in treated cells. Of a number of suggested functions for the labile protein (among them, the role of intracellular free cholesterol carrier), we are attracted most by the one illustrated in Fig 11–7,A, (p. 194) i.e., a facilitation of the binding of free cholesterol to P450$_{scc}$ at the inner membrane of the mitochondrion. P450$_{scc}$, which is often described as rate-limiting for the entire process of cortisol synthesis, is present in sufficiently high concentration to increase cortisol synthesis if it is supplied with cholesterol substrate. It is therefore more correct to say that the rate limitation is a function of the amount of hormone precursor that is delivered to P450$_{scc}$.

If P450$_{scc}$ is examined immediately after adrenal cells have been treated with ACTH, more cholesterol is bound to it than one can demonstrate in untreated preparations. We conclude that the earliest effect of ACTH or cAMP on steroidogenesis is the facilitation of binding of cholesterol to P450$_{scc}$. Under resting

TABLE 11–1.

Levels of Circulating ACTH*

CONDITION	PLASMA ACTH pg/ml
Hypopituitarism	Undetectable
Diurnal fluctuation	
10 P.M.–2 A.M. (lowest)	< 10
8 A.M. (highest)	50–80
1° adrenal insufficiency	> 300
ACTH adenoma (Cushing's)	40–200
Ectopic ACTH (lung tumor)	200–12,000
Severe stress	200–1,000 +

*Adapted from Daughaday WH, in *Williams Textbook of Endocrinology,* ed 7. Philadelphia, WB Saunders Co, 1985.

conditions, most mitochondrial cholesterol is in the *outer* mitochondrial membrane, while $P450_{scc}$ is associated with the *inner* membrane. How the translocation of cholesterol across the membrane is accomplished is not clearly understood, though one suggestion is that the phospholipid environment of both outer and inner membranes may be altered by labile protein in such a way that cholesterol and enzyme are more freely accessible to each other.

There is enough cholesterol in the outer mitochondrial membrane to respond to ACTH or dbcAMP stimulation, for purified labile protein has been shown to increase pregnenolone synthesis in mitochondria isolated from unstimulated cells. In the intact cell, however, even as the initial stimulation of steroidogenesis occurs at the side chain cleavage step, the free cholesterol pool (the source of mitochondrial membrane free cholesterol) is being replenished in multiple and interesting ways. Large amounts of cholesterol ester are stored in lipid droplets in adrenal cells (as well as in Leydig cells, corpus luteum cells, and other steroidogenic cells). The enzyme cholesterol ester hydrolase (CEH), which frees cholesterol from its associated long chain fatty acid, is a substrate for cAMP protein kinase. In its phosphorylated state, it is activated and is able to mobilize free cholesterol from lipid droplets. Although the adrenal cell is demonstrably able to synthesize free cholesterol de novo from acetyl CoA via HMG CoA, this pathway contributes only minimally to the free cholesterol pool in stimulated cells because it is inhibited by cholesterol derived from ester hydrolysis.

In sustained ACTH stimulation the most important source of steroid hormone precursor is the almost limitless amount in the circulation in the form of lipoproteins. Although there are species differences in the particular lipoprotein used by the adrenal (low-density lipoprotein [LDL] in the human; high-density lipoprotein [HDL] in the rat), the design of the system is the same. The plasma membrane of the steroidogenic cell contains specific receptors for LDL or HDL. When the cell is stimulated by ACTH, the cholesterol ester-containing lipoprotein, bound to its specific membrane receptor, is internalized by the process of endocytosis and the endocytotic vesicle, containing lipoprotein lipid and protein as well as receptor, fuses with one or more lysosomes to form a phagolysosome, a microdigestion sac. Catabolic lysosomal enzymes then digest the macromolecules (salvaging digestion products for use by the stimulated cell) and split cholesterol esters, adding to the free cholesterol pool. Free cholesterol not immediately used for steroid hormone synthesis can be reesterified and incorporated into existing lipid droplets. We do not understand the mechanism by which an occupied ACTH receptor communicates (either directly or indirectly) with the part of the membrane that contains an LDL receptor. However, this is one phase of the action of ACTH that involves both Ca^{2+} and cytoskeletal structures, microtubules, and microfilaments.

Although the business of the adrenal cell does not seem to resemble that of a thyroid cell, it is instructive to reflect on similarities in the ways in which the two cells respond to hormonal stimulation. Glucose transport is stimulated by ACTH as it is by TSH. The increased influx of glucose is necessary to provide energy for biosynthetic processes, organelle movement, etc., and specifically to provide NADPH (via the pentose phosphate shunt) which is essential for some of the many hydroxylations that are necessary for the synthesis of cortisol from cholesterol. (The same cofactor, as we have seen in Chapter 10, served peculiarly thyroid cell functions when its production was elicited by TSH.) Shunt-generated NADPH specifically supports endoplasmic reticulum hydroxylations; mitochondrial hydroxylation reactions (side chain cleavage and 11β) are sustained by NADPH which is generated in the mitochondrion by reverse electron transport.

The role of Ca^{2+} in ACTH-stimulated steroidogenesis appears to be pervasive, though still incompletely understood. As we have seen, Ca^{2+} affects ACTH binding to its receptor, and Ca^{2+} Calmodulin are involved in the function of cytoskeletal elements, microtubules, and microfilaments. Ca^{2+} is also believed to be necessary for the transmembrane translocation of cholesterol that must precede side chain cleavage (though the cytoskeletal structures are not involved in this maneuver). The increase in cellular $[Ca^{2+}]$ produced by ACTH stimulation results in Ca^{2+} sequestration by mitochondria and ER. What effect this has on steroid metabolism in those organelles is unknown. That Ca^{2+} may have effects on the adrenal cell similar to those of cAMP is suggested by the fact that γ MSH has been shown to simulate the effect of ACTH or dbcAMP on cholesterol ester hydrolase by a mechanism that does not involve cAMP.

2. Subacute (Intermediate) Effects of ACTH: Specific Enzyme Induction (Fig 11–7,B)

Following hypophysectomy (ACTH deprivation), there is a striking decrease in the activities of all of the P450 enzyme systems involved in steroidogenesis. Continuous treatment with ACTH restores them to normal or supernormal levels in 12–24 hours. Adrenocortical cells in culture exposed to ACTH show dramatically increased rates of synthesis of cyto-

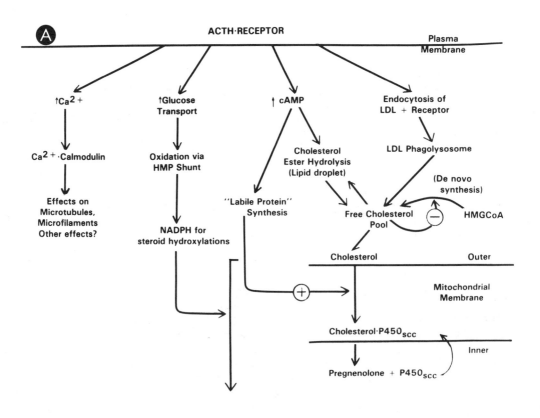

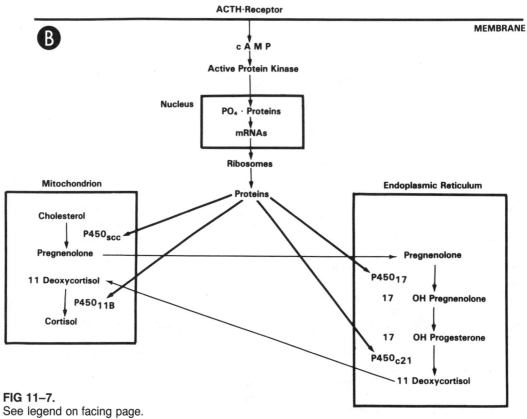

FIG 11–7.
See legend on facing page.

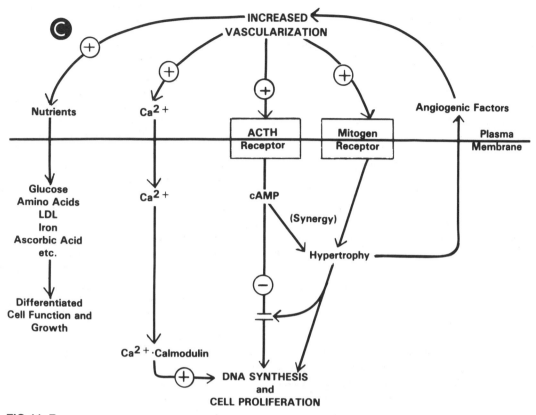

FIG 11–7.
A, acute effects of ACTH. **B,** pattern of induction of steroid hydroxylase enzyme complexes by ACTH. **C,** ACTH-mitogen relationships in chronic effect of ACTH on adrenal hypertrophy and hyperplasia. (Adapted and modified from Gill GN *Pharmacol Ther* 1976; 2:313.)

chromes $P450_{scc}$ and $P450_{11\beta}$ by immunoprecipitation, demonstrating that the increase in activity is due to the appearance of new protein units. As in the case of induced P450 enzymes in the liver by drugs, the ACTH effect on steroidogenic enzymes is based on increased transcription of new mRNAs for the respective proteins. Studies by two-dimensional polyacrylamide gel chromatography indicate that only a few species of proteins are induced by ACTH in adrenal cells during the first few hours of treatment, a selective effect on gene transcription that is reminiscent of others we have discussed in connection with steroid and thyroid hormones.

The synthesis of both mitochondrial and microsomal (ER) steroidogenic enzymes is induced not only by ACTH but also by dibutyryl cAMP and cholera toxin. This strongly suggests that one or more protein substrates phosphorylated by cAMP-dependent protein kinase are vital in eliciting the increase in mRNA synthesis necessary for the increase in P450 enzymes.

While all of the hydroxylase enzyme complexes necessary for cortisol production are induced, the extent of induction is not precisely the same for each. Unfortunately, the mechanisms by which cAMP affects transcription in the adrenal are less known than the mechanisms of induction of the lac operon in *E. coli* by cAMP. Cyclic AMP is also involved in the induction of gluconeogenic enzymes in the liver (see Chapter 14), possibly by mechanisms that resemble its mode of action in the adrenal.

3. Cellular Hypertrophy and Proliferation (Fig 11–7,C)

If adrenal cells are treated long enough (hours, days) with ACTH, generalized cellular hypertrophy (in addition to selective enzyme induction) and cellular proliferation occur. These effects are not due primarily to ACTH alone but to a collaboration between ACTH and certain mitogenic growth factors. Indeed, in order for cellular replication to occur under the influence of growth factors, cells must first become resistant to the *anti*replication effects of ACTH or of other agents that stimulate production of cAMP. Sustained production or administration of cAMP is characteristically associated with *inhibition* of cell division.

Figure 11-7,C illustrates that the hypertrophy-hyperplasia response is the result of a complex interplay of hormonal, nutritional, and vascular processes. Cyclic AMP and a mitogen (the most studied one is fibroblast growth factor) synergize to produce hypertrophy. When that process is far enough advanced, a mysterious event occurs that makes the cell refractory to the inhibitory effect of cAMP on mitogenesis. In all cases of normal and pathological growth, increased vascularization occurs, though agents responsible for this have been studied most extensively in tumor growth. The effect on blood vessel proliferation and increased blood flow is to bring more nutrients, metals, Ca^{2+}, etc., as well as more hormones, to the cells.

As Gill has emphasized, ACTH participates in this process not only by facilitating the influx of glucose, amino acids, and LDL, but also by establishing and maintaining *differentiated* steroidogenic function in the adrenal cell, i.e., by insuring that the correct P450 enzymes are present for the synthesis of cortisol and not some other steroid. As we saw in Chapter 9 (see Fig 9-7), the pattern of steroid produced in the fetal adrenal is quite different from that of the fully differentiated postnatal adrenal; the major steroid product in the fetus is dehydroepiandrosterone•SO_4, while in the fully differentiated adrenal, it is cortisol (human) or corticosterone (rat). ACTH, which is secreted copiously perinatally, induces the full complement of P450 enzymes necessary for cortisol production. Its presence during hypertrophy and hyperplasia insures that these enzymes will be maintained.

Compensatory hypertrophy of one adrenal after the contralateral one has been removed was considered to be the purest example of the operation of the CRF-ACTH feedback system. It is, however, more complex than that because such hypertrophy can occur to a measurable (but not complete) extent even in the hypophysectomized animal or in the animal treated with anti-ACTH antiserum. The suggestion has been made that there is an efferent neural component involved in this response (see Engeland and Dallman).

REGULATION OF SECRETION

Just as the adrenal cortex is dependent on stimulation by ACTH, the pituitary corticotrophic cell is driven by CRF. The peptidergic neuron in turn responds to multiple neurotransmitter substances. This general pattern conforms with the model description presented in Chapter 5. The CRF-ACTH-cortisol system has a number of distinctive features.

In the first place, adrenalectomy in animals (or primary Addison's disease in human beings) is associated with high circulating levels of ACTH. Thus, a decrease in target hormone concentration eliminates its tonic negative feedback influence, and more CRF, and therefore ACTH, is summoned. If exogenous glucocorticoid is administered to an individual with a normally functioning pituitary-adrenal axis, ACTH secretion is effectively shut off. Thus, this system exhibits the expected target organ hormone negative feedback control.

The opposing effects of CRF and glucocorticoids on ACTH synthesis and secretion have now been demonstrated at the level of gene transcription both by in vivo treatment and by rat anterior pituitary cells in primary culture (Gagner and Drouin). CRF has been shown to *stimulate* the rate of transcription of the proopiomelanocortin (POMC) gene within 15 minutes, and a glucocorticoid, dexamethasone, *inhibited* transcription of the POMC gene within 30 minutes. The highly selective action of glucocorticoid on gene transcription is illustrated by the fact that transcription of a number of genes is stimulated by the steroids (growth hormone in the pituitary, α2u globulin, tyrosine aminotransferase, tryptophan oxygenase in the liver, for example) while that of two (POMC in the pituitary and α fetoprotein in the liver) is inhibited.

The negative feedback system, however, can be overridden by a second control system with a higher priority. When the animal or man is subjected to a variety of challenges, which are collectively referred to as "stress" (e.g., trauma, burns, hypoglycemia, exercise, infection, chemical intoxications, hemorrhage, pain, psychologic stress), ACTH secretion is more or less vigorously stimulated *in spite of the fact that circulating cortisol levels are much higher than those required to inhibit ACTH production completely in the unstressed condition*. Either the sensitivity of the CNS neurons that participate in feedback inhibition is dulled, or the "normal" feedback inhibitory system is bypassed by an emergency circuit that takes precedence over it. In addition to these control mechanisms, there is, as we have seen, a set of rhythmic or episodic controls as well as a diurnal, sleep-related pattern of control.

It is not possible to assign the appropriate central neurotransmitter to each of the many stimuli that may elicit CRF secretion. We can only cite the scheme of

Jones (Fig 11–8), who has suggested that serotonin (5-HT) and acetylcholine (AcCh) may be involved in communicating stimulatory signals to the CRF neuron, whereas norepinephrine and gamma aminobutyric acid (GABA) may play inhibitory roles.

Although the monoaminergic control mechanisms for CRF are not explicitly known, it is interesting that drugs that interfere with the action of putative transmitters in this system have already been tried clinically with some success. Cyproheptadine, a serotonin antagonist that probably has some anticholinergic and antihistaminergic activity as well, has proved to be effective in blocking ACTH secretion in certain patients with hypercorticotrophic Cushing's disease.

The important conceptual point here is that the neural connections used to communicate such factors as the presence of pain, emotion, hemorrhage and hypoglycemia may arise in different regions of the brain, but they converge on the CRF peptidergic neuron and are thus able to initiate a stereotyped response.

Suppressibility of ACTH secretion by exogenously administered glucocorticoid is the basis for a diagnostic maneuver that is sometimes helpful in differentiating a normal individual with a suspiciously high output of glucocorticoids from a person with Cushing's disease or ectopic ACTH production. The synthetic steroid dexamethasone (see synthetic glucocorticosteroids below) regularly suppresses ACTH and glucocorticoid production below empirically derived limits. In individuals with partial or complete autonomy of ACTH-producing cells, it fails to do so. (Dexamethasone is such a potent glucocorticoid compared with cortisol that it does not interfere chemically with the analysis of excretion products of the naturally occurring steroids.)

There is unequivocal evidence for the fact that steroids can inhibit ACTH secretion by the pituitary by acting directly on the pituitary. Studies in which the quantity of CRF in the hypothalamus was measured as an indicator of glucocorticoid feedback effect are difficult to interpret but suggest that part of cortisol's feedback effect may be exerted at the hypothalamic level or even on suprahypothalamic neurons that control hypothalamic function. In addition to long-loop feedback control by cortisol, there is a possibility that ACTH can back-inhibit CRF-secreting neurons by a short loop.

ACTH, CORTISOL AND STRESS

One of the dominant themes in adrenocortical physiology has been the theory that the pituitary-adrenal axis participates prominently in the "nonspecific systemic reactions of the body, which ensue upon long exposure to stress." In 1946, Selye called attention to the fact that "diverse noxious agents" produced a rather stereotyped response in rats. At the time, the main features of this response were adrenal hypertrophy, atrophy of the lymphoid tissue of the body, and lymphopenia. Subsequently it was found that the earliest detectable change following trauma, heavy muscular exercise, infections, hemorrhagic shock, cold exposure, hypoxia, burns, and even severe psychologic trauma is a depletion of cholesterol and ascorbic acid in the adrenals, which is associated with an increased output of 11-oxygenated adrenal corticoids in adrenal vein blood. There also may be some degree of sodium retention and an increased excretion of potassium. A negative nitrogen balance is characteristic of the response, but this can be largely inhibited in many instances by force feeding carbohydrate. The sequence of events cannot occur in the absence of the hypophysis, and hypophysectomized or adrenalectomized animals and human beings are notoriously vulnerable to such stresses as those enumerated above. Figure 11–9 is a graphic summary of many factors that elicit CRF secretion. (For a recent discussion of the interaction of some hormones involved in responses to stress, see the review by Axelrod and Reisine, 1984.)

The alarm reaction aspect of the general adaptation syndrome has proved to be an enormously valuable

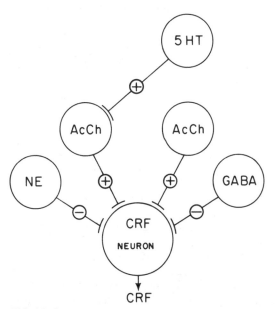

FIG 11–8.
Control of CRF secretion (after Jones). *5-HT* = serotonin; *AcCh* = acetylcholine; *GABA* = gamma aminobutyric acid: *NE* = norepinephrine.

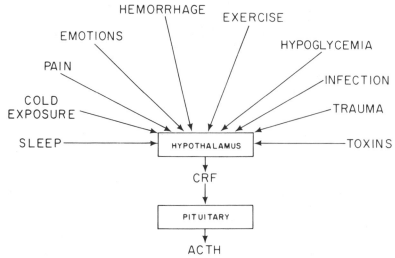

FIG 11–9.
Factors that elicit CRF secretion.

construct, and it has stimulated much useful experimental work and fruitful dialogue. It is a remarkable fact that the pituitary-adrenal axis is activated by such a variety of potentially harmful stimuli, and it is certainly possible, though not yet proved, that the increased amount of cortisol secreted immediately after injury, or even in anticipation of injury, may assist in the vital redistribution of amino acids that must occur in order for repair to proceed. A possible locus of participation of cortisol in the nonspecific injury response as well as the possible evolutionary survival value of a generalized injury response is suggested by the following quotation from Cuthbertson:

From teleological considerations the present writer early suggested that the general reaction by which labile protein is catabolized as a result of injury may serve to provide energy, or amino acids, or both, for the healing process, and that this is a primitive response independent of food, for a wounded animal is necessarily reduced in its capacity to feed itself.

(For a discussion of the role of hormones in the trauma-induced efflux of amino acids from skeletal muscle, see Lund and Williamson, 1985.)

The stereotyped response to stress may be imagined as the equivalent, on a macroscale, of the stereotyped tissue response to an inflammatory stimulus. As we shall see, the inflammatory response occurs in three phases: (1) immediate, (2) stage of proteolysis, and (3) repair of damage and reconstitution. At the level of organization of the whole animal or person, similar phases may be perceived in the response to stress or trauma. The *immediate* responses are mediated by way of the CNS by way of the hypothalamus. These responses are very largely concerned with insuring continued blood supply to the vital organs, particularly the heart, lung, and brain. Other tissues, such as skeletal muscle (50% of body weight), kidneys, gastrointestinal tract, and reproductive apparatus, are not accorded the same high priority. The major effort appears to be a defense of fluid volume and blood pressure and in this enterprise the CRF-ACTH-adrenal glucocorticoid system collaborates with catecholamines, the ADH and the renin-angiotensin-aldosterone systems.

Analogous with the *proteolysis* stage of inflammation is the *redistribution of substrates* both for energy supply and for anabolic processes to be instituted during the repair phase. During this phase the glucocorticoids collaborate with the hormones of the endocrine pancreas (decreased insulin, increased glucagon) and with the amines of the autonomic nervous system and the adrenal medulla. Insulin secretion is inhibited by epinephrine, whereas that of glucagon is stimulated. Glucagon secretion is also enhanced by treatment with glucocorticoids.

During the *repair* phase the hormonal mix and the pool of energy-yielding substrates and protein precursors together provide a climate of protein synthesis and cell proliferation. This is achieved by an increasing emphasis on insulin, growth hormone and thyroid hormones with, one suspects, important contributions by the family of growth factors discussed in Chapter

5 in connection with somatomedins. Figure 11–10 is a graphic summary of this conception of a generalized response to trauma. ADH was discussed in Chapter 6; the renin-angiotensin-aldosterone system will be described in Chapter 12, the catecholamines in Chapter 13 and the hormones of the endocrine pancreas in Chapter 14.

Selye's theory that hyperactivity of the adrenals incident to stress resulted in "diseases of adaptation," among which he included rheumatoid arthritis, became untenable when Hench and Kendall discovered the anti-inflammatory effects of pharmacologic doses of cortisone in patients with that disease. The subsequent discoveries that glucocorticoids *inhibit* the synthesis and/or actions of many mediators of inflammation, including arachidonic acid metabolites, kinin production and effects, various mediators of immune responses, etc., were difficult to reconcile with the need for large quantities of adrenal hormones to combat stress. According to Munck's (1984) refreshing new hypothesis, "pharmacologic" quantities of glucocorticoids are not so much required to combat the initial stress as to prevent the body's responses to stress from overshooting, and thus damaging the organism. This is an interesting suggestion that at least confronts head-on the paradox of physiological hyperadrenocorticism in stress, but it requires the large assumption that the "governor" or "brake" effect of glucocorticoids does not take effect until the initial defense mechanisms have been activated. This still leaves room for a metabolite redistribution function for the adrenal hormones in stress.

"ECTOPIC" ACTH PRODUCTION

Wide application of radioimmunoassay methods for peptide hormones has led to the discovery that cancer cells may synthesize and secrete many different peptide and amine hormones (15 different hormones by more than 20 different tumor types). We have already seen one instance of this in our discussion of inappropriate ADH. One of the most extensively studied hormones overproduced by cancer cells is ACTH, which stimulates adrenocortical cells to hyperactivity.

The mechanisms involved in the turning on of the biochemical machinery for ACTH synthesis and release in an oat cell carcinoma of the lung or in an

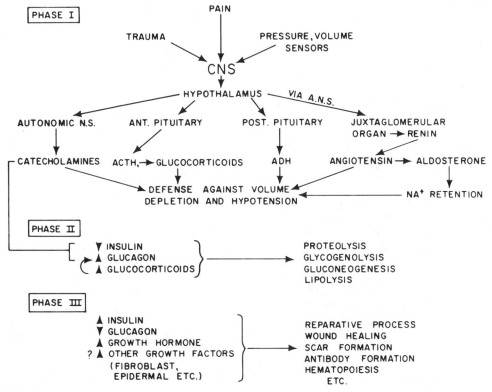

FIG 11–10.
Summary of generalized, phasic response to trauma.

adenocarcinoma cell of the colon are not evident. It has generally been regarded as an opening of specific DNA sequences, for transcription, by some unknown feature of the neoplastic process. It is likely to occur in cells that already have some capability for synthesizing amines, such as the cells of neuroectodermal origin designated as APUD by Pearse.

Inappropriate ACTH production by a tumor may yield diagnostic and therapeutic opportunities. Since the hormone secreted in excess by the tumor is usually indistinguishable immunologically or biologically from that secreted by the pituitary, it can be measured readily by radioimmunoassay. Such measurement may help with the original diagnosis, and moreover, assaying the venous blood draining the region in which the tumor is suspected may help to localize the source of the ACTH. If the tumor is treated surgically or chemotherapeutically, serial determinations of ACTH may indicate the efficacy of the therapy and later signal a recurrence.

BEHAVIORAL EFFECTS OF ACTH-RELATED PEPTIDES

In 1964 De Wied reported that the acquisition of avoidance behavior was impaired in hypophysectomized rats but that the deficit could be corrected by ACTH administration. He then discovered that α MSH or fragments of ACTH *devoid of adrenotrophic effect* were capable of correcting the defect. Moreover, neither adrenalectomy nor glucocorticoid treatment had any effect on the animal's ability to acquire a conditioned response.

Since that time, much work has been done on the behavioral effects of ACTH and related peptides. They have been found to delay extinction of a variety of conditioned behaviors as well as promoting their acquisition. Attempts have been made to categorize the peptide effects into "motivational" and "learning and memory" aspects of behavior. The peptide fragment $ACTH^{4-10}$ (also $\alpha\ MSH^{4-10}$) is the most active naturally occurring compound studied in these tests, although some synthetic peptides with substituted amino acids are many times more active than $ACTH^{4-10}$. The amino acid sequence $ACTH^{4-10}$ occurs not only in ACTH and MSH but also in β MSH and β LPH.

The route by which these injected peptides reach the brain is not known. It does not seem probable that parenterally injected peptides could cross the blood brain barrier. Possibly the suggestion of Bergland and Page is pertinent to the solution of this problem. These investigators have challenged the conventional wisdom that the direction of blood flow from the median eminence to the pituitary is invariably undirectional toward the latter. They present evidence to suggest that there is a kind of circular flow within the hypophyseal-portal system that makes possible the delivery of molecules of pituitary origin to the brain and cerebrospinal fluid as well as the passage of hypothalamic regulatory factors to the pituitary. If this proves to be the case, it may provide the communications link between the pituitary and those parts of the brain that are involved in the behavioral effects described by De Wied. Incidentally, it would also add credibility to the case for ultra-short-loop feedback regulation of peptidergic neurons.

The development of a radioimmunoassay for CRF has resulted in the demonstration of CRF or some similar substance in many parts of the brain other than the hypothalamus. Moreover, intraventricular injections of CRF cause an increase in plasma catecholamines, especially norepinephrine, together with cardiovascular responses that suggest stimulation of the autonomic nervous system. Studies with CRF generally show that the peptide causes evidence of general arousal or activation, both in EEG pattern and behavior. From these and other observations, an impression has grown that CRF magnifies the internally perceived stress of unpleasant challenges. Accordingly, Vale and others (1983) have suggested that CRF all over the central nervous system, not just in the hypothalamus, may have an integrative role in the response to stress, which includes both recruitment of biological responses as well as modification of behavior appropriate to the stress.

Cortisol

TRANSPORT OF CORTISOL IN BLOOD

Glucocorticoids are transported in the circulation by corticosteroid-binding globulin (CBG, or transcortin). This protein binds cortisol noncovalently with a high affinity and a low capacity. Cortisol also can bind loosely to albumin. The concentration of CBG in the blood is affected by gonadal hormones. Castration of male animals resulted in a striking increase in CBG concentration, which was restored to precastration values by androgen treatment. On the other hand, estrogen treatment increases CBG without inducing any evidence of hypercorticism, since the concentration of free hormone is not changed in spite of the increase in total circulating hormone. The glucocorticoid carrier protein is increased in the pregnant woman and in women treated with contraceptive pills containing estrogens.

METABOLISM AND EXCRETION

The major metabolic alteration of cortisol occurs in the liver (Fig 11–11). The molecule is serially reduced, first to dihydrocortisol and then to tetrahydrocortisol. Since it is possible for small amounts of cortisol to be converted to cortisone, parallel reductions of cortisone occur. The tetrahydro-derivatives are conjugated with glucuronide at the 3 position and easily excreted in the urine. The very first reduction product, dihydrocortisol, has no glucocorticoid activity, nor do any of the other metabolically modified products of the active hormone. (Cortisone must be reduced to cortisol in order to be activated.)

A minor quantity of cortisol may yield 17-KS by cleavage of its side chain, and thus contribute to the total 17-KS pool, which is mainly derived from adrenal and/or testicular androgens. It has sometimes been the practice, in measuring urinary steroids, deliberately to convert C_{21} steroids to 17-ketosteroids. If a suitable color test is done before and after such conversion, a reasonable estimate of adrenal glucocorticoids is obtained. This is the origin of the designation *"17-ketogenic steroids"* as indicators of glucocorticoid secretion. The measurement of *"17-hydroxysteroids"* (Porter-Silber reaction) is a direct measure of the $CHOH \cdot CO \cdot CH_2OH$ side chain present in both cortisol and cortisone. *"17-ketosteroids"* is the designation for those steroids in the urine that give a positive meta-dinitrobenzene reaction *before* oxidation of the cortisol side chain.

Knowledge of the chemistry of cortisol's excretion products can be used in estimating daily secretion rates. If a tracer amount of radioactive cortisol is given and it is assumed that the tracer mixes uniformly with the total body pool, isolation of the excretion products from a 24-hour urine sample and estimating their specific radioactivity (i.e., the extent of dilution of the isotope by endogenously produced "cold" cortisol) can give a fair estimation of the cortisol contribution of the adrenals over the period of the urine collection.

A minor pathway of cortisol metabolism (and inactivation) is that of 6-hydroxylation. This pathway may assume quantitative significance if the enzyme, 6β-hydroxylase, is induced either by a drug (phenobarbital) or by estrogens, as in pregnancy. This hydroxylation reaction, which occurs in the liver, uses a P450 cytochrome system similar to that required for steroid hormone biosynthesis in the adrenals and gonads.

BIOLOGIC EFFECTS

Cortisol is the prototype of the so-called glucocorticoid, or adrenal steroid, whose predominant function is in organic metabolism, as opposed to the "mineralocorticoid" or salt-retaining steroid hormone, whose main function is sodium conservation and defense of the body's fluid volume. As we have already seen, each type of steroid hormone has effects in the traditional domain of the other. The secretion

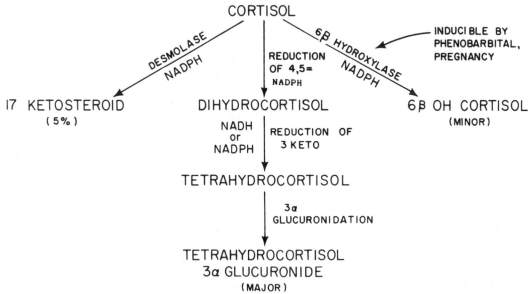

FIG 11–11
Patterns of cortisol metabolism.

rate and plasma concentrations of cortisol and aldosterone are very different. Cortisol is secreted at a rate of 20–25 mg/day, whereas aldosterone is secreted at a rate of 0.125 mg/day. Plasma concentrations of cortisol vary diurnally from about 4 to 16 μg/dl. The corresponding value for aldosterone is 0.01 μg/dl.

An inventory of the effects of glucocorticoids touches practically every aspect of physiology and biochemistry. If cortisol is not directly involved in a biochemical process, it frequently affects the responsiveness of cells to other hormones or neurotransmitters. It is necessary to distinguish between *physiologic* or *replacement* doses of cortisol and *pharmacologic* or *anti-inflammatory* doses. The former are doses that are adequate to restore to normal all those functions impaired by adrenal insufficiency; in the unstressed human being, for example, a dose a little larger than the daily secretion rate, 25–37.5 mg/day of cortisol, or its equivalent in a more potent steroid, is sufficient. Pharmacologic doses may be the equivalent of 80–200 mg of cortisol/day. If replacement doses are administered to a deficient individual undergoing stress, the requirement for the hormone is increased to 80–100 mg of cortisol equivalent. Under these circumstances, these are not pharmacologic doses; they simply reflect the fact that hormone requirement is increased by stress (e.g., surgical trauma).

In replacement doses, cortisol corrects all of the organic metabolic defects associated with adrenal insufficiency. If the associated sodium loss is mild, it can correct that too, since cortisol does have some aldosterone-like action on sodium reabsorption by the renal tubule. If salt loss is severe, a mineralocorticoid (usually a synthetic fluorinated analogue of cortisol) is given as well.

The following *defects* associated with cortisol deficiency are *corrected* by replacement doses of glucocorticoids:

1. Insulin hypersensitivity
2. Failure to maintain tissue glucogen stores
3. Hypoglycemia on food deprivation
4. Inadequate mobilization of peripheral protein
5. Inadequate gluconeogenesis
6. Poor response of fat cells to usual lipolytic stimuli
7. Failure of feedback inhibition of ACTH and β LPH.
8. Hypotension
9. Growth failure in rapidly growing animals
10. Diminished capacity to excrete a water load
11. Muscle weakness and easy fatigability
12. Psychologic and emotional difficulties; EEG abnormalities; abnormal susceptibility to convulsive seizures

GLUCOCORTICOID EXCESS

As we have seen, inappropriately large amounts of thyroid hormones, or ADH, essential for normal function when available in appropriate amounts, cause disease and disability. Similarly, too much cortisol may cause disease. Excessive cortisol may be produced by autonomous adrenal tumors, by ACTH-producing pituitary tumors (Cushing's disease) and by ACTH-producing ectopic tumors, e.g., cancer of the lung. In all cases many manifestations of the disease may be similar. In addition to these naturally occurring diseases, hypercortisolism is often induced by the physician during anti-inflammatory treatment of a chronic disease, e.g., rheumatoid arthritis. Since large doses of glucocorticoids are required to produce an anti-inflammatory effect, it is not surprising that many unwanted side effects occur, which collectively resemble the clinical picture of iatrogenic or physician-induced Cushing's disease.

Musculoskeletal System

Weakness of muscles, particularly of the arms and shoulder girdles, is sometimes seen. This probably is a manifestation of the antianabolic effect of glucocorticoids on skeletal muscle, a caricature of the desirable amino acid-mobilizing effect of corticoids during starvation. This is a serious complication, which may necessitate stopping treatment.

Osteoporosis, which may declare itself as a vertebral compression fracture or fracture of a long bone as a result of minimal trauma, is sometimes seen in people, particularly postmenopausal women, who receive large amounts of cortisol. A discussion of the pathophysiology of this condition will be found in Chapter 17.

Gastrointestinal Complications

Peptic ulceration (particularly in the stomach) has often been seen. Although the role of glucocorticoids in initiating peptic ulcers has recently been challenged, steroids are certainly ulcerogenic in experimental animal models. Since PGs (prostaglandins) inhibit gastric acid secretion and protect against experimental ulcers, it is possible that inhibition of PG synthesis by high doses of glucocorticoids might contribute to vulnerability of gastric mucosa to ulceration.

Pancreatitis, peritonitis due to a ruptured viscus or other *infections* may occur without the usual indications of severe inflammation in naturally occurring or iatrogenic Cushing's disease. This is due to the anti-inflammatory effect of glucocorticoids, which suppress the production of pain-generating signals, fever, and leukocytosis that would be expected to announce the event. Infections in other locations can similarly gain a foothold.

Central Nervous System

Psychiatric disorders, ranging from unusual to psychotic behavior, are sometimes seen in people treated with anti-inflammatory doses of steroids. Presumably the steroids act in this way in people who have a predisposition to these manifestations. In many people, steroids produce a welcome feeling of well-being, which may be due partly to alleviation of annoying symptoms and partly to effects of glucocorticoids on the CNS. In some individuals, excessive food intake may result from steroid therapy.

Ophthalmic

Glaucoma may be brought into relief by steroid treatment. Rarely, posterior subcapsular *cataracts* may occur during such treatment.

Cardiovascular-Renal

Hypervolemia and *hypertension* may occur, although the risk of sodium and water retention is minimized by the use of synthetic steroids, which have very little aldosterone-like effect while being powerfully anti-inflammatory.

Hypokalemic alkalosis occurs rarely, but almost never in people given the 16α substituted synthetic glucocorticoids. It is due to the potassium excretion-promoting action of steroids, which is associated with their sodium-retaining action.

Endocrine Pancreas-Related Effects

A *diabetes-mellitus-like* picture may occur, again in people with a predisposition to this condition. The steroids can inhibit peripheral glucose utilization, exaggerate peripheral protein breakdown, overstimulate hepatic gluconeogenesis, cause hyperglucagonemia, cause secondary hyperinsulinism, induce hyperlipidemia and cause centripetal obesity. Many of these effects would be appropriate as positive adaptive responses to starvation, but they are clearly inappropriate in people in the fed condition.

Other Endocrine Disorders

Although replacement doses of cortisol in adrenally insufficient animals are growth promoting, pharmacologic amounts are *growth inhibiting,* an effect seen in some severely asthmatic children. Again, this effect is related to the protein catabolic power of the steroids in pharmacologic doses.

Secondary amenorrhea is commonly observed in naturally occurring forms of hypercortisolism. Endogenous overproduction of glucocorticoids is accompanied by increases in secretion of adrenal androgens, some of which may serve as precursors of extraovarian estrogens (see Chapter 9). These steroids inhibit gonadotropin production and disrupt the menstrual cycle. To the extent that the surfeit of adrenal androgens generates testosterone, *virilization* (hirsutism, acne) may be seen.

One of the most important endocrine effects of chronic steroid therapy is *adrenal insufficiency on withdrawal.* Chronic suppression of the hypothalamopituitary-adrenal axis with exogenous steroids results in atrophy of the whole system. If treatment is withdrawn abruptly, the individual is a victim of iatrogenic Addison's disease. Such a person may have all of the manifestations of adrenal insufficiency, but especially an inadequate capacity to withstand traumatic or other stress. Moreover, the staged recovery from prolonged suppression may take a very long time—up to 12 months, in some instances. It is therefore essential to be aware of this possibility and to prevent it if possible.

One maneuver that is sometimes recommended (see Melby) is treatment with relatively short-acting steroids, e.g., prednisolone, on *alternate days,* which is said to minimize the complete suppression of the CRF-pituitary apparatus and facilitate withdrawal. Steroids that have a longer duration of action, e.g., betamethasone and dexamethasone, are not suitable for this purpose.

Inhibition of Fibroplasia

The most obvious consequence of inhibition of fibroblast function and proliferation by glucocorticoids is *impairment of wound healing*. Not only do glucocorticoids impair glucose utilization by fibroblasts, they also inhibit DNA synthesis, and therefore cell division (see Henderson and Loeb). The combination of decreased collagen-producing capacity and impaired cell division seriously interferes with the reparative phase of a mechanically induced inflammatory process, such as a surgical incision.

The Immune Response

Corticosteroids are of value in many circumstances characterized by hypersensitivity reactions, due either to exogenous or endogenous antigen-antibody reactions. At one time it was believed that the lymphocyte-destroying action of cortisol was the basis for impairing antibody production. Now it is apparent that even large doses of glucocorticoids probably do not affect circulating antibody titers. They do, however, inhibit the inflammatory responses (cell-mediated) that are initiated by hypersensitivity reactions. In other words, they function primarily as anti-inflammatory agents in hypersensitivity situations exactly as they do in inflammatory reactions elicited by other agents. This is why they are valuable adjuncts in management of severe allergic reactions and, with immunosuppressive drugs, are important tools in the prevention of heterologous graft rejection.

ANTI-INFLAMMATORY EFFECTS

The anti-inflammatory effect of *pharmacologic* doses of adrenal glucocorticoids was discovered empirically by Hench and Kendall in 1949. The remarkable ability of glucocorticoids to inhibit the inflammatory response has been intensively studied ever since, but there still is no single satisfying mechanistic hypothesis that "explains" the phenomenon. However, since anti-inflammatory glucocorticoids and nonsteroidal anti-inflammatory agents are among our most frequently used drugs, it is pertinent here to examine briefly the process of inflammation.

Although the stereotyped sequence of events that occurs when tissue is injured appears to us to be a mobilization of resources to contain the injury and to repair damage, the inflammatory process itself can inflict injury, pain and loss of function. This is particularly true when the original injury is perpetrated by an autoimmune mechanism, a blurring of the distinction between "self" and "not-self." In this case, the enemy to be contained is not an invading microorganism or a wood splinter; rather, the immune system generates inappropriate antibodies, which interact with antigens to set in motion an inflammatory response. Once the response is initiated, it tends to perpetuate itself and the resulting chronic inflammation may result in tissue destruction and disability. It is this apparently pointless kind of inflammation that may require intervention with an anti-inflammatory agent. We must emphasize that inhibition of the inflammatory response, which may ameliorate symptoms such as pain and impaired function, does not

affect the underlying disease process. It merely suppresses one of its manifestations. In some circumstances this suppression may be extremely dangerous, since the symptoms of inflammation (pain, fever, malaise) are important signals that warn of impending danger, e.g., bacterial infection. People under treatment with anti-inflammatory doses of steroids have been known to develop severe infections without suspecting their presence.

The inflammatory process has fascinated biologists for centuries, and the anti-inflammatory effect of glucocorticoids has been investigated intensively since 1949. It has only been recently, however, that the central role of eicosanoids (arachidonic acid metabolites) in inflammation has been appreciated. Figure 11–12 shows a skeletal concept of the process of inflammation which includes the locus of action of three different types of anti-inflammatory agents, including glucocorticoids. Some of these ideas were discussed in Chapter 4.

Like the generalized response to trauma summarized in Figure 11–10, the inflammatory process may be divided into three phases: (1) the *earliest* events, characterized by vasodilation, leukocyte adhesion to the endothelium of microvessels, and an extravascular convention of polymorphonuclear leukocytes at the site of injury; (2) an *intermediate* phase, when local proteolysis is the dominant theme; and (3) the *repair* phase when protein synthesis, cell replication, and revascularization occur. The process may be entrained by a variety of injurious stimuli, including bacterial, mechanical, chemical, and thermal, as well as by tissue hypoxia (as in coronary thrombosis, for example). If the source of the inflammation is removed (for example, by an antibiotic in the case of a bacterial infection, by removal of a splinter, or by aseptic closure of a surgical wound), the inflammatory process proceeds successfully through phase 3. If, however, it is initiated by an autoimmune response, it may perpetuate itself (see Fig 11–12) to the point of destruction of tissue and loss of function. All of the molecular mediators of the inflammatory process are ubiquitously present, as products of membrane phospholipids (eicosanoids); as secretory granules in mast cells (histamine, serotonin or 5HT); or as high molecular weight precursors of locally produced proteolytic products (kinins, chemotactic factors, vasoactive substances, products of the complement cascade—not shown in Fig 11–12).

Figure 11–12 was drawn to emphasize the prominence of the role of phospholipase A_2 in initiating the inflammatory response. The importance of prostaglandin generation in the process was realized when Vane observed that aspirin (and later, other *nonste-*

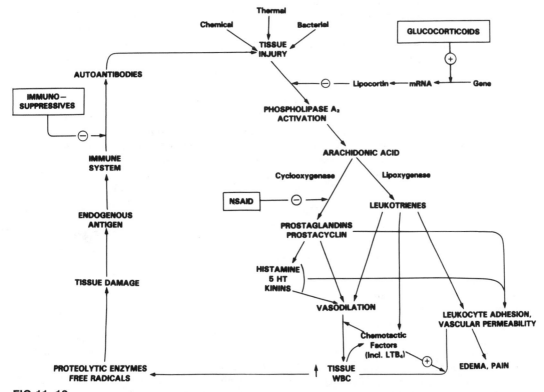

FIG 11–12.
The central role of arachidonic acid metabolites in the initiation and maintenance of inflammation: sites of action of three categories of anti-inflammatory drugs. NSAID = nonsteroidal anti-inflammatory drugs. Note that prostaglandins affect both secretion and action of histamine, serotonin (5-HT), and the kinins.

roidal *anti-inflammatory drugs* [NSAID]) is an inhibitor of cyclooxygenase. When the lipoxygenase products were characterized, LTB$_4$ turned out to be an extremely potent chemotactic agent, and the slow-reacting substance of allergy (SRS-A) proved to be the peptidolipid leukotrienes (Chapter 4).

The central role of polymorphonuclear leukocytes (PMNL) in inflammation is important. Over a century ago, Metchnikoff described the escape of PMNL from the circulation into the region of inflammation and announced that there could be no inflammation without leukocytes. Later, it was shown that dogs rendered unable to produce PMNL by an inhibitor of the developmental process could not respond to an inflammatory challenge in the usual manner. At the earliest visible stage of inflammation, when histamine and 5HT are released from stored granules in mast cells, leukocytes are seen to adhere to the endothelial surfaces of the dilated microvessels. The spaces between adjacent endothelial cells enlarge, and protein-rich transudate and PMNL traverse the vessel wall and en-

ter extravascular spaces. There, the PMNL are stimulated by leukotriene B$_4$ and by chemotactic peptides to secrete lysosomal enzymes and, if indicated, to phagocytose microorganisms. In the process, the PMNL generate noxious free radicals which, though a formidable weapon against microbial invaders, may, with locally secreted proteolytic enzymes, contribute to tissue injury.

The prostaglandins and leukotrienes pervade the whole process of inflammation. Prostaglandins both influence the secretion of histamine and 5HT by mast cells and magnify their effects in microvessels. They also inhibit the production of kinins. Leukotriene B$_4$ is chemotactic and stimulatory to PMNL, while the peptidolipid leukotrienes have prolonged vasodilatory effects, as well as simulatory effects on bronchial smooth muscle. The prostaglandins also synergize with kinins to stimulate pain receptors.

Figure 11–12 represents only a simple cartoon of the intricate process of inflammation. It does not include many simultaneous events that are important parts of the program of inflammation. Among these are *activation of the complement cascade,* which results in the generation of many bioactive substances, including chemotactic peptides, vasoactive materials, and chemicals that trigger the production of *lymphokines* by B lymphocytes. The lymphokines function as mediators and coordinators of later stages of inflammation. In addition, the *clotting system* is activated, fibrin is formed, and the anticlotting system, the *plasmin-fibrinolysin* apparatus, is recruited.

In an adaptively successful inflammation, the proteolytic phase is followed by repair and rebuilding. Now the emphasis is on protein synthesis, cell growth, and cell replication. Collagen is laid down and new blood vessels form; finally scar tissue formation (cicatrization) occurs.

MECHANISM OF THE ANTI-INFLAMMATORY EFFECT OF GLUCOCORTICOIDS

Practically all phases of the inflammatory process are inhibited by glucocorticoids in doses that exceed the daily maintenance requirement for an adrenalectomized animal or person. Microvessel dilation, leukocyte stickiness and migration, histamine and 5HT secretion, kinin production, complement proteolysis, clotting system, and plasmin-fibrinolysin activation are all inhibited. So are all of the events in the repair phase: fibroblast growth and proliferation, collagen synthesis, neovascularization, and cicatrization.

With the implication of prostaglandins in the inflammatory process, the foundation of a new hypothesis for the mechanism of the anti-inflammatory action of glucocorticoids emerged. For it was quickly demonstrated that glucocorticoids, like the NSAIDs, inhibited prostaglandin synthesis in vivo. However, they do not inhibit cyclooxygenase; rather they decrease the availability of arachidonic acid for the synthesis of *both* prostaglandins and leukotrienes by inhibiting the action of phospholipase A_2.

The mechanism of phospholipase A_2 inhibition by glucocorticoids has been elucidated only recently. In 1980, Blackwell et al. discovered a glucocorticoid-induced protein (called "macrocortin") that inhibited phospholipase A_2. In the same year, Hirata et al. discovered a similar protein (called "lipomodulin") produced by leukocytes. A short time thereafter, proteins with similar properties were found in kidney tissue ("renocortins"). While the molecular weights of the purified materials were rather disparate, the investigators believe that the disparity is probably due to preparation artifacts, and that all of the proteins are related (monomer: dimer:trimer). Since the prolifera-

tion of names threatened to confound the interested public the investigative teams involved in the discoveries described above have now agreed to abandon the earlier names and to refer to all of these PLA_2 inhibitors as *lipocortins*. All of these substances are glycoproteins whose rates of synthesis and secretion are dramatically increased by glucocorticoids in many different cell types. The purified proteins inhibit eicosanoid production across the board by most intact cells, and this effect is reversed by excess phospholipid substrate. Lipocortins are inactivated by phosphorylation and reactivated by alkaline phosphatase treatment. In all cases studied, the increased rate of synthesis and secretion induced by glucocorticoid depends on an increased rate of transcription of the lipocortin gene by a receptor-mediated process (see next section). It is gratifying to have a molecular explanation for Hench and Kendall's "miracle" of 1949!

CELLULAR MECHANISM OF ACTION OF GLUCOCORTICOIDS

Cortisol (or corticosterone in some species) acts on a variety of cells and elicits many different responses. In some cases, it is the major agonist, while in others, it "permits" another hormone to exert its typical effect. In many instances, it stimulates primarily *catabolic* events: for example, *lymphocytolysis* in animals and in human leukemic lymphocytes; *skeletal muscle,* inhibition of protein synthesis; *skin,* decreased protein synthesis, including collagen; *fibroblast,* decreased metabolism, growth, and replication; *adipocyte,* anti-insulin effect; permits lipolytic hormones to function; and *pituitary,* inhibition of POMC synthesis.

On the other hand, the same molecular signal can elicit *anabolic* responses, such as the induction of the synthesis of specific enzymes, or even (in the case of the liver) hypertrophy of an organ. The following are examples of such anabolic responses to glucocorticoids: *pituitary,* stimulation of growth hormone synthesis; *many cells,* stimulation of lipocortin synthesis (see section on anti-inflammatory effects above); *liver,* induction of gluconeogenic enzymes, glycogen synthesis and liver hypertrophy, inhibition of DNA synthesis; *embryonic retina,* induction of glutamine synthetase; *embryonic lung,* increase in choline incorporation into lecithin, surfactant synthesis; *brain cells,* synthesis of unknown substances that affect excitability of neurones.

The reason for this apparently unrelated array of effects is in the responding cells. At the time of its final differentiation, each cell type "decided" to express not only genes whose products are involved in recognizing the hormone (receptor and ancillary proteins) but also to order its chromatin in a configuration that would allow the hormone-receptor complex to enhance selectively the transcription of a distinctive collection of mRNAs. *Both catabolic and anabolic responses are ultimately dependent upon gene transcription.* We have already examined a similar set of apparently paradoxical responses to the thyroid hormones.

Thus, the general mechanism of action of glucocorticoids conforms to the all-purpose steroid hormone action model presented in Chapter 2:

Hormone (H) + Receptor (R)—HR
HR + Nuclear Acceptor(s) (NA)—HR:NA

In an unknown way, HR:NA leads to the transcription of specific mRNAs that code for a battery of proteins. These translation products together effect the coordinated response to the hormone.

Glucocorticoid receptors are similar in size and other characteristics to other steroid hormone receptors. They are shaped more or less like fat cigars and have a molecular weight of 94 kd. These are the first steroid receptors that have been described to occur in different types in different tissues (Funder). As in the case of catecholamine receptors, the glucocorticoid receptors are classified according to their affinity for different ligands. Thus, *Type I* receptors have a high affinity for naturally occurring glucocorticoids (cortisol, corticosterone) and a lower affinity for the synthetic, dexamethasone. When they occur in the central nervous system, it has been suggested that they may be involved in periodic and cyclic (diurnal) changes in CRF output. (Receptors indistinguishable from Type I, in the renal tubule, are aldosterone receptors. We try to explain how aldosterone is able to commandeer Type I receptors in renal tubular cells, even in the presence of thousandfold higher concentrations of cortisol, in Chapter 12.) *Type II* receptors, much more extensively studied, are widely distributed. By definition, they have a moderately high affinity for dexamethasone and a *lower* affinity for the naturally occurring hormones.

The glucocorticoid receptor has been shown by controlled proteolysis to consist of three domains: (1) at one end, a steroid-binding domain (meroreceptor) which interacts with both surfaces of the flat steroid and constitutes about 25% of the intact monomer; (2) at the other end, a DNA binding site (about the same size as the meroreceptor) which binds DNA even more avidly than the intact monomer; and (3) an intermediate immunoreactive domain (half the weight of the intact monomer) which has been called the "specifier." The last contains major antigenic determinants and may guide the HR complex to appropriate gene sites by interacting with protein constituents of chromatin. Mutants that lack the "specifier" show increased DNA binding and steroid hormone insensitivity.

The receptor can exist either as an oligomer or a monomer, and the hormone can bind to either. The monomeric form of HR is the one that interacts with its nuclear acceptors.

The Receptor Cycle

Recent studies of the glucocorticoid receptor underscore the point that the standard steroid hormone action model described in Chapter 2 does not begin to suggest the subtlety and complexity of the mechanism of action of these molecules. Rousseau (1984) has summarized a large amount of experimental data by constructing a model of the glucocorticoid receptor cycle. It is instructive to contemplate this model because there are indications that some features of it may apply not only to glucocorticoids but also to other steroids as well, notably, androgens and progesterone.

In addition to the fact that the receptor can exist either as an oligomer or a monomer, it has been demonstrated that (1) the receptor can exist either in the phosphorylated or the dephosphorylated state; (2) that it contains S which can exist either as SH or S-S; and (3), there is at least one factor, F, of unknown composition, that stabilizes the HR complex. "Activation" is defined as a change in the receptor that enables it to bind steroid. "Transformation" is defined as that conformational change in the HR complex that renders it competent to interact with chromatin components.

The glucocorticoid receptor can exist in *five* distinguishable states (or shapes), as follows:

A. Oligomeric, SH + P + F (activated).

B. Glucocorticoid hormone bound to A.

C. B Dissociated into monomers; loss of P (i.e., *de*phosphorylation) and F (transformed).

D. C bound to DNA and other chromatin components.

E. D dissociated from DNA in S-S state.

Treatment of E with protein kinase, ATP, and F restores condition A, i.e., it activates the system to a steroid-binding capability. As we suggested, this model may be important as a generalized one for other steroids. In fact, Liao (Chapter 8) has constructed a similar one for androgen.

The Nuclear Events

As we mentioned briefly in Chapter 2, the demonstration of selective HR binding to known sequences of DNA was first achieved by students of glucocorticoid action (see Ringold review, 1985). In 1971, McGrath observed that glucocorticoids stimulated the production of mouse mammary tumor virus (MMTV) in cultures of mouse mammary carcinoma cells. MMTV is a retrovirus, i.e., it is a single-stranded RNA virus that replicates via reverse transcriptase by synthesizing a proviral DNA. The provirus is integrated into the host cell's genome and proceeds to transcribe viral RNA and other viral components. When the nucleotide sequence of the virus was determined, it was found that the continuous sequence coding for viral constituents was surrounded by two long, untranscribed regions, called long terminal repeats, or LTR, 1350 base pairs in length. Using restriction enzymes as molecular scalpels, the investigators concluded that there are two distinguishable base sequences in the LTR upstream from the transcription initiation site: one, a *promoter* site, relatively near the initiation site, and another, a *regulatory* site, 140–190 bases upstream from the initiation site. By working with fragments of different sizes generated by a battery of restriction enzymes, the experimenters found that the -140 to -190 site corresponded to both the preferential *binding* region for glucocorticoid-receptor complex and the *regulatory* region for eliciting transcription of viral RNA. By constructing recombinant plasmids containing the LTR of MMTV followed by insertions of cDNAs for three enzymes not normally inducible by glucocorticoids, each of the enzymes was rendered inducible. Similar selective HR binding was demonstrated for glucocorticoid-inducible genes in liver: tyrosine aminotransferase and tryptophan oxygenase. All DNA binding sites to which glucocorticoid-receptor complex binds with highest affinity in vitro contain the same hexanucleotide sequence:

T-G-T-T-C-T

It is puzzling that the same sequence and correspondingly high affinity binding of HR by DNA occurs in the middle of the viral genome and far upstream in the LTR, but the significance of binding in these regions, if any, is not known. DNA binding may be important for the initiation of transcription at specific sites, but it cannot account for the whole story. A protein has been found which itself does not bind to DNA but enhances binding of glucocorticoid-receptor to MMTV DNA. Also, we must reserve the possibility that the "specifier," immunoreactive half of the receptor monomer may have a probing role in locating regulatory DNA sequences similar to that of the specific acidic protein-binding subunit of the chick progesterone receptor.

Chromatin Structure and Hormone-Receptor Accessibility to DNA

In Chapter 2 we commented on various orders of chromatin structure and noted that the complex structure of chromatin may participate in directing the transaction between HR and DNA. One approach to this problem (by M.M. Ip et al.) was to study DNA binding of the glucocorticoid receptor to mononucleosomes (from a glucocorticoid-responsive lymphosarcoma) containing both core DNA (183 base pairs) and linker DNA (168 base pairs). Different types of protein are associated with each of these domains. The HR complex bound selectively to DNA associated with core nucleosomes which are depleted of histone H_1. We mention this study to emphasize the complex nature of the nuclear environment in which HR must navigate before it arrives at its destinations: the regulatory sequences of DNA where it can initiate transcription of a few genes.

Selective Gene Activation by Glucocorticoids

The major consequence of binding of the hormone-receptor complex in the nucleus is the accumulation of specific messenger RNAs. The study of this problem with glucocorticoids was extremely difficult because generally the target cells express only about 10% of their complement of DNA and, of this, glucocorticoids influence the synthesis of only 0.5%–1%. In spite of this formidable handicap, glucocorticoid-stimulated mRNA accumulation has been described for the following: tyrosine aminotransferase, tryptophan oxygenase, phosphoenolpyruvate carboxykinase, glutamine synthetase, and progrowth hormone.

The first three of these are in the category of gluconeogenic enzymes inducible by cortisol in the liver or in minimal deviation hepatoma cells in tissue culture. Glutamine synthetase is inducible in embryonic chick retina.

The studies on pro-GH synthesis in a tumor-derived strain of anterior pituitary cells are among the most interesting because they illustrate a partnership between a thyroid hormone (T_3) and a synthetic glucocorticoid. Either hormone alone was capable of inducing the appearance of mRNA for a higher molecular weight precursor of GH, pro-GH. However, the response to the two combined was greater than additive.

Genetic Analysis of Glucocorticoid Action

Many of the postulated features of glucocorticoid action have been validated by the genetic experiments of Yamamoto et al., who were able to isolate mutants of S49 lymphoma cells (normally killed by glucocorticoids) that were defective either in hormone binding or in hormone-receptor binding in the nucleus. Other mutants (called ''deathless'') resisted killing by the steroid in spite of nuclear binding of the complex. In these the mutation must have involved some event beyond nuclear binding. These studies may prove of considerable interest to oncologists, since glucocorticoid-resistant lymphomas have been described that lack receptors. This approach to characterizing tumors and predicting their biologic responses is of course reminiscent of work on breast cancer, discussed previously.

Effect of Glucocorticoids on Growth

One of the most interesting effects of cortisol and related compounds is growth inhibition in rapidly growing experimental animals and children, a subject that has been studied by Loeb and colleagues. These investigators have used the incorporation of radioactive thymidine as an indicator of DNA synthesis in two different kinds of tissues: (1) those in which DNA synthesis represents new cell accretion (liver, heart, skeletal muscle, kidney) and (2) those in which DNA synthesis is a reflection of cell turnover (intestinal and gastric mucosa, testis, spleen). In group 1 cells, low doses of glucocorticoid *stop* DNA synthesis. This occurs in liver, a tissue in which the selective *transcription* of DNA is stimulated at the same time. Group 2 cells, which share rapid turnover of their populations, appear to be immune to glucocorticoid inhibition of DNA synthesis. The molecular mechanisms involved in these effects are not known.

DEVELOPMENTAL EFFECTS

As we have seen, steroid hormones and thyroid hormones function as developmental signals during embryogenesis. Although much investigative effort has been expended on the general problem of hormone action, little is known about how hormones influence the process of differentiation.

One extensively studied model of a developmental effect of glucocorticoids is the induction of the enzyme *glutamine synthetase* (GS) in embryonic chick retina. The enzyme level is extremely low but rises abruptly about five days before hatching. Cortisol can induce the enzyme prematurely in organ culture of intact retina. A lag period of two hours is required.

A similar developmental effect of cortisol is of great interest to neonatologists and others who must manage infants with the *respiratory distress syndrome* (RDS). This condition, seen frequently in premature infants, is related to failure of development of the capacity to synthesize *surfactants,* surface tension-reducing lecithins that coat the alveolar surfaces of the lung and permit its expansion and aeration. The successful transition from the nonbreathing, intrauterine state to the breathing neonatal condition requires synthesis of these phospholipids.

On the basis of experiments with fetal lambs, a role for glucocorticoids in maturation of the lung was postulated. Since then, acceleration of lung maturation by glucocorticoid administration has been demonstrated in a number of species, including the human. It has been found that oral administration of glucocorticoids to women between 28 and 32 weeks of gestation results in a higher lecithin-sphingomyelin ratio in amniotic fluid than in that of control women. This ratio is generally conceded to be an indicator of surfactant production, and therefore a predictor of susceptibility to RDS. Application of this kind of information may lead to prevention of this condition by exploiting the ability of cortisol to induce enzymatic machinery that is capable of synthesizing surfactant phospholipids.

Recent studies of the *differentiation of mammary glands* have revealed that differentiation of these structures and development of their capacity to synthesize and secrete milk is the product of a very complex consortium of hormones, cortisol among them. Differentiation of mammary gland explants in organ culture requires insulin, prolactin, and cortisol. Epithelial cells of the explant cannot differentiate into alveolar cells without a prior cell division. Insulin performs a mitogenic function and stimulates cell division in this system. Cortisol acts on the first generation daughter cells by inducing a whole battery of enzymes involved in the process of lipogenesis. The glucocorticoid effect must precede the ability of the cells to respond to prolactin by synthesizing milk proteins. Cortisol's role in this complex process is particularly strange in view of the fact that, in *liver,* the very enzymes induced by glucocorticoid in mammary gland explants are *repressed*. (See the review by Turkington et al.)

In addition to these positive manifestations of cortisol's participation in developmental processes, pharmacologic doses of glucocorticoids given to pregnant animals may result in *developmental malformations,* most notably cleft palate and harelip.

In order for the palate to develop normally, precisely timed and localized secretion of lysosomal enzymes must occur. These destructive enzymes cause a breakdown of the epithelium on the leading, medial edges of the two sides of the developing palate that are destined to fuse. Glucocorticoids prevent this breakdown and therefore inhibit fusion. Following the discovery that this teratogenic effect of glucocorticoids can be corrected significantly by arachidonic acid in an organ culture system, Gupta et al. demonstrated that the glucocorticoid effect could be duplicated by a purified phospholipase A_2 inhibitory protein which they called *phospholipase A_2 inhibitory protein*, or PLIP, before the consensus designation *lipocortin* was adopted for similar proteins (see discussion above). This exciting discovery makes one wonder how many other glucocorticoid effects can be reproduced by lipocortin.

SYNTHETIC GLUCOCORTICOIDS

The widespread use of adrenocortical steroids as anti-inflammatory agents has stimulated searches for compounds that have certain desirable qualities exaggerated and undesirable ones suppressed or eliminated. Organic chemists synthesized many analogues of cortisol, each of which was subjected to bioassay in experimental animals for glucocorticoid potency (glycogen deposition), salt-retaining potency (urinary $Na^+ : K^+$ ratio, or some variant) and anti-inflammatory potency (inhibition of experimentally induced inflammation). Promising compounds generated by this screening procedure were then tested in human beings. Many valuable compounds have been developed by this empirical method.

The *halogenated steroids* were originally prepared as intermediates in laboratory synthesis of cortisone from naturally occurring steroid precursors. When cortisol was fluorinated at the 9α position, both salt-retaining potency and glucocorticoid activity were remarkably enhanced. In fact, one of the fluoro derivatives, 2-methyl-9α-fluoro cortisol is more than three times as potent as aldosterone in salt-retaining activity, and it is effective as replacement for aldosterone deficiency in human beings at a dose of only 25 µg/day by mouth. The halogenated compounds owe some of their potency and long duration of action

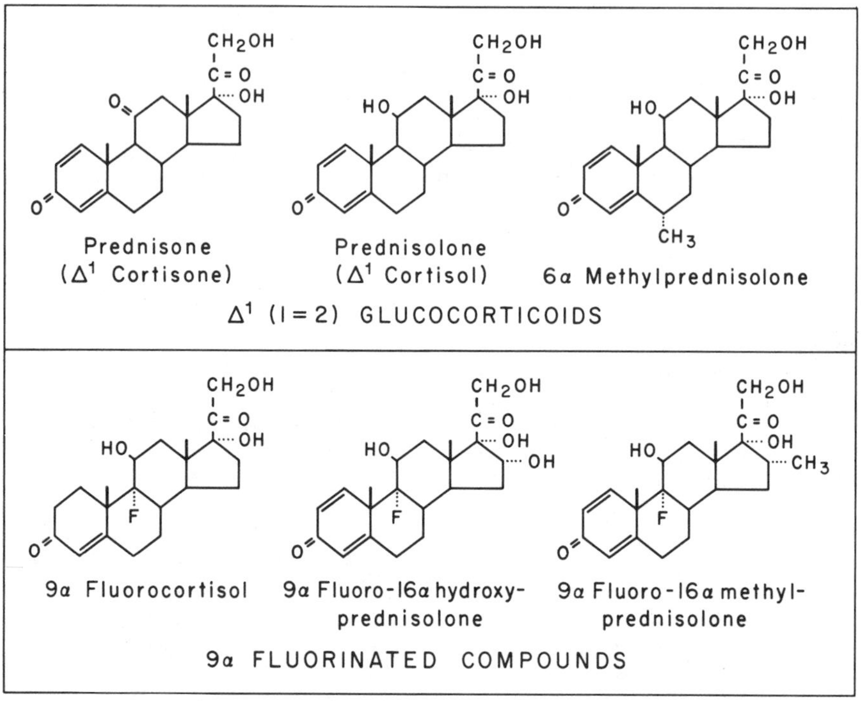

Δ^1 (I = 2) GLUCOCORTICOIDS

Prednisone (Δ^1 Cortisone) — Prednisolone (Δ^1 Cortisol) — 6α Methylprednisolone

9α FLUORINATED COMPOUNDS

9α Fluorocortisol — 9α Fluoro-16α hydroxyprednisolone — 9α Fluoro-16α methylprednisolone

FIG 11–13.
Synthetic analogues of adrenocortical steroids. 9α-Fluorocortisol is powerfully salt-retaining, but the 16α-hydroxy substituted compound (triamcinolone) and the 16α-methyl substituted compound (dexamethasone) are predominantly anti-inflammatory glucocorticoid substances.

TABLE 11–2.
Biologic Activity Profiles of Synthetic Analogues of Cortisol

STEROID	POTENCY (PER MG) ANTI-INFLAMMATORY	EQUIV. DOSE (mg)	SODIUM RETENTION	BIOL. EFFECT* (hr)
Cortisol	1.0	20	1.0	8–12
9α-Fluorocortisol	10	—	125	—
Short-acting analogues				
Prednisolone	4	5	0.8	12–36
6α-Methylprednisolone	5	4	0.5	12–36
Triamcinolone	5	4	0	12–36
(9α-F,16α-OH prednisolone)				
Long-acting analogues				
Betamethasone	25	0.6	0	36–54
(9α-F,16β-methylprednisolone)				
Dexamethasone	25	0.6	0	36–54
(9α-F,16α-methylprednisolone)				

*Biol. effect = duration of action.

when administered orally to the fact that they resist metabolism in the liver.

Long before the receptors for cortisol and aldosterone were studied, it was possible to infer that they were able to discriminate between glucocorticoids and mineralocorticoids. The Δ^1 compounds (Fig 11–13)—prednisone and prednisolone—differ from cortisol and cortisone by a 1,2 double bond in the A ring. This modification changes the characteristics of these substances so that their glucocorticoid activity is enhanced by a factor of 3–5, but there is a slight *decrease* in salt-retaining potency. Since early clinical experience with cortisone and cortisol revealed the dangers of salt and water retention in many people who were being treated with anti-inflammatory doses of the steroids, the discovery of the Δ^1 compounds was a substantial advance. These compounds are still very valuable, for they are prototypical short-acting steroids, which are recommended for alternate-day steroid therapy (see above). They are useful for this type of treatment because the biologic half-life of glucocorticoids is proportional to their feedback potency on the hypothalamo-pituitary CRF-ACTH complex. The shorter half-life of these compounds permits some recovery of the trophic complex, which is not possible when steroids with a longer duration of action (betamethasone and dexamethasone) (Table 11–2) are used.

Although there has been some success in dissociating anti-inflammatory effect from salt-and-water retention, there has been no successful dissociation of anti-inflammatory effect from all of the side effects described above as iatrogenic Cushing's disease. If a steroid such as betamethasone or dexamethasone is 25 times as potent an anti-inflammatory agent as cortisol, it is also 25 times as potent a producer of cortisol's unwanted side effects.

One of the most striking features of the anti-inflammatory steroids is that they are extremely active when applied locally. This approach can often be made with minimal risk of systemic toxicity. Diseases of the eye and of the skin are often treated with glucocorticoid preparations, usually a 9α fluorinated compound. Monoarticular arthritis or severe bursitis can also be managed successfully with locally applied steroids.

When the anti-inflammatory effects of steroids were first discovered in 1949, they were hailed as universal panaceas. As clinical experience accumulated, some of their limitations became apparent and they were used, particularly for symptom suppression in chronic diseases, with more discrimination than they had been. Now they are respected as therapeutic fall-back positions when less toxic nonsteroid anti-inflammatory agents have ceased to be effective.

BIBLIOGRAPHY

Anderson DC, Winter JSD (eds): *Adrenal Cortex*. London, Butterworths, 1985.

Atkinson JP, Frank MM: Effect of cortisone therapy on serum complement components. *J Immunol* 1973; 111:1061.

Axelrod J, Reisine TD: Stress hormones: Their interaction and regulation. *Science* 1984; 224:452.

Baxter JD, Ivarie RD: Regulation of gene expression by glucocorticoid hormones: Studies of receptors and responses in cultured cells, in O'Malley BW, Birnbaumer L (eds): *Receptors and Hormone Action,* vol 2. New York, Academic Press, 1978, pp 251–295.

Bergland RM, Page RB: Pituitary-brain vascular relations. *Science* 1974; 204:18.

Bondy PK: Disorders of the adrenal cortex, in Wilson JD, Foster DW (eds): *Williams Textbook of Endocrinology,* ed 7. Philadelphia, WB Saunders Co, 1985.

Bonta IL, Bray MA, Parnham MJ (eds): *The Pharmacology of Inflammation, Handbook of Inflammation,* vol 5. New York, Elsevier North-Holland, Inc, 1985.

Buckingham JC: Hypothalamo-pituitary responses to trauma. *Br Med Bull* 1985; 41:203.

Cheitlin R, Buckley DI, Ramachandran K: The role of extracellular calcium in corticotropin-stimulated steroidogenesis. *J Biol Chem* 1985; 260:5323.

De Wied D: Behavioral effects of neuropeptides related to ACTH, MSH and β LPH. *Ann NY Acad Sci* 1977; 297:263.

Engeland WC, Dallman MF: Neural mediation of compensatory adrenal growth. *Endocrinology* 1976; 99:1659.

Funder JW: Glucocorticoid receptors and the physiological roles of glucocorticoid hormones, in Labrie F, Proulx L (eds): *Endocrinology.* Excerpta Medica ICS 655. New York, Elsevier North-Holland, Inc, 1984.

Gagner J-P, Drouin J: Opposite regulation of proopiomelanocortin gene transcription by glucocorticoids and CRH. *Mol Cell Endocrinol* 1985; 40:25.

Gardner LI (ed): *Endocrine and Genetic Diseases of Childhood and Adolescence,* ed 2. Philadelphia, WB Saunders Co, 1975.

Gaunt R: History of the adrenal cortex, in Blaschko H, Sayers G, Smith AD (eds): *Handbook of Physiology, Endocrinology,* vol 6. Washington, DC, American Physiological Society, 1975.

Gerwirtz G, Yalow RS: Ectopic ACTH production in carcinoma of the lung. *J Clin Invest* 1974; 53:1022.

Gill GN: ACTH regulation of the adrenal cortex. *Pharmacol Ther* 1976; 2:313.

Gill GN, Crivello JF, Hornsby PJ, et al: Growth, function, and development of the adrenal cortex: Insights from cell culture, in Sato G, Pardee AB, Sirbasko DA (eds): *Growth of Cells in Hormonally Defined Media,* vol 9. Cold Spring Harbor, New York, Conference on Cell Proliferation, 1982.

Gospodarowicz D, Hornsby PJ, Gill GN: Control of bovine adrenal cortical cell proliferation by fibroblast growth factor: Lack of effect of epidermal growth factor. *Endocrinology* 1977; 100:1080.

Gupta C, Katsumata M, Goldman AS, et al: Glucocorticoid-induced phospholipase A_2-inhibitory proteins mediate glucocorticoid teratogenicity in vitro. *Proc Natl Acad Sci USA* 1984; 81:1140.

Gwynne JT, Mahaffee D, Brewer HB, Jr, et al: Adrenal cholesterol uptake from plasma lipoproteins: Regulation by corticotrophin. *Proc Natl Acad Sci USA* 1976; 73:4329.

Hall PF: Trophic stimulation of steroidogenesis: In search of the elusive trigger. *Recent Prog Horm Res* 1985; 41:31.

Haynes RC, Jr: Theories on the mode of action of ACTH in stimulating secretory activity of the adrenal cortex, in Blaschko H, Sayers G, Smith AD (eds): *Handbook of Physiology, Endocrinology,* vol 6. Washington, DC, American Physiological Society, 1975.

Hirata F: Lipomodulin: A modulator of cellular phospholipid metabolism, in Cheung WY (ed): *Calcium and Cell Function,* vol 5. New York, Academic Press, 1984, pp 279–290.

Hornsby PJ: The regulation of adrenocortical function by control of growth and structure, in Anderson DC, Winter JSD (eds): *Adrenal Cortex.* London, Butterworths, 1985, pp 1–32.

Ip MM, Milholland RJ, Shea WK, et al: The glucocorticoid receptor complexes to the nucleosomal core in P1798 mouse lymphosarcoma. *Mol Cell Endocrinol* 1985; 41:45.

Jones MT, Hillhouse EW: Neurotransmitter regulation of corticotropin-releasing factor in vitro. *Ann NY Acad Sci* 1977; 297:536.

Kerepesi T, Aranyi P: Low levels of glucocorticoid binding sites in circulating lymphocytes of premature infants suffering from hyaline membrane disease. *J Steroid Biochem* 1985; 22:151.

Krieger DT: Regulation of circadian periodicity of plasma ACTH levels. *Ann NY Acad Sci* 1977; 297:561.

Krieger DT, Ganong WF (eds): ACTH and related peptides: Structure, regulation and action (monograph). *Ann NY Acad Sci* 1977; 297.

Lerner AB, Buettner-Janusch J: The structure of human corticotropin (adrenocorticotropic hormone). *J Biol Chem* 1961; 236:2970.

Leung K, Munck A: Peripheral actions of glucocorticoids. *Ann Rev Physiol* 1975; 37:245.

Lewis DA: Endogenous anti-inflammatory factors. *Biochem Pharmacol* 1984; 33:1705.

Liggins GC, Howie RN: A controlled trial of antepartum glucocorticoid treatment for prevention of the respiratory distress syndrome in premature infants. *Pediatrics* 1972; 50:515.

Loeb JN: Corticosteroids and growth. *N Engl J Med* 1976; 295:547.

Lund P, Williamson OH: Intertissue nitrogen fluxes. *Br Med Bull* 1985; 41:251.

Melby JC: Systemic corticosteroid therapy: Pharmacology and endocrine considerations. *Ann Intern Med* 1974; 81:505.

Munck A, Guyre PM, Holbrook NJ: Physiological functions of glucocorticoids in stress and their relation to pharmacological actions. *Endocr Rev* 1984; 5:25.

New MI, Dupont B, Grumbach K, et al: Congenital adrenal hyperplasia and related conditions, in Stanbury B, Wyngaarden JB, Fredrickson DS, et al (eds): *The Metabolic Basis of Inherited Disease,* ed 5. New York, McGraw-Hill Book Co, 1983, pp 973–1000.

Parente I, DiRosea M, Flower RJ, et al: Relationship between the antiphospholipase and anti-inflammatory effects of glucocorticoid-induced proteins. *Eur J Pharmacol* 1984; 99:233.

Ringold GM: Steroid hormone regulation of gene expression. *Ann Rev Pharmacol Toxicol* 1985; 25:529.

Rousseau GG: Structure and regulation of the glucocorticoid hormone receptor. *Mol Cell Endocrinol* 1984; 38:1.

Schleimer RP: The mechanisms of anti-inflammatory steroid action in allergic diseases. *Ann Rev Pharmacol Toxicol* 1985; 25:381.

Selye H: General adaptation syndrome and diseases of adaptation. *J Clin Endocrinol* 1946; 6:117.

Simpson ER, Waterman MR: Regulation by ACTH of steroid hormone biosynthesis in the adrenal cortex. *Can J Biochem Cell Biol* 1983; 61:692.

Svec F: Glucocorticoid receptor regulation. *Life Sci* 1985; 36:2359.

Turkington RW, Majumder GC, Kadohama N, et al: Hormonal regulation of gene expression in mammary cells. *Recent Prog Horm Res* 1973; 29:417.

Vale W, Rivier C, Brown MR, et al: Chemical and biological characterization of corticotropin releasing factor. *Recent Prog Horm Res* 1983; 39:245.

Weincove C, Anderson DC: Interactions between adrenal cortex and medulla, in Anderson DC, Winter JSD (eds): *Adrenal Cortex*. London, Butterworths, 1985, pp 208–234.

Yamamoto KR, Gehring V, Stampfer MR, et al: Genetic approaches to steroid hormone action. *Recent Prog Horm Res* 1976; 32:3.

12

The Renin-Angiotensin-Aldosterone System

Hypophysectomy is not fatal, but bilateral adrenalectomy is. The life-maintaining principle supplied by the adrenal cortices is the salt-retaining steroid, aldosterone, which is produced by cells in the glomerulosa, or subcapsular layer, of the cortex. Aldosterone deficiency, whether it occurs in an experimental animal or in a patient, results in failure of the renal tubule to retrieve sodium from the glomerular filtrate and therefore in a net loss of sodium from the body. At the same time, potassium *retention* occurs that results in an increase in potassium concentration of the blood and extracellular fluid. If the Na^+ loss continues, there is loss of water, at first from the extracellular fluid compartments, but later from intracellular stores as well. Finally, the combined effects of potassium retention, peripheral circulatory failure, and renal failure lead inexorably to death. This sequence does not occur in the hypophysectomized individual because the adrenal glomerulosa (G) cell, unlike the fasciculata cell, can function sufficiently in the absence of ACTH to prevent it. However, ACTH may be required for optimal function of the G cell. In this chapter, we examine the information system that is primarily responsible for controlling G cell function.

The renin-angiotensin-aldosterone regulatory system was discovered by two different groups of investigators, who did not realize that they were collaborators in a single enterprise. The demonstration by Bauman and Marine of salt loss in the urine of adrenalectomized dogs was the point of departure for the long search for an adrenal salt-retaining hormone. The first potent salt-retaining steroid was the synthetic steroid, deoxycorticosterone acetate (DCA), which effectively corrected the salt-losing defect in adrenalectomized animals and in patients with Addison's disease. The work with DCA stimulated many searches for the "physiologic" DCA, whose existence was inferred from the finding by Luetscher et al. of a very active salt-retaining factor in the urine of some patients. Aldosterone was isolated and identified as the long-sought salt-retaining hormone of the adrenal cortex by Simpson and Tait in 1952.

Parallel with these developments, another group of investigators was attempting to elucidate the role of the kidney in the cause of hypertension. In 1934, at a time when the life of patients with Addison's disease was being prolonged by salt administration, Goldblatt showed that constriction of the renal arteries resulted in high blood pressure in dogs. In 1939, Page in the United States and Braun-Menendez and Leloir in Argentina independently showed that renin, the substance of renal origin that produced hypertension, was an enzyme that split the vasoactive material from a circulating substrate. Not long after the amino acid sequencing of vasopressin and insulin, the sequence of angiotensin II was described and the octapeptide was synthesized (1958).

In the same year (1958) Gross, in Germany, described an inverse relationship between salt balance and renal renin content in rats. In 1960, the two lines of investigation converged when Laragh in New York and Genest in Canada independently demonstrated that angiotensin infusion increased the secretion of aldosterone. This made possible (1) the development of contemporary concepts of the role of aldosterone in maintaining water and electrolyte balance, and (2) a reexamination of the problem of hypertension, which promises to provide a rational basis for individualizing therapy in that group of disorders. Having started with Goldblatt's renal hypertension in dogs, we appear to have come full circle.

Chemistry

The renin-angiotensin-aldosterone system has many of the features of a pituitary-target organ system, since it uses a pair of prohormone-derived peptides, angiotensins II and III, which are trophic to the adrenal G cell in almost the same way that ACTH controls the adrenal fasciculata cell. As in the cases of ACTH and LH, a steroid hormone is secreted by the target cell.

PEPTIDES

Peptides of the renin-angiotensin-aldosterone system are shown in Figure 12–1. *Renin substrate* is a globulin secreted by the liver. A decapeptide, angiotensin I, is produced by action of the enzyme, renin, at a leucyl-leucine bond of the globulin. *Angiotensin II* (A II) is an octapeptide generated by the action of converting enzyme on angiotensin I. Angiotensin III (A III) is des-Asp-angiotensin II, a heptapeptide.

Many synthetic and naturally occurring peptides have been examined for their effects on this system. A sample peptide converting enzyme inhibitor and a competitive antagonist of angiotensin, saralasin, are shown at the bottom of Figure 12–1.

STEROIDS

The structures of a few mineralocorticoids, or salt-retaining steroids, are shown in Figure 12–2. *Deoxycorticosterone* was important historically as the first widely studied mineralocorticoid. It lacks a hydroxyl group at carbon 2 and is therefore devoid of glucocorticoid activity. *Aldosterone* is the major hormonal product of the adrenal G cell. Its salt-retaining potency is 30–50 times that of deoxycorticosterone. It does have appreciable glucocorticoid activity, but it is so powerful a salt-retaining hormone that a replacement dose for adrenal insufficiency in the human being is of the order of 100–200 μg/day. In contrast, the replacement dose for cortisol is about 25 mg/day. Therefore, the glucocorticoid potential of aldosterone has no practical significance. The biosynthesis of aldosterone from cholesterol is described in Chapter 11.

The *spirolactones* are synthetic analogues of aldosterone, which in high enough doses can bind to the

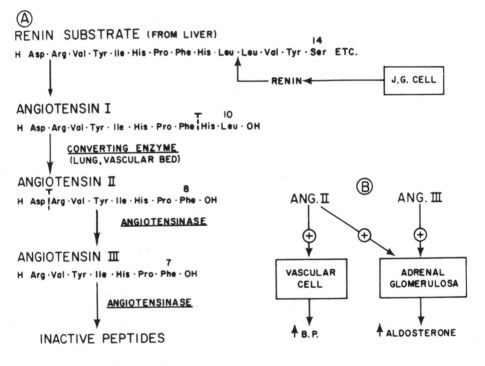

FIG 12–1.
Structures and biosynthesis of angiotensins II and III, and structures of certain important inhibitors of the system.

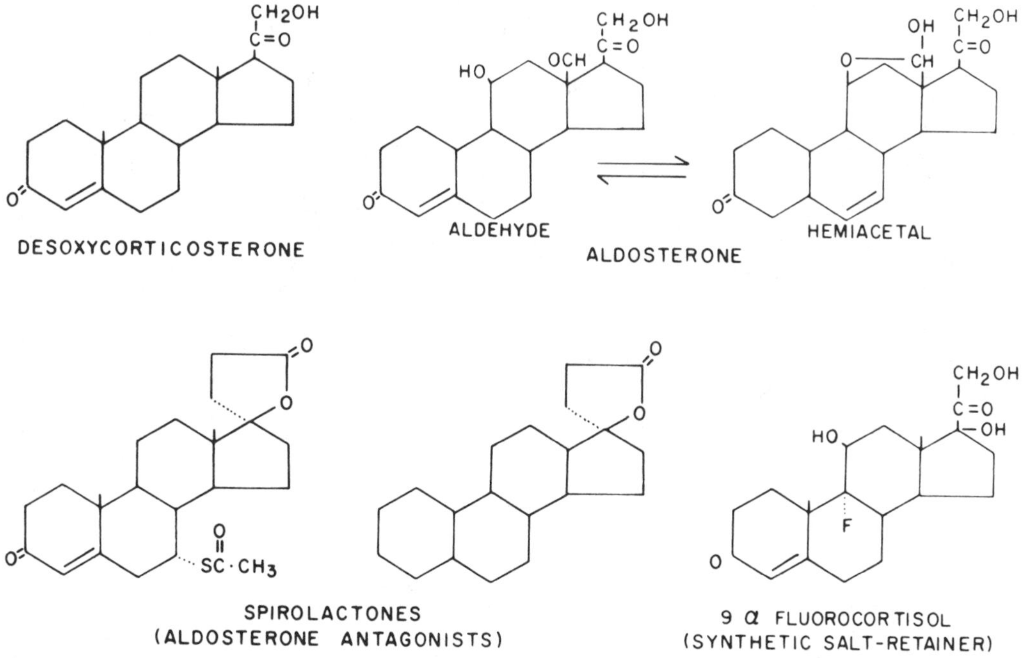

FIG 12–2.
Steroids related to aldosterone.

aldosterone receptor without initiating a biologic response and therefore inhibit the effect of aldosterone at its end-organ. Their use will be discussed later.

A representative synthetic 9α *fluorinated steroid* is shown in Figure 12–2. Some of these synthetic compounds are more potent salt-retainers, on a weight basis, than is aldosterone itself. This, together with their greater resistance to metabolic inactivation than the parent compound, enabling them therefore to be given orally, probably explains why synthetic mineralocorticoids, and not aldosterone, are used for replacement of aldosterone deficiencies.

Design of the System

The design of the renin-angiotensin-aldosterone system is shown in Figure 12–3. The juxtaglomerular (JG) cells of the afferent arterioles store the enzyme renin in secretory granules, which resemble the granules seen in other secretory cells. In this case, the granules may be categorized as specialized lysosomes whose contents are secreted on signal into the circulation. These cells are probably modified smooth muscle cells. Maintaining animals on a salt-free diet causes the population of JG cells to increase.

Renin is a glycoprotein with a molecular weight of about 40,000 daltons. It is assayed by its ability to generate angiotensin II from renin substrate, the angiotensin II being detected by radioimmunoassay (or bioassay).

The major variables that are continuously monitored by the JG apparatus are blood pressure and volume. In addition, it receives information about the Na^+ concentration of tubular urine at the level of the macula densa, and it is innervated by sympathetic nerves via β receptors. The sequence in Figure 12–3 is a deliberate oversimplification to illustrate the closed-loop nature of the renin-angiotensin system. A decrease in blood pressure or volume or both is sensed by the JG cell, which responds by secreting renin. The enzyme encounters an α_2 globulin of hepatic origin, which is already in circulation where it functions as a prohormone reservoir for angiotensin. The released renin cleaves the decapeptide, angiotensin I, from the precursor globulin, and a converting enzyme, mainly in the lung but also present in other vascular beds, cleaves the two terminal amino acids from *angiotensin* I to produce angiotensin II. This octapeptide is one of the most potent known vasoconstrictor substances, and it acts primarily as an arteriolar vasoconstrictor. It also acts as a trophic hormone for the glomerulosa cells, which synthesize and secrete *aldosterone*. The aldosterone-secreting cells of the adrenal are under complex control, which includes

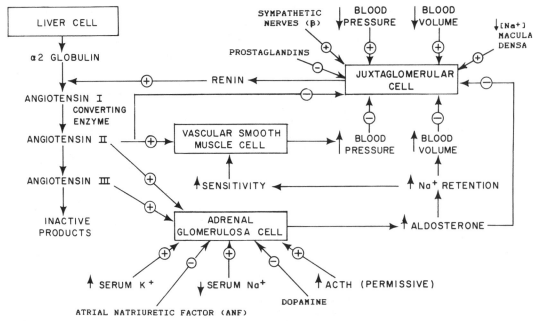

FIG 12–3.
Physiologic regulation of the renin-angiotensin-aldosterone system.

responses to ambient electrolyte concentrations as well as to ACTH. In some species, ACTH is the primary stimulus for aldosterone secretion, but in the human being it appears to play a more supportive role. Apparently it maintains the capability of the G cell to respond to the effects of angiotensin.

Recently a metabolic product of angiotensin II, des-Asp-angiotensin II, or angiotensin III, has been found to be a very potent stimulator of aldosterone secretion. Apparently it has none of angiotensin II's vasoconstricting effect. Angiotensins II and III are equipotent as stimulators of aldosterone secretion. However, in humans A II is more important quantitatively than A III since the plasma concentration ratio of A II to A III is 5:1. In addition, adrenal cells appear to have a population of receptors that selectively bind the heptapeptide (III).

The consequences of aldosterone secretion in man and toad are the same: conservation of Na^+ and preservation of circulating fluid volume. A deficiency of aldosterone, as seen in the adrenalectomized experimental animal or the patient with Addison's disease, is expressed as Na^+ loss in the urine (natriuresis) and retention of K^+. Aldosterone reverses the situation: retrieval of Na^+ from the glomerular filtrate in the kidney tubule is stimulated and K^+ excretion in the urine is encouraged.

The effect of retaining Na^+ is expressed in at least two ways: (1) water retention, and therefore, volume restoration, is enhanced, and (2) the presence of increased Na^+ concentration renders the arteriolar muscle cells, which contribute to the maintenance of blood pressure, more sensitive to the vasoactive substances that stimulate them. The arteriolar and adrenal effects of the angiotensins collaboratively help to restore blood pressure to the equilibrium level.

In addition to these effects, which constitute closing the loop by restoring the monitored variables to their original levels, aldosterone is believed to have a direct negative feedback influence on the JG cell in much the manner of a steroid hormone exerting feedback inhibition on the pituitary or hypothalamus. The coalition of restored blood pressure, restored blood volume, and direct feedback inhibitory effect of aldosterone effectively inhibits renin secretion. In addition to these feedback controls, there is some evidence that renin secretion is inhibited by angiotensin II.

Actions of Angiotensin

ADRENAL GLOMERULOSA CELL

As stated in the preceding chapter, the glomerulosa and fasciculata "zones" of the adrenal cortex are functionally discrete glands that secrete different products and are controlled by different stimulators and inhibitors.

Stimulators of Aldosterone Secretion

The glomerulosa cell is stimulated to synthesize and secrete aldosterone not only by angiotensins II and III but also by ACTH, prostaglandin E, high $[K^+]$ and low $[Na^+]$.

Angiotensins II and III have distinguishable receptors (on the basis of ligand affinities), but we are not aware of differences in their modes of action. A II receptors are unusual in the fact that, unlike most peptide hormone receptors, they are up-regulated, or induced, by their hormonal ligand. They do not articulate with the adenylate cyclase system and, therefore, do not stimulate synthesis of cyclic AMP as ACTH does. They bring about activation of aldosterone synthesis by increasing intracellular Ca^{2+} concentration ($[Ca^{2+}]_c$) and by switching on polyphosphatidyl inositol (PIP_2) turnover (Fig 12–4). Current evidence suggests that PIP_2 turnover is stimulated via a G protein. Influx of Ca^{2+} from extracellular fluid via a Ca^{2+} channel is also stimulated, but the connec-

tion between receptor occupancy and increased Ca^{2+} uptake is presently unknown. The stimulation of phospholipase C or PIP_2 phosphodiesterase (not to be confused with cAMP phosphodiesterase) results in the accumulation of inositol triphosphate (IP_3) and diacylglycerol (DAG). As in the model we described in Chapter 3, IP_3 mobilizes Ca^{2+} from intracellular stores and DAG sensitizes C kinase to the activating influence of Ca^{2+}. Note that in this case $[Ca^{2+}]_c$ is increased both by Ca^{2+} influx (or inhibited efflux) *and* by the action of IP_3. The increase in $[Ca^{2+}]_c$ directly stimulates some functions and indirectly (via Ca_4-Calmodulin) others.

The steroidogenic response to A II is biphasic, i.e., an initial sharp increase in aldosterone output within a few minutes is followed later by a more gradual and sustained increase. On the basis of ingenious experiments, Kojima et al. have demonstrated that the early sharp peak is associated with Ca_4-Calmodulin mediated events, while the sustained aldosterone secretory response is dependent on the activation of C kinase. (The fast response can be duplicated by a Ca^{2+} ionophore which quickly raises $[Ca^{2+}]_c$. The slower response can be reproduced by administering a DAG-like C kinase sensitizer. When both reagents are pre-

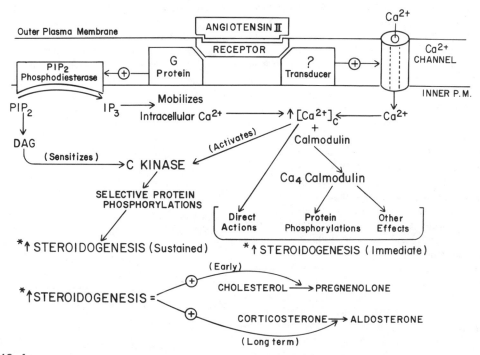

FIG 12–4.
Mechanism of action of angiotensin II on the adrenal granulosa cell. It is still uncertain whether the observed increase in cytosolic Ca^{2+} concentration is due to increased influx (as shown here) or inhibited efflux. (Adapted from Kojima I, Kojima K, Rasmussen H: *J Biol Chem* 1985; 260:9171.)

sented simultaneously, the cell's secretory response is the same as it is to A II.) As in the case of ACTH's action on the fasciculata cell, the A II response is achieved via phosphorylation of proteins involved in the process of feeding cholesterol into the steroidogenic process, and the major site of action is at the desmolase or side chain cleavage step. Just as persistent stimulation with ACTH affects the P450 hydroxylating enzyme complement of the fasciculata cell, continued A II stimulation of the glomerulosa cell induces and sustains $P450_{c18}$ (and, no doubt, antecedent P450s as well).

Another parallel between the effects of ACTH on the fasciculata cell and A II on the glomerulosa cell involves the provision of a continuing supply of cholesterol for hormone biosynthesis. Leitersdorf et al. have demonstrated, in primary cultures of zona glomerulosa cells, that A II stimulates receptor-mediated uptake of low-density lipoproteins (LDL) 200%–300% after 12–16 hours of incubation. At this time, there is a demonstrable increase in LDL receptor number.

Glomerulosa cells also respond to ACTH by increasing both aldosterone and cortisol secretion. In this case, both cyclic AMP and Ca^{2+} are mediators of the response, but the increase in $[Ca^{2+}]_c$ is achieved by stimulated influx and not by intracellular mobilization. While the renin-angiotensin-aldosterone system can function well enough to sustain life in a hypophysectomized (i.e., ACTH-less) animal, the glomerulosa cell of the intact animal is more responsive to A II. Although ACTH is not the primary glomerulosa cell stimulator, it has a secondary maintenance function in aldosterone secretion.

Increased K^+ concentration also elicits aldosterone synthesis and secretion by depolarizing the glomerulosa cell membrane and thereby opening voltage-dependent Ca^{2+} transport channels. Curiously, this depolarization also activates the adenylate cyclase system and a modest increase in cAMP occurs. The net effect of K^+, therefore, is similar to that of ACTH: an increase in $[Ca^{2+}]_c$ without mobilization of intracellular stores and phosphorylation of proteins by cAMP-dependent protein kinase.

One's general impression of the glomerulosa cell is that it is not particularly fastidious about what happens to stimulate it. It contains redundant capacities to respond to Ca^{2+}, cAMP, and DAG $+ Ca^{2+}$, and it dutifully synthesizes and secretes aldosterone in response to multiple second messengers which, under different circumstances, may be present in different patterns. Ca^{2+} and the products of PIP_2, however, are the major messengers for A II.

Inhibitors of Glomerulosa Cell Secretion

Inhibitors of aldosterone synthesis and secretion include: dopamine, atrial natriuretic factor (ANF), and high $[Na^+]$.

That inhibition by dopamine is physiologically important is suggested by the observation (Aguilera and Catt) that secretion of aldosterone, either in vivo or in vitro, is stimulated by the dopamine antagonist, metoclopramide. The mechanism of dopamine's inhibitory action on aldosterone secretion is unknown.

Atrial natriuretic factor (ANF) is a powerful diuretic and natriuretic peptide that is extractable from mammalian atrial muscle (de Bold). Generally, ANF is a physiological antagonist to A II, for instead of causing vasoconstriction and (through stimulated aldosterone secretion) sodium retention, ANF is a vasodilator and salt-*losing* hormone. Both glomerulosa cells and fasciculata cells carry receptors for ANF which inhibits the aldosterone secretory response to A II in the former as well as that of cortisol to ACTH in the latter. Evaluation of the physiological importance of ANF is ongoing. Whatever the result, the existence of a receptor-mediated inhibitory response to ANF in the glomerulosa cell suggests a coordinately controlled, interacting, Claude Bernardian balance of salt-retaining and salt-losing mechanisms.

High extracellular $[Na^+]$, as it occurs in salt-loading, renders the glomerulosa cell insensitive to the stimulatory effect of A II by a mechanism that is unknown to us. In the intact animal, volume expansion secondary to Na^+ retention inhibits the system at the juxtaglomerular cell level, but a local inhibitory effect on the glomerulosa cell operates as well. It is certainly eminently sensible, from a teleonomic point of view, to shut off the secretion of a salt-retaining hormone in the presence of a plethora of salt.

Smooth Muscle

Angiotensin is a stimulant of smooth muscle, particularly vascular smooth muscle. It is more active on arterial and arteriolar smooth muscle than on venous smooth muscle. There is no evidence that cAMP is involved in the stimulatory effect of angiotensin on vascular smooth muscle. It acts by increasing $[Ca^{2+}]_c$ by a mechanism unknown to us.

Central Nervous System

Since Fitzsimons described the induction of drinking behavior by angiotensin and attributed a dipsogenic function to it, much evidence has accumulated that suggests that the octapeptide may be an important thirst signal (see Fregly). Since water intake is so obviously involved in volume regulation, a hormone that works to restore depleted volume by eliciting aldosterone secretion would aid its cause by stimulating drinking behavior. The localization of angiotensin, renin and converting enzyme activity in the CNS makes a role for angiotensin in mediating thirst and drinking behavior seem plausible.

Angiotensin II may also play a role in the stimulation of NaCl appetite in the rat. NaCl appetite is assessed by measuring preference for NaCl solution over water when both are presented simultaneously to rats. After bilateral adrenalectomy, and also in other circumstances in which rats prefer NaCl solution to water, the renin-angiotensin-aldosterone system is clearly involved. Although the mechanisms in NaCl appetite regulation are complex (for example, aldosterone counteracts the stimulatory effect of A II on NaCl preference) the idea of concurrent regulation of thirst and NaCl appetite to restore volume is certainly a teleonomically attractive one (Fregly and Rowland).

THE MECHANISM OF ACTION OF ALDOSTERONE

Aldosterone has three important actions: (1) it increases Na^+ reabsorption in the renal tubule; (2) it increases secretion of K^+; and (3) it increases H^+ (proton) secretion.

These actions have been studied most frequently in the mammalian kidney, but important insights have been acquired from experiments on the isolated toad bladder, which, fortunately, responds to aldosterone much the way cortical collecting duct renal tubular cells do. Ussing discovered that half a toad bladder mounted between two chambers transported Na^+ from the mucosal (urine) side to the serosal (blood) side and the extent of Na^+ transcellular transport was directly proportional to the "short circuit current" (SCC); i.e., the measured amount of current that had to be applied to the system to nullify the potential difference set up on the two sides of the membrane by Na^+ migration. Crabbé found that aldosterone added in vitro to the serosal side of the bladder increased Na^+ transport markedly after a 60–90 minute lag period. One attractive feature of this method was the fact that the other hemibladder could be used as a control. Our understanding of aldosterone mechanism, therefore, requires attention both to the renal tubule and to the toad bladder model preparation,

which, historically, inspired many experiments on the tubule.

Aldosterone has effects on Na^+ conservation and K^+ loss not only in the kidney and toad bladder, but also in salivary glands, distal colon, and sweat glands. Under most circumstances, its effects on the kidney are quantitatively most important, but in humans who adapt successfully to the massive loss of Na^+ in sweat due to hot ambient temperatures, enhanced secretion of aldosterone plays a crucial role in the adaptation. (Conn was interested in this phenomenon at about the time he discovered primary aldosteronism.)

The following brief summary of the mechanisms involved in aldosterone's actions is based on a large number of experiments by many investigators who applied a large repertory of methods to the problem. In addition to the bioelectric method mentioned above, *some* of these were: *renal clearances* and other methods applied to more or less intact animals and humans; *microperfusion* of renal tubules and specific segments of tubules (sometimes with SCC measurements); *autoradiography* of tritiated aldosterone-treated tubules or toad bladders; *electron microscopy* to identify morphological responses to hormone treatment; two-dimensional *gel electrophoresis* of aldosterone-sensitive cells before and after stimulation; measurements of *enzyme activity* and of *rates of enzyme synthesis and degradation; inhibitor studies* (amiloride, actinomycin D, etc.), etc.

In the amphibian bladder and in the mammalian nephron, two different cell types are programmed to respond to aldosterone in different ways. The predominant one in both cases is mainly devoted to Na^+ reabsorption and K^+ extrusion. The other, which contains the enzyme *carbonic anhydrase* (CA) (the enzyme that catalyzes the reaction

$$CO_2 + H_2O \rightarrow H^+ + HCO_3^-,$$

secretes H^+ in response to aldosterone. In both types of cell, the response must be sustained by a continuing supply of ATP. Also, in both types of cell, aldosterone induces extensive membrane remodelling and rearrangement. It is not clear whether the proton-secreting cell contains an H^+-ATPase *in addition* to all of the response elements present in the "main" responsive cell and only secretes protons because it expresses the enzyme CA or whether it is highly specialized to secrete H^+.

Aldosterone Receptor

Circulating glucocorticoids are measured in mg/dl; aldosterone, in µg/dl. The aggregate mass of glucocorticoid-producing cells in the adrenal cortex is much greater than that of aldosterone-secreting cells. One might predict, on this basis, that the aldosterone receptor must be a particularly discriminating one. However, it is somewhat surprising to discover that adrenal steroid receptors (compared with those of estrogen and vitamin D metabolites) are a somewhat promiscuous lot.

Many different adrenal steroid-binding proteins have been described: (1) Type I glucocorticoid receptors (also known as aldosterone receptors), which occur in certain regions of the brain, in specific distal regions of the renal tubule, in the mammary gland, in sweat glands, salivary glands, and distal colon; (2) Type II receptors, which occur ubiquitously and have been studied most extensively as "the" glucocorticoid receptor; and (3) corticosteroid-binding globulin (CBG), alias transcortin, also called Type III receptor, although there is no evidence that it is, in fact, a receptor that mediates a biological response. CBG is the circulating carrier protein for glucocorticoids, but a similar protein is found in kidney cells (see below).

These proteins have been classified according to their ligand-binding properties. Type I binds naturally-occurring glucocorticoids (cortisol, corticosterone) *or* aldosterone with approximately equal (and high) affinity and the synthetic glucocorticoid, dexamethasone (DEX), with lower affinity. Type II binds DEX with medium affinity and cortisol and corticosterone much less well. CBG binds cortisol with very high affinity and aldosterone minimally, if at all.

If the concentration of circulating glucocorticoids is several hundredfold higher than that of aldosterone, how can aldosterone possibly affect renal tubular function? Type II glucocorticoid receptors are present throughout the length of the renal tubule, including that part (late distal convoluted tubule–collecting duct) where aldosterone acts. Type I receptors, however, are confined to the aldosterone target region. According to the most plausible current hypothesis, aldosterone, in spite of its low concentration, can succeed in occupying Type I receptors in its sensitive cells because these cells contain a binding protein (sometimes called Type III) which is not distinguishable from circulating transcortin or CBG. This intracellular molecular sponge, which is distributed along the renal tubule in parallel with the Type I receptor, soaks up glucocorticoids that enter cells, spares the aldosterone, and thereby enables it to compete successfully for a receptor that binds both classes of adrenal hormones with equal affinity. Indeed, when the circulating concentration of glucocorticoid is very high, the intracellular buffering capacity of Type III binder may be overwhelmed, and glucocorticoid can

bind to the "aldosterone" receptor and mimic the renal effect of aldosterone. Progesterone and the spironolactones (or spirolactones) bind to the Type I receptor but are unable to transform it into a biologically active form. Therefore, they function as *anti*aldosterones, or natriuretic agents.

Like the target cells of other steroid hormones, aldosterones respond to their hormone by enhancing the transcription of a small number of mRNAs, possibly as few as six. At the same time, as has been demonstrated by two-dimensional gel electrophoresis, a small number of proteins are present in *decreased* amounts after aldosterone. The small amounts of induced proteins and the cellular heterogeneity of the organs in which aldosterone has its principal action have tended to inhibit much of the molecular biology-gene cloning sort of action we have seen with other steroids.

Given the fact that aldosterone induces proteins selectively at the gene level, can we identify them? No, but we can point to several potential candidates.

Proteins That May Be Induced by Aldosterone

Figure 12–5 is a model of the action of aldosterone on a transcellular Na^+-transporting cell in either renal tubule or toad bladder. It shows the now familiar stimulation of RNA synthesis by the hormone-receptor complex. Na^+ enters through a specific Na^+ channel ("permease," transporter) on the luminal side of the tubular or bladder cell. It goes down a concentration gradient and is extruded on the contraluminal, or blood, side of the cell by Na^+K^+ATPase which is powered by ATP generated in mitochondria. Aldosterone also causes a change in the pattern of membrane phospholipids. Theoretically, Na^+ transport could be stimulated by an effect at the permease step, at the energy-producing locus, or at the Na^+ pump. (Circled numbers below refer to Figure 12–5.)

There is good evidence for the induction of an increased number of permease elements into the luminal membrane by aldosterone. The drug amiloride binds selectively to the Na^+ transporter and amiloride-binding has been used to estimate the increase in number of transporters in membranes of aldosterone-treated cells (Cuthbert and Shum). The effect on the *number* of surface units cannot be the *primary* effect of the hormone because an effect on transcellular Na^+ transport can be detected *before* the increase in number of surface transporters can be detected.

Aldosterone, therefore, appears to improve the performance of preexisting Na^+ transporters, and this seems to be its earliest detectable effect. Following the discovery by Goodman et al. that one of aldoste-

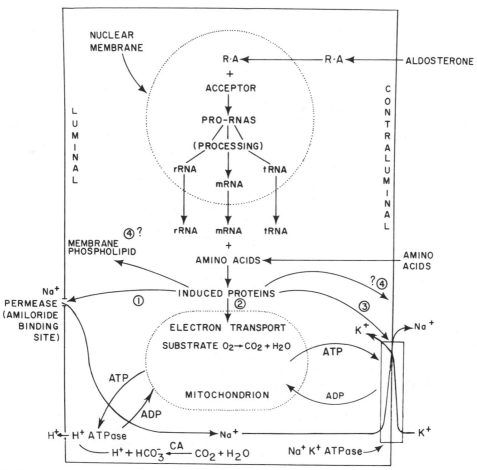

FIG 12–5.
A composite view of many theories of the mechanism of action of aldosterone. A = aldosterone; R = receptor; r = ribosomal; m = messenger; t = transfer; CA = carbonic anhydrase. The H^+ extrusion system (proton pump), shown in the lower left corner, is demonstrable in some aldosterone-sensitive cells.

rone's effects is to change the ratio of phosphatidyl choline (PC) to phosphatidyl ethanolamine in membranes of sensitive cells ④, Wiesmann et al. discovered that aldosterone stimulated methylation reactions involved in PC synthesis as well as carboxymethylation of proteins. Interestingly, administration of a methyl donor (S-adenosylmethionine) to aldosterone-sensitive cells stimulated Na^+ transport and inhibitors of transmethylation prevented the effect of aldosterone on Na^+ transport. While the molecular details of the consequences of stimulated methylation for Na^+ transporter function are entirely speculative, this new finding points to new possibilities for the induction by aldosterone of proteins which, though perhaps not intrinsic components of the permease itself, may be related to the remodelling of the membrane in such a

way as to enhance the efficiency of the transporter.

② Stimulated Na^+ transport must be supported by the oxidation of substrate. In this connection, Kirsten et al., having demonstrated a sharp (50%) decrease in the activity of the mitochondrial enzyme, citrate synthase, within days after adrenalectomy in the rat, showed that aldosterone could restore the activity to normal in three hours. In the toad bladder, the activity of citrate synthase and transepithelial Na^+ transport fluctuated in parallel, and induction of citrate synthase and related mitochondrial enzymes was inhibited by an RNA synthesis inhibitor. That the enzyme induction was not secondary to increased Na^+ flow through the cell was shown by the persistence of aldosterone's ability to induce citrate synthase even when Na^+ transport was blocked by amiloride.

Both in kidney and toad bladder, new $Na^+K^+ATPase$ molecules are synthesized and inserted into the contraluminal membrane in response to aldosterone treatment. This is a relatively late event in the action of aldosterone, but it is necessary for a sustained response to the hormone. Thus, the old argument about whether Na^+ pump hypertrophy "pulls" Na^+ through the cell or increased Na^+ flux is the earlier event appears now to be settled in favor of the view that, although increased transport of Na^+ through the cell occurs first, induction of the sodium pump occurs even when Na^+ transport is blocked by amiloride.

The details of aldosterone's effect on proton-secreting cells in kidney and toad bladder have not been worked on much, no doubt because of the extreme technical difficulty of the problem. But, on the basis of what we know about the response of the Na^+ transporting cell, we can predict confidently that a pattern similar to the one we have described—membrane remodelling, proton pump activation, and enhanced ATP-generating capacity—will emerge eventually.

One aspect of aldosterone's action has puzzled observers for many years. On the basis of several lines of evidence, a number of investigators have suggested that the effects of aldosterone on Na^+ reabsorption and K^+ secretion are dissociable, and that different mechanisms may be involved in achieving them. On the other hand, more recent students of the problem are more impressed by the coordinate nature of the Na^+ and K^+ effects and suggest that the latter are linked to primary influences on Na^+ transport. For the quality of the evidence on both sides of this controversy, see Marver, 1985.

Pharmacology of Renin-Angiotensin-Aldosterone System

When the design of a complex regulatory system becomes apparent, it is possible to modify the system at many points with drugs. In some cases, the intervention is calculated and beneficial, whereas in others the system may be affected by a drug that is being given for some purpose unrelated to fluid and electrolyte regulation.

The *liver cell* is the source of renin substrate, the prohormone of the angiotensins. Renin substrate is a globulin, which, like other globulins secreted by the liver (cortisol-binding, sex steroid-binding), appears in higher concentration as a result of estrogen presence or administration. Although the amount of available renin substrate is not rate limiting under ordinary circumstances, an increase in its concentration may lead to the production of inappropriately high amounts of angiotensin, and therefore stimulation of the adrenal glomerulosa. Almost all pregnant women show a slight increase in blood pressure and some, presumably with an inherent predisposition to hypertension, show a considerable rise, which often reverts to the prepregnancy level after delivery. Oral estrogen-containing contraceptive pills, postmenopausal estrogen therapy and pharmacologic amounts of glucocorticoids can also elevate renin substrate concentration. In severe liver disease or adrenocortical insufficiency, plasma renin substrate concentration may be low.

The *juxtaglomerular secretory cells* (JG cells) contain droplets of material identified as renin. The JG cell responds to a variety of ionic, humoral, paracrine and neural signals and is therefore a site of pharmacologic intervention when renin production and release are inappropriately high. The JG cell is stimulated by catecholamine β agonists, and its secretion is inhibited by β blocking agents (e.g., propranolol). This action of propranolol is one of the bases for its use in diagnosis and treatment of high renin hypertension. Prostacyclin is a stimulator of renin release, and there is some evidence that the prostacyclin synthesis inhibitor, indomethacin, decreases renin production when it is being released in excess, as in Bartter's syndrome (JG cell hyperplasia). The inhibitory effect of ADH on renin release is another example of the close functional relationship between the complementary hypothalamic-pituitary-ADH system and the renin-angiotensin-aldosterone system.

Since angiotensin I is biologically inactive, the effects of excessive production of renin can be neutralized by *preventing angiotensin II synthesis by the converting enzyme*. Peptides with this effect have been described (Fig 12–6). These peptides are useful as diagnostic agents in characterizing the contribution of the renin system to the hypertension of individual patients. Ondetti et al. have introduced modified amino acid inhibitors of converting enzyme that are effective when taken orally. These have proven important for therapy of hypertension (see Gavras et al.).

The peptide *saralasin* has also been studied extensively as a diagnostic agent in analysis of hypertension. Although it binds to the stereospecific plasma membrane-receptors for angiotensins I and II, it cannot initiate a biologic response. It therefore competitively inhibits the angiotensins from stimulating blood vessel cells or adrenal glomerulosa cells.

Finally, the *spirolactones*, structural analogues of aldosterone, compete with aldosterone for the recep-

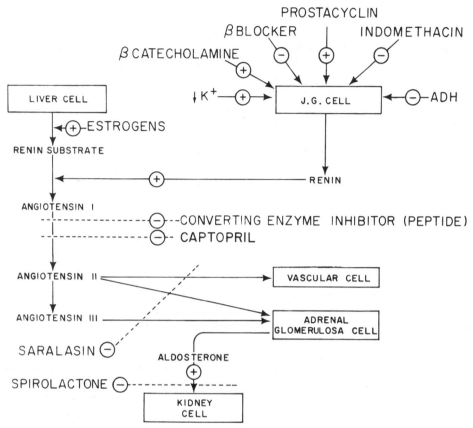

FIG 12–6.
An outline of the pharmacology of the renin-angiotensin-aldosterone system.

tor, which participates in aldosterone's effect in the renal tubular cell and other aldosterone-sensitive cells. The spirolactones (e.g., aldactone) are effective when given by mouth, and their effect persists for some hours. It is for this reason that they are useful as therapeutic agents in edematous states.

Primary and Secondary Hyperaldosteronism

Inappropriate secretion of aldosterone occurs in a group of disorders collectively called Conn's syndrome (primary hyperaldosteronism). Excessive secretion of sodium-retaining steroid hormone is seen in individuals with either aldosterone-producing tumors or diffusely hyperplastic adrenal glands. Increased aldosterone production is manifested by hypertension (often mild), potassium loss, sodium retention, and almost total suppression of plasma renin activity.

Aldosterone, like glucocorticoids, is produced in a recurrent diurnally variable pattern. In recumbent individuals, aldosterone levels in the circulation tend to parallel those of cortisol, the highest levels being seen in the early morning. However, in the case of aldosterone, a *postural* determinant of secretion rate is superimposed on the basic rhythm. A normal individual who changes from the recumbent to the upright posture and stands for four hours shows a two- to fourfold increase in plasma aldosterone concentration. This is demonstrably related to function of the renin-angiotensin system.

In contrast, a person with an autonomously functioning aldosterone-producing tumor and a virtually nonfunctioning renin-angiotensin system may actually show a paradoxical *fall* in plasma aldosterone concentration on assuming the upright posture.

The postural response test is helpful in estimating the competency of the renin-angiotensin system. It works because a redistribution of body fluid occurs on assuming the upright posture. This is sensed by the JG apparatus as a decrease in the "effective" or "perceived" blood volume.

In many clinical conditions, notably those characterized by accumulation of edema fluid (e.g., cirrhosis of the liver, heart failure), aldosterone is overproduced (secondary hyperaldosteronism). This, of course, is maladaptive and tends to perpetuate the edema by promoting sodium retention. As in the posturally induced increase in aldosterone secretion in normal individuals, edematous people, although they contain an excess of fluid, may have a decreased "effective" or "perceived" blood volume to which the JG apparatus makes its line-of-duty response. Thus, unless the cycle is broken by promoting excretion and limiting intake of sodium, the accumulation of edema fluid can only become progressively greater. This is an example of a "normal" response of a monitoring device to garbled signal.

In the case of secondary hyperaldosteronism associated with severe liver disease, there may be not only inappropriate overproduction of aldosterone but also a failure of the liver to metabolize it to its tetrahydro form in preparation for its excretion. Thus, salt retention may be promoted by the combination of overproduction and decreased inactivation of the primary mineralocorticoid.

Renin-Angiotensin-Aldosterone: Role in Hypertension

At one time "anemia" was considered a disease. Now we understand that anemia is a symptom of many diseases. Similarly, high blood pressure or hypertension is defined as the sustained elevation of blood pressure above empirically determined limits. Since regulation of blood pressure is so complex, it is not surprising that different components of the blood pressure-maintenance equipment can fail, with resulting hypertension.

Some of the many major contributory factors to a person's ability to regulate blood pressure within the range of normality are as follows:

1. Sympathetic nervous system, particularly by way of the catecholamines
2. Locally produced prostaglandins
3. Vasodilating substances (e.g., bradykinin)
4. Salt intake
5. Sodium excretion by the kidneys
6. *Renin-angiotensin-aldosterone system*

Since it is now clear that the life expectancy of a population of hypertensive persons is significantly improved by control of the hypertension, the desirability of improving such control is obvious. Since uncontrolled hypertension is statistically associated with a high incidence of stroke, coronary heart disease, congestive heart failure, retinal disease, kidney disease, and dissecting aneurysms of the aorta, an im-

proved understanding of the causes of various hypertensive states is obviously desirable.

A few hypertensive patients—between 10% and 15%—have curable hypertension. One type of hypertension is due to *pheochromocytoma,* or a catecholamine-producing tumor (see Chapter 13). The other two types directly involve the renin-aldosterone system:

1. *Primary aldosteronism,* which is due to inappropriate and uninhibited production of aldosterone by either an adrenal tumor or diffusely hyperplastic adrenal glands. This (as we have seen) is characterized by high aldosterone production rates and low levels of renin-angiotensin.

2. *Renovascular hypertension,* which is caused by a compromised arterial blood supply to one kidney, with normal function in the contralateral kidney. In this instance, renal vein renin measurements on the two sides may be made for diagnosis and guidance in formulating therapeutic strategy. In fortunate circumstances, removal of the ischemic kidney may eliminate the hypertension.

If 10%–15% of hypertension is due to correctable defects, 85%–90% is in the category of "essential." Yet the large majority of hypertensive patients do not constitute a homogeneous group. It is this group in which an analysis of the renin-angiotensin system can provide valuable clues for successful management.

Laragh et al., Streeten et al., and other groups of investigators have developed methods of triage of hypertensive patients on the basis of their renin status. It is now widely known that, in any large population of hypertensive individuals, some will have high circulating renin levels, some will be in the normal range, and others will have low renin levels. The analysis developed by Laragh et al. is reminiscent of our discussion of the inappropriate ADH syndrome in which we stressed that measuring a hormone level is meaningful only if a regulated function is measured simultaneously. In Figure 12–7 are shown two correlations: (1) between urinary sodium excretion and plasma renin activity, and (2) between urinary sodium and aldosterone excretion. Patients *A* and *B* have the same plasma renin level, but *B* is considered hyperreninemic, since his level is inappropriately high for his urinary sodium excretion. Similarly, patient *C* has a subnormal aldosterone excretion rate for his level of sodium excretion.

It is important to measure an individual person's renin levels relative to his sodium excretion because rational management may be suggested by the result. In any population of hypertensives, there is a spectrum from those (15%) with a very high renin level to those (30%) with low renin, i.e., it is not essential to have a high renin output to sustain high blood pres-

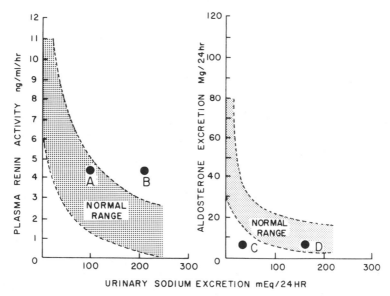

FIG 12–7.
Plasma renin and aldosterone excretion related to urinary sodium excretion in patients *A, B, C,* and *D.* (After Laragh JH, Sealey JE: *Cardiovasc Med* 1975; 2:1053.)

sure. The majority, 55%, represents a gradient of diminishing renin excess from rather high to rather low.

In general, high-renin hypertension responds favorably to β blocking drugs, such as propranolol, whereas low-renin hypertension improves on salt-restriction and use of diuretic agents. Moreover, the high-renin group contains a population of treatable renal hypertensives who can be identified by renal vein catheterization.

BIBLIOGRAPHY

Aguilera G, Catt KJ: Dopaminergic modulation of aldosterone secretion in the rat. *Endocrinology* 1984; 114:176.

Bartter FC, Gill JR, Froehlich JC, et al: Prostaglandins are overproduced by the kidneys and mediate hyperreninemia in Bartter's syndrome. *Trans Assoc Am Physicians* 1976; 89:77.

Baxter JD, Tyrrell JB: The adrenal cortex, in Felig P, Baxter JD, Broadus AE, et al (eds): *Endocrinology and Metabolism.* New York, McGraw-Hill Book Co, 1981, pp 285–510.

Biglieri EG, Baxter JD: The endocrinology of hypertension, in Felig P, Baxter JD, Broadus AE, et al (eds): *Endocrinology and Metabolism.* New York, McGraw-Hill Book Co, 1981, pp 551–598.

Cuthbert AW, Shum WK: Effects of vasopressin and aldosterone on amiloride binding in toad bladder epithelial cells. *Proc R Soc Lond (Biol)* 1975; 189:543.

deBold AJ: Atrial natriuretic factor: A hormone produced by the heart. *Science* 1985; 230:767.

DeLéan A, Racz K, Gutkowska J, et al: Specific receptor-mediated inhibition by synthetic atrial natriuretic factor of hormone-stimulated steroidogenesis in cultured bovine adrenal cells. *Endocrinology* 1984; 115:1636.

Devynck M-A, Pernollet MG, Matthews PG, et al: Specific receptors for des-Asp^1-angiotensin II ("Angiotensin III") in rat adrenals. *Proc Natl Acad Sci USA* 1977; 74:4029.

Enyedi P, Büki B, Mucsi I, et al: Polyphosphoinositide metabolism in adrenal glomerulosa cells. *Mol Cell Endocrinol* 1985; 41:105.

Fregly MJ (ed): Angiotensin-induced thirst: Peripheral and central mechanisms (symposium). *Fed Proc* 1978; 37:2667.

Fregly MJ, Rowland NE: Role of renin-angiotensin-aldosterone system in NaCl appetite of rats. *Am J Physiol* 1985; 248 (*Reg Integ Comp Physiol* 17): R1.

Funder JW: On mineralocorticoid and glucocorticoid receptors, in Anderson DC, Winter JSD (eds): *Adrenal Cortex.* London, Butterworths, 1985, pp 86–95.

Geering K, Claire M, Gaeggeler H-P, et al: Receptor occupancy vs induction of Na$^+$K$^+$ATPase and Na$^+$ transport by aldosterone. *Am J Physiol* 1985; 248 (*Cell Physiol* 17): C102.

Gibbons GH, Dzau VJ, Farhi ER, et al: Interaction of signals influencing renin release. *Ann Rev Physiol* 1984; 46:291.

Gilman AG, Goodman LS, Rall TW, et al (eds): *The Pharmacological Basis of Therapeutics,* ed 7. New York, Macmillan Publishing Co, 1985.

Goodman DBP, Wong M, Rasmussen H: Aldosterone-induced membrane phospholipid metabolism in toad urinary bladder. *Biochemistry* 1975; 14:2803.

Horisberger J-D, Diezi J: Inhibition of aldosterone-induced anti-natriuresis and kaliuresis by Actinomycin D. *Am J Physiol* 1984; 246 (*Renal Fluid Electrolyte Physiol* 15): F201.

Kinne RKH (ed): *Renal Biochemistry: Cells, Membranes, Molecules.* New York, Elsevier North-Holland, Inc, 1985.

Kirsten E, Kirsten R, Sharp GWG: Effects of sodium transport stimulating substances on enzyme activities in the toad bladder. *Pfluegers Arch* 1970; 316:26.

Kojima I, Kojima K, Rasmussen H: Characteristic of angiotensin II-, K^+-, and ACTH-induced calcium influx in adrenal glomerulosa cells. *J Biol Chem* 1985; 260:9171.

Kojima I, Kojima K, Rasmussen H: Role of calcium fluxes in the sustained phase of angiotensin II-mediated aldosterone secretion from adrenal glomerulosa cells. *J Biol Chem* 1985; 260:9177.

Laragh JH, Sealey JE: Renin-sodium profiling: How, when, why in clinical practice. *Cardiovasc Med* 1975; 2:1053.

Leitersdorf E, Stein O, Stein Y: Angiotensin II stimulates receptor-mediated uptake of LDL by bovine adrenal cortical cells in primary culture. *Biochim Biophys Acta* 1985; 835:183.

Lewis SA: Control of Na^+ and water absorption across vertebrate "tight" epithelia by ADH and aldosterone. *J Exp Biol* 1983; 106:9.

Ludens JH, Fanestil DD: Aldosterone stimulation of acidification of urine by the isolated urinary bladder of the Columbian toad. *Am J Physiol* 1974; 226:1321.

Marver D, Kokko JP: Renal target sites and the mechanism of action of aldosterone. *Miner Electrolyte Metab* 1983; 9:1.

Marver D: The mineralocorticoid receptor, in Litwack G (ed): *Biochemical Actions of Hormones*, vol 12. New York, Academic Press, 1985, pp 386–431.

Oates JA, Whorton AR, Gerkens JF, et al: The participation of prostaglandins in the control of renin release. *Fed Proc* 1979; 38:72.

Ondetti MA, Rubin BM, Cushman DW: Design of specific inhibitors of angiotensin-converting enzyme: New class of orally active antihypertensive agents. *Science* 1977; 196:441.

Re RN: Cellular biology of the renin-angiotensin systems. *Arch Intern Med* 1984; 144:2037.

Reid IA: The renin-angiotensin system and body function. *Arch Intern Med* 1985; 145:1465.

Rossier BC, Paccolat MP, Verrey F, et al: Mechanism of action of aldosterone: A pleiotropic response. *Horm Cell Reg* 1985; 9:209.

Schmidt U, Schmid J, Schmid H, et al: Sodium and potassium-activated ATPase, a possible target of aldosterone. *J Clin Invest* 1975; 55:655.

Stone DK, Kokko JP, Jacobson HR: In vitro stimulation of proton secretion by aldosterone. *Kidney Int* 1982; 21:240.

Streeten DH, Anderson GH, Freiberg JM: Use of an angiotensin II antagonist (saralasin) in the recognition of "angiotensinogenic" hypertension. *N Engl J Med* 1975; 292:657.

Wiesman WP, Johnson JP, Miura GA, et al: Aldosterone-stimulated transmethylations are linked to sodium transport. *Am J Physiol* 1985; 248 (*Renal Fluid Electrolyte Physiol* 17):F43.

13

Catecholamines

Epinephrine was the first hormone to be chemically identified and synthesized. Cyclic AMP was discovered by an investigator whose point of departure was the glycogenolytic effect of epinephrine. Many of our modern concepts of stimulus-secretion coupling in cells that store hormones in membrane-wrapped granules were initiated by a student of adrenal medullary secretion. Experimental studies of the catecholamine receptors and their blocking agents have resulted in significant contributions to receptor theory. Practical applications of these investigators' findings have led to advances in the therapy of such diseases as hypertension, hyperthyroidism, angina pectoris, allergic states and bronchial asthma.

Like the posterior pituitary, the adrenal medulla is a functional extension of the nervous system. It may be regarded as a specialized sympathetic ganglion, innervated by a long preganglionic, cholinergic neuron that forms synaptic connections with chromaffin cells. When the preganglionic neuron is stimulated, the chromaffin cells discharge the contents of their secretory granules directly into the blood.

Although the adrenal chromaffin cell and the adrenergic postganglionic neuron are both stimulated by preganglionic neurons in similar fashion, the main secretory product of the chromaffin cell in most species is epinephrine. Although the medullary cell secretes from 10% to 50% of its catecholamines as norepinephrine, depending on the species, most of the norepinephrine in the body acts as a neurotransmitter in the central and autonomic nervous systems.

The sympathetic, or adrenergic, division of the autonomic nervous system has two main distinguishing features: (1) it is designed to respond quickly and its mediators are inactivated or sequestered in preganglionic nerve endings soon after they are released, and (2) the catecholamine chemical alert signal is received all over the body. A single preganglionic neuron may synapse with as many as 25,000 postganglionic neurons. The sympathetic nervous system operates over a wide range of circumstances, from the unobtrusive fine-tuning of equilibrium states in organs and organ systems to life-threatening emergencies. The adrenal medulla is called upon in many (but not all) stressful situations.

The responses of the sympathetic nervous system and adrenal medullae are not necessarily parallel, for each stress has a character of its own. The sympathetic nervous system is most important in the response to cold stress, exercise (in humans), and in counteracting hypotension on changing from recumbant to upright posture. Epinephrine secretion is elicited by anxiety or the performance of mental tasks in humans, by hypoxia and most especially in response to hypoglycemia. Indeed, during fasting, adrenal medullary secretion (mainly epinephrine) is increased and the activity of the sympathetic nervous system (which is mainly responsible for thermogenesis) is depressed. This is an admirable arrangement, for epinephrine is useful for blood glucose maintenance and suppression of a tonic thermogenic influence conserves needed calories. The important lesson implicit in this is the fact that the nervous system is organized in such a way that individual components of the sympathetic nervous system, including those responsible for controlling the secretory activity of the adrenal chromaffin cells, can be called upon singly or in any appropriate combination.

In our discussion of stress in Chapter 11, we tried to emphasize the interaction among the catecholamines, ACTH and adrenal glucocorticoids, the renin-angiotensin-aldosterone system, and ADH in stress responses. The catecholamines, norepinephrine and epinephrine, can be considered a first line of defense. The others prolong the defensive reaction over a longer time scale.

Synthesis of Catecholamines

The pathway for synthesis of catecholamines (Fig 13–1) was first proposed by Blaschko in 1939. Tyrosine is converted to 3,4-dihydroxylphenylalanine (DOPA), which in turn is decarboxylated to dopamine (D). This amine enters the chromaffin granule and is oxidized to norepinephrine by the granule-limited enzyme, dopamine β hydroxylase. Norepinephrine returns to the cytosol for methylation to epinephrine by phenylethanolamine N-methyltransferase (PNMT). Epinephrine then reenters the chromaffin granule for storage in preparation for secretion. Three compounds in this series are biologically active, either as hormones (epinephrine) or as neurotransmitters (norepinephrine, dopamine).

The enzymes of this pathway have been well characterized. *Tyrosine hydroxylase* requires molecular O_2, tetrahydropteridine and NADPH or an NADPH-generating system. This is the rate-limiting enzyme in the sequence and it is back-inhibited by its remote product, norepinephrine (Fig 13–2). *DOPA decarboxylase* is apparently present in sufficient excess to function over the whole range of synthesis rates demanded of the gland. *Dopamine β hydroxylase* is the granule-limited enzyme; purified preparations contain 2 M of Cu^{2+} per mole of enzyme. PNMT is present mainly in the adrenal medulla, though very small amounts of activity may be associated with nerve endings. It uses S-adenosylmethionine as a methyl donor.

REGULATION OF SYNTHESIS

Regulation of catecholamine synthesis, both in the adrenal medulla and in sympathetic nerves, occurs within two different time frames: (1) acute (no change in the number of enzyme molecules is required), and (2) as a result of *chronic* stimulation (synthesis of enzymes of the biosynthetic pathway occurs and more enzyme molecules appear).

Acute regulation occurs mainly at the rate-limiting step, tyrosine hydroxylase. Nerve stimulation has two major consequences: (1) hormone secretion by exocytosis, and (2) an increased rate of catecholamine synthesis from readily available tyrosine. Tyrosine hydroxylase (TH) exists in two states: inactive and active. Nerve stimulation causes a marked increase in the proportion of activated TH molecules. The molecular mechanism of activation is still incompletely understood in spite of much work on the problem. The enzyme can be phosphorylated by cyclic AMP-dependent protein kinase, but this is unlikely to be the physiological phosphorylating enzyme since acetyl choline, the major chromaffin cell stimulant, is an inhibitor of adenylate cyclase in some tissues and cAMP does not stimulate catecholamine secretion. We can only speculate that TH is indeed activated by phosphorylation but that the probable activator is a non-cAMP-dependent kinase, possibly Ca_4Calmodulin-dependent. We are unaware of experimental support for this guess.

Chronic stimulation (for 12 hours or more) results

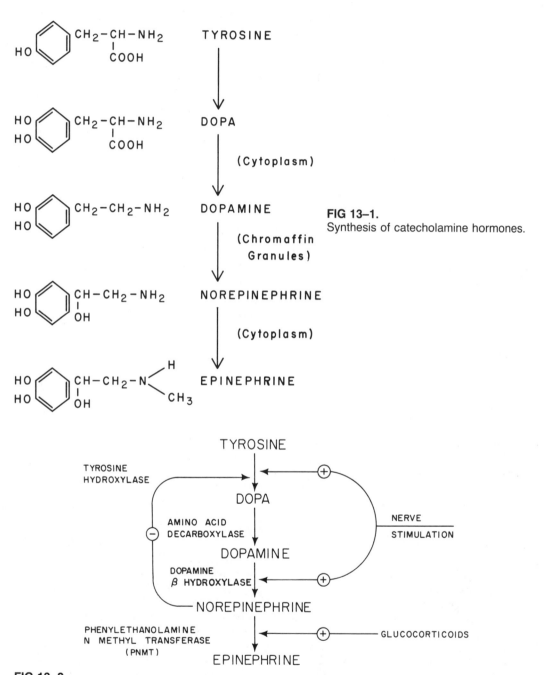

FIG 13–1.
Synthesis of catecholamine hormones.

FIG 13–2.
Regulation of catecholamine synthesis in the adrenal medulla. (Modified from Axelrod J., Weinshilboum R: *N Engl J Med* 1972; 287:237.)

in selective induction of TH by a mechanism that involves gene transcription and protein synthesis. Accompanying the induction of TH, there is a less marked induction of dopamine β hydroxylase after prolonged stimulation.

The adrenal cortex and adrenal medulla are related not only anatomically but functionally as well. Blood from the sinusoids of the cortex traverses and perfuses the adrenal medulla before entering the general circulation. The chromaffin cells, therefore, are exposed to a high concentration of glucocorticoids. In human extra-adrenal chromaffin cells, only NE is formed, and in hypophysectomized rats, PNMT is sharply reduced with the consequence that E synthesis is markedly impaired.

The decrease in PNMT activity after hypophysectomy is related primarily to an accelerated degradation rate of the enzyme. An interesting mechanism by which glucocorticoid administration may restore PNMT to (but not above) normal levels after hypophysectomy is suggested by Ciarenello's findings that (1) S-adenosylmethionine (SAM, which functions as a methyl donor in the conversion of NE to E) stabilizes PNMT against thermal or enzymatic inactivation and (2) the amount of SAM in the adrenal medulla is sharply reduced after hypophysectomy. The restoration of SAM levels by glucocorticoids could then stabilize the enzyme and permit the reestablishment of a normal level of PNMT even if there were no change in the rates of transcription of its mRNA or translation of its message.

Storage and Release of Epinephrine and Norepinephrine

The most obvious feature of the adrenomedullary chromaffin cell is its complement of "chromaffin granules," which resemble the storage and secretory granules of other endocrine and exocrine gland cells (Fig 13–3). These are osmiophilic, electron-dense, membrane-limited particles, which are smaller than mitochondria. They can be prepared in relatively pure form and have been studied more extensively than granules from other types of secretory cells.

Chromaffin granules are highly specialized, complex organelles that consist of an enveloping membrane and its soluble contents. The *membrane* contains a variety of proteins and glycoproteins, including: a proton (H^+) pump ATPase; a catecholamine carrier protein; a nucleotide carrier protein; cytochrome b 561; actin; assorted glycoproteins (inwardly oriented); and dopamine β hydroxylase. We will attempt to demonstrate the functional significance of some of these later.

Among the major constituents of the *granule contents,* expressed as per cent of *total* dry weight, are the following:

Catecholamines (mostly epinephrine in most species)	20
Nucleotides (70% ATP)	15
Chromogranin A (protein)	25
Ascorbic acid	0.8
Enkephalins	< 0.5

When the granule membrane fuses with the plasma membrane and discharges its contents, all of them are secreted. Whether substances other than the catecholamines are physiologically important is unknown. Chromogranin A is a major component of the soluble granule contents, but no function has been assigned to it. Enkephalins may or may not be involved in the well-known hypoalgesia that has been described in athletes injured at the height of competition.

The organization of the adrenomedullary cell requires that catecholamines be stored in granules at a concentration of 0.55 M, or 10,000x their concentration in the surrounding cytosol. Moreover, since dopamine β hydroxylase is in the granule (mostly membrane-bound), dopamine must be transported into the granule; but, since the methylating enzyme PNMT is in the cytosol, NE must be exported from and E must be recaptured by the granule for storage. Recent studies make it possible to describe some of the beautiful mechanisms involved in the biosynthesis and storage of catecholamines.

The transport of catecholamines (DA and NE) into the storage granule is an energy-requiring process. The energy is supplied by the flow of protons down an electrochemical proton gradient from the interior of the granule. The proton gradient is established and maintained by the action of an H^+-ATPase that hydrolyzes ATP on the exterior surface of the granule membrane and injects H^+ into the granule, thus making the granule contents more acid (pH 5.7), and more positively charged, than the cytosol. Thus, the proton gradient represents a mechanism for storing energy used to power the uptake of catecholamines and ATP into the granule.

The large catecholamine concentration difference between the interior of the granule and the surrounding cytosol suggests that there must be a mechanism for trapping the hormones in the granule. At least part of this function is assigned to the high intragranular concentration of ATP. Binding of ATP to catecholamines and possibly to matrix proteins within the granule has the effect of preventing the egress of stored hormone, although NE must be at least partially exempt from such sequestration since it must escape to be methylated to E.

The H^+ pump that establishes the in→out proton

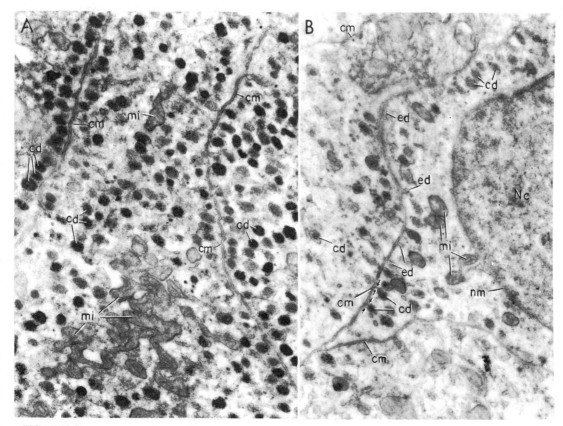

FIG 13–3.
Electronmicrographs (×41,000) of (rabbit) adrenal medulla. **A** before and **B** after stimulation of splanchnic nerve: *cd* = catechol-containing droplets; *cm* = cell membrane; *mi* = mitochondria; *ed* = empty droplets; *Nc* = nucleus; *nm* = nuclear membrane. Note that the stimulated cell is nearly free of *cd,* and those that remain are at the periphery of the cell. Several *ed* may be observed attached to cell membrane (*arrows* in **B**). (From DeRobertis EDP, Sabatini DD: *Fed Proc* 1960; 19(Suppl 5):70. Reprinted with permission.)

gradient is also important as a source of energy for importing electrons into the granules. This is necessary because intragranular ascorbate acts as a one electron donor in the dopamine→NE reaction which is catalyzed by dopamine β hydroxylase. One of the products of this reaction is semidehydroascorbate, which must be recharged to ascorbate in order to be recycled back into the reaction, since there is no evidence for an exchange of ascorbate between granule and cytosol. This is accomplished by the inward transport of an electron coupled to the outward transport of a proton, an exchange that is mediated by the vesicle membrane-bound protein, cytochrome b 561.

These proton gradient-powered transport mechanisms, imaginatively elucidated in the chromaffin cell granule, have wider implications, for similar ones have been described in adrenergic neurons, platelets, the neurohypophysis, the hepatocyte, the parotid gland and in other secretory tissues (see Njus et al. for documentation).

STIMULUS-SECRETION COUPLING

When a muscle cell contracts in response to a neural stimulus, the molecular events that intervene between release of acetylcholine at the motor endplate and the contraction are collectively subsumed under the term "stimulus-contraction coupling." The redistribution of Ca^{2+} among the various organelles of the muscle cell represents the main connection between stimulus and contraction.

When an adrenomedullary cell mobilizes chromaffin granules at the cell surface and when these granules discharge their contents into the pericellular fluid in response to an acetylcholine stimulus, the secretory response is related to the stimulus by events called "stimulus-secretion coupling." Douglas and colleagues have presented convincing evidence that calcium influx secondary to membrane depolarization produced by acetylcholine is the central event in stimulus-secretion coupling. These studies have been confirmed and extended by many investigators of a variety of secretory cells, most recently by the demonstration, by means of the fluorescent probe, Quin 2, that the intracellular Ca^{2+} concentration of chromaffin cells increased when they were stimulated to secrete catecholamines either by acetyl choline or by a high K^+ (i.e., depolarizing) medium (Knight and Kesteren). No one now doubts that Ca^{2+} is both necessary and sufficient to elicit exocytotic secretion of catecholamines.

The choreography of secretory granule movement, interaction with the inner plasma membrane, and discharge of its contents by exocytosis is far from simple. The granule must move to the plasma membrane but this need not be a long journey, since extensions of the plasma membrane may be invaginated into the cell. Granules may aggregate into a sort of secretory collective. On the one hand, demonstrable cross-linking between granular membranes and actin (a component of cytoskeletal structures) suggests that the cytoskeleton may be involved in granule movement. On the other hand, one of the effects of an increase in $[Ca^{2+}]_c$ is a *decrease* in the viscosity of actin-granule gels. This has led to the suggestion that an increase in $[Ca^{2+}]_c$ could free granules from binding to cytoskeletal structures that occurs at low $[Ca^{2+}]_c$, thus permitting their movement to the membrane by an unspecified mechanism.

When the granule is closely approximated to the plasma membrane, some force must overcome the mutually repulsive effect the two membranes have on one another. Then, a sharply localized breakdown and reorganization into a new lipid bilayer must occur. It has long been assumed that Ca^{2+} is involved in these events, and recently, Burgoyne and Geisow have demonstrated that Calmodulin can bind to granule membrane and induce selective phosphorylation of granular membrane proteins. Although the Calmodulin inhibitor, trifluoperazine, failed to block stimulated exocytosis, Kengsberg and Trifaro succeeded in inhibiting stimulated exocytosis by the microinjection of anti-Calmodulin antibody into cultured chromaffin cells. These not entirely congruent findings suggest a role for Ca_4Calmodulin in the exocytotic process.

Another dimension was added to the study of exocytotic mechanisms with the discovery (see Creutz et al.) of *synexin,* a 47,000-dalton protein which polymerizes into large aggregates in the presence of Ca^{2+}.

These polymers cause the aggregation of dispersed, single secretory granules. Moreover, they bind preferentially to certain phospholipids. Synexin could well represent one of the molecular machine tools involved in Ca^{2+}'s pleiotropic action on secretory cells.

Inevitably, when the mechanisms linked to polyphosphatidyl inositol turnover were described, attempts were made to discover a role for protein kinase C in the stimulated chromaffin cell. Although C kinase is present in catecholamine-secreting cells, its function is not known.

If exocytosis were to be stimulated over a period of minutes to hours, the fusion of granule membrane to plasma membrane would result in a very redundant plasma membrane. Since the plasma membrane does not expand indefinitely in the stimulated cell, there must be a mechanism for excising segments from it and either recycling them through the Golgi packaging factory or breaking them down in phagolysosomes and scavenging their products for reuse. In fact, both of these processes take place in the chromaffin cell. The clipping of plasma membrane segments for recycling by one method or the other is impressively nonrandom. By preparing fluorescent antibodies to distinctive granular membrane proteins, it has been found that the segments of granular membrane that are inserted into the plasma membrane at the time of exocytosis are *selectively* identified, excised, and endocytosed in the form of small vesicles, and the plasma membrane rejoined. Thus, there is a recycling of granular membrane to and from the plasma membrane. The molecular mechanisms involved in this exquisitely precise chemical microsurgery are unknown to us.

One of the most significant results of work begun on stimulus-secretion coupling in the chromaffin cell has been the realization that the granule secretory mechanism in all cells so far studied is operationally similar. This is true whether the secretory response is elicited by nerve stimulation or by hormonal stimulation. Organelle movement, membrane fusion and recycling are features of secretory responses generally, and Ca^{2+} appears to play the central role in the process, whatever the cell type.

Metabolism and Inactivation of Catecholamines

Epinephrine and norepinephrine can be measured in blood by a variety of difficult methods, which depend either on fluorescence measurement or on enzymatic conversion of radioactively labeled catecholamines to recognizable products. The methods are in use mainly in research laboratories. Many clinical laboratories, however, are capable of measuring the catecholamines and their metabolic products in 24-hour samples of urine. Much work has been done by ingenious bioassay methods, which depend either on measuring blood pressure in the rat or on measuring contractile responses of various smooth muscle preparations in vitro (see Vane).

The half-life of injected catecholamines has been estimated to be less than 20 seconds, or about one total circulation time. The plasma concentration of epinephrine in normal people is of the order of 0.05 ng/ml and that of norepinephrine is typically about four times that of epinephrine, or 0.2 ng/ml. Severe stress (e.g., myocardial infarction) produces levels of 0.27 and 4.1 ng/ml for epinephrine and norepinephrine, respectively. Severe psychologic stress may result in urinary levels of catecholamine excretion as high as those found in catecholamine-producing tumors (pheochromocytoma, see below). Surgical anesthesia regularly causes pronounced hypercatecholemia.

Characteristically, neurotransmitters and related substances have a very evanescent effect because they are so quickly removed or inactivated. Hypersecretion increases concentrations of amines at nerve ends or at peripheral receptors because the secretion rate is high enough to overwhelm the inactivating mechanisms.

The catecholamines are inactivated by reuptake into

nerve endings or by metabolism either in or near the postsynaptic cell or in the liver. When the sympathetic nerves are stimulated, some of the norepinephrine released leaks into the general circulation. Indeed, the major part of circulating norepinephrine comes from this source and not from the adrenal medullae. Catecholamines secreted by the adrenal are partly taken up in sympathetic nerve endings and partly metabolically altered in the liver according to the scheme illustrated in Figure 13–4. The same enzymes that metabolize catecholamines in liver occur in the postsynaptic neuron, where they dispose of the norepinephrine that is not removed by reuptake of amine into the presynaptic nerve terminal (Fig 13–5). In the nervous system, the approximate proportion of norepinephrine subjected to reuptake versus that metabolized is estimated to be about 80:20.

The reuptake process is stereospecific, although it operates not only on norepinephrine but also on epinephrine, dopamine and certain chemically related synthetic compounds such as amphetamine. Reuptake blockade by tricyclic antidepressants (see below) is central in the chemotherapy of depression. Cocaine and amphetamine also work in part by blocking reuptake of catecholamine.

Most of the catecholamine that is produced appears in the urine as vanillylmandelic acid (VMA) plus 3-methoxy, 4-OH phenyl glycol (see Fig 13–4). These are products of the activity of both catechol-O-meth-

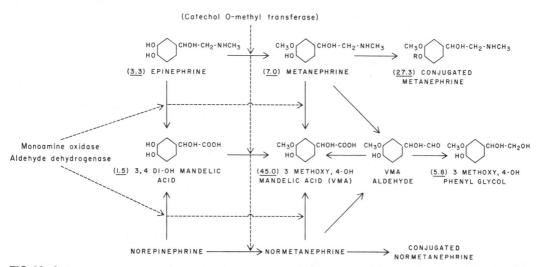

FIG 13–4.
Metabolic fate of catecholamine hormones. Numbers in parentheses signify percentage of administered dose of labeled epinephrine that appeared in urine in the form indicated. Monoamine oxidase and aldehyde dehydrogenase *both* participate in reactions indicated by *upper* and *lower* *dashed arrows.* (From Axelrod I, in Vane JR, Wolstenholme GEW, O'Connor M [eds]: *Adrenergic Mechanisms,* Ciba Foundation Symposium. Boston, Little, Brown & Co, 1960. Reproduced with permission.)

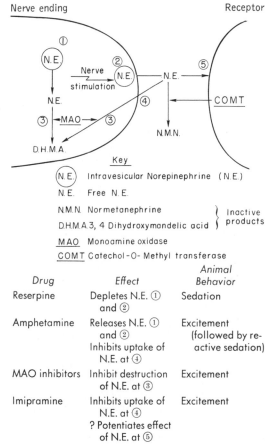

Key

N.E. — Intravesicular Norepinephrine (N.E.)

N.E. — Free N.E.

N.M.N. — Normetanephrine } Inactive

D.H.M.A. — 3, 4 Dihydroxymandelic acid } products

MAO — Monoamine oxidase

COMT — Catechol-O-Methyl transferase

Drug	Effect	Animal Behavior
Reserpine	Depletes N.E. ① and ②	Sedation
Amphetamine	Releases N.E. ① and ② Inhibits uptake of N.E. at ④	Excitement (followed by reactive sedation)
MAO inhibitors	Inhibit destruction of N.E. at ③	Excitement
Imipramine	Inhibits uptake of N.E. at ④ ? Potentiates effect of N.E. at ⑤	Excitement

FIG 13–5.
Presumed loci of action of drugs that affect catecholamine metabolism in brain. (Suggested by Schildkraut JJ: *Am J Psych* 1965; 122:509, and by Axelrod J: *Pharmacol Rev* 1966; 18:95.)

yltransferase and monoamine oxidase. Although they are present in smaller concentrations, the 3-methoxy amines, metanephrine and normetanephrine, are regarded as better indicators of total catecholamine produced than are the deaminated compounds.

Adrenergic Receptors and Cellular Mechanism of Action of Catecholamines

Although Paul Ehrlich's lock-and-key hypothesis of drug-cell interaction was the beginning of receptor theory, Langley's experiments with adrenal extracts mark the beginning of the application of the receptor idea of endocrinology. A. J. Clark deduced the existence of receptors (in 1937) because drugs evoked specific responses, slight changes in their structure produced drug antagonistic effects and different tissues showed variable response patterns to individual drugs. Most modern work on receptors represents a set of variations on Clark's themes.

In the 1930s epinephrine effects were described as stimulatory or inhibitory, and Cannon and Rosenblueth deduced that there were two different molecular species of "sympathin," which caused either stimulation (sympathin E) or inhibition (sympathin I). On the basis of analysis of the effects of six different, closely related catecholamines in a variety of tissues, Ahlquist (1948) concluded that there were two types of *receptor,* which responded to *one* hormone. Ahlquist's concept of α and β receptors, together with the operational classification of receptors by *rank-ordering responses to a series of agonists,* is still one of the main criteria for classifying adrenergic receptors.

Among the thousands of catecholamine analogues synthesized by many organic chemists were a few which, sharing some similarity in shape with the naturally occurring hormones and neurotransmitters, acted as their *competitive antagonists.* While they were able to bind noncovalently to receptors, they were unable to initiate biological responses. Some of these were so selective in their blocking actions that they were extremely helpful in assigning receptors to one or another subgroup. The same massive program of synthesizing and screening compounds yielded some that were more discriminating in their effects on individual receptor types than were the naturally occurring substances. (Between these and the "pure" antagonists, there was a whole spectrum of partial agonists.) As more was learned about the multiplicity of catecholamine receptors, synthetic analogues, both agonist and antagonist, became molecular markers or indicators of their individuality.

As new information accumulated about the mechanisms by which biologic effects were achieved, certain patterns began to emerge. It was apparent that catecholamine receptors of one subtype initiated biologic responses by recruiting a different set of second messengers than did those of another. As a result, we can now sort out a variety of catecholamine receptors that can be described in three ways: (1) by rank ordering their responses to different agonists, and particularly by their preference for certain empirically discovered synthetic agonists; (2) by determining whether their effects are blocked by distinctive synthetic antagonists; and (3) whether they act by either stimulating or inhibiting adenylate cyclase, or by stimulating polyphosphatidyl inositol turnover.

On the basis of these criteria, four well-defined types of catecholamine receptors have been described: α_1, α_2, β_1, and β_2 (Fig 13–6). Each of these shows a

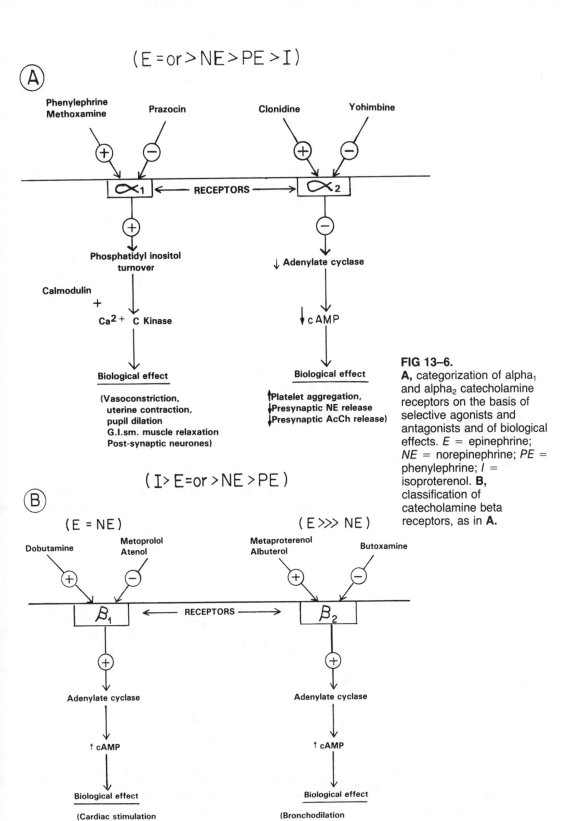

$(E = or > NE > PE > I)$

A

Phenylephrine
Methoxamine   Prazocin   Clonidine   Yohimbine

α_1 ← RECEPTORS → α_2

Phosphatidyl inositol
turnover

Calmodulin
+
Ca^{2+} C Kinase

↓ Adenylate cyclase

↓ cAMP

Biological effect

(Vasoconstriction,
uterine contraction,
pupil dilation
G.I.sm. muscle relaxation
Post-synaptic neurones)

Biological effect

↑Platelet aggregation,
↓Presynaptic NE release
↓Presynaptic AcCh release)

FIG 13–6.
A, categorization of alpha$_1$
and alpha$_2$ catecholamine
receptors on the basis of
selective agonists and
antagonists and of biological
effects. *E* = epinephrine;
NE = norepinephrine; *PE* =
phenylephrine; *I* =
isoproterenol. **B,**
classification of
catecholamine beta
receptors, as in **A.**

$(I > E = or > NE > PE)$

B

$(E = NE)$ $(E >>> NE)$

Dobutamine   Metoprolol   Metaproterenol   Butoxamine
              Atenol   Albuterol

β_1 ← RECEPTORS → β_2

Adenylate cyclase   Adenylate cyclase

↑ cAMP   ↑ cAMP

Biological effect   **Biological effect**

(Cardiac stimulation   (Bronchodilation
Adipocyte lipolysis   Vasodilation
GI Sm muscle relaxation   Uterine relaxation)

237

preference for one or more distinctive agonists and one or more antagonists. All four receptors have been solubilized and purified by a variety of methods, including affinity chromatography and photoaffinity labelling with a radioactive ligand (for details, see Caron et al. and Benovic et al.) They are all glycoproteins of similar size, from 60–80,000 d. Moreover, they are *different* glycoproteins and therefore must represent products of different genes. In the case of the β receptors, the purified glycoprotein has been inserted into phospholipid vesicles that were then fused with amphibian erythrocytes containing G_s protein and adenylate cyclase but no catecholamine receptor. The result was an isoproterenol-stimulatable adenylate cyclase.

It is helpful to imagine each of the receptor subtypes as displaying an outwardly-facing domain that binds its particular ligand and an inwardly-facing surface which, when ligand is bound, recognizes and interacts with its own transducing protein. This, in turn, either activates adenylate cyclase, inhibits it, or activates phospholipase C phosphodiesterase. In Chapter 3, we described models for the participation of G_s protein in cyclase-activating responses and G_i protein in cyclase-inhibiting responses. Both β_1 and β_2 receptors initiate responses via G_s, while α_2 (as we have seen) causes the dissociation of G_i into $G_{i\alpha}$ and $G_{i\beta}$. The plethora of free $G_{i\beta}$ then inhibits the dissociation of G_s into its subunits, and, therefore, inhibits even tonic stimulation, resulting in a decrease in cAMP concentration in the cell. (The α and β designations for G protein subunits have nothing to do with the α and β classification of catecholamine receptors!)

Following the discovery that, in rat liver, epinephrine does not stimulate glycogenolysis via an increase in cAMP, it was established that the process was stimulated as a result of a Ca_4Calmodulin-mediated phosphorylation of phosphorylase (Exton). When the details of the phosphatidyl inositol turnover cycle were elucidated, it became clear that occupied catecholamine α_1 receptor stimulated polyphosphatidyl inositol-specific phosphodiesterase (phospholipase C), resulting in all of the events outlined in Chapter 3. There is now circumstantial evidence that a G protein (i.e., GTP-requiring and activatable by a stable analogue of GTP) communicates the information that the α_1 receptor is occupied to phospholipase C, thereby causing its activation (Wallace and Fain).

The tissue distribution of catecholamine receptor subtypes and the variety of biological effects that are elicited through them reminds us once again of the significance of target cell differentiation in hormone responses. In order to be competent to respond to a particular catecholamine in a certain way, the target cell must insert precisely the correct receptor into its membrane, together with the appropriate transducer elements and enzyme amplifiers. Then, depending on the mix of messengers generated, it must display the proper protein substrates for phosphorylation. These are weighty decisions to make for a cell when it "decides" to be a liver cell or an adipocyte or a muscle cell.

RECEPTOR REGULATION: DESENSITIZATION OR TACHYPHYLAXIS

Receptors, which participate so intimately in regulating metabolic processes in cells, are themselves regulated. This is illustrated by the down-regulation of plasma membrane receptor populations in the continuing presence of agonist. Down-regulation of receptors is one aspect of the more general problem of *desensitization (or tachyphylaxis),* which can be defined as *the decreased responsiveness of a cell to stimulation when it is continuously exposed to its stimulant.* The phenomenon of desensitization has been described in many different species, from bacteria to human. Students of the β adrenergic-G protein-adenylate cyclase system have constructed mechanistic models of desensitization that may have general applications (Sibley and Lefkowitz).

Desensitization to a cell's natural ligand (homologous desensitization) occurs in definable stages. First (seconds to a few minutes), *uncoupling* of receptor from the G_s-adenylate cyclase complex occurs without a decrease in the number of surface receptors. There is some evidence that phosphorylation of the receptor by a cAMP-independent protein kinase causes uncoupling to occur. Over a longer time scale, *sequestration* of receptor (*without* G protein or adenylate cyclase) away from the cell's surface occurs. It is not entirely clear whether the receptor in the endocytosed vesicle is phosphorylated. Phosphorylation may, in fact, be a precondition for endocytosis. Following sequestration, the receptor-containing vesicles are *processed* either in the Golgi for recycling back to the plasma membrane or in phagolysosomes where they are degraded. Finally, *resensitization* occurs when Golgi-processed receptors are reinserted into the plasma membrane. During short exposures, this whole process does not require protein synthesis. After longer exposures, when a larger proportion of endocytosed receptors has been digested in phagolysosomes, protein synthesis is necessary to restore the full complement of surface receptors.

Another type of desensitization (heterologous) occurs in cells whose G protein-adenylate cyclase complex responds to more than one hormone. If hormone

A is administered, the response to hormone B is decreased although there is no decrease in B's surface receptor number. In this case, it has been shown that G_s, the transducing protein, has been rendered less competent to function in a reconstructed membrane system (i.e., when it is inserted into a G_s-deficient membrane). The molecular nature of G_s's "lesion" is not certainly known, but it may be phosphorylated. It *is* known that the receptor itself is phosphorylated (it is a substrate for almost all protein kinases, including cAMP-dependent and C kinase), and that this impairs its ability to communicate with G_s.

REGULATION OF CATECHOLAMINE RECEPTOR-RESPONSE SYSTEM BY OTHER HORMONES

Thyroid hormone has striking effects on the sensitivity of tissues to β adrenergic stimulation (Chapter 10). In some tissues, but not in others, T_4 treatment results in an increased number of β receptors in the plasma membrane. Even in tissues that show no change in receptor number, sensitivity to β agonists varies with thyroid status. In hypothyroidism, decreased catecholamine responsiveness (i.e., decreased cAMP accumulation in response to a standard stimulus) occurs without alteration in receptor number. This has been interpreted to mean that thyroid hormone deficiency has an uncoupling effect on the receptor-G-cyclase system.

Glucocorticoids have striking effects on the responsiveness of many tissues to β adrenergic stimulation (reviewed by Davies and Lefkowitz). In some tissues, treatment with glucocorticoids increases receptor density and agonist affinity. Enhanced coupling and increased adenylate cyclase activity have also been described. Generally, adrenalectomy causes reverse changes. Recovery from desensitization is impaired in the absence of glucocorticoids and stimulated when the deficiency is corrected. Although effects on G protein (amount? alteration in efficiency?) have been noted, there are no mechanistic explanations for these phenomena.

Effects of Adrenomedullary Hormones

The effects of epinephrine and norepinephrine are ubiquitous; there is scarcely a field of physiology that does not have its own private preoccupations with these agents. Their effects on the brain; heart and circulation; smooth muscle of the gastrointestinal tract, uterus, eye, and bronchi; CNS; skeletal muscle; blood clotting; spleen; redistribution of stored calories in the body; and many other physiologic functions are so rich and varied that they can scarcely be known in detail by any single person. There is, however, a discernible theme in many of these effects. Although people who are disturbed by teleologically "impure" thinking in biology are sometimes made uncomfortable by Cannon's "fight-flight" characterization of the sympathoadrenomedullary discharge, the fact is that the overall effect of such a discharge is to mobilize the individual to meet an emergency. One can often recall what epinephrine does to an organ or tissue by reflecting on whether a particular response serves a useful adaptive purpose in a "fight-flight" emergency.

The overall response to the effects of simultaneous sympathetic discharge and adrenomedullary secretion involves cardiocirculatory responses that are qualitatively similar to those seen at the beginning of exercise—increase in cardiac output, increase in pulse rate, rise in blood pressure. In addition, after a brief initial period of apnea, there is an increased minute volume of respiration. Splanchnic vascular constriction (including a reduction in renal blood flow) and dilatation of the skeletal muscle vessels produce a redistribution of the enlarged cardiac output that anticipates muscle work. The CNS arousal effect of the catecholamine substances results in alertness and quick responsiveness. Hepatic glycogenolysis, its attendant hyperglycemia and mobilization from the fat depots of a large supply of free fatty acids (FFA), all collaborate to provide a quick charge of readily available energy to muscles that may be called on. Chemical changes in the muscles themselves increase their capacity for work and possibly diminish the generation of a fatigue signal by the muscle. The CNS effects of the substances may at the same time diminish central perception of fatigue. As if in anticipation of blood loss, the spleen contracts and adds volume and red cells to the circulation while the coagulability of the blood increases.

Too much emphasis on the massive "fight-flight" aspects of catecholamine function obscures the fact that the sympathetic nervous system and adrenal medulla, as we suggested above, respond to different challenges by selective recruitment of subsystems. All 88 keys on the piano are not ordinarily struck at once; rather, chords appropriate to the circumstances are played.

An inventory of catecholamine effects can occupy many pages. We propose to give an abbreviated account of a few of them that will suffice to illustrate the pervasive influence of these ubiquitous substances. The responses of individual cells depend, as we have stressed, on the type and proportion of receptors they display on their surfaces and on their response potential (second messengers, kinase substrates, etc.). Many cells have more than one type of receptor-response complex, and it is often possible to bring a latent response capability into relief only by blocking a dominant one with the appropriate specific receptor blocking agent; for example, the β stimulation of insulin release can be seen best in the presence of an α blocker. Not only do certain cells change their receptor patterns as they go from one phase of their life cycle to another (intestinal crypt cell), but also other cells of the same type (vascular smooth muscle cells, adipocytes) exhibit different receptors in their fully differentiated state in different anatomical positions.

CENTRAL NERVOUS SYSTEM: CATECHOLAMINES AND AFFECTIVE DISORDERS

It is useful to imagine that so complex a variable as emotion, mood or affect is regulated homeostatically as is blood glucose or serum calcium. Mood swings around some imaginary equilibrium "value" are present in nearly everyone to a degree. However, in some individuals the amplitude of the swing may be very large, and there may be sustained periods of incapacitating depression or uninhibited mania. Studies in experimental animal models showed that reserpine, a drug that causes striking depletion of catecholamines, is associated with sedation and hypoactivity. When the same drug is given to people, they report feelings of depression. On the other hand, other drugs (e.g., monoamine oxidase inhibitors) prevent catecholamine destruction and cause stimulation in animals and reversal of depression in human subjects. Because of these and similar observations, Schildkraut and Kety proposed the "catecholamine hypothesis of affective disorders." Although the original hypothesis has been modified to include other neurotransmitters, it is still the conceptual basis for chemotherapy of mood disturbances, decompensations of the mood-regulatory apparatus. The loci of action of some drugs that affect mood disorders are summarized in Figure 13–5.

Norepinephrine and serotonin are believed to be involved in mood disorders that are collectively described as depression. In some depressed individuals, changes in urinary excretion of catecholamine metabolites correlate well with subjective estimations of severity of depression. In others with so-called serotonin depression (Berg et al.), the spinal fluid concentration of 5-hydroxyindoleacetic acid, a metabolite of serotonin, was low in depressed individuals.

Disordered dopamine regulation, on the other hand, has been linked with psychoses, particularly schizophrenia, and with Parkinson's disease, which is characterized by motor incoordination. In the former case symptoms are ameliorated by a variety of compounds that function as dopaminergic blocking agents. The motor disability of Parkinson's disease is believed to be related to depressed dopaminergic function. The modification of central neurotransmitter function by drugs is important for therapeutic, toxicologic and social reasons. (See Baldessarini.)

Tricyclic Antidepressants

As a group, tricyclic antidepressants block reuptake of bioamines from the synaptic cleft into the nerve ending of the presynaptic neuron (Fig 13–7). This increases the effective concentration of the amine involved in the region of its receptors on the postsynaptic neuron. Thus, if there is a functionally inadequate amount of neurotransmitter, prevention of its destruction by the reuptake mechanism (estimated to be about 80% for norepinephrine) has the effect of compensating for the deficiency. While reuptake block was once considered the major mechanism for the antidepressant action of these agents, it is now recognized that this was a simplistic view.

Although the tricyclic compounds are chemically related, they differ with respect to their amine reuptake-blocking capabilities. Table 13–1 shows a spectrum of effects, from practically pure serotonin (5-HT) reuptake blocking (amitriptyline) to pure norepinephrine blocking (desipramine). Nortriptyline and imipramine block both serotonin and norepinephrine reuptake. This comparison is an oversimplification of a very complicated subject, as the table does not deal with the fact that the tricyclics have varying degrees of anticholinergic activity, which may be important in the mechanism of their ameliorating effect in clinical depression. Although the role of cholinergic mechanisms in depression is not clear, there are indications that anticholinergic activity may contribute to the antidepressant effects of tricyclic compounds. It is entirely possible that future studies of the etiologic factors of depression will involve one or more of the following: histamine, excitatory amino acids (e.g., glutamate and aspartate), inhibitory amino acids (GABA), opiate-like peptides, other peptides (e.g., hypothalamic-releasing factors and ACTH fragments) and prostaglandins. The tricyclic antidepressants, like most drugs, have undesirable side effects, including precipitation of arrhythmias and myocardial infarction (see Baldessarini).

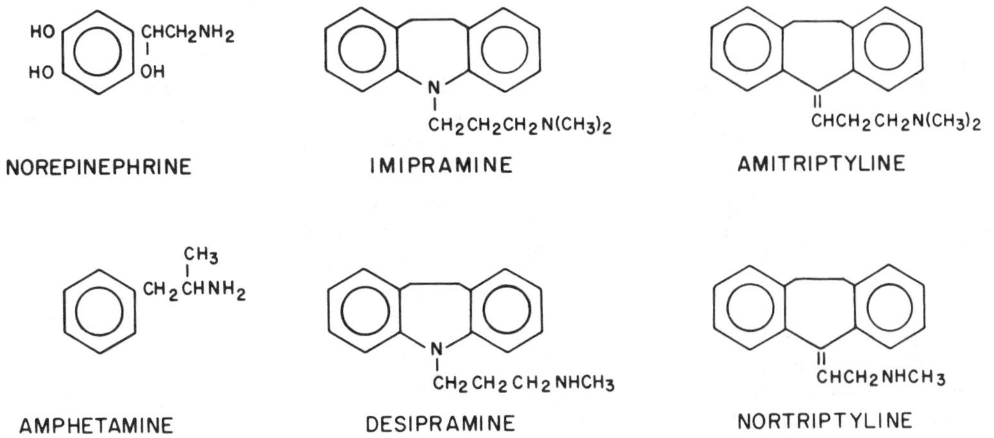

FIG 13–7.
Imipramine, amitriptyline, desipramine, nortriptyline, norepinephrine, and amphetamine.

Monoamine Oxidase Inhibitors

If the mitochondrial enzyme, monoamine oxidase (MAO) is inhibited and the reuptake mechanism is intact, most of the retrieved amine is available for repackaging and subsequent discharge. This is another way of making a little amine go a long way. MAO inhibitors have been studied extensively in depressed people; they do indeed alleviate depression in some. However, their use has been limited by widespread acceptance of the tricyclic compounds (see Lake and Ziegler).

HEART AND BLOOD VESSELS

NE is the more important of the catecholamines in the minute-to-minute fine adjustment of cardiac function and regulation of blood pressure. E makes its contribution in stressful circumstances, including psychological stress associated with fear and anxiety. Through β_1 receptors, the catecholamines *increase*

TABLE 13–1.

Comparison of Inhibitory Effects of Tricyclic
Antidepressants on Reuptake of Neurotransmitters*

COMPOUND	NEUROTRANSMITTER†	
	5-HT	NE
Amitriptyline	+ + + +	0
Nortriptyline	+ +	+ +
Imipramine	+ + +	+ +
Desipramine	0	+ + + +

*Adapted from Maas JW: *Arch Gen Psychiatry* 1975; 32:1357.
†5-HT = serotonin; NE = norepinephrine.

heart rate (positive chronotropic effect); *increase the force of contraction* (positive inotropic effect); *increase conduction velocity;* and *increase oxygen consumption.* They also *sensitize the heart to rhythm disturbances* induced either by chlorinated hydrocarbons or by exertion. (The combination of cold exposure and shovelling snow seems to be particularly dangerous.)

The effects of E on the coronary circulation are complex, but dilation of the vessels is predominant. This may be both direct (β effects on the vascular smooth muscle) or indirect (secondary to the local release of adenosine caused by the stimulation of metabolism related to increased cardiac work).

Accompanying the increased cardiac output due to the positive chronotropic and inotropic effects, NE, as well as E, via α receptors, cause peripheral vasoconstriction in selected vascular beds, notably in the skin, mucosae, kidneys, and veins. The pattern of redistribution of blood flow generally favors heat conservation. The vasodilatory effects (β_2) of these agents can be exposed either by giving an α blocker or by infusing very low doses of E, since the β_2 receptor-equipped vascular smooth muscle cells are more sensitive than α_1 cells. Under these conditions (α blocker or low dose), E may actually cause a *fall* in blood pressure rather than a rise. The usual rise in blood pressure is marked by an increase in pulse pressure, since there is a more marked effect on systolic than on diastolic pressure (also true in hyperthyroidism which is characterized by increased sensitivity to catecholamines).

When catecholamines are administered to experimental animals over a period of days (or in some humans with catecholamine-producing tumors), vascular cells and heart muscle cells show severe damage that can be prevented by Ca^{2+} channel-blocking drugs. This phenomenon has been attributed to sustained elevation of intracellular Ca^{2+} concentration.

LUNGS

Both hormones accelerate the rate and increase the depth of respiration after a brief period of apnea, which is believed to be induced by way of the carotid sinus mechanism as a result of rising blood pressure.

Epinephrine, via β_2 receptors, is a powerful bronchodilator, and has long been used in the management of human bronchial asthma. In Chapter 4 we mentioned the intense bronchial constriction that occurs in that condition as a result of the local release of the sulfido-peptide leukotrienes.

SMOOTH MUSCLE

The variable effects of epinephrine and norepinephrine on the vascular smooth muscle in different parts of the circulatory system are seen again in an analysis of the responses of other kinds of smooth muscle to their administration. Much of the smooth muscle of the body—including the nonsphincteric muscle of the gastrointestinal tract, the bronchioles and the urinary bladder—is relaxed by epinephrine or by sympathetic nerve stimulation. Many other types of smooth muscle—including that associated with the splenic capsule, sphincters of the gastrointestinal tract, ureters, erectores pili apparatus of the skin, nictitating membrane of the cat, dilator pupillae of the iris—are stimulated by epinephrine.

Some structures, like the uterus, vary in their response according to species and presence or absence of pregnancy. Uterine smooth muscle has both β and α receptors: stimulation of α receptors increases contractions, whereas stimulation of β receptors promotes relaxation. Estrogens increase sensitivity to α stimulation, and progesterone brings about dominance of a β receptor response.

SKELETAL MUSCLE

It was shown long ago that the contractions of a stimulus-driven skeletal muscle could be markedly prolonged by epinephrine, and that this substance had the capacity to increase the force of contraction in a fatigued muscle preparation. That these effects are at least partially independent of the neuromuscular

transmission apparatus is shown by the fact that they are obtainable even when the stimulus is applied directly to the muscle cells in in vitro preparations. One of the most prominent metabolic effects of epinephrine is seen in skeletal muscle as well, namely, a rapid glycogenolysis with the accumulation of sufficient lactic acid to raise the level of lactate that is carried to the liver, where it is resynthesized into glycogen and recirculated as glucose. It also travels to the heart, which uses lactate very efficiently as an energy source.

Epinephrine has been found to cause lipolysis of intracellularly stored triglyceride in muscle, as it does in fat cells, by a cAMP-mediated mechanism.

LIVER

The glycogenolytic effect of epinephrine was the point of departure for the discovery of cyclic AMP (Chapter 3). It is principally responsible for the acute hyperglycemia produced by the hormone, but the sustained elevation in blood glucose and the maintenance of blood glucose during fasting mainly depends on glucagon-stimulated gluconeogenesis as well as on inhibited insulin secretion. There are some species (dog, rabbit) in which epinephrine (β_1) stimulates glycogenolysis by activating phosphorylase via a cAMP-dependent mechanism. In others (rat), it does so via the α_1 receptor, Ca^{2+}, Calmodulin, and stimulated polyphosphatidyl turnover. In both cases the final result is the activation of the rate limiting enzyme of glycogenolysis, phosphorylase.

ADIPOSE TISSUE

One of the largest target tissues for catecholamines is the aggregate adipose tissue organ, which consists of a number of more or less discrete depots. E and NE stimulate lipolysis via β_1 adrenergic receptors which, acting through the cAMP mechanism, activate (i.e., phosphorylate) triacylglycerol ("hormone-sensitive") lipase. Free fatty acids (FFA) and glycerol are released into the circulation. As we shall see in Chapter 14, the lipolytic effect of E and NE is assisted (permitted) by their coordinate *inhibition* of insulin secretion (via an α receptor). In fact, insulin, by its antilipolytic action, can override the lipolytic action of catecholamines.

In addition to β_1 receptors, adipocytes also display α_2 receptors. The ratio of $\beta_1 : \alpha_2$ not only varies from species to species in similar cells but also within a single individual, from one fat depot to another. α_2 and β_1 receptors both stimulate glucose uptake by adipocytes, but they have *opposite* effects on lipolysis, α_2 being *anti*lipolytic and β_1, lipolytic. In other words, catecholamines acting via α_2 receptors are, in a sense, insulin-mimetic. The higher the proportion of β_1 to α_2 receptors, the more rapid is the turnover of triglycerides in adipocytes and the greater the load of FFA presented to the circulation for disposal. The possible implications of these findings in regional obesity (β_1 dominant abdominal versus α_2 dominant gluteal-thigh obesity) will be discussed in Chapter 16.

NE, released in adipose tissue, both directly stimulates adipocytes and controls blood flow. It is not possible to assign a preponderant role in FFA mobilization to circulating E versus locally released NE in all circumstances. We believe that the innervation of adipose tissue is most important in meal-to-meal regulation. In prolonged fasting, however, the combination of circulating catecholamines, glucagon, and low-insulin levels is responsible for FFA export from fat cells. In cold exposure, as indicated above, locally released NE is the main lipolytic stimulus.

CELL GROWTH

The catecholamines are even growth hormones, of a sort. There is a growing list of tissues that are stimulated to undergo hypertrophy and hyperplasia (cell division) by catecholamines. Among them are the parotid gland, intestinal crypt cells, and erythropoietin-producing cells. In addition, the following paired organs fail to show compensatory hypertrophy after unilateral removal if sympathetically denervated: adrenal cortex and ovary. Intestinal crypt cells are particularly interesting because they are stimulated to grow via α_2 receptors but their growth is inhibited via α_1 and β receptors. This suggests that, at different stages of its life history, as it migrates from crypt to surface, a cell may express a different combination of receptors on its plasma membrane.

The mechanisms by which growth and cell division are stimulated by way of a receptor that causes a reduction in cAMP are not known. However, high cAMP levels have often been observed to *inhibit* cell division. Perhaps it is advantageous for cAMP to abandon the terrain to one or another mitogen.

INTERACTIONS WITH OTHER HORMONES

We have already discussed some effects of other hormones (notably, thyroid hormone and glucocorticoids) on catecholamine synthesis and action. Also, we have referred to the stimulatory effect of E and NE on glucagon secretion and melatonin synthesis as well as their inhibitory effect on insulin secretion. We also mentioned the inhibitory effect of dopamine on aldosterone secretion.

The catecholamines have effects on many other hormone-producing cells, in most of which they stimulate secretion by way of β receptors. In some, they increase cAMP in imitation of a primary stimulator. Some examples are the following: they (1) mimic TSH in thyroid follicular cells; (2) stimulate calcitonin secretion in thyroid C cells; (3) stimulate parathyroid hormone secretion (major stimulus, low Ca^{2+}) (2 and 3 will be discussed in Chapter 17); (4) stimulate gastrin secretion in the stomach; (5) stimulate renin secretion (JG apparatus); and (6) stimulate erythropoietin secretion (kidney).

This laundry list is calculated to make the point that, although we separate our discussions of hormones into pedagogically convenient compartments, there are complex relationships among many of them in intact animals and people.

Clinical Applications: Some Selected Examples

CATECHOLAMINE-PRODUCING TUMORS

Just as tumors of the thyroid may produce thyroid hormone and tumors of the pancreatic β cells may produce insulin, tumors of chromaffin tissue—in or out of the adrenal—may secrete inappropriately large amounts of catecholamines. *Pheochromocytoma,* a tumor of chromaffin cells, is rare but, if it is recognized, an almost certainly fatal disease can be cured. Fewer than 0.1% of hypertensive patients have pheochromocytoma.

Pheochromocytoma is often, but not invariably, expressed as recurring paroxysms or "attacks," characterized by headache, sweating, palpitations, chest pain, anxiety, pallor, and hypertension. Some patients have hypertension only during a paroxysm. If a sustained output of excessive catecholamine secretion occurs, the clinical picture may resemble that of hyperthyroidism. The symptoms are due to secretion by the tumor of excessive amounts of catecholamine.

The diagnosis of pheochromocytoma is made by measuring free catecholamines, metanephrines, and VMA in the urine. Normally 20–100 μg of total catecholamines are excreted daily, but patients with catecholamine-producing tumors may excrete 300 μg or more per day. Separate estimation of epinephrine and norepinephrine is helpful because the presence of large amounts of epinephrine suggests that the tumor is of adrenal medullary origin. These measurements are all that is needed to identify 90% of patients with pheochromocytoma.

If measurements of urinary catecholamines yield equivocal results, or if they happen to be done in an individual who excretes normal amounts of catecholamines between paroxysms, two other types of tests may be done by experienced observers: (1) the *adrenolytic test,* which involves administering an α blocking agent, phentolamine, to see whether or not a fall in blood pressure occurs, and (2) *provocative test* to determine whether administration of histamine, glucagon or tyramine causes a rise in blood pressure. Provocative tests are hazardous, and results are sometimes difficult to interpret.

Once the presence of a pheochromocytoma is established, management based on established principles of catecholamine physiology and pharmacology is instituted. Alpha blockade is established but this is likely to result in tachycardia; therefore, low-dose β blockade (propranolol) is added. This has the effect of protecting against cardiac arrhythmias that may be precipitated by anesthesia and surgery. Following studies (angiography, tomography) to establish the anatomical location of the tumor, surgery is performed. The efficacy of surgery can be judged by serial measurements of urinary catecholamines and by following blood pressure.

Both chromaffin cells and sympathetic ganglion cells have their embryologic origin in primitive neural crest cells known as *sympathogonia,* which are precursors of *sympathoblasts* (sympathetic ganglion cell precursors) and *pheochromoblasts* (chromaffin cell precursors). As we have seen, chromaffin cells may give rise to pheochromocytoma. Similarly, a type of catecholamine-producing neural crest-derived tumor may arise, as follows (Fig 13–8).

1. Sympathicoblast → sympathicoblastoma
2. Pheochromoblast → pheochromoblastoma
3. Sympathetic ganglion cell → ganglioneuroma

Numbers 1 and 2 are *neuroblastomas,* whereas 3 is a *ganglioneuroma.*

This type of tumor occurs in neonates and children and rarely in young adults. The most common symptom is diarrhea, and hypertension is infrequent. The cause of the diarrhea is not known and, since it is not a common feature of other hypercatecholamine states, it may be due to some secretory product of the tumor that is not catecholamine. Some of these tumors, especially in young children, metastasize early, but when metastases are confined to the abdomen, they can sometimes be controlled by surgery, radiotherapy and chemotherapy.

Again, basic knowledge of catecholamine metabolism and excretion is indispensable in managing these patients. The major diagnostic tool is urinary catecholamine measurement. Some information about the relative malignancy of the tumor may be obtained by comparing the excretion of dopa and dopamine with that of norepinephrine and its metabolites. In general, the more malignant tumors produce relatively more "unfinished" hormone, whereas those that produce

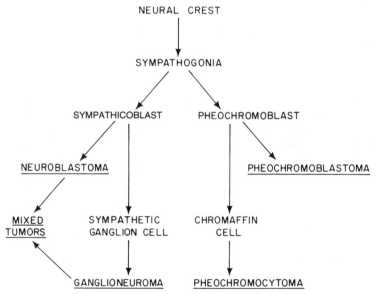

FIG 13–8.
Origins of neural crest-derived tumors.

very little dopa and dopamine are likely to be benign or less malignant. Again, measurement of urinary catecholamines reflects the success or failure of treatment, whether surgical, radiologic, or chemotherapeutic. The reappearance of excessively large amounts of urinary catecholamines heralds a recurrence of tumor growth.

SOME CLINICAL USES FOR ADRENERGIC AGONISTS AND ANTAGONISTS

We have referred to the importance of the catecholamines in depression, Parkinson's disease and neural crest-derived tumors. They are involved also in a variety of other circumstances, either as etiologic factors, as the basis for drug therapy or as diagnostic agents.

There is a vast literature on the role of the sympathetic nervous system in causation of *hypertension*. The catecholamines are related to blood pressure homeostasis in two main ways: (1) via their stimulation of the renin-angiotensin-aldosterone system and (2) because of their stimulatory effects on the heart and small vessels. Propranolol, the most commonly used β blocker, is prominent among antihypertensive agents, both in categorizing the type of hypertension and in management.

Cardiac arrhythmias may be precipitated by catecholamines, especially during anesthesia and surgery. Anticipation of this possibility and the use of appropriate blocking agents is an important responsibility of the anesthesiologist.

Angina pectoris is effort-related pain of cardiac origin. The positive inotropic effect of epinephrine and norepinephrine may contribute to cardiac hypoxia and pain. Amelioration of angina can sometimes be achieved by judicious use of propranolol.

The association between catecholamines and *thyrotoxicosis* was discussed in Chapter 10. The introduction of β blockade as an adjunctive, symptomatic treatment in this condition was an important advance.

The emergency use of catecholamines may be lifesaving in a variety of emergencies, including *traumatic shock, allergic reactions to drugs* and other forms of *peripheral circulatory failure*.

Bronchial dilation by catecholamines is the basis of their use in *bronchial asthma*, both in acute, emergency situations and in long-term management of the condition.

Finally, catecholamines, their congeners and derivatives are constituents of a vast number of over-the-counter remedies for *nasal congestion* due to the *common cold*.

(See Weiner for detailed discussion.)

BIBLIOGRAPHY

Ahlquist RP: A study of adrenotropic receptors. *Am J Physiol* 1948; 153:586.

Axelrod J: Biogenic amines and their impact in psychiatry. *Semin Psychiatr* 1972; 4:199.

Axelrod J, Weinshilboum R: Catecholamines. *N Engl J Med* 1972; 287:237.

Baldessarini RJ: Drugs and the treatment of psychiatric disorders, in Gilman AG, Goodman LS, Rall TW, et al (eds): *Goodman and Gilman's The Pharmacological Basis of Therapeutics*, ed 7. New York, Macmillan Publishing Co, 1985, pp 387–495.

Benovic JL, Shorr RGL, Carson MG, et al: The mammalian $β_2$-adrenergic receptor: Purification and characterization. *Biochemistry* 1984; 23:4510.

Blaschko H, Sayers G, Smith AD (eds): *Handbook of Physiology, Sect 7, Endocrinology, vol 6, Adrenal Gland*. Washington, DC, American Physiological Society, 1975.

Burgoyne RD, Geisow MJ: Specific binding of ^{125}I-Calmodulin to and protein phosphorylation in adrenal chromaffin granule membranes. *FEBS Lett* 1981; 131:127.

Carmichael SW, Winkler H: The adrenal chromaffin cell. *Sci Am* 1985; August:40.

Caron MG, Cerione RA, Benovic JL, et al: Biochemical characterization of the adrenergic receptors: Affinity labeling, purification and reconstitution studies. *Adv Cyclic Nucleotide Protein Phosphorylation Res* 1985; 19:1.

Christensen NJ, Galbo H: Sympathetic nervous activity during exercise. *Ann Rev Physiol* 1983; 45:139.

Ciaranello RD: Regulation of phenylethanolamine N-methyl transferase synthesis and degradation: I. Regulation by rat adrenal glucocorticoids. *Mol Pharmacol* 178; 14:478.

Creutz CE, Pazoles CJ, Pollard HB: Identification and purification of an adrenomedullary protein (synexin) that causes calcium-dependent aggregation of isolated chromaffin granules. *J Biol Chem* 1978; 253:2858.

Davies AO, Lefkowitz RJ: Regulation of β adrenergic receptors by steroid hormones. *Ann Rev Physiol* 1984; 46:119.

Douglas WW: Secretomotor control of adrenal medullary secretion: Synaptic, membrane, and ionic events in stimulus-secretion coupling, in Blaschko H, Sayers G, Smith AD (eds): *Handbook of Physiology*, vol 6. Washington DC, American Physiological Society, 1975, pp 376–388.

Eliasson K: Stress and catecholamines. *Acta Med Scand* 1984; 215:197.

Elks ML, Manganiello VC: Effects of thyroid hormone on regulation of lipolysis and adenosine 3',5'-monophosphate metabolism in 3T3 L1 adipocytes. *Endocrinology* 1985; 117:947.

Exton JH: Mechanisms involved in α adrenergic phenomena. *Am J Physiol* 1985; 248 (*Endocrinol Metab* 11):E633.

Fain JN, García-Sáinz JA: Role of phosphatidyl inositol turnover in Alpha$_1$ and of adenylate cyclase inhibition in Alpha$_2$ effects of catecholamines. *Life Sci* 1980; 26:1183.

Geisow MJ, Burgoyne RD: Recruitment of cytosolic proteins to a secretory granule membrane depends on Ca^{2+}Calmodulin. *Nature* 1983; 301:432.

Kengsberg RL, Trifaro JM: Microinjection of Calmodulin antibodies blocks catecholamine secretion in response to stimulation. *Neuroscience* 1985; 14:335.

Kennedy MFG, Tutton PJM, Barkla DH: Adrenergic factors involved in the control of crypt cell proliferation in jejunum and descending colon of mouse. *Clin Exp Pharmacol Physiol* 1983; 10:577.

Knight DE, Kesteren NT: Evoked transient intracellular free Ca^{2+} changes and secretion in isolated bovine adrenal medullary cells. *Proc R Soc Lond (Biol)* 1983; 218:177.

Lake CR, Ziegler MG (eds): *The Catecholamines in Psychiatric and Neurologic Disorders.* London, Butterworths, 1985.

Landsberg L, Young JB: Catecholamines and the adrenal medulla, in Wilson JD, Foster DW (eds): *Williams Textbook of Endocrinology,* ed 7. Philadelphia, WB Saunders Co, 1985.

Limbird LE: Adrenergic receptors and regulation of adenylate cyclase activity: Methodological approaches and interpretation of data in terms of receptor-cyclase coupling, in Agarwal MK (ed): *Principles of Recepterology* (sic). Berlin, W de Gruyter, 1983, p 593.

Maas JW: Biogenic amines and depression: Biochemical and pharmacological separation of two types of depression. *Arch Gen Psychiatry* 1975; 32:1357.

Manger WM: *Catecholamines in Normal and Abnormal Cardiac Function.* Basel, S Karger AG, 1982.

Mendels J, Stern S, Frazer A: Biochemistry of depression. *Dis Nerv Sys* 1976; 37:3.

Njus D, Kelley PM, Harnadek GJ: The chromaffin vesicle: A model secretory organelle. *Physiologist* 1985; 28:235.

Pollard HB, Ornberg R, Levine M, et al: Regulation of secretion from adrenal chromaffin cells. *Physiologist* 1985; 28:247.

Rubin RP: The role of calcium in the release of neurotransmitter substances and hormones. *Pharmacol Rev* 1970; 22:389.

Schildkraut JJ, Kety SS: Biogenic amines and emotion. *Science* 1967; 156:21.

Schildkraut JJ: Norepinephrine metabolites as biochemical criteria for classifying depressive disorders and predicting response to treatment: Preliminary findings. *Am J Psychiatry* 1973; 130:695.

Sibley DR, Lefkowitz RJ: Molecular mechanisms of receptor desensitization using the β-adrenergic receptor-coupled adenylate cyclase system as a model. *Nature* 1985; 317:124.

Smith U (ed): Adrenergic control of metabolic functions (symposium). *Acta Med Scand* 1983; (Suppl) 5:671–676.

Ungar A, Philips JH: Regulation of the adrenal medulla. *Physiol Rev* 1983; 63:787.

Usdin E, Carlsson A, Dahlström A, et al (eds): *Catecholamines,* vol 3. New York, Alan R Liss, 1984.

Voorhess ML, Gardner LI: Urinary excretion of norepinephrine, epinephrine and 3-methoxy-4-hydroxymandelic acid by children with neuroblastoma. *J Clin Endocrinol* 1961; 21:321.

Wallace MA, Fain JN: Guanosine 5'-O-thiotriphosphate stimulates phospholipase C activity in plasma membrane of rat hepatocytes. *J Biol Chem* 1985; 260:9527.

Weiner N: Norepinephrine, epinephrine, and the sympathomimetic amines, in Gilman AG, Goodman LS, Rall TW, et al (eds): *Goodman and Gilman's The Pharmacological Basis of Therapeutics,* ed 7. New York, Macmillan Publishing Co, 1985, pp 145–180.

PART VII

Body Fuel Metabolism

14

Endocrine Function of the Pancreas

SOME LANDMARKS IN DIABETES AND INSULIN CHRONOLOGY*

DATE		INVESTIGATOR(S)
c. 10 A.D.	Clinical description	Celsus
c. 20 A.D.	Name "diabetes" introduced	Aretaeus
c. 1000	"Degenerative disease" complications	Avicenna
1679	Noted sweet taste of urine in "the pissing evil"	Thomas Willis
1788	Pathology of pancreas in association with diabetes	Cawley
c. 1850 et seq.	Dietary restriction in treatment of diabetes	Bouchardat; von Noorden; Naunyn; Allen and others
1869	Discovery of pancreatic islets	Langerhans
1870	Glycogenic function of liver (rabbit), hyperglycemia of diabetes	Bernard
1874	Hyperpnea of diabetic acetonemia	Kussmaul
1889	Experimental diabetes after pancreatectomy (dog)	Von Mering, Minkowski
1895	Hereditary nature of diabetes; distinction between juvenile and late-onset diabetes	Naunyn
1900	Islet lesions in diabetics	Opie, Ssobolov, Stangle, Weichselbaum
1909	Hypothetical hormone of islets named "insuline"	deMeyer
1910–1920	Insulin "almost" discovered	Zuelzer, Scott, Knowlton, etc.
1921	Insulin discovered (dog)	Banting and Best, Paulesco
1923	Amelioration of pancreatic diabetes by hypophysectomy (toad)	Houssay
1925–	Elucidation of metabolic pathways	Emden, Meyerhof, Parnas, Cori, Lipman, Krebs, Dickens, Ochoa, Leloir, Lynen, etc.
1936	Amelioration of pancreatic diabetes by adrenalectomy (cat)	Long, Lukens
1937	Permanent diabetes by pituitary extract injection (dog)	Young
1955	Structure of insulin elucidated	Sanger
1967–	Proinsulin discovered; structure established	Steiner, Chance
1969–	New role for glucagon	Unger et al.
1969–	Three-dimensional structure of insulin discovered	Hodgkin et al.

*Adapted from Best CH, in Williams RH (ed): *Diabetes*. New York, Paul B Hoeber, Inc, 1960.

The history of diabetes, insulin, its counterregulatory hormones, and the control of body fuel metabolism (see chronology) is nothing less than a minihistory of biology and medicine. Insulin, which is essential for the synthesis and conservation of body carbohydrate, fat, and protein, is both a powerful therapeutic agent and an endlessly fascinating object of contemplation for serial generations of investigators. The discovery of insulin's primary structure was a major event in the history of biology (see Fig 1–1). It played a central role in the development of radioligand assay methods, which have revolutionized modern endocrinology. The discovery of proinsulin was a landmark in the study of protein biosynthesis. Most recently, insulin became the second material of mammalian origin (after somatostatin) to be synthesized by the recombinant DNA technique in *E. coli*.

Insulin

STRUCTURE

In Figure 1–1, we suggested that Sanger's elucidation of the amino acid sequence of the insulin molecule was a central event in the history of biology. Insulin consists of two amino acid chains, A and B, joined by two disulfide bridges. An additional disulfide bridge connects cys 6 and cys 11 of the A chain (Fig 14–1). The S-S bridges do not participate directly in the interaction between insulin and its receptor, but they are important in determining the three-

dimensional configuration of the molecule that is essential for receptor binding and biological activity (see below).

Insulin is a phylogenetically ancient molecule. A substance that is bound by antiinsulin antibody and can mimic the biological activity of insulin in mammalian fat cells has been found in bacteria and yeast, but its function in those forms, if it has one, is not known (Roth). An insulin molecule similar to that of mammals has been synthesized by the hagfish beta cell for the past 500,000,000 years.

Sanger's interspecies comparisons of the amino acid sequences of insulin marked the beginning of the science of molecular evolution. Some insulins found in different species are remarkably similar; for example, porcine and human insulins differ by only one amino acid substitution at B30. At the other extreme, guinea pig insulin (which evolved in South America) differs from human insulin at 17 amino acid loci. Remarkably, all insulins share a highly conserved region that contains the receptor binding site (see three-dimensional structure below).

For many decades, the only source of insulin was the slaughterhouse: insulin was (and is) extracted from the pancreases of countless cattle, pigs, and sheep. Even after the extraction methods were refined enough to yield highly purified insulin preparations, practically all diabetic patients who received cattle or sheep insulin developed anti-insulin antibodies. Since pork insulin differs so little from human insulin, it is much less antigenic than the others. This is why pork insulin is now the preferred agent for replacement

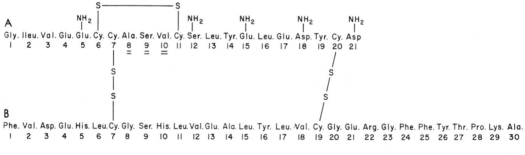

FIG 14–1.
A and **B,** amino acid chains. Structure of insulin in various species. (Adapted from Sanger F: *Br Med Bull* 1960; 16:183.)

therapy among those extracted from animal pancreases.

Insulin has been synthesized de novo from individual amino acids, but the method is not cost effective. Human insulin can be prepared in two ways: (1) by removing amino acid B30 (alanine) from pork insulin and substituting the human B30 residue, threonine; and (2) by recombinant DNA technology. Following the successful production of somatostatin by the recombinant DNA method, insulin was synthesized in this manner by two groups. One (Villa-Komaroff et al.) inserted the proinsulin (see below) gene into *E. coli*, recovered the proinsulin from the medium, and produced insulin by proteolytic cleavage. Another team (Goeddel et al.) chemically synthesized individual genes for the insulin A and B chains, inserted them into separate *E. coli* cultures, retrieved the separate chains, and established S-S bonds between them by oxidation. Insulin produced by the latter method, as well as by modifying porcine insulin, is now being used successfully in the management of insulin-dependent diabetics.

Three-Dimensional Structure

In 1969, Hodgkin and associates at Oxford announced the construction of a three-dimensional model of the insulin molecule derived from x-ray diffraction studies of porcine 2 zinc-insulin crystals. (The structure was solved independently by a group working in Peking, China. Investigators in both countries, together with a Japanese group, have continued to refine it.) This brilliant achievement, a first for a protein hormone, will one day make it possible to give a precise molecular description of the interaction of insulin with its receptor.

Insulin may exist as a monomer (Fig 14–2), a dimer, or a hexamer (3 dimers). In some species, it is possible to see, with the electron microscope, that hexameric crystals are the storage form of insulin in its secretory granule. Analyses of insulins from a variety of species (see Hodgkin) showed that the most highly conserved amino acids are A1, A19, A20, A21 as well as B23, B24, and B25. This does not seem very illuminating when one inspects a standard sequence map, but as one can see in Figure 14–2, all of the conserved residues cluster within a boundary on one side of the three-dimensional reconstruction of the molecule. Indeed, this is the region that articulates with the insulin receptor, and this arresting finding suggests the reason for the biological response of tissue of one species even to phylogenetically remote insulins.

The importance of the terminal B chain is under-

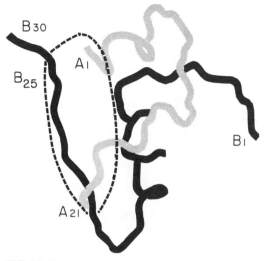

FIG 14–2.
Arrangement of A and B chains in an insulin monomer. Receptor-interactive domain is indicated by the dotted oval. (See Hodgkin.)

scored by the finding that amputation of *five* amino acids (B26–B30) does not reduce biological activity. Removal of *six* amino acids (B25–B30) reduces receptor binding to about 2%, but leaves 40% of biological activity. Removal of *one additional acid* (B24–B30) results in a molecule that neither binds to the receptor nor initiates a biological response.

The fact that receptor binding and initiation of biological response can be dissociated has suggested to some observers the idea that one or several associated amino acids can direct insulin to its binding site on the receptor (the ''address'') while another amino acid, positioned by the binding (even when binding is only a small fraction of total binding capacity), can initiate the biological response (the ''message;'' see Zhang).

These discoveries have already been applied practically, for Haneda et al. have described a new syndrome—familial hyperinsulinemia—which is based on the substitution of an ''incorrect'' amino acid either in position B24 or B25 in translated insulin. Family members with one of these genetic defects present with mild hyperglycemia since their tissues do not respond normally to their own insulin. However, they do show normal sensitivity and responsiveness to exogenously administered insulin.

Another interesting consequence of Sanger's characterization of the insulin molecule has been the base-sequencing of the human proinsulin gene (Bell et al.) and its localization to the distal end of the short arm of chromosome 11 (Harper et al.).

Insulin Preparations

The widespread use of insulin in treatment of diabetic patients has stimulated the development of many insulin preparations, which are designed to permit the hormone to enter the circulation at different rates. Characteristics of some of these are given in Table 14–1. Although these preparations were developed in the hope that appropriate mixes could be tailored to the needs of individual patients, this hope has not been universally realized (see discussion to follow on control of diabetes and experimental insulin delivery systems).

BIOSYNTHESIS: PROINSULIN AND PREPROINSULIN

In 1967 Steiner discovered that radioactive leucine, added to slices of a human insulin-producing tumor in vitro, was incorporated into a larger protein than insulin at first, and only later into insulin itself. Subsequent experiments with isolated rat islets of Langerhans (Fig 14–3) led to the isolation of the precursor protein, which was called proinsulin. Within a remarkably short time, Chance and colleagues established the amino acid sequence of porcine proinsulin shown in Figure 14–4. The sequences of other proinsulins, including human, are now known. The connecting peptides (CPs) of proinsulins generally show far more interspecies variability than do the corresponding insulins.

When proinsulin synthesis was studied in reconstructed, cell-free, ribosomal protein-synthesizing systems, an even larger protein, called *pre*proinsulin was discovered. In this molecule an amino acid sequence (pre) was present at the N terminal end of the proinsulin sequence, thus: pre-β chain-connecting peptide-α chain. The function of the pre sequence is believed to be related to discharge of the nascent

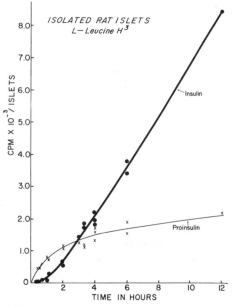

FIG 14–3.
Incorporation of radioactive leucine into proinsulin and insulin by isolated rat islets of Langerhans. (Courtesy of Donald Steiner.)

proinsulin molecule into the lumen of the endoplasmic reticulum (ER) on which it is synthesized. Similar introductory sequences are present on other proteins destined for secretion (see Chapter 17). Readers interested in this aspect of the subject should consult Steiner's Banting Lecture.

When proinsulin is reduced (i.e., the S–S bonds are reduced to SH) and then permitted to reoxidize spontaneously, almost all of the original proinsulin is recovered. If the same experiment is done with insulin, almost no insulin is recovered. This suggests that the CP is necessary for the positioning of the α and β chains to permit the disulfide bonds, so necessary for "correct" affiliation of the two chains, to form readily.

The methods of pulse-labeling of proteins with a radioactive amino acid, quantitative electron microscopy autoradiography, and immunocytochemistry have been used to elucidate the events involved in the synthesis, processing and storage of hormone in the beta cell. Most recently, the use of a highly specific monoclonal antibody against proinsulin that was produced by the recombinant DNA method has made it possible for Orci et al. to trace proinsulin's fate in the cell from the time it is synthesized in the rough endoplasmic reticulum to the secretory granule awaiting exocytosis.

TABLE 14–1.

Classification of Insulin Preparations*

EFFECT	TYPE OF INSULIN	PEAK ACTIVITY (HR)
Short-acting	Regular crystalline	2–4
	Semilente	2–4
Intermediate	NPH†	6–12
	Lente	6–12
Prolonged	Protamine zinc	14–24
	Ultralente	18–24

*From Bressler R, Galloway JA: *Ration Drug Ther* 1971; 5:5. Used by permission.
†NPH = isophane.

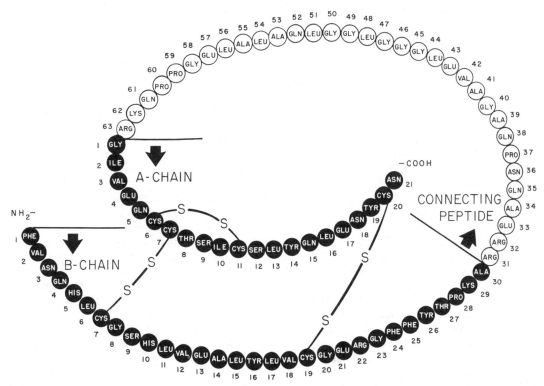

FIG 14–4.
Proinsulin molecule and insulin structure: primary structure of porcine proinsulin. The insulin sequence is represented by amino acids *(dark circles)*. Connecting peptides are indicated by *light circles*. (From Shaw WN, Chance RR: *Diabetes* 1968; 17:737. Reproduced with permission.)

Proinsulin (the pre sequence having been quickly removed) is concentrated in immature (i.e., clathrin-coated) granules within 10 minutes after a pulse of ^{3}H leucine, some 20 minutes before it is detectable in mature (i.e., noncoated) granules. As the coated granules traverse the Golgi, practically all of the proinsulin is processed to insulin and CP by an intra-granular trypsin-like thiol protease that excises two basic amino acids at each end of the CP (Doherty et al.). Insulin and CP are stored in stoichiometric quantities within the granule and are so released when ex-ocytosis occurs. Little or no processing occurs in the mature granule. Secreted proteins are marked "for export only." Lysosomal packages are designated for retention within the cell, while vesicles containing plasma membrane constituents (receptors, transport devices, enzymes) are given suitable instructions to remain within the membrane when the vesicle membrane fuses with the plasma membrane. Presumably, the latter products are not secreted because their lipophilic amino acid domains are already embedded in the lipid bilayer of the vesicle when it opens at the cell surface.

Applications of basic studies on insulin biosynthesis came quickly (Robbins et al.). The development of a specific radioimmunoassay for CP made it possible to measure the ability of the beta cell to respond to a glucose challenge even in diabetics who were taking exogenous insulin, and to discover that many of them whose diabetes was especially difficult to control ("brittle") had virtually no CP response to a glucose load. Moreover, a new disease—familial hyperproinsulinemia—was described, in which the patients showed abnormally high levels of circulating proinsulin that was more resistant to tryptic digestion than porcine proinsulin.

The Regulation of Proinsulin Biosynthesis

Proinsulin synthesis is strongly stimulated by *glucose, mannose, and leucine,* all of which happen to be powerful secretory stimulants as well. Operationally, then, synthesis and secretion are often effectively coupled, but this does not mean that they are controlled by the same intracellular signals, for the secretory response can be elicited when synthesis is blocked and vice versa. Moreover, the threshold glucose concentration required for stimulation of synthesis is only about half that required for secretion stimulation (4–6 mmole).

Other stimuli to synthesis include *growth hormone,* as well as *glucagon* (and related hormones) that increase cyclic AMP. Glucagon, or dibutyryl cAMP, stimulates proinsulin synthesis only in the presence of glucose. Synthesis is *inhibited* by epinephrine (which decreases cAMP and also decreases responsiveness to cAMP), and by sulfonylureas (discussed below) which stimulate insulin secretion, at least in the first phase of the glucose response.

The mechanisms by which glucose stimulates transcription of the proinsulin gene and an increase in its mRNA or that by which cAMP apparently facilitates this process are presently unknown. We can say only that the glucose must be metabolized to have the effect (indeed, certain intermediary metabolites of glucose also stimulate proinsulin synthesis, but less than glucose). Whether the change in redox potential NAD(P)H:NAD(P) or energy charge (ATP:ADP:AMP) brought about by glucose oxidation contribute to the stimulatory signal is conjectural.

Over a longer term (days to weeks), a persistently high or low level of proinsulin synthesis may be seen. This is associated with either hypertrophy or atrophy of the aggregate beta cell mass. Proinsulin synthesis is markedly *decreased* by starvation or by feeding a low carbohydrate, high fat diet; it is *increased* by a high carbohydrate diet, in experimental and clinical obesities, in pregnancy, and in circumstances of chronic growth hormone excess. The increase in pregnancy may be due to a combination of increased food (including carbohydrate) intake and high somatomammotrophin (placental GH-like hormone) levels. Difficulty in compensating for these stimuli may result in pregnancy-related hyperglycemia and glycosuria.

INSULIN SECRETION

The pancreatic β cell conforms to the general model of cells that synthesize peptide or amine hormones and store them in electron-dense secretory granules, poised for secretion. Indeed, the elegant work of Lacy on the ultrastructure of the β cell importantly contributed to the construction of the model. The general features of Douglas' stimulation-secretion model are applicable. This model defines Ca^{2+} as the proximate stimulus for the secretory process, whatever the stimulus for secretion. Experiments with microtubule inhibitors (e.g., colchicine) suggest that microtubule participation is required for insu-

lin secretion, as it is for that of many other hormones.

With the advent of radioimmunoassay methods for measuring insulin, it became possible to obtain a minute-to-minute measure of the secretory activity of β cells (as well as α cells and D cells). When such studies are done in intact human beings or animals, sudden changes in hormone concentration are nearly always due to changes in secretory rate, since they occur much too fast to be influenced by hormone removal rate. Hormone secretion studies can be done on the perfused pancreas of animals as small as the rat, on isolated islets in incubation vessels and on perifused isolated islets, i.e., on islets held on a porous platform under a continuous drip of suitable fluid and mounted over an automatic fraction collector. Whether one studies the secretory response of the β cell to a glucose stimulus in an intact human being or a perifused preparation of rat islets, the pattern of secretory response is the same: (1) there is a sharp spike of hormone release within 2–5 minutes of application of the stimulus; (2) if the glucose stimulus is continuously present, there is a slow, gradually rising increase in insulin content of the blood or perifusate. The initial phase of release may occur without protein synthesis, but the prolonged secondary phase shows a progressive requirement for protein synthesis as time passes.

The two phases of release have been interpreted to signify the existence of two pools of insulin in the β cell: one readily releasable and one less readily releasable. The two pools may merely reflect the fact that some granules are already at the plasma membrane of the cell poised for secretion, whereas others must be moved from the interior of the cell and still others may contain newly synthesized hormone. In any case, even β cells in culture show a typical biphasic hormone release pattern when stimulated with glucose.

Stimulus-Secretion Coupling in the Beta Cell

We can only give a progress report on the cytophysiology of insulin release since the experts in this field, though they have done many ingenious experiments, confess that there is much about glucose-stimulated insulin secretion that we do not know. (This is probably no more true of this subject than of most others discussed in this book.)

The beta cell is a glucose sensor just as a thermostat is a heat sensor. When the temperature rises, the air-conditioning apparatus is activated to lower it. When blood glucose rises, insulin is secreted to restore it to an equilibrium level. At one time, some investigators believed that the primary glucose-sensing device was in the plasma membrane, but most now believe that glucose (or mannose) must be oxidized within the beta cell in order to elicit insulin secretion. A long search for "the" intermediary glucose metabolite that activates the secretory switch has resulted in a cornucopia of hypotheses but no universal agreement. Each of them may contain a fragment of the truth.

The beta cell has a distinctive glucose metabolism: like the liver cell, it contains a highly specific glucokinase and a less fastidious (but lower capacity) hexokinase. Lacking the enzyme fructose 1,6 biphosphatase, it is incapable of gluconeogenesis. However, since it does possess the enzyme phosphoenolpyruvate carboxykinase (PEP CK), the metabolite PEP accumulates when glucose traffic through the Emden-Meyerhof glycolytic pathway is heavy. This metabolite has been reputed to participate in signalling for insulin release (Hedeskov).

In addition to PEP, several other potential signals that may be generated by glucose oxidation have been identified, including: a redox potential shift—an increase in the NAD(P)H:NAD(P) ratio; increased ATP availability; and a shift to an acid pH. There is circumstantial evidence that all of these may participate in mediating glucose-induced insulin secretion.

Some event or combination of events associated with beta cell glucose oxidation also activates adenylate cyclase and causes an increase in cyclic AMP; increases cytosolic $[Ca^{2+}]$ (directly demonstrated by increased Quin 2 fluorescence); and activates polyphosphatidyl inositol turnover, thereby generating inositol polyphosphates and diacylglycerol. There is good evidence that Calmodulin is involved in insulin release, and both tubulin aggregation into microtubules and microfibrillary contraction have been demonstrated to participate in granule movement. The activation of the PIP_2 system is unique in this instance since it is one of the consequences of glucose oxidation, and is not the result of a primary plasma membrane perturbation as it is so frequently. (Such a perturbation *is* induced by another stimulant of insulin release, acetylcholine, which also activates PIP_2 turnover, via a membrane receptor, with the usual consequences). Thus, cAMP, Ca_4Calmodulin and C kinase must phosphorylate many regulatory proteins in a manner calculated to produce an increase in $[Ca^{2+}]_c$ and exocytosis. The only ones identified so far are tubulin (phosphorylation promotes aggregation into microtubules), microtubule-associated protein (MAP) and myosin kinase (important in microfibrillar contraction). Ca^{2+} may also have direct effects; i.e., those not mediated via Calmodulin.

A considerable amount of glucose oxidation—up to 25% of capacity—can occur without stimulation of insulin release. When this threshold is exceeded there is a *sharp* increase in insulin secretion. This explains why fructose, which is phosphorylated too slowly by hexokinase to attain the threshold oxidation rate, cannot by itself stimulate insulin release. It can, however, potentiate the glucose signal, since its metabolites, redox potential changes, ATP, etc., though produced at a subthreshold rate, are additive with those of glucose. In other words, pretreatment of a beta cell with fructose lowers its threshold for glucose.

When we discussed the stimulation of aldosterone biosynthesis and secretion by angiotensin II (Chapter 12), we described experiments by Rasmussen's group which indicated that Ca_4Calmodulin is responsible for the *early* secretory response, while the C kinase system, sensitized by diacylglycerol, is primarily responsible for the *sustained* secretory response. The same group (see Zawalich et al.) have done similar experiments on glucose-stimulated insulin secretion and have come to a similar conclusion, adding the observation that, in order to mimic the effect of glucose, it was necessary to increase cyclic AMP production (by forskolin) in addition to simulating the early and late effects of glucose (by means of a sulfonylurea drug and a diacylglycerol-like phorbol ester, respectively).

In this, as in most other secretory granule-exocytosis forms of secretion, Ca^{2+} is the major second messenger. The presumption is that the exocytotic process involves selective phosphorylation of granule membrane proteins, microfibrillar and microtubule-associated proteins and, possibly, inner membrane proteins as well (see discussion of adrenal medullary secretion in Chapter 13). The identity of these proteins, their functions, and which of the protein kinases are responsible for their phosphorylation are subjects that will engage students of this problem in the future.

Glucagon

Only two years after the discovery of insulin, Murlin et al. described the hyperglycemic effects of aqueous extracts of pancreas. For many years it was known simply as hyperglycemic-glycogenolytic factor, or HGF. Investigative work on glucagon was overshadowed by dramatic advances in the field of insulin research and it was not until the late 1950s, when glucagon was purified and its structure was learned, that interest in this hormone began to spread. Some of the early radioimmunoassays for glucagon failed to differentiate between pancreatic glucagon and enteroglucagon (gut glucagon), a larger molecule of gastrointestinal origin, which shares some amino acid sequences with the pancreatic material. With the development of a highly selective antibody for pancreatic glucagon by Unger and the central role of glucagon in the cyclic nucleotide revolution of the 60s, glucagon came into its own. (See Unger, 1976.)

CHEMISTRY

Glucagon is a 29 amino acid peptide with a molecular weight of 3,485. The sequence of amino acids is invariant in most mammalian species. Glucagon and three gastrointestinal hormones, secretin, vasoactive inhibitory peptide (VIP) and gastric inhibitory peptide (GIP), are homologous in many respects in their amino acid sequences, particularly at amino acids 6, 10, 13, 14, 19, 22, 23, 25, 26, and 27. Yet, although all of these hormones share certain features (e.g., potentiation of the stimulatory effect of glucose on β cell insulin secretion), they also have distinctive features. Many glucagon analogues have been synthesized, including some that competitively inhibit the effect of the natural hormone. Glucagon exists in the secretory granules as a crystal trimer.

From studies with synthetic analogues, it has been determined that the N terminal and central portions of the molecule are most crucial for binding and for adenylate cyclase activation. The tyrosines at positions 10 and 13 are also important. Studies on glucagon binding to its receptor and adenylate cyclase activation by Rodbell and associates were fundamental in the development of contemporary ideas about the receptor-adenylate cyclase complex (see Chapter 3).

BIOSYNTHESIS AND SECRETION

Like insulin, glucagon is the proteolytic product of a prohormone, which in turn is a fragment of a larger preprohormone. Shortly after synthesis in the rough ER the pre sequence is cleaved, leaving the prohormone *glicentin* (Fig 14–5). In the granule, glicentin undergoes proteolysis into an amino terminal peptide called glicentin-related pancreatic peptide, or GRPP (1–30), GLUCAGON (designated (1)–(29) in capital letters), and a carboxyterminal hexapeptide. When granules are examined by immunofluorescence microscopy with antibodies specific for glicentin and glucagon, the former occurs mainly near the granule membrane and the latter mainly in the central core of the granule. When the A cell is stimulated to secrete, a small amount of glicentin and much larger amounts of its constituent peptides are released into the circulation by exocytosis. GRPP and the terminal hexapeptide have no known biological functions. In individuals with A cell tumors (glucagonoma), and in a very rare condition called familial hyperglucagonemia, circulating glicentin levels are supernormal.

The biosynthesis, processing and packaging of glucagon and its storage in electron-dense granules is analogous to similar events that occur in the B cell. The highly efficient, tightly packed crystalline arrangement in the B cell is repeated in the A cell as a Δ-shaped crystal with each side of the equilateral triangle representing the 1–29 linear sequence of glucagon.

Just as we have become comfortable with the concept that Ca^{2+} mediates exocytotic secretion in the B cell and in many other kinds of cells, we are rudely

```
1                                    10
Arg-Ser-Leu-Gln-Asn-Thr-Glu-Glu-Lys-Ser-Arg-Ser-Phe-Pro-Ala-

          20                                      30
Pro-Gln-Thr-Asp-Pro-Leu-Pro-Asp-Pro-Asp-Gln-Met-Thr-Glu-Asp-

       (1)                              40
Lys-Arg-HIS-SER-GLN-GLY-THR-PHE-THR-SER-ASP-TYR-SER-LYS-TYR-

          50                                      60
LEU-ASP-SER-ARG-ARG-ALA-GLN-ASP-PHE-VAL-GLN-TRP-LEU-MET-ASN-

 (29)                          69
THR-Lys-Arg-Asn-Lys-Asn-Asn-Ile-AlaCOOH
```

FIG 14–5.
Amino acid sequence of porcine glicentin (1–69), showing the embedded sequence of GLUCAGON [(1)–(29)] and the proteolytic cleavage sites, *Lys-Arg.* (Adapted from Thim L, Moody AJ: *Regul Pept* 1981; 2:139.)

confronted with the idea that Ca^{2+} can also *inhibit* secretion (Leclerq-Meyer and Malaisse). Glucose, which stimulates insulin secretion, inhibits glucagon secretion. In both the B and the A cell, oxidation of glucose is necessary for the response to occur, and, in both cases, intracellular $[Ca^{2+}]$ rises as a consequence of glucose metabolism. However, in the A cell the increase in $[Ca^{2+}]$ has the effect of shutting off glucagon secretion. This idea is somewhat unsettling until we recall that there are other circumstances (for example, parathyroid hormone secretion, Chapter 17) in which increased $[Ca^{2+}]$ is associated with inhibited secretion. We are not aware of convincing explanations for this paradoxical effect of Ca^{2+}.

A population of cells in the upper gastrointestinal tract secretes a substance that is indistinguishable from pancreatic glucagon and reacts positively to immunofluorescent probes specific for pancreatic glucagon. In some species (example: the dog), a significant amount of circulating glucagon in response to an arginine stimulus is derived from these gastrointestinal (GI) A cells. In humans, however, the physiological significance of these cells has not been established.

METABOLISM AND CLEARANCE

A confusing variety of molecular species that bind antiglucagon antibody is found in the circulation. These include a 2.0K (apparent) degradation product, a 3.5K glucagon monomer, a 9.0K glicentin, and much larger aggregates that may be polymers or monomers attached to high molecular weight circulating proteins.

The liver removes about a third of an injected dose of labelled glucagon by endocytosing receptor-bound hormone. The material preferentially removed by the liver is the 3.5K monomer. The kidney, on the other hand, preferentially extracts the 9.0K material from its blood perfusate. Markedly elevated levels of glicentin may be found in the blood in renal failure.

ACTIONS

The primary site of action of glucagon is the liver, where it stimulates glycogenolysis acutely and gluconeogenesis and ketogenesis over a longer time scale. The purified glucagon receptor of rat and human tissue is a 60K glycoprotein (Livingston et al.). Glucagon interacts with its receptor and activates adenylate cyclase via G_s protein (as described in Chapter 3) to increase the production of cyclic AMP. The biological effects of glucagon are generally attributed to activation of cyclic AMP-dependent protein kinase, but, in this age of proliferating second messengers, this may prove to be an oversimplification. Glucagon is a catabolic hormone not only for glycogen but also for protein and triglyceride. Protein synthesis is inhibited and lysosomal activity is stimulated by it. Glucagon promotes lipolysis by causing the phosphorylation, and, therefore, activation of triacylglycerol lipase ("hormone sensitive"), and also by actively inhibiting lipogenesis by multiple mechanisms (see below). This, together with the metabolic changes that occur as a result of decreased glucose oxidation which often accompanies glucagon action (again, see below), results in ketogenesis.

Glucagon, one of insulin's principal physiologic antagonists, is most effective when insulin is in short supply. On the other hand, it is often difficult to demonstrate a biologic effect of insulin on the liver unless the liver is under the influence of glucagon. We will return to the insulin-glucagon contest later in this chapter.

Glucagon is an extremely potent hormone; its concentration in blood is measured in *pico*grams per ml (10^{-12} M). As little as 0.01 μg of the hormone produces an intense glycogenolysis in the isolated, perfused liver. In contrast, the molar concentration of epinephrine required to produce a comparable effect is 30–50 times that found in the blood after insulin-induced hypoglycemia. This does not rule out a role for catecholamines in glycogenolysis, for they may have an effect by simultaneously stimulating glucagon secretion and inhibiting insulin secretion.

There are similarities, as well as significant differences, in the responses of A and B cells to amino acid stimulation. Arginine and leucine stimulate secretion in cells of both types, but alanine, a major gluconeogenic substrate, selectively stimulates the secretion of glucagon and does *not* elicit insulin secretion. This is a convenient arrangement, for alanine is the major circulating amino acid in starvation. (Incidentally, glucocorticoids, which also appear in starvation, sensitize the A cell to the stimulatory effect of alanine.)

Somatostatin

The story of the discovery of somatostatin (somatotropin release inhibiting hormone, SRIH), its chemistry, its tissue distribution, and its presence in the pancreatic islet D cell was told in Chapter 5. Its short plasma half-life (about five minutes) and the lack of a trustworthy assay for plasma somatostatin concentration measurement have inhibited studies in intact people and animals. Most available information on somatostatin secretion has been obtained from studies on islets or perfused pancreas preparations.

Most stimulants of insulin secretion, including glucagon and sulfonylureas (see below), also stimulate somatostatin secretion. As we noted in Chapter 5, somatostatin inhibits not only insulin and glucagon secretion, but also the secretion of many other hormones in addition to growth hormone with which it was first associated. The only mechanisms suggested to explain the generally inhibitory effect of somatostatin on secretory processes are: (1) an inhibitory effect on the action of cyclic AMP (apparently, it does not influence the stimulated generation of cyclic AMP); and (2) an inhibitory effect on Ca^{2+} transport (Griffey et al.).

The discovery that somatostatin inhibits both insulin and glucagon secretion led to the use of the agent as *an investigative tool in the study of metabolic processes*. It was postulated that adding back either insulin or glucagon by infusion into a somatostatin-blockaded person or animal would permit evaluation of the relative contribution of each to the state that existed prior to the blockade. For example: is ketosis due to insulin deficiency, glucagon excess, or a combination of the two? Or, to put it another way, is glucagon necessary for the full expression of insulin deficiency?

A typical example of the usefulness of somatostatin blockade was the demonstration by Gerich et al. that human diabetic ketoacidosis could be prevented or interrupted by somatostatin. In other studies, diabetic hyperglycemia was corrected by somatostatin. Although the effects of somatostatin in this circumstance are complex (it decreases glucose absorption from the GI tract as well as glucagon secretion and growth hormone secretion), these data, along with others, helped to establish the importance of glucagon as a major contributor to the pathophysiology of human diabetes mellitus and, in the nondiabetic human or animal, as a first line defender against hypoglycemia. It is, however, only one of a number of counterregulatory hormones arrayed against insulin. Glucocorticoids (Chapter 11), pituitary growth hormone (Chapter 5), and catecholamines (Chapter 13) are all involved in the hormonal regulation of metabolism in feast or famine. This formidable team of fail-safe, backup controls underscores the point that the immediate consequences of hypoglycemia are far more life-threatening than those of hyperglycemia. It is not surprising, therefore, that insulin, which lowers the blood glucose, is a solo performer, while its counterregulatory antagonists that protect against hypoglycemia are a quartet. *Sustained* elevation of blood glucose, the result of unopposed action of the quartet, may have life-threatening pathophysiological consequences, some of which we mention later.

The "Islet-as-Mini-Organ" Concept

Demonstration by immunofluorescence of somatostatin in the D cells of the islets by Orci et al. led to a reexamination of the microanatomy of the islets. It was found that α, β, and D cells are characteristically distributed in human and rat islets. In a shallow peripheral cortex, glucagon (α)- and somatostatin (D)-containing cells are interspersed among one another, and both are adjacent to the outer layer of insulin-producing (β) cells. The "medulla" or core of the islet consists entirely of β cells. Most cells in normal islets (60%) are beta cells; α cells constitute 25% and D cells 10% of the population. The proportional representation of the cell types is altered in some circumstances. Hypertrophic islets associated with obesity or chronic glucocorticoid treatment show a relative increase in β cell number and a relative decrease in the other types. In juvenile-onset diabetes β cell number is low, whereas the proportions of glucagon and somatostatin secreting cells are high. On the other hand, in adult-onset diabetes, there are few somatostatin-secreting cells.

A fourth peptide appears in the cortical layer of islet cells in islets near the duodenum. This substance is called pancreatic polypeptide (PP), and it has a molecular weight of about 4,200 daltons. The function of PP is unknown but hyperplasia of PP-producing cells occurs in diabetes.

The architecture of the islet at the light microscope level is intriguing, but Orci's observation of the ultrastructure of islet cells, especially by the freeze-fracture method, has revealed another layer of complexity. Islet cells show extremely complicated cell-cell relationships: some form tight junctions with adjacent ones, whereas others form gap junctions with their neighbors. Gap junctions are low resistance pathways, which represent continuity of cytoplasm between adjacent cells. These connections are sufficiently large to permit the passage of substances with MW 800 to pass freely from cell to cell. Surprisingly, these connections have been seen between similar cells (β–β) as well as dissimilar ones (α–D; α–β). Their existence suggests that many cells may share information simultaneously and respond as a syncytium, or community of cells. Electrophysiologic studies of islet cells suggests that waves of depolarization can pass readily from one cell to another. In a recent study, Kohen et al. injected individual islet cells in monolayer culture with fluorescent dye. When the glucose concentration of medium was high, the dye spread into more adjacent cells than when glucose concentration was low. This suggests that cell-cell communication is enhanced in the presence of a secretory stimulus.

The significance of the tight junctions is unknown, but it is fair to guess that the functional separation of extracellular fluid pools achieved by tight junctions (e.g., Sertoli-Sertoli cell junctions in the testis) has some physiologic meaning. Perhaps the arrangement of tight junctions channels secretory products into the venous effluent draining the islet. Or possibly the secretory signals and substrates of the cells are presented preferentially to one face of the cell. In any case it is difficult to believe that these elaborate architectural features are simply decorative.

To anticipate our discussion of islet hormone-releasing signals, it should be mentioned here that the islet cell hormones have powerful effects on the secretory activity of their neighbors.

The well-established potentially paracrine effects are as follows (Fig 14–6).

> *Insulin* inhibits α cell secretion.
> *Glucagon* stimulates β cell and D cell secretion.
> *Somatostatin* inhibits α and β cell secretion.

On the basis of the morphologic and functional relationships of islet cells, Orci, Unger and their colleagues have proposed that the islet of Langerhans is a small organ that is programmed to respond to many secretory and inhibitory stimuli by the coordinated activity of its cells. According to this view, the pattern of hormones released by the islet represents an integrated response by all of the islet cells, not only to the humoral and neural signals that reach them but also to the paracrine influences that they exert on each other. The physiological significance of the paracrine intercommunication of islet cells is controversial, though the arguments for paracrine regulation seem convincing to us.

Although it is presently impossible to give a more precise definition than this of the "islet-as-mini-organ" concept, it is esthetically appealing to think of islet function in this way. It is interesting to look first at a photograph of the roomful of equipment that Albisser et al. used (e.g., glucose analyzer, computer, pumps, reservoirs) to construct a successful "artificial pancreas" able to regulate blood glucose in insulin-deficient diabetics and then to look at an islet of Langerhans, which not only works better than the artificial pancreas but in most individuals gives maintenance-free, microminiaturized service for a lifetime.

Islet Hormone Release and Release-Inhibiting Signals

Gastrointestinal Endocrine Cell: Early Warning Device

Although the word "hormone" was first used to describe a substance produced in the gastrointestinal

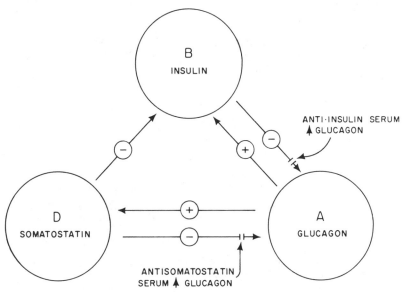

FIG 14–6.
Possible paracrine effects of islet cells.

tract, gastrointestinal hormones have been associated with digestive processes (secretion, motility) and therefore have been considered in the domain of gastroenterology rather than that of endocrinology. In recent years, a new concept of gastrointestinal hormone function has been advanced, largely as a result of studies on hormone release by pancreatic endocrine cells. One of the major stimuli for this development was the demonstration that oral ingestion of a glucose load produced higher serum insulin concentrations and lower serum glucose concentrations than did intravenous administration of a similar dose of glucose. Fujita and colleagues describe the relationship between gastroenteric cell and islet cell function as a gastroentero-pancreatic (GEP) system. Unger and Eisentraut use the term "entero-insular axis" to describe the same concept. Students interested in this aspect of endocrinology are referred to monographs edited by Fujita for ultrastructural and biochemical data on which the GEP concept is based, and to an essay by Unger and Eisentraut.

The gastrointestinal tract is by far the largest endocrine organ in the body. Interspersed among columnar epithelial cells polarized for absorption and among exocrine secretory cells, which discharge into the gastric or intestinal lumen, there are highly specialized cells that present a sensor face to the lumen and secrete granule-stored hormones back into the blood (Fig 14–7). By means of immunocytochemical techniques and electron microscopy, it has been possible to identify many cells of this type. Each is stimulated to secrete by a different combination of chemical messages (e.g., glucose, amino acids, fatty acids, acid or alkaline pH). The secreted hormone then travels to the endocrine pancreas and sensitizes an appropriate endocrine cell to respond to its customary nutrient stimuli. The process of sensitization occurs *before* the incoming nutrient reaches the pancreas in high concentration. Thus the endocrine pancreas is prepared to play its role in disposing of the incoming nutrient because the gastroenteric endocrine cell was able to sample intraluminal contents and to warn the appropriate endocrine cell of its impending responsibility.

When glucagon was discovered to have a potentiating effect on the β cell's response to glucose stimulation, other gastrointestinal hormones (gastrin, secretin, cholecystokinin-pancreozymin [CCK-PZ]) were found to have a similar effect. More recently, with the development of radioimmunoassay methods for GIP, increases in circulating levels of this peptide have been observed following glucose ingestion. Moreover, in obese middle age-onset diabetic patients, who show exaggerated insulinemia after glucose taken by mouth, serum GIP responses to glucose were also found to be exaggerated (Crockett et al.; Ebert et al.). Investigators of GIP have concluded that insulin has an inhibitory effect on GIP secretion, and that the delayed secretion of insulin in diabetic patients may permit a higher degree of GIP sensitization of the β cell's response to secretory stimuli. GIP now appears to be the principal gastrointestinal hormone to potentiate insulin release.

Although fewer studies have been done on the

FIG 14–7.
Intestinal endocrine cell, an early warning device.

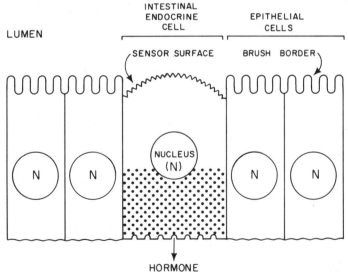

modulation of α cell secretion by gastrointestinal hormones, such effects have been described. Pancreozymin, whose secretion is stimulated by amino acids, powerfully potentiates glucagon secretion by the stimulated α cell. This may, in fact, be part of the mechanism of stimulated glucagon secretion in response to a protein meal.

The relationship between the gastrointestinal tract and the endocrine pancreas is not unidirectional; important signals generated in the islets of Langerhans (in addition to inhibition of GIP secretion) may feed back to the intestinal epithelium. For example, somatostatin, whose secretion from the islet D cell is stimulated by almost all of the known stimuli for insulin secretion, has the effect of *decreasing* glucose absorption by the gastrointestinal tract. This may be a mechanism by which the rate of entry of an incoming nutrient can be slowed down. Perhaps locally secreted somatostatin in the gastrointestinal mucosa may have a similar paracrine function. (For a recent review, see Creutzfeldt and Ebert on the incretin concept.)

CONTROL OF ISLET CELL SECRETORY ACTIVITY

Islet cells are sensors that respond to changes in their nutrient and hormonal environment either by secreting stored hormone or by withholding hormone. Endocrine pancreatic cells secrete into the portal circulation; therefore, the concentrations of these hormones are higher in portal blood than in peripheral venous or arterial blood.

The availability of radioimmunoassay methods has permitted study of minute-to-minute changes in secretion by islet cells in response to a wide variety of stimuli and secretion inhibitors. Table 14–2 represents an attempt to summarize some of the features of the signal-response systems of β and α cells.

The first noteworthy point is the fact that islet *hormones* influence hormone secretion by their neighbors. This is deemed to be physiologically important because treatment of an islet preparation with either antiglucagon serum or antisomatostatin serum results in patterns of hormone secretion that suggest that the α cell and D cell tonically modulate each other's secretory activity. Moreover, in some experimental and clinical obesity conditions, hyperinsulinemic responses to glucose are associated with decreased numbers of D cells in the islets.

The *fuels*, whose disposition is controlled by the islet hormones, are major determinants of islet cell secretion. Glucose is a major signal for insulin secretion, and insulin reserve is widely assessed by the *glucose tolerance test*. This test involves ingestion (or, in some circumstances, injection) of a test dose

TABLE 14–2.

Stimulation (↑) and Inhibition (↓) of Insulin and Glucagon Secretion

	SECRETION	
SIGNAL	INSULIN	GLUCAGON
Islet hormone		
Insulin	?	↓
Glucagon	↑	?
Somatostatin	↓	↓
Fuels		
Glucose	↑	↓
Amino acids	↑	↑
Fatty acids	?	↓
Gastrointestinal hormones*		
GIP	↑	↑
Gastrin	↑	↑
Secretin	↑	↑
PZ-CCK	↑	↑
Neurotransmitters		
Acetylcholine	↑	↑
Catecholamines	↓	↑
Stresses		
Exercise	↓	↑
Trauma, etc.	↓	↑
Ions		
Low calcium	↓	↑
High calcium	↑	↓
Drugs		
Sulfonylureas	↑	?
2-Deoxyglucose	↓	?
D-Mannoheptulose	↓	?
Diazoxide	↓	?

*GIP = gastric inhibitory peptide; PZ-CCK = pancreozymin-cholecystokinin.

of glucose and observation of serum glucose over a fixed period of time. Empirically set serum glucose levels are established at one and two hours after administration of the test dose.

A protein meal or an amino acid mixture signals for *both* insulin and glucagon. This is fortunate, since insulin secretion alone would probably cause hypoglycemia, whereas simultaneous secretion of glucagon compensates for the effect of insulin by stimulating glycogenolysis and gluconeogenesis. When a mixed meal is fed, glucose inhibits glucagon secretion and prevents amino acid-stimulated glucagon secretion.

The significance of the *gastrointestinal hormones* has been discussed. They act primarily by amplifying the response of the β cell to glucose.

There is much evidence to suggest that the neurotransmitters are involved in modulating pancreatic endocrine function. Vagus nerve section causes a decrease in insulin release, whereas acetylcholine and its congeners stimulate insulin release. Acetycholine also stimulates glucagon release. The catecholamines, epinephrine and norepinephrine, inhibit insulin release by way of the α receptor and stimulate glucagon release. It is probable that some of the glycogenolytic effect of exogenously administered epinephrine is due to its glucagon-stimulating action.

In stress responses the inhibitory effect of sympathetic stimulation and circulating catecholamine on insulin secretion was discussed in Chapter 11. This is part of the complex, stereotyped response to trauma and is important during the catabolic phase of the stress response, which precedes repair.

Many drugs stimulate or suppress secretion of insulin. There is much less information available about the pharmacology of the α cell. Sulfonylureas stimulate primarily the first peak of the biphasic insulin response; they will be referred to below. 2-Deoxyglucose is a competitive inhibitor of glucose, which prevents glucose stimulation of insulin release but cannot itself initiate release. D-Mannoheptulose also prevents insulin release, as does diazoxide.

Pancreatic somatostatin release is stimulated by glucose, amino acids, gastrointestinal hormones and cAMP. It is inhibited by epinephrine and diazoxide. Generally, insulin-releasing signals and inhibitors also affect somatostatin release. The biologic significance of somatostatin in this circumstance is unknown.

The main point of enumerating these forces, which either tonically or episodically control pancreatic islet hormone release, is to emphasize the fact that α and β cells, as well as D cells, are under the continuous influence of a complex battery of stimuli and inhibitors that normally work together, primarily in meal-related episodes. That an inhibitor of insulin release may be elicited by glucose, or that glucagon stimulates secretion of its antagonist, can probably be explained as being examples of the generation of both a positive signal and a turn-off signal by the same stimulus.

Cellular Mechanism of Action of Insulin

Although an enormous amount of investigative effort has been expended on the problem of insulin action, it is not yet possible to give more than a status report of progress. If we divide the process of insulin action into (1) hormone-receptor interaction; (2) propagation of signals that are initiated by 1; and (3) biologic effects of signal generation, it is apparent that some progress has been made in the first area and good descriptive accounts exist for the last. However, the links between the binding of insulin to its receptor

and the biologic consequences of the binding are still incompletely known. For some idea of the amount of investigative ingenuity and energy expended on this problem, see Czech.

Metabolic control systems in liver, adipose tissue, and muscle are regulated by insulin and by its counterregulatory hormones: glucagon, catecholamines, glucocorticoids and growth hormone. In general, when insulin is ascendant, secretion of the antagonists is suppressed and, when insulin is in short supply, the antagonists tend to be abundant. Insulin dominance favors anabolic processes, i.e., glycogen synthesis, fatty acid and triglyceride synthesis, protein synthesis, whereas dominance of the antagonists favors catabolic processes, i.e., triglyceride hydrolysis, fatty acid oxidation, ketogenesis, proteolysis, glycogenolysis (Table 14–3). One should note that insulin, in addition to stimulating anabolic processes, also increases the proportion of carbohydrate to fat in the fuel mixture, particularly in muscle and adipose tissue.

The Insulin Receptor

Giant advances in the field of insulin receptorology have been made since the fourth edition of this book was published in 1980. We now know the subunit structure of the insulin receptor, as well as something about its autophosphorylation (reviewed in Czech). New information has been added to our knowledge of the internalization of the hormone-receptor complex, receptor recycling, and surface regulation (Bergeron et al.). As if that were insufficiently impressive, *two* groups have now deduced the entire 1,370–82 amino acid sequence of the human insulin receptor from cloned complementary DNA (Ullrich et al.; Ebina et al.).

STRUCTURE

The accepted heterotetrameric structure of the receptor can be represented as follows:

$$\beta \text{ s-s } \alpha \text{ s-s } \alpha \text{ s-s } \beta$$
(Total molecular wt 360K)

The α subunit has a molecular weight of 125K; the β, 90K. Both subunits are glycoproteins with outwardly oriented sugars. The receptor is synthesized as a continuous peptide as follows: signal sequence (pre sequence)—α subunit—proteolytic cleavage site—β subunit. The prorecceptor is processed in the Golgi apparatus and the naked individual subunits are glycosylated. The α subunit contains the major insulin

TABLE 14–3.

Effects of Insulin Excess and Deficiency and Correlative Conditions*

INSULIN EXCESS OR ANTAGONIST DEFICIENCY OR LOW CYCLIC AMP CONC.		INSULIN DEFICIENCY OR ANTAGONIST EXCESS OR HIGH CYCLIC AMP CONC.
	Anabolic Processes	
	Lipid synthesis	
	Protein synthesis	
	Glycogen synthesis	
	Catabolic Processes	
	Lipolysis	
	Fatty acid oxidation	
	Ketogenesis	
	Glycogenolysis	
	Proteolysis	
	Gluconeogenesis	

*From Fritz IB: *Insulin Action*. New York, Academic Press, 1972.

binding domain; the β subunit is a transmembrane protein that contains a 23 amino acid lipophilic sequence that anchors the whole assembly in the membrane.

RECEPTOR PHOSPHORYLATION

The β subunit of the insulin receptor is a tyrosine kinase. When the α subunit is occupied by insulin, the β subunit kinase is activated and autophosphorylation of the β subunit occurs (Kasuga et al.). Activated β kinase, in addition to phosphorylating itself, can also phosphorylate a variety of other proteins. In broken cell preparations, only tyrosine is phosphorylated on the β subunit, but in intact cells exposed to insulin, serine and threonine residues are also phosphorylated by kinases other than the β subunit. (Parenthetically, tyrosine kinase activity, though rare, has been identified as an intrinsic property of several growth factor (g.f.) receptors, including those of epidermal g.f., platelet-derived g.f., and insulin-like g.f. I (somatomedin C), as well as several peptide oncogene products that are also involved in stimulating growth.)

These intriguing observations have been pursued energetically in many laboratories, but there is no satisfactory answer to the following questions: (1) is tyrosine phosphorylation of the β subunit an essential (possibly initiating) event in the transmembrane signalling that results in all or part of the pleiotropic insulin response? (2) if it is, how does it work?

While there are many experiments in which biological effects correlate well with β subunit receptor phosphorylation, there are others that suggest that the biological response to receptor occupancy can be dissociated from receptor phosphorylation. Among the most interesting in the latter category are those in which anti-insulin receptor antibody can mimic insulin's biologic effects in the absence of β subunit phosphorylation. However, even if one disregards this evidence and accepts the proposition that phosphorylation is the primary event that initiates the complex cellular response to insulin, no one has suggested how this could occur.

One interesting aspect of β subunit phosphorylation is the fact that the nontyrosine phosphorylations (ser and thr) can be catalyzed by cyclic AMP-dependent protein kinase. Here is a pretty example of counterregulation at the molecular level, for the effect of serine and threonine phosphorylation of the subunit is a reduction in the affinity of the α subunit for insulin; in other words, insulin resistance is produced by an elevation of [cAMP] within the cell. Not to be outdone, insulin can decrease the production of cAMP, accelerate its destruction by phosphodiesterase, and interfere with its activation of cAMP-dependent protein kinase. The β subunit of the insulin receptor is a tiny arena in which the hormonal gladiators, insulin and glucagon, do battle.

RECEPTOR REGULATION

The action of the receptor can be modified acutely or chronically by alterations in the *affinity* of the receptor for its ligand, or chronically by *changes in receptor density* in the membrane.

Affinity changes do not necessarily parallel insulin sensitivity, although they may do so as in the reduction in both affinity and sensitivity described in the last paragraph. For example, starvation may result in a paradoxical *increase* in affinity and a *decrease* in sensitivity and responsiveness to insulin due to post-receptor adaptations. (Sensitivity decrease means that the insulin dose-response curve is shifted to the right, i.e., it takes more insulin to produce the same half-maximal response, but enough insulin can be added to achieve a full response. A decrease in responsiveness means that the full biological response to insulin cannot be achieved with *any* dose of insulin.)

Since the affinity of insulin for its receptor decreases progressively as insulin concentration increases, DeMeyts et al. suggested that site-site interactions resulted in negative cooperativity. Now that we know that β subunit phosphorylation results in decreased affinity of the α subunit for insulin, we guess that DeMeyts' negative cooperativity may be one manifestation of β sununit phosphorylation.

Interest in the chronic regulation of receptor density or number was stimulated by the pioneering studies of Roth, Kahn, and their associates on the effect of obesity on the insulin receptor population of cells in experimental and clinical obesities. They found (1) that there were fewer insulin-binding sites on adipocytes and monocytes of obese individuals than on those of lean controls; and (2) that this reduction in receptor number was associated with hyperinsulinemia. (This led to the demonstration of down-regulation of receptors in cultured cells incubated with insulin, and indeed to the study of down-regulation of their receptors by many other peptide and amine hormones and neurotransmitters.) If obese animals or people were subjected to weight reduction, insulin receptor number increased toward control levels.

Subsequently, it was found that the *occupied* insulin receptor (and those of practically all other peptide and amine hormones) is internalized by the process of endocytosis. Although they are taken into the cell as a hormone-receptor complex, insulin and receptor have different fates within the cell. The former is rapidly degraded (T ½, 30 minutes), while some of the receptors are conserved, reprocessed, and reinserted into the membrane. Others are degraded with a T ½ of about 10 hours. Although many attempts have been made to associate insulin-receptor internalization with its biological actions, most evidence suggests that insulin need not enter the cell to produce most of its usual effects. This is certainly true of insulin-mimicking antireceptor antibodies. (For a reveiw of this field, see Bergeron et al.)

SPARE RECEPTORS

Many, but not all, insulin-sensitive cells demonstrate the spare receptor phenomenon, since a maximum biologic effect can be achieved with only 2%–5% occupancy of available surface binding sites. The presence of spare receptors makes it possible for cells to respond to insulin even at relatively low insulin concentrations. The liver cell does not have very many receptors to spare, i.e., biologic effects and receptor occupancy parallel each other. Perhaps this is related to the anatomical location of the liver in the path of the venous effluent from the pancreas, where it is exposed to much higher concentrations of insulin than are cells in the periphery.

Cellular Mechanisms of Action of Insulin

The history of research on the mechanisms of action of insulin is nothing less than a minicourse in the history of contemporary cell biology. Investigators have examined the problem from many vantage points with every conceivable methodologic instrument. As a result, we now have mountains of information about insulin-receptor interactions (see above), a huge data bank on the biochemical consequences of insulin action, but only a fragmentary idea about how the two may be connected. Individual responses need not be connected in exactly the same way, since different biological effects of insulin can be elicited at very different insulin concentrations, and many of them occur at different times after insulin administration. In addition, as in all other hormone actions, the mechanism of action of insulin is determined by the capacity of the sensitive cell to respond; for example, the hormone has different effects in liver cells and fat cells that are specialized to perform different functions. Eventually, we will be obliged to specify which effects are brought about by X mechanism, which by Y, and which are secondary to antecedent events. Unfortunately, it is not yet possible to do this.

At the outset, it is helpful to categorize insulin's biological effects into four groups: (1) *very fast* (seconds): membrane hyperpolarization in some cells, changes in membrane transport of glucose and ions; (2) *fast* (minutes): activation or inhibition of many enzymes with the effect of accentuating anabolic actions; i.e., glycogenesis, lipogenesis, and protein synthesis. There is a coordinate inhibition of the opposing catabolic actions; (3) *slower* (minutes to hours): increased amino acid influx, selective induction or repression of enzyme synthesis (induced enzymes are rate-limiting to anabolic reaction sequences; repressed ones are key enzymes in the opposing catabolic ones.); (4) *slowest* (hours to days): mitogenesis and cell replication.

IMMEDIATE EFFECTS OF INSULIN ON PLASMA MEMBRANE FUNCTION

As we have seen, interaction of insulin with the α subunit of the receptor results in the immediate autophosphorylation of the β subunit. Other membrane changes occur very soon after insulin stimulation; a catalogue of some of these is worth contemplating.

Hyperpolarization of the membrane of many insulin-sensitive cells (other than liver) (Zierler)

H^+ extrusion, Na^+ uptake; increase in cell pH

Ca^{2+} retention (inhibition of Ca^{2+} pump)

K^+ uptake, Na^+ extrusion (Na^+ K^+ ATPase)

Increased glucose transport.

The impression is that the insulin-receptor interaction causes a profound change in the physical state of the membrane that may itself qualify as a transducing message that results in the simultaneous activation of multiple transport systems.

Activation of glucose transport is particularly interesting because, for a decade or so following Levine's demonstration of insulin's stimulatory effect on glucose transport, it was widely taught that all of insulin's effects were secondary to glucose transport stimulation. When certain insulin effects were demonstrated in the absence of glucose, this theory became untenable. Recently, there has been a renaissance of interest in insulin's effect on glucose transport because two investigators (Kono and Cushman), using different methods, have shown independently that insulin treatment of fat cells causes a recruitment of glucose transporters from some cryptic, interior pool to the plasma membrane. When insulin is withdrawn, the majority of transporters leave the plasma membrane and return to their hidden compartment. This insulin-induced membrane remodelling happens practically instantaneously and can account (practically) quantitatively for increased glucose transport in response to insulin. The rapidity of the response suggests that the transporters, waiting in the wings to be inserted, may be just under the plasma membrane, possibly in apposition to it.

Insulin may cause membranes to *lose* components as well as to gain them, for Kono et al. have described the dissociation of insulin-sensitive phosphodiesterase away from the membrane and into the cell in response to insulin. In adipocytes, this is one way in which insulin lowers previously elevated cyclic AMP.

Clearly, the fast membrane effects of insulin are an important part of its action, for they result in an influx of glucose and a marked change in the ionic microenvironment within the cell. Whatever else insulin does

via its receptor must be added to its effect at the plasma membrane. However, we must leave open the possibility that some membrane effects (for example, increased amino acid transport) may prove to be mediated by identifiable messengers other than membrane hyperpolarization.

ENZYME REGULATION

The discovery of cyclic AMP, with its emphasis on metabolic control by reversible phosphorylation of key enzymes, stimulated investigators to study possible effects of insulin on the phosphorylation-dephosphorylation patterns of solubilized, dispersed proteins on two-dimensional gels. It was found that insulin treatment resulted in highly selective phosphorylation of a few proteins and dephosphorylation of others. Although reaction velocities at specific enzymic sites are controlled by many variables (substrate, coenzyme, ATP/ADP availability, ionic environment and others), control by phosphorylation-dephosphorylation has become one of the major themes of contemporary biochemical control theory (Cohen).

In Chapter 3 we described the coordinate control of the two opposing enzymes of glucogen metabolism. *Glucagon,* through cyclic AMP, causes phosphorylation (activation) of phosphorylase and phosphorylation (inhibition) of glycogen synthase, thus permitting the phosphorylase to act unopposed. *Insulin* has precisely the opposite effects: it brings about the activation of a phosphatase that *de*phosphorylates both enzymes, thus facilitating glycogen synthesis and inhibiting its breakdown.

This theme—simultaneous facilitation of one pathway and inhibition of the corresponding reverse pathway—recurs often throughout the lipogenesis reaction sequence in liver and adipocyte. For example, insulin treatment has the effect of favoring

(Lipogenic)		(Gluconeogenic)
1. Phosphofructokinase (PFKI)	>	Fructose 1,6 bisphosphatase
2. Pyruvate kinase	>	Phosphoenol pyruvate carboxykinase
3. Triacylglycerol synthase	>	Triacylglycerol lipase

Currently, there is a great deal of attention being paid to number 1, and we will attempt to summarize recent advances in this field later. However, enthusiasm for the new should not be allowed to obscure the fact that insulin has *simultaneous* effects at many biochemical loci, both lipogenesis-enhancing and gluconeogenesis-inhibiting, and therefore establishes nothing less than a *total biochemical climate* for lipogenesis. For, in addition to exerting the controls listed above, insulin also stimulates enzymes involved in generating

NADPH, the obligatory cofactor for lipid synthesis; namely, glucose-6-phosphate dehydrogenase and NADP malic enzyme. It also controls the entry of glucose into the hepatocyte by its effect on glucokinase and causes stimulation of the action of the crucial lipogenic enzymes, acetyl CoA carboxylase, and fatty acid synthase.

It is not surprising that the interest in hormone second messengers stimulated by the discovery of cyclic AMP, which also affects many reactions in cells in a coordinate way, inspired Larner to search for "a" second messenger for insulin. In 1979, he and his coworkers demonstrated that material (Fraction II) extracted from insulinized rat muscle inhibited cyclic AMP protein kinase activity and stimulated glycogen synthase-PO_4 phosphatase activity. Independently, Jarett et al. showed that coincubation of plasma membrane, insulin, and mitochondria resulted in activation of PDH—the first demonstration of an effect of insulin in a cell-free system. In collaboration with Larner, the Jarett group showed that Larner's Fraction II also activated PDH when added to mitochondria. It was later shown that the putative second messenger activates the phosphatase component of PDH and causes activation of the enzyme by dephosphorylating it (Gottschalk and Jarett review).

In addition to the enzymes already mentioned, the factors produced by membranes in response to insulin stimulate insulin-responsive cAMP phosphodiesterase, $Ca^{2+}Mg^{2+}$ATPase, and acetyl CoA carboxylase. One of them also inhibits adenylate cyclase. Thus, the activity conforms perfectly to the pattern of response of these enzymes when insulin acts in an intact cell.

In spite of much effort, "the" insulin second messenger has not yet been identified chemically. More than one messenger may be produced in response to insulin, for inhibitory substances also appear at high insulin concentrations. The lack of progress in the effort to purify and characterize these substances has resulted in some waning of the enthusiasm that was shown in 1979. We count ourselves among the believers; in a variety of circumstances of insulin resistance (fat feeding, glucocorticoid treatment, diabetes), the generation of PDH activator by membranes exposed to insulin is decreased. In one condition, insulin hypersensitivity induced by physical exercise, a supernormal amount of PDH activator is released from insulin treated membranes. The congruence of activator production in response to insulin with the physiologic state of the cells from which test membranes were obtained suggests to us that the mediators, though not yet chemically characterized, are physiologically significant. This is not to say that they

are the *only* mechanism involved in insulin's action. For example, they do not affect glucose transport or glucose oxidation by fat cells. In our view, insulin will ultimately be shown to act by way of a network of interconnected mechanisms that will include the Larner-Jarett second messengers.

Insulin has rapid effects on *protein synthesis* that do not involve increased synthesis of mRNA. It has been known for some time that insulin causes the aggregation of ribosomes into polysomes, and that it stimulates the *initiation* of translation as well as the elongation of nascent peptide chains. While the molecular mechanism of this action is incompletely understood, we can now make a plausible connection between a highly specific protein, phosphorylated in response to insulin treatment, and insulin's stimulatory effect on the translation process. Rosen and her colleagues discovered that ribosomal protein S6 is one of the cell's proteins that is serine phosphorylated following insulin treatment. This protein, in its phosphorylated state, is involved in the initiation of translation. In fact, a tight temporal relationship has been described relating an enhanced rate of initiation to the phosphorylation of r.p. S6 following insulin stimulation (Hansson and Ingelman-Sundberg). Ribosomal protein S6 is another molecular battleground for insulin and glucagon, for it is phosphorylated at another site by cyclic AMP *de*pendent kinase, which has the effect of *decreasing* the initiation rate of protein synthesis. The kinase, or kinases, stimulated by insulin are cyclic AMP *in*dependent ones, either protein kinase C or protease-activated protein kinase II (PAPK II). This is an example of an important regulatory molecule (there are others) that can be activated by phosphorylation at one site and inhibited by phosphorylation at another site (Burkard and Traugh).

Enzyme Synthesis and Repression Affected by Insulin

So far, we have been discussing insulin's effects on enzyme regulation that do not involve a change in the number of enzyme molecules. We have emphasized the effects of insulin on the activation of substrate traffic-controlling, rate-limiting enzymes in the glycogenic, lipogenic, and protein synthetic pathways and the coordinate inhibition of opposing enzymes in the gluconeogenic pathway. We failed to mention that insulin has also been shown to oppose the action of proteolytic systems that are balanced in opposition to protein synthetic ones.

If insulin stimulation persists for hours to days, the

following enzymes (in liver) increase not only in *activity* but also in *number of molecules* of catalytic protein: glucokinase, ATP citrate lyase, acetyl CoA carboxylase, fatty acid synthase, L-type pyruvate kinase, glucose-6-phosphate dehydrogenase, and NADPH malic enzyme. It is apparent that members of this team of enzymes are activated acutely by insulin treatment and that they are all involved in the lipogenic pathway. Coordinate with the induction of these enzymes, their physiological opponents, key enzymes in the gluconeogenic pathway, are repressed. The phenomenon of enzyme induction and repression by insulin has been studied extensively in intact animals, as well as in a variety of cells in culture.

In all cases of induction examined so far, an *increased rate of transcription (mRNA synthesis)* has been demonstrated following insulin administration. In the case of one extensively studied gluconeogenic enzyme, phosphoenol pyruvate carboxykinase (PEP CK), insulin has been shown to *decrease* the rate of mRNA transcription. In the case of PEP CK, cyclic AMP *induces* new enzyme mRNA synthesis.

The mechanisms by which insulin induces the selective transcription of a few genes is unknown. The fact that fructose, a sugar that can be metabolized by the liver cell without insulin, can induce many of the same enzymes in diabetic animals suggests that insulin's effect on the genetic apparatus is secondary to the increased metabolism of glucose that occurs under its influence. This impression is strengthened by the ability of glycerol to induce pyruvate kinase in the absence of insulin. The great mystery is the nature of the selective transcription stimulus that is generated by the metabolism of substrates either in the presence or absence of insulin. While we can describe the induction of the lac operon in *E. coli* by cyclic AMP in some molecular detail, we cannot do as well with the induction of PEP CK by cyclic AMP in the hepatocyte. (See Czech and Sasaketal.)

MITOGENIC EFFECT OF INSULIN

Insulin's stimulatory effects on growth and cell replication are well documented both in vivo and in vitro. The in vivo effects of the hormone are complex and partly indirect: while the metabolic effects of insulin no doubt contribute to the overall growth stimulatory effect of the hormone, there is good evidence that it also facilitates the growth hormone-stimulated synthesis of somatomedin (IGF I) in the liver and, possibly, in other tissues as well. Moreover, it may act synergistically with somatomedin, in the stimulation of growth. Somatomedin, however, is the senior partner of the pair, since human Laron dwarfs, African pygmies and toy poodles, all of whom have an inability to make somatomedin, have no obvious shortage of insulin.

Insulin also acts as a *mitogen* in many different cell types in culture. A commonly used indicator of this effect is stimulation of ^{3}H thymidine incorporation into DNA. In some cells (fibroblasts), much higher concentrations of insulin are required to stimulate DNA synthesis than are needed to enhance glucose transport, or other acute metabolic indicators of insulin action. In these cells, blocking the insulin receptors with fragments of antireceptor antibody (themselves incapable of mimicking insulin's biologic effects) does not interfere with insulin's ability to stimulate DNA synthesis. It has been concluded that, in these cells, insulin elicits its mitogenic effect by cross-reacting with IGF I (som C) receptors. In other types of cells (liver, many tumor cells), insulin clearly acts as a mitogen by binding to its own high affinity receptor.

The most appealing (though still somewhat vague) hypothesis to explain insulin's mitogenic effect (as well as that of other growth factors such as EGF, PDGF, FGF, IGF I) states that persistent stimulation of protein synthesis via phosphorylation of ribosomal protein S6 eventually results in the synthesis of an evanescent protein that is essential to arouse cells arrested in the G_1 phase of the mitotic cycle into the DNA-synthesizing state. The other well-known growth factors resemble insulin (1) in having a common molecular ancestor (see discussion above); (2) in interacting with receptors that are tyrosine autokinases; and (3) in stimulating the serine phosphorylation of ribosomal protein S6. (The mechanistic link between (2) and (3), if it exists, is not obvious to us.) Insulin synergizes (effects of each hormone pair more than additive) with all of the others in stimulating mitogenesis, a fact that suggests that, though they may all share mechanisms, they do not act precisely the same way.

This field of investigation is now being explored energetically, not least because phorbol esters, which are analogues of diacylglycerol, stimulate C kinase, which in turn phosphorylates ribosomal protein S6 and potentiates the effects of tumor-forming agents. The peptide products of oncogenes, like insulin and growth factor receptors, are tyrosine kinases. We can predict that further elucidation of these mechanisms will shed new light on both normal and abnormal growth (Straus).

Macroregulation of Body Fuel Distribution: Interorgan Collaboration in Starvation and Refeeding

Restriction of blood glucose (BG) concentration within narrow limits is achieved by a consortium of neural and hormonal mechanisms. A *rising* BG level stimulates insulin secretion but inhibits secretion of insulin's physiologic antagonists, particularly glucagon and growth hormone (Fig 14–8).

ADAPTATION TO STARVATION: FORCES THAT TEND TO ELEVATE BLOOD GLUCOSE

Food deprivation sets in motion an intricate set of adaptive responses, which have the overall effect of conserving the body's substance and redistributing its chemical resources. Adaptations to changes in the food environment operate on two time scales: (1) acutely, when time is measured in minutes, and (2) chronically, when time is measured in hours and days. In general, the earlier changes are accomplished largely through the acute effects of hormones and nutrients without changes in the amounts of intracellular enzymes. The chronic adjustments may involve elaborate resetting of cellular enzyme levels. It is increasingly evident that these changes in enzyme pattern are the results of collaborative effects of hormones and

the metabolic substrate mixtures to which cells are exposed.

It has been customary to discuss BG regulation during starvation and refeeding and its hormonal regulation. Emphasis on BG regulation alone does a vast injustice to the extraordinarily complex set of control mechanisms that operate in starvation and refeeding in all areas of metabolism simultaneously—carbohydrate, fat, and protein metabolism—as well as in that of water and electrolytes. The most impressive single fact about metabolic control mechanisms, whether examined at the level of organization of the whole animal or within the cell, is their coordinate nature. The metabolism of all three foodstuffs (carbohydrate, fat, protein) is controlled simultaneously by the same set of signals.

Hunger

One of the symptoms of a rapidly falling BG level is hunger. Teleologically, this is an appropriate response, for hunger usually leads to food-seeking behavior and food ingestion. The inclusion of hunger among the forces that tend to elevate BG is an attempt to reemphasize the point made by Richter and others: metabolic events often have behavioral expression, and the behavioral projection of metabolic need that involves interaction of an animal with its environment

RAISE [B.G.]	LOWER [B.G.]
Hunger	Satiety
Glucose absorption	
Glucose injection	[Glucose diffusion through body water]
Hepatic glycogenolysis **GLUCAGON (G)** **EPINEPHRINE (E)**	
	INSULIN
Gluconeogenesis **G, E, CORTISOL**	↓hepatic glucose output ↑glucose oxidation ↑glycogen deposition ↑lipogenesis
↓Glucose utilization **FATTY ACIDS** **GROWTH HORMONE** **CORTISOL**	
[Dehydration]	[Glycosuria]

FIG 14–8.
Outline of forces that tend to raise and lower blood glucose *(BG)* concentration. (Hunger increases food intake. Satiety limits food intake.)

is just as much a part of "homeostasis" as are the adjustments that take place within the body.

Routes of Entry of Glucose into Blood

There are only three ways by which glucose can enter the bloodstream. The *first* (which is not the usual way) is by *injection*, either intravenously or by another parenteral route. This route may be especially important in diagnosis and treatment of patients and in certain types of experimental analysis. The *second* (and customary) route is by *absorption* from the gastrointestinal tract. In ordinary circumstances men and animals have two main depots of ready calories on which to draw: the adipose tissue and the contents of the gastrointestinal tract. It is easy to see how malabsorption of glucose or other carbohydrates could interfere with the proper maintenance of BG, and this, in fact, is what happens in certain human diseases.

The *third* route by which glucose enters the blood is that discovered by Bernard—the "internal secretion" of glucose into the blood by the liver. Some years ago it was demonstrated that even in the absence of obvious hormonal influence, the liver has a certain degree of autonomous control over the amount of sugar it releases into the hepatic vein and the amount it retains. But this autonomous control is modulated by a number of hormonal forces. In time of need, and in response to appropriate hormonal signals, the liver can maintain an adequate level of BG even in the absence of absorption of glucose from the gastrointestinal tract.

There are two principal processes involved in the liver's ability to secrete glucose into the blood. The first, *glycogenolysis,* happens in minutes, and the second, *gluconeogenesis,* occurs over hours and days. Glycogenolysis is simply the breakdown of existing glycogen in the liver, ultimately to G-6-P. This compound is split by a specific phosphatase, which occurs in the liver, but not in muscle, with the liberation of free glucose into the circulation.

The glycogenolytic release of glucose from the liver seems well adapted to acute emergencies, but the BG could not be maintained for long if the liver glycogen were quantitatively delivered to the bloodstream as glucose. If a 1,500-gm human liver contained as much as 4% glycogen, only 60 gm of glucose (or a paltry 240 calories) would be delivered to the blood as glucose on total glycogenolysis. In circumstances of prolonged glucose deprivation, as in starvation, or if there is a failure of renal reabsorption of glucose, as in phlorhizin diabetes, some other mechanism must come into play if the BG level is to be effectively maintained. The other, or long-range,

hepatic maneuver for maintaining BG concentration is called *gluconeogenesis,* which, though defined variously, is used here to signify the transformation of deaminated residues of amino acids, glycerol and lactate, into glucose in the liver. Operationally this process actually includes the delivery of the newly formed glucose to the bloodstream at a very high rate, because those physiologic conditions that are characterized by a high rate of gluconeogenesis are also characterized by a "hypertrophy" of the hepatic enzyme glucose-6-phosphatase (G-6-Pase), which is the equivalent of stamping a larger than usual number of G-6-P molecules "for export only." The liver has an extraordinary capacity for absorbing certain amino acids from its incoming blood, as one can readily demonstrate by infusing large amounts of protein hydrolysate intravenously. It is difficult, in fact, to maintain an elevated blood concentration of amino acids, even with rapid infusion rates. The sources of the amino acids that are used for long-term maintenance of BG in starvation and in other conditions are the protein tissues of the body, principally the muscle mass, which constitutes about 50% of the body's net weight. Adrenal cortical steroid hormones of the glucocorticoid type play an important role in mobilization of peripheral tissue protein to the liver as amino acids, most of which are used for gluconeogenesis. Of course, some of the amino acids must be used to support protein synthetic activities going on in the liver and elsewhere.

If, under conditions of carbohydrate deprivation or chronic renal tubular loss, the glucose utilization rate of tissues other than the CNS remained as high as it is in the "fed" state, the problem of maintaining a continuing supply of glucose to the brain would be more demanding than it is. For in starvation, the peripheral tissues adapt in such a way that they use less glucose than before. This is partly due to the fact that adaptation to starvation includes a fall in total metabolism. A true tissue adaptation can also be demonstrated in the muscles of starved or fat-fed rats. Such muscles, incubated in vitro with glucose and a radioactively labeled fatty acid, burn less glucose and more fatty acid than do muscles taken from normal fed controls. There is in fact a demonstrable block in peripheral carbohydrate oxidation, and a tendency for the tissues to shift their "preference" to fatty acids. This, of course, makes the liver's job of supplying BG by way of gluconeogenesis far easier, since, viewed in the light of the overall economy of the animal, more of the newly formed glucose remains available for the critical tissues, that need it most.

The nature of the hormonal effects on the *blockade of peripheral glucose oxidation* in starvation is not known with certainty. We do know that both adrenal glucocorticoids and pituitary growth hormone have been alleged to have "braking" effects on glucose use by muscle.

An experimental demonstration of the effect of acute lowering of the BG on plasma concentrations of two insulin antagonists is shown in Figure 14–9.

Glucose-Amino Acid Cycle

In recent years, Cahill and Felig and their colleagues, whose point of departure was Benedict's monumental 1915 study on the metabolism of fasting man, have added important new information to the subject of human adaptation to long-term starvation. After confirming that nitrogen excretion of starvation (a measure of protein breakdown) is very high in early starvation but diminishes gradually over a period of many days, they calculated that in prolonged starvation the protein catabolized was insufficient to supply adequate glucose to the brain. It was evident that the brain, long believed to be an obligatory glucose burner, was extracting its energy from another metabolic fuel. Later studies showed that man's brain can adapt to burn ketone bodies, and that this capacity develops concomitantly with a decrease in general protein catabolism and a decrease in glucose production from amino acids by the liver. Smith, Satterthwaite, and Sokoloff described an adaptive increase in β-hydroxybutyrate dehydrogenase activity in rat brain during starvation. The concurrent adaptation of the brain and the decrease in protein breakdown that occurs with prolonged starvation have obvious survival value, since the fully adapted human can survive at a cost of only 3–4 gm of his own protein per day. Part of the sharp reduction in protein requirement during fasting is due to an adaptive decrease in total metabolism that results from an absence of food intake. The basal metabolic rate of a starved human being may diminish to 50% of the prestarvation level.

During fasting (Fig 14–10,A), no amino acids are absorbed from the gastrointestinal tract. The muscle exports a mixture of amino acids that does not resemble a hydrolysate of skeletal muscle protein but, rather, contains a preponderance of *alanine* and *glutamine*. Alanine is returned to the liver, where it is

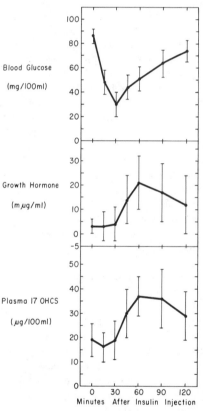

FIG 14–9.
Responses of plasma 17-hydroxycorticosteroids and plasma growth hormone (GH) to insulin-induced hypoglycemia in normal subjects. Insulin in a dose of 0.1 units/kg body weight was injected intravenously at "0" time. The response indicates the presence of intact GH and the ACTH-releasing capacity of hypothalamic-pituitary system. (Courtesy of Myron Miller; unpublished.)

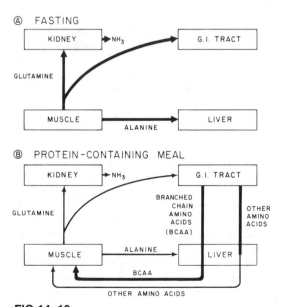

FIG 14–10.
A and **B,** amino acid disposal in fasting and feeding.

the preferred substrate for gluconeogenesis. Glutamine is taken up by the kidneys and by the gastrointestinal tract. In the kidneys glutamine is a precursor of NH_3, which is generated at a high rate during starvation. This is teleonomically advantageous, since ketoacid excretion occurs during starvation and the increased NH_3 availability for excretion has the effect of decreasing sodium loss in the urine.

Alanine is generated in muscle from other amino acids, which donate amino groups to carbohydrate-derived pyruvate. Pyruvate may be generated primarily from muscle glycogen, since utilization of circulating glucose is low in this circumstance. This arrangement is a feature of the primary end of gluconeogenesis—to provide new glucose for the brain and other obligatory glucose-oxidizing tissues.

The importance of alanine as the principal gluconeogenic substrate is indicated by the fact that it is a prime stimulator of secretion of an important gluconeogenic hormone, glucagon. Another hormone long identified with the gluconeogenic process, cortisol, renders the α cell highly sensitive to the stimulatory effect of alanine. This combined control of an important biologic process by substrate availability and stimulation of secretion of appropriate hormones is an excellent example of interlocking control systems.

The interorgan trade in amino acids that follows ingestion of a protein meal is equally interesting. Felig and others have been able to estimate the extent of abstraction of individual amino acids from the portal blood mixture, which represents a hydrolysate of the protein in the meal. The liver retains a large fraction of most of the amino acids in the portal blood mixture, but it permits most of the branched chain amino acids—valine, leucine, isoleucine—to pass through to the general circulation. Thus the mixture abstracted from the blood by skeletal muscle contains a preponderance of branched chain amino acids. Even during absorption of the protein meal from the gastrointestinal tract, when insulin secretion is stimulated and protein synthesis is occurring in muscle cells, the muscle still releases alanine and glutamine. The alanine is returned to the liver where it helps to sustain gluconeogenesis, which prevents the hypoglycemia that might otherwise occur because of stimulation of insulin secretion by amino acids. Thus, during absorption of a meat meal digest, the usually antagonistic hormones, insulin and glucagon, work in tandem—the former to promote storage of the components of the meal and the latter to prevent hypoglycemia.

Many investigators have shown unmistakably that the circulating insulin levels decrease sharply on starvation, that insulin release in response to many re-leasing signals is diminished on starvation and that both adipocytes and muscle of the starved individual are relatively insulin resistant. In fact, starvation resembles a sort of mild diabetes. Cahill stresses insulin withdrawal as a critical feature of the adaptation to starvation. This would account for fatty acid mobilization from adipose tissue, ketosis, and diminished protein synthesis in muscle. It is stated that glucocorticoids may play a largely permissive role in the control of substrate traffic during starvation, since they tend to be excreted in diminishing amounts as starvation is prolonged.

Recent work by Gerich, by McGarry and Foster, and by Unger and associates has indicated that some of the manifestations of the response to starvation or to insulin deprivation (as in diabetes) can be blocked by somatostatin, which blocks glucagon secretion. Sherwin and Felig and their colleagues have questioned the importance of glucagon excess relative to insulin deficiency largely on the grounds that the blood sugar-lowering effect of glucagon is only transitory. Moreover, they suggest that some of the improvement in diabetes brought about by somatostatin in Gerich's studies is caused by somatostatin's inhibition of glucose absorption from the alimentary tract.

The participants in this dialogue are not really in serious disagreement. All agree that insulin deficiency is important, and few doubt that elimination of glucagon (1) decreases ketogenesis and (2) decreases hepatic gluconeogenesis. The peripheral effects of insulin on glucose utilization and on lipolysis are not powerfully antagonized by glucagon. It is perhaps unfair to expect glucagon to oppose insulin without its allied hormones. In fact, the apparently transitory effect of glucagon on blood sugar lowering may be due to the recruitment of catecholamines and other blood sugar-raising hormones by the transitory blood sugar-lowering effect of somatostatin. Gerich et al. have shown that treatment of an insulin-deficient diabetic for five days with somatostatin certainly causes amelioration of the diabetic state.

Glucose-Fatty Acid Cycle

It has long been known that starvation or feeding fat-rich, carbohydrate-poor diets results in impaired glucose tolerance and comparative insensitivity to insulin in intact animals and men. In fact, increased rates of oxidation of fatty acid and correspondingly decreased rates of glucose oxidation have been described in diaphragms obtained from either diabetic or fat-fed rats. It had been widely assumed that these effects were mainly attributable to the fact that the rate of insulin release from the pancreas is diminished in starvation and fat feeding.

Randle and colleagues, among others, have emphasized the fact that fatty acids can modify the pattern of metabolism of carbohydrate in muscle in a striking way in a very short time. Such acute effects of fatty acids can even be seen in isolated tissues in vitro, particularly in the isolated perfused heart and the diaphragm. In such tissues, acute insulin insensitivity, impaired ability to oxidize glucose to lactic acid and a diminished rate of oxidation of pyruvic acid can all be elicited simply by perfusing the tissue with fatty acids or ketone bodies.

The carbohydrate-sparing action of fatty acids and their metabolic products also illustrates how an effect of hormone deprivation in one type of cell can powerfully influence events in a distant cell of another type. If too much FFA is released from the fat cells, it can function as a signal to inhibit carbohydrate metabolism in muscle cells in the manner described. In fact, there is evidence obtained from studies on maturity-onset diabetic patients that carbohydrate and insulin intolerance may occur despite adequate or even supernormal amounts of insulin in the blood in response to a glucose challenge. Randle and colleagues have mustered evidence to suggest that the serum FFA levels of these insulin-resistant diabetics are inappropriately high both in the fasting state and for some time after a glucose load. They suggest that some of the carbohydrate and insulin intolerance of this group of people may be attributed to the glucose-sparing effect of too much FFA in the blood. Fatty-acid-as-signal, which is the fundamental message of Randle's glucose-fatty acid cycle postulate, illustrates that metabolic control occurs simultaneously at many levels and that concentrations of normally occurring metabolites constitute part of the information system of a cell and may determine substrate traffic patterns in the cell.

Insulin (see below) is a protein that is inactivated in certain tissues, especially the liver. As indicated above, insulin binding precedes internalization and destruction of the insulin molecule by the liver cell. Variations in the rates of insulin inactivation and breakdown could conceivably affect glucose tolerance.

There are certain conditions and processes that have only an apparent effect on BG; a few of these are indicated in Figure 14–8 in brackets. Dehydration appears to elevate the BG only because the concentration of all blood solutes is increased by virtue of a diminution in the volume of the fluid in which they are dissolved. The very elevated BG concentrations found in severely acidotic diabetics owe some of their height to coexisting hemoconcentration. These, then, are some of the influences that tend to raise the BG concentration.

ADAPTATION TO REFEEDING: FORCES THAT TEND TO LOWER BLOOD GLUCOSE

The response to refeeding may begin before any food is actually ingested. The sight, smell or even anticipation of eating initiates the cephalic phase of the digestive process. Secretory and motor activity of the gastrointestinal tract may be stimulated, and indeed these responses can be conditioned, as Pavlov showed.

The nature of the food mixture that is introduced into the stomach determines to some extent the progression of assimilation of nutrients by eliciting specific gastrointestinal hormones. For example, fat ingestion prolongs gastric emptying time, whereas a fat-free sucrose-containing drink enters the duodenum very quickly. Even the nature of the carbohydrate affects the rate of assimilation from the gastrointestinal tract. Monosaccharides derived from a mixture of starch and fiber enter the circulation more slowly than glucose or the products of sucrose hydrolysis.

As we have seen, gastrointestinal hormones, whose secretion is elicited by stimuli in the intestinal contents, alert the endocrine pancreas to its imminent nutrient disposal problem. Depending on the metabolic mixture absorbed, insulin, glucagon, and somatostatin are secreted in varying ratios. If pure carbohydrate is taken, insulin (and somatostatin) is secreted selectively and the combination of glucose and insulin inhibits glucagon secretion. A protein meal elicits all three islet hormones.

The major processes promoted by the endocrine pancreatic hormones during feeding are synthesis and storage. Under the influence of insulin, liver, muscle, and adipose tissue take up carbohydrate and oxidize or store it as glycogen or fat. About 55% of an ingested dose of glucose is taken up by the liver; only 15% is taken up by insulin-dependent tissues (adipose tissue and skeletal muscle); and 25% is abstracted by insulin-independent tissue (brain, nerves, formed elements of the blood, renal medulla and germinal epithelium of the testis) (Fig 14–11).

In the refeeding situation the liver conserves carbohydrate as glycogen or fat, and secretion of glucose by the liver is suppressed. In some species, including human beings, the liver is the major lipogenic organ; triglyceride synthesized in the hepatocyte is exported as VLDL to the adipocyte for storage. The adipocyte is able to store the lipid of VLDL because insulin stimulates the enzyme lipoprotein lipase (sometimes

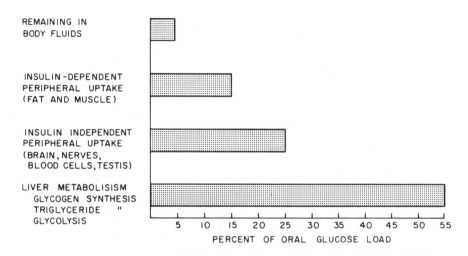

(DATA FROM FELIG, WAHREN AND HENDLER, 1975)

FIG 14–11.
Pattern of disposal of oral glucose load.

called clearing factor lipase). At the same time, insulin promotes retention of triglyceride in the adipocyte by inhibiting lipolysis. Although insulin does lower the cAMP of adipocytes, lipolysis inhibition can be demonstrated when there is no change in cAMP concentration. The precise mechanism of insulin's antipolytic effect in adipocytes is not known.

The most prominent events in skeletal muscle during refeeding are glycogen deposition and a shift from protein catabolism to protein synthesis. This involves not only positive stimulation of protein synthesis but also coordinate inhibition of protein catabolism.

An example of the coordinate responses of pancreatic β and α cells to a carbohydrate meal is shown in Figure 14–12. Figure 14–13 is an attempt to suggest that the nervous system, gastrointestinal hormones, incoming substrates and islet hormones all participate in the overall response of the islet. To the positive and negative influences shown, we can now add inhibitory effects of somatostatin on both α and β cell secretion.

Microhomeostasis: Examples of Intracellular Control Mechanisms

Having examined the coordinate control of substrate traffic in the intact organism, it is pertinent to inspect some mechanisms involved in the control of substrate flow within the liver cell. Before we proceed to a detailed account of specific biochemical pathways, it is necessary to make a few general points about control mechanisms.

1. It is impossible separately to describe control

mechanisms that are operative in gluconeogenesis, ketogenesis, and lipogenesis because all of these processes are under simultaneous control by the same set of signals. An intracellular substrate and hormonal "climate" that favors gluconeogenesis and ketogene-

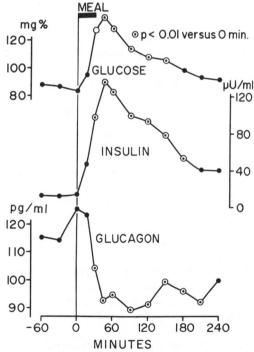

FIG 14–12.
Suppression of glucagon secretion by carbohydrate meal in 11 normal subjects. (From Unger R: *N Engl J Med* 1970; 283:109.)

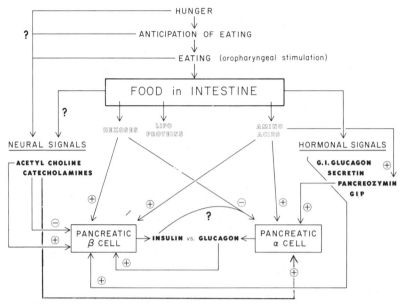

FIG 14–13.
Coordinate control of insulin and glucagon secretion by neural, hormonal, and substrate signals. *GIP* = gastric inhibitory peptide.

sis actively discourages lipogenesis, and vice versa.

2. Control occurs at certain points in a metabolic pathway in two different time scales: (a) *acutely*, when no change in the population of enzyme molecules occurs, and (b) *chronically,* when there may be large changes in the equilibrium concentrations of certain rate-limiting enzymes.

3. *Acute control* may involve any or all of the following:

a. Change in the *quantity of available substrate* or of substrate removal.

b. Change in the *availability of* a necessary *coenzyme* (e.g., NAD, NADH, NADP, NADPH).

c. *Change in energy level* (e.g., ATP, ADP, GTP, GDP).

d. *Change in ionic environment,* which may affect the kinetic capability or behavior of a rate-limiting enzyme.

e. *Covalent* modification of the enzyme (e.g., protein phosphorylation by cAMP-dependent, Ca^{2+}Calmodulin-dependent, C kinase and others).

f. *Allosteric* activation or inhibition by noncovalently bound metabolites, e.g., phosphorylated intermediates of glucose metabolism, ATP, citrate, fatty acids and fatty acyl CoAs (coenzyme A).

4. *Chronic* control mechanisms involve the resetting of the equilibrium concentrations of key enzymes. These adaptive changes in populations of enzyme molecules often occur at metabolic switch points that are most obviously under (often multiple) acute controlling influences. They involve changes in the rates of synthesis and of degradation of enzyme protein. Studies on a few enzyme proteins by purifying the enzyme in question; raising an antibody to it; and studying the rate of synthesis (by immunoprecipitation of enzyme protein) by comparing the rate of enzyme synthesis with that of general protein synthesis have permitted the conclusion that, in some instances (G-6-PD, NADP malic enzyme, acetyl CoA carboxylase, fatty acid synthetase, gluconeogenic enzymes inducible by glucocorticoids), gene transcription is involved in the induction. Examples of enzyme induction were discussed in Chapters 2, 10, and 11.

5. Rate-limiting, controlling enzymes are most likely to occur when two *different* enzymes or enzyme systems catalyze the forward and backward reactions.

KETOGENESIS

A decrease in insulin availability and an excess of insulin antagonists, most notably glucagon and catecholamines, result in (1) lipolysis and FFA mobilization and (2) a direct effect on the liver cell, which favors ketone body production.

The carnitine acyltransferase carrier system escorts fatty acids across the mitochondrial membrane to the interior of the mitochondrion where fatty acyl CoA is re-formed and carnitine diffuses out to participate in the transport of additional fatty acid (Fig 14–14). The most striking feature of this system is that it is regulated in large part by the availability of carnitine and not by changes in the apoprotein of the transferase enzyme. Thus when ketogenesis rates are high, the carnitine content of the liver is high; conversely, in the lipogenically active liver (i.e., the liver dominated by insulin) carnitine concentration is low (see McGarry and Foster).

Ketogenesis occurs when the insulin:glucagon ratio is low, as in starvation and diabetic ketoacidosis. Cyclic AMP is elevated and its protein kinase substrates are phosphorylated. Catabolic events (glycogenolysis, lipolysis) are dominant, and anabolic processes (general protein synthesis, lipogenesis) are inhibited. Gluconeogenesis is coordinately stimulated.

Carnitine is a trimethylated product of the amino acid lysine, its methyl groups having been donated by S-adenosyl methionine (see Hulse et al.). Owing to the extensive protein breakdown that occurs in starvation, lysine availability is great when the need for high concentrations of carnitine is present. Whether the extremely complex system of enzymes responsible for synthesizing carnitine adaptively increases at times of ketogenesis is unknown to us.

Another example of the exquisite coordination of events in the liver cell is the fact that malonyl CoA, a prime intermediate in the synthesis of fatty acids, is an allosteric inhibitor of carnitine acyltransferase (see McGarry et al.; see Fig 14–14). Thus, when lipogenesis is inhibited (as it notoriously is in starvation and insulin deficiency), the malonyl CoA concentration falls; carnitine acyltransferase is released from inhibition, and fatty acid transport into the mitochondrion is facilitated. Cyclic AMP, which is high in the ketotic liver cell, stimulates triglyceride lipolysis by activating a lipase (Fig 14–14, ①) and simultaneously inhibits the formation of malonyl CoA via the rate-limiting step in fatty acid synthesis, acetyl CoA carboxylase (Fig 14–14, ②). Additionally, the process of fatty acid synthesis is inhibited by high concentrations of fatty acids. It is the combination of FFA mobilized from the periphery and the dominance of lipolysis over lipogenesis in the liver cell that is responsible for generating the acetyl CoA that forms the ketone bodies, acetoacetate and β-hydroxybutyrate. Since fatty acid oxidation provides a reducing environment (NADH > NAD) and since conversion of acetoacetate to β-hydroxybutyrate requires NADH, most of the ketone body mixture exported from the liver is in the form of β-hydroxybutyrate.

GLUCONEOGENESIS

In Figure 14–15,A, we have tried to describe the conditions in a hepatocyte that is poised for ketogenesis (see preceding section) and for gluconeogenesis.

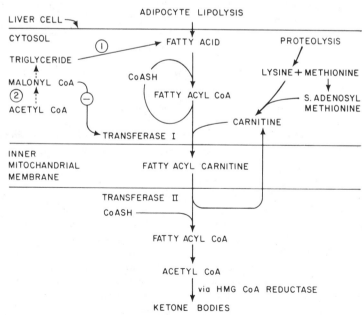

FIG 14–14.
Ketogenesis. (Largely after McGarry J and Foster DW.)

A. GLUCONEOGENESIS

B. LIPOGENESIS

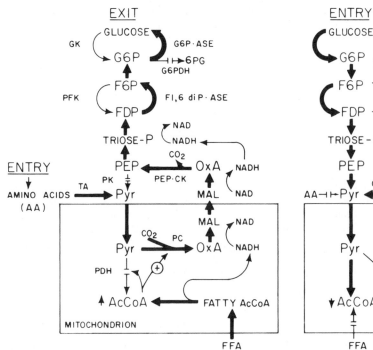

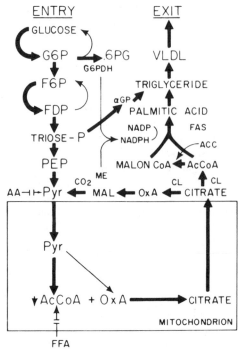

FIG 14–15.

A, gluconeogenesis. **B,** lipogenesis. *Substrates: G6P* = glucose 6 phosphate; *F6P* = fructose 6 phosphate; *FDP* = fructose diphosphate; *PEP* = phosphoenol pyruvate; *AcCoA* = acetyl coenzyme A; *OxA* = oxalacetic acid; *MAL* = malic acid; Malon CoA = malony CoA; *VLDL* = very-low-density lipoproteins. *Enzymes: GK* = gluco-kinase; *PFK* = phosphofructokinase; *PK* = py- ruvate kinase; *TA* = transaminase; *PDH* = pyruvic dehydrogenase; *PC* = pyruvic carboxylase; *PEPCK* = PEP carboxykinase; *F1,6 dl P·ASE* = fructose 1,6 diphosphatase; *G6PDH* = glucose 6 phosphate dehydrogenase; *G6P·ASE* = glucose 6 phosphatase; *ME* = NADP malicenzyme; *CL* = citrate lyase; *ACC* = acetyl CoA carbox-ylase; *FAS* = fatty acid synthase.

The point of entry is the increased rate of delivery of gluconeogenic substrate to the liver from the periphery, predominantly from skeletal muscle and principally as alanine (see glucose-amino acid cycle). This occurs when insulin availability is low and insulin antagonists are dominant. The hepatocyte cAMP concentration in this circumstance tends to be high.

Alanine is transaminated (via *TA*) to pyruvate, which enters the mitochondrion. There it encounters conditions that are mainly caused by the delivery of large amounts of FFA to the liver, again owing to the dominance of counterregulatory hormones over insulin in the fat cell. Increased oxidation of FFA, besides causing ketogenesis (see preceding section) has two consequences: (1) concentration of acetyl CoA (*AcCoA*) in the mitochondrion increases markedly and (2) NADH is generated from NAD. The *AcCoA* in-

hibits the pyruvate dehydrogenase (*PDH*) complex and, simultaneously, allosterically activates pyruvate carboxylase (*PC*). *PDH* is under complex control, but one of its controlling influences is a cAMP-*in*dependent protein kinase, which phosphorylates it to an inactive form when the hepatocyte is under glucagon's influence. The dephospho form, which predominates in insulin-dominated cells, is active. In the gluconeogenic condition, pyruvate is "steered" to oxalacetate (*OxA*) but, owing to the large excess of NADH over NAD (generated by β oxidation of fatty acyl CoA), malate (*MAL*) is formed. This turns out to be a fortunate event because the mitochondrial membrane is equipped to transport malate to the cytoplasm but is unable to transport *OxA*.

When malate encounters the cytosol, NAD predominates over NADH, since little NADH is generated by the Emden-Meyerhof pathway in this circumstance. Therefore, *OxA* is re-formed, and reducing equivalents generated by fatty acid oxidation are shuttled out of the mitochondrion into the cytosol where they are required for the gluconeogenic process at the triose level.

OxA is decarboxylated to phosphoenolpyruvate (*PEP*) by the key gluconeogenic enzyme phosphoenolpyruvate carboxykinase (*PEP CK*). Recently, several groups of investigators (see Pilkis et al.) have discovered that the enzyme pyruvate kinase (*PK*) is phosphorylated to an inactive state by cAMP-dependent protein kinase and is thus inactivated under gluconeogenic conditions. This encourages the disposal of *PEP* upward toward triose phosphates. This is an elegant design, since if *PK* remained unidirectionally patent, *PEP* generation from alanine, once begun, would become an elaborate wheel-spinning, futile cycle. (See next section for discussion of PFK-F1,6P$_2$ control.)

The final control point is at the G-6-Pase step, which hydrolyzes phosphate from glucose phosphate and permits secretion of glucose into the bloodstream. G-6-Pase is assisted in performing its function because the high concentration of fatty acids and fatty acyl CoAs in the liver cell under these conditions inhibits a number of enzymes, among them glucokinase (*GK*) and G-6-PD (glucose-6-phosphate dehydrogenase), as well as the major enzymes of fatty acid synthesis, acetyl CoA carboxylase (*ACC*) and fatty acid synthetase (FAS).

The beauty of the system is obvious. Control operates at critical switch points. The oxidation of fatty acids, in addition to furnishing fatty acid-derived substrates in the form of ketone bodies for use by peripheral tissues, provides the reducing equivalents to sustain gluconeogenesis. Also, this process illustrates how intramitochondrial events are correlated with events that occur in the cytosol.

Regulation of gene expression by glucocorticoids was discussed in Chapter 11.

LIPOGENESIS

When refeeding occurs and the organism is confronted with the problem of storing incoming nutrients because they are being absorbed in far greater amounts than those required for current use, insulin is secreted and the secretion of counterregulatory hormones—particularly glucagon and growth hormone—is suppressed. The insulin is delivered directly to the liver in a concentration that exceeds that in peripheral arterial blood. Glucose is also present in portal venous blood in high concentration. The liver cell there-

fore is confronted with a drastic shift in hormonal dominance and in proportions of glucose, amino acids and fatty acids in its metabolic mixture. Insulin encourages protein synthesis and inhibits protein breakdown in skeletal and cardiac muscle and in other tissues, thus reducing the amino acid supply of the liver from those sources. Similarly, the antilipolytic effect of insulin in fat cells inhibits the release of FFA from adipose tissue and thus decreases FFA concentration of the liver perfusate.

By acting directly on the liver cell (which contains readily demonstrable insulin receptors), insulin promotes glycogen deposition (see Chapter 3) and inhibits glucose release. The liver, in fact, responds to much smaller concentrations of insulin than are necessary to produce certain biologic responses in skeletal muscle or adipose tissue (see Rabinowitz and Liljenquist).

Figure 14–15,B represents a simplified account of the response of the hepatocyte to glucose and insulin and to a decrease in counterregulatory hormone influence. The control points are the same as those discussed in the section on gluconeogenesis, but the substrate flow is in the opposite direction.

Glucose encounters no permeability barrier in liver cells as it does in muscle and adipocytes: the plasma membrane is freely permeable to glucose. However, whether or not glucose can enter the Emden-Meyerhof pathway depends on the outcome of the contest between *GK* (glucokinase) and G-6-Pase. Insulin controls the equilibrium concentration of *GK*: in diabetes, *GK* concentration falls and, with insulin treatment, it rises. The mechanism for this is not entirely understood: it may be due, at least in part, to the decreased concentration of fatty acids in insulinized liver cells. This same fall in fatty acid and fatty acyl CoA concentration relieves the inhibition of the pentose phosphate pathway (G-6-PDH). This has the effect of siphoning off G-6-P and therefore denying substrate to G-6-Pase. Glucokinase is the clear winner.

Fructose-2,6 Bisphosphate: A Third Messenger

The information processing that occurs in cells following the delivery of the *first* message (hormone) to its receptor is transduced into a variety of *second* messages (cyclic AMP, Ca^{2+}, Ca^{2+}Calmodulin, inositol triphosphate, diacylglycerol, insulin second messengers, etc.). Now, as a result of discoveries by Hers and coworkers and by S. J. Pilkis and colleagues (see El Maghrabi et al.), we can describe a control mechanism that operates at the phosphofructokinase (PFK) versus fructose-1,6 bisphosphatase (F-1,6 P$_2$ase) couple. In Figure 14–16 we have attempted to

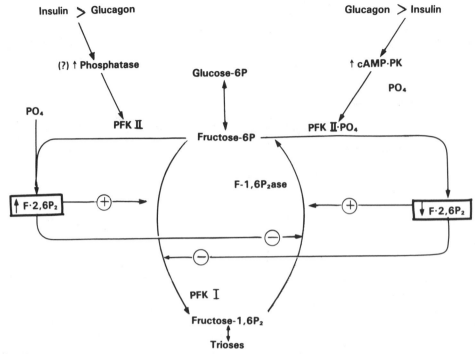

FIG 14–16.
The role of fructose 2,6 bisphosphate (F-2, 6P₂) in the regulation of phosphofructokinase I (PFK I) and fructose 1,6 bisphosphatase (F-1,6P₂ase). Substrate flow (glycolysis versus gluconeogenesis) is regulated by controls exerted on these enzymes. (From the data of Hers HG: *Biochem Soc Trans* 1984; 11:411, and El-Maghrabi, et al. J.B.C. 1982; 257:7603.)

depict the elegant symmetry of control exerted by a *third* messenger, fructose-2,6 bisphosphate, or F-2,6 P₂.

The key to understanding this mechanism is the recognition that [F-2,6 P₂] in the liver cell *increases* in the fed state; i.e., in the presence of glucose, when the molar ratio of insulin:glucagon is high. Its concentration *decreases* when the hormone ratio is reversed, i.e., in starvation and diabetes. The enzyme PFK II, which catalyzes the formation of F-2,6 P₂, is oddly bifunctional; that is to say, when it is phosphorylated, it functions as a phosphatase and *diminishes* the concentration of F-2,6 P₂, but when it is *de*phosphorylated, it acts as a kinase and *increases* the production of F-2,6 P₂ and therefore its concentration.

The phosphorylation state of PFK II is controlled by cyclic-AMP-dependent protein kinase and an insulin-dependent phosphatase (we are not exactly sure of the last point, but we know that insulin activates other phosphatases and we guess that it activates this one as well).

F-2,6 P₂, the third messenger, markedly stimulates PFK I (the original PFK 6 PF-1 kinase) at catalytic concentrations, and it coordinately inhibits the opposing enzyme, F-1,6 P₂ase. This has the effect of directing substrate traffic downward to the triose level. A *decreased* F-2,6 P₂ concentration has a meaning of its own: by reversing the effect of the third messenger on the downward flow of substrates through the glycolytic pathway, upward flow is facilitated. Thus, high F-2,6 P₂ favors lipogenesis from glucose, and low F-2,6 P₂ permits gluconeogenesis from trioses.

Understandably, elucidation of this mechanism has generated much interest and comment (for example, see Foster). However, its esthetic appeal should not obscure the fact that *simultaneous* adjustments are being made at other paired enzyme loci as we suggested in our discussion of the cellular mechanism of action of insulin. Regulation at the PFK I–F-1,6 P₂ase reaction is part of a grand regulatory design that pervades the cell when it is dominated by either insulin or glucagon.

Again, *PK* (pyruvate kinase), whose blockade was so critical in sustaining the flow of pyruvate to glucose, is now *de*phosphorylated because cAMP protein kinase is relatively inactive. This permits the flow of large amounts of pyruvate into the mitochondria.

There, *PDH* (pyruvate dehydrogenase) is not only released from inhibition because the *AcCoA* concentration is low, it is also dephosphorylated because insulin causes activation of its phosphatase (see discussion above). PC (pyruvate carboxylase) is relatively less active because of the low concentration of *AcCoA*.

Citrate is generated in large quantities and readily enters the cytosol via a tricarboxylic acid transport system, which, in starvation and diabetes, is inhibited by fatty acyl CoAs but is now uninhibited. Citrate is cleaved by citrate-lyase into *AcCoA* and *OxA*. The *AcCoA* is carboxylated to malonyl CoA by *AcCoA* carboxylase (*ACC*) and, together, they enter the FAS (fatty acid synthesis) pathway. As we have seen, malonyl CoA inhibits fatty acid oxidation at the carnitine acyl transferase I locus.

The fate of *OxA* in the cytosol is interesting because it appears to be so teleonomically useful. Since the Emden-Meyerhof pathway is now extremely active, much NADH is generated. Therefore, *OxA* goes promptly to malate. The enzyme that decarboxylates malate—malic enzyme (*ME*)—requires NADP and generates NADPH. The whole reaction sequence, then, is a mechanism for transferring reducing equivalents from NADH to NADPH. This is the co-factor that is required for lipogenesis, just as NADH is required for gluconeogenesis. Additional NADPH for lipogenesis is generated by the first two reactions of the pentose phosphate pathway (the first of which is shown in Fig 14–15, B).

Stimulation of lipogenesis by insulin is the result of three simultaneous events: (1) provision of lipogenic substrate in the form of cytosolic AcCoA; (2) establishment of the proper coenzyme environment (NADPH generation); and (3) *removal* of inhibitory influences on the lipogenic process in starvation and diabetes. These inhibitory influences include the following:

1. Inhibition of glucokinase, G-6-PD, acetyl CoA carboxylase, fatty acid synthetase and egress of citrate from the mitochondria by high fatty acyl CoA concentrations.

2. Decreased activity of pyruvate kinase, acetyl CoA carboxylase and pyruvate dehydrogenase (PDH) (insulin dephosphorylates PDH). The first two of these enzymes are believed to be substrates for cAMP-dependent protein kinase.

3. A low concentration of F2,6P$_2$.

Other possible contributions of decreased cAMP generation are (a) activation of intrahepatic triglyceride lipase is decreased, and (b) the mitochondrial membrane may contain cAMP-sensitive constituents, which participate in establishing the selective permeability of the membrane to metabolites generated in the mitochondrion.

Fatty acid synthesis in starvation and diabetes is inhibited by fatty acids partly owing to a lack of α glycerophosphate (α GP), which is low when gluconeogenesis is active. However, when the Emden-Meyerhof pathway is in heavy use, α GP is generated and therefore becomes available for esterifying new synthesized fatty acyl CoAs.

PROTEIN SYNTHESIS AND BREAKDOWN

It has long been recognized that protein synthesis and positive nitrogen balance are promoted by insulin and that the counterregulatory hormones—glucagon, catecholamines and cortisol—have generally opposite effects on overall protein synthesis. One member of the counterregulatory group, growth hormone, is an anabolic agent, like insulin.

Regulation of protein synthesis and breakdown in skeletal and cardiac muscle has been the subject of many studies by Wool et al., Morgan et al., and Goldberg et al.

Protein synthesis in muscle is stimulated by insulin, by branched chain amino acids (leucine, isoleucine, valine), by glucose, by ketone bodies and, most particularly, by repeated contractions. Protein synthesis can be measured by studying the rate of incorporation of a radioactively labeled amino acid into protein. Protein degradation can be measured by prelabeling muscle protein with a radioactive amino acid and then following the disappearance of the label from the protein over time. Synthesis and breakdown of protein, like that of glycogen, are coordinately controlled; i.e., when synthesis is stimulated, breakdown is inhibited, and vice versa.

Effects of insulin on phosphorylation of ribosomal protein S6 and initiation of translation, as well as its effect on enzyme induction, were discussed above under cellular mechanism of action of insulin.

Insulin Deficiency and Excess

ETIOLOGY OF DIABETES MELLITUS: GENETIC AND ENVIRONMENTAL FACTORS

There are many animal models (chiefly rodents and hamsters) of hereditary syndromes that resemble human diabetes mellitus. Although the patterns of expression of the disease are quite variable from one model to another, there is no doubt about the genetic transmission of the disorder. In some of these models, genetic analysis suggests a single gene mutation.

It is interesting to recall attitudes toward the etiology of human diabetes mellitus in the light of these studies on experimental animal models. Before 1950 or so, diabetes mellitus in man was regarded as a single disease, which occurred in more severe form in children and young adults than in middle age. It was all one disease and equally hereditary in all respects. Although there was some hedging on the single gene hypothesis (e.g., "incomplete penetrance"), few investigators voiced any serious disagreement with it.

The concept that diabetes is a group of diseases, differing in etiology, biochemical features, and natural history, began to develop around 1950. The classification into juvenile-onset, ketosis-prone, insulin-dependent (Type I) and maturity-onset, ketosis-resistant, insulin-independent (Type II) came into general use and was formalized in 1979. Since many diabetics do not fit precisely into either group (example: maturity onset diabetes of youth, MODY), the 1979 classification is now being reexamined. The newly discovered syndromes of anti-insulin receptor antibody diabetes, genetically modified insulin diabetes, and familial proinsulinemia go beyond the old (1979) categorization. When radioimmunoassay methods for insulin and C peptide became available, it was clear that Type I diabetics are divisible into two general groups: one that secretes little or no C peptide in response to a glucose challenge and another whose C peptide secretory response (and, therefore, presumably insulin secretion) is present but variably impaired. It was also found that many Type II diabetics were not insulin deficient at all, but rather showed supernormal (though delayed) elevations of serum insulin following stimulation by glucose or other secretagogues. In retrospect, many observations suggested multiple etiologies for diabetes mellitus. Some of these were the following:

Extensive studies on identical (monozygote) twins have revealed the interesting fact that, whereas the concordance rate in adult-onset diabetes is virtually 100%, it is only about 50% in twins whose disease began before they were 45 years of age. Thus, although these high incidence rates certainly confirm the presence of some genetic factor, the lower rate in the younger group indicates the play of environmental factors as well.

It has recently been established that predisposition to Type I diabetes is linked to the HLA-D locus on the short arm of chromosome 6. This region has been associated with the determination of immune responses. Patients with certain alterations of genes in this region are susceptible to autoimmune destruction of their beta cells in response to various environmental factors that need not necessarily be present in the same proportions. Though this precise histocompatibility antigen association holds for Type I diabetes and not Type II, there are certainly strong genetic components in the etiology of the latter, though no clearcut genetic markers have been identified. Some authorities believe that the primary defect in Type II diabetes is in the beta cell, while others are more impressed by target cell resistance to insulin as the major problem. We are inclined to believe that these views are not really mutually exclusive (reviewed in Efendić et al.).

Antibodies against proteins of islet cells (ICA) are often found in insulin-dependent diabetics, suggesting an autoimmune component of the disease. In fact, the few patients with insulin-*in*dependent diabetes in whom ICAs are detected are likely to progress, in time, to insulin dependence.

For decades a number of *chemical agents* have been used to produce destruction of pancreatic β cells. Alloxan and streptozotocin have been the principal betacytotoxic agents in general use in experimental animals. The disease induced by these substances closely resembles insulin-dependent diabetes in man.

That the β cells may be selectively damaged by *betacytotrophic viruses* has been convincingly demonstrated by Craighead and others. A long list of such viruses has been compiled (e.g., Coxsackie B, measles, cytomegalovirus, Epstein-Barr virus, mumps virus) but only the last has been shown to enter the pancreatic β cell in vitro.

When we add to all of these observations the fact that *epidemiologic associations* have been made between the incidence of mumps and other viral infections and of juvenile diabetes mellitus, the parallel between certain animal models and the human condition becomes more evident. In fact, one animal model has been described (see Rossini et al.) in which a chemical intoxication of the β cells, a virus infection and cell-mediated immunity all collaborated to produce diabetes.

The frequent association of *obesity* with diabetes in people was observed often in the 19th century. Obesity coexists frequently in many of the genetic obesities in experimental animals, and striking insulin resistance occurs in hypothalamic obesity in rodents. (See discussion of insulin receptor above.)

Perhaps the fairest way to summarize the emerging view is to suggest that the *expression* of the syndrome of diabetes in any individual may be the integrated response to multiple factors (e.g., genetic predisposition, environmental chemical and infectious agents, autoimmune events, nutrition, physical activity and psychologic stress), which may be operative in different proportions.

A graphic summary of these ideas is given in Figure 14–17.

PATHOPHYSIOLOGY OF DIABETIC KETOACIDOSIS

There is no better way to appreciate what insulin means to the economy of the body than to study the effect of acute insulin deprivation. When insulin is withdrawn acutely from a severely diabetic animal or man, a remarkable sequence of intricately interconnected events is begun and, if there is no intervention, the inevitable outcome is coma and death. These events involve not merely carbohydrate metabolism but fat, protein, electrolyte and water metabolism as well. The repercussions of insulin lack appear in the CNS, the respiratory system, the cardiovascular system, the renal excretory system and the gastrointestinal system. Insulin withdrawal permits the unopposed action of the counterregulatory hormones.

What happens in the insulin-deprived diabetic patient is a ghastly caricature of the normal adaptation to starvation. Many of the same kinds of changes occur, but the responses are inappropriately violent. Moreover, it is often difficult for the beginning stu-

dent to understand the interrelations of many things that are happening more or less simultaneously. For this reason we have elected to make an arbitrary division of our description into three fragments, and then to show how all of these processes are related. This discussion is concerned with the level of organization of the whole animal or person.

"CARBOHYDRATE" METABOLISM

The primary event is relative insulin withdrawal. In diabetic patients, this may not necessarily mean an absolute decrease in the amount of insulin the patient takes but rather a sudden and unexpected increase in his requirement. An attack of acidosis may be precipitated by an infection, by physical trauma, by emotional stress—all of which tend to increase the need for insulin. Or it may be initiated by the omission of insulin. Often, there are nausea and vomiting, which are associated with failure of food and water intake.

With insulin lack, there is decrease in glucose use by the peripheral tissues, mainly muscle and adipose tissue. This contributes to the developing hyperglycemia, and liver and muscle glycogenolysis contributes more. (Gluconeogenesis, too, adds to the increase in blood sugar.) When the BG level rises above the renal threshold for glucose, glycosuria appears and an osmotic diuresis is instituted. This is the

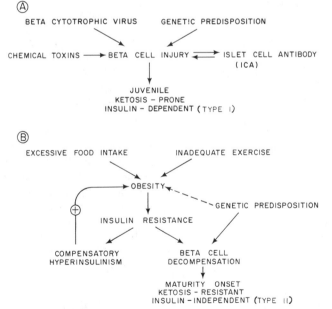

FIG 14–17.
A and **B**, composites of contemporary theories of the etiology of diabetes.

basis of the polyuria of diabetes, the first symptom of the disease to be recognized in antiquity.

The loss of water and electrolytes in the urine, especially in view of the fact that intake by mouth has usually ceased, leads to dehydration and hemoconcentration. This in turn leads to peripheral circulatory failure because of the marked reduction in circulating blood volume or shock. One of the characteristic features of shock is hypotension followed by diminished renal blood flow, which may progress to the point of anuria. Generalized tissue anoxia, with a consequent shift to anaerobic metabolism, results in increasing concentrations of lactic acid in the blood. Coma appears some time after the appearance of peripheral circulatory failure. Death is inevitable in the untreated individual. Figure 14–18 is a diagrammatic summary of this sequence of events.

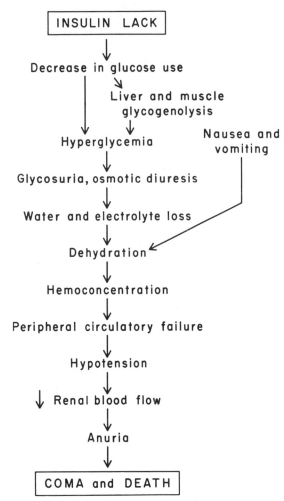

FIG 14–18.
Effect of insulin lack on carbohydrate metabolism.

"Fat" Metabolism

The relative insulin lack and decrease in glucose use by the adipose tissue of the body result in a large-scale mobilization of depot fat into the blood. This may result in a secondary hypertriglyceridemia as the FFAs are synthesized into very low-density lipoproteins by the liver.

The liver is flooded with fat, much of which, for reasons discussed, it can oxidize only as far as the acetyl CoA stage. The 2-carbon fragments then generate acetoacetic acid and β-hydroxybutyric acid, in which form they appear in hepatic venous blood in increasing concentrations. The developing ketonemia has two prominent effects: (1) It leads to a progressive metabolic acidosis, which in turn initiates the characteristic deep and rapid (Kussmaul) breathing that is one of the diagnostic signs of diabetic acidosis. (2) As ketonemia exceeds the renal threshold for ketone body reabsorption, ketone bodies appear in the urine. In the process of being excreted by the kidneys, they deplete the body of fixed base. This contributes to the net sodium loss, which means in effect that the ionic "skeleton" of extracellular water is diminished and can therefore "support" progressively smaller volumes of fluid. These developments are summarized in Figure 14–19.

"Protein" Metabolism

Withdrawal of insulin and impaired use of glucose cause a decrease in protein synthesis and therefore have the effect of promoting net protein catabolism, at first in insulin-sensitive tissues and especially in muscle. This process is accompanied by a net loss of nitrogen from the body. It is also accompanied by release of K^+ and other intracellular ions into the blood and by K^+ excretion in the urine.

Besides the impairment of protein metabolism, there is interference with cell function by other effects of insulin lack. For example, progressive water loss eventually causes intracellular dehydration, which favors catabolic processes and adds to the diffusion of intracellular electrolytes into extracellular water. As long as urine flow continues, there is an opportunity for K^+ to be lost to the body in cumulatively dangerous amounts. A summary of these developments is given in Figure 14–20.

Insulin Resistance of Acidosis

Severely ketoacidotic patients and experimental animals are resistant to the action of insulin. Even the

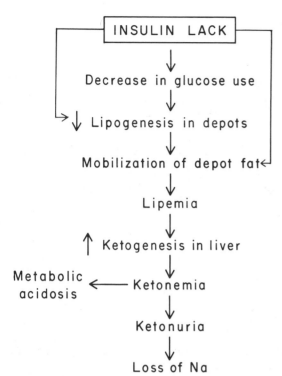

FIG 14–19.
Effect of insulin lack on fat metabolism.

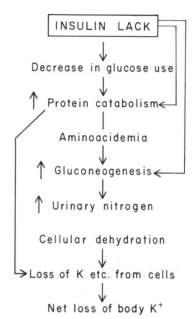

FIG 14–20.
Effect of insulin lack on protein metabolism.

"low-dose" insulin treatment of diabetic ketoacidosis produces levels of circulating insulin that are 4–15 times higher than those found in normal individuals. Many possible mechanisms have been suggested to account for insulin resistance in this circumstance, among them: (1) high levels of circulating FFA; (2) the presence of high concentrations of hormones that are physiologic antagonists of insulin (glucocorticoids, glucagon, catecholamines, growth hormone); (3) the acidosis itself.

Cuthbert and Alberti, on the basis of experiments with severely acidemic diabetic rats, have concluded that the hydrogen ion itself is the probable cause of most of the insulin resistance of diabetic ketoacidosis. They base their conclusion on (1) reversal of the insulin resistance by administration of sodium bicarbonate and (2) duplication of the condition of insulin resistance in nondiabetic rats made acidotic with ammonium chloride. The acidosis interferes with the action of insulin both by affecting hormone-receptor interaction at the plasma membrane and by inhibiting glycolysis at the phosphofructokinase step. Sodium bicarbonate was used in this study as an experimental probe. Obviously it cannot correct all of the metabolic and circulatory abnormalities of diabetic ketoacidosis,

though it may be used as adjunctive treatment (see Ginsberg). Figure 14–21 is a composite summary of the events we have discussed.

Effect of Ketoacidosis on Hemoglobin Function

Figure 14–22 is a diagrammatic syllogism, which describes the effects of acidosis and dehydration on the oxygen-carrying function of hemoglobin. Glycolysis-derived 2,3-diphosphoglyceric acid (2,3-DPG) is an allosteric modulator of hemoglobin (one in Fig 14–22). When its concentration in the red blood cell falls, the affinity of hemoglobin for oxygen is increased and the ability of the hemoglobin to unload O_2 in the tissues is decreased. Among the factors that regulate 2,3-DPG production by the red cell is PO_4 availability: When PO_4 is in short supply, 2,3-DPG levels are low; when PO_4 is abundant, 2,3-DPG levels can rise.

The combination of acidosis and dehydration has the effect of reducing red cell 2,3-DPG concentration. This results in high affinity of hemoglobin for O_2 and decreased delivery of O_2 to the tissues in the microcirculation. Thus, in addition to inadequate perfusion of the tissues because of peripheral circulatory failure, tissue oxygenation is further compromised (two in Fig 14–22),

When ketoacidosis is conventionallly treated (three in Fig 14–22), repletion of fluid volume and correc-

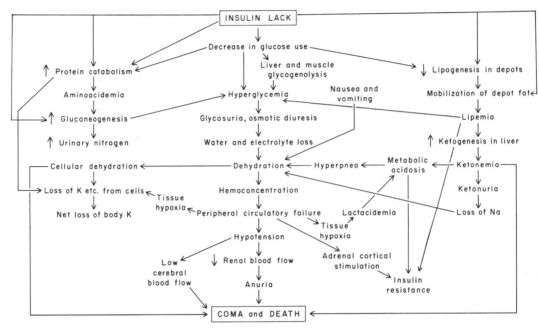

FIG 14–21.
Composite summary of pathophysiology of diabetes acidosis. Note particularly the connections among the three general areas of metabolism.

tion of the insulin deficiency may occur, but one of the consequences of insulin's action is to *lower* serum phosphate concentration. The low serum PO_4 may prevent regeneration of 2,3-DPG in the RBC, and therefore O_2 delivery to the tissues may be persistently impaired. However, if PO_4 is added to the treatment regimen and serum PO_4 is normalized (four in Fig 14–22), normal hemoglobin function may be restored (see Ditzel and Standl).

Summary

When all of these sequential events are united into a single diagram (see Fig 14–21), certain important points become obvious. In the first place, the common starting place for the disturbance can be seen clearly. Second, the intricate interrelations of carbohydrate, fat, protein, electrolyte and water metabolism are well shown in Figure 14–21. Finally, this

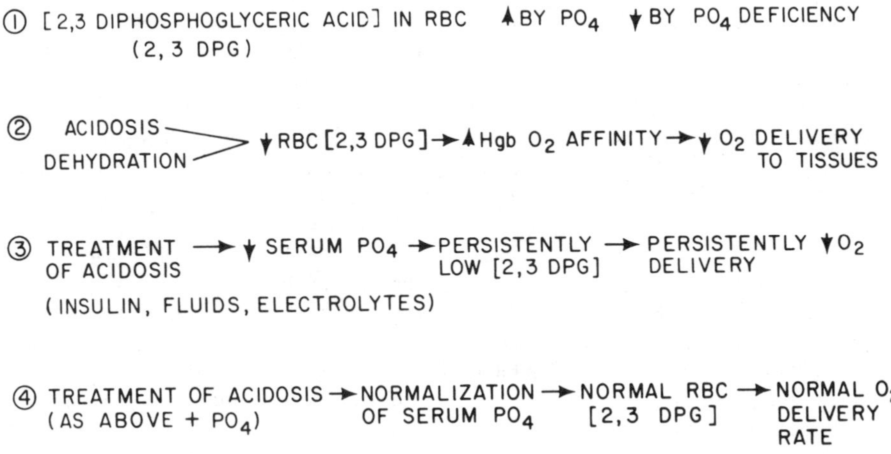

① [2,3 DIPHOSPHOGLYCERIC ACID] IN RBC ▲ BY PO_4 ▼ BY PO_4 DEFICIENCY
  (2, 3 DPG)

② ACIDOSIS————→ ▼ RBC [2,3 DPG] → ▲ Hgb O_2 AFFINITY → ▼ O_2 DELIVERY
  DEHYDRATION   TO TISSUES

③ TREATMENT ——→ ▼ SERUM PO_4 → PERSISTENTLY ——→ PERSISTENTLY ▼ O_2
  OF ACIDOSIS   LOW [2,3 DPG]   DELIVERY
  (INSULIN, FLUIDS, ELECTROLYTES)

④ TREATMENT OF ACIDOSIS → NORMALIZATION → NORMAL RBC → NORMAL O_2
  (AS ABOVE + PO_4)   OF SERUM PO_4 [2,3 DPG]   DELIVERY
                                                            RATE

FIG 14–22.
Effect of ketoacidosis on hemoglobin function.

chart shows the cause-and-effect relationships that have been discussed; it gives some idea of the complexity of the disturbance, and it suggests that many of these interrelated events are occurring at the same time. Proper management of the acidotic patient is almost obvious from the outline given above. If shock is present, measures to increase the effective circulating blood volume should be instituted. This involves the administration of fluid and electrolytes. Acidosis is reversed by administration of sodium bicarbonate. Since insulin lack triggered the whole disturbance, insulin must be given—by vein, if shock is profound and the likelihood of its being picked up from a subcutaneous depot is small. In spite of the fact that the BG level may be very high, depletion of muscle and liver glycogen stores has usually been so extensive that carbohydrate must be infused soon after the beginning of treatment. In recent years, more and more attention has been paid to the net K^+ deficit that develops in some people, and K-containing infusion mixtures are used (with caution) in repairing the electrolyte disturbance. After the acute phase of treatment, when the patient begins to take fluids by mouth, K-containing substances, such as fruit juices, are often given. As treatment proceeds, the general condition of the patient is carefully observed, and blood pressure records are kept. The efficacy of the management can be assessed by tests of blood glucose, blood CO_2-combining power, serum K, and nonprotein nitrogen. Electrocardiographic tracings are often made for the purpose of guiding K administration. As the quantitative data come from the laboratory, the physician's therapeutic plan may be modified. Before this condition was as well understood as it is now, the results of treatment were disappointing

and mortality was high. Now, at one representative teaching hospital, the mortality is given as 1.5%

LONG-RANGE COMPLICATIONS OF DIABETES

Understanding the pathophysiology of diabetic ketoacidosis has sharply reduced the number of diabetic patients who die in an episode of acidosis. However, in spite of the fact that insulin has been available for treatment of diabetes since 1922, diabetic persons of all ages—but especially young diabetic patients— have a shorter life expectancy than do age-matched nondiabetic individuals. One of the causes of excess mortality is illustrated in Figure 14–23 (see Goodkin). Most of these deaths are attributable to one or more of the long-range complications of diabetes:

1. *Macrovascular disease*, usually expressed as atherosclerotic disease of the brain, heart or kidney vessels or of vessels of the extremities (especially legs and feet).

2. *Microvascular disease,* particularly of kidney microvessels or those of the retina.

3. *Neuropathy*, impairment of nerve conduction in peripheral or autonomic nerves or both.

Macrovascular Disease

The atherosclerosis that occurs prematurely in diabetic patients is indistinguishable from age-related atherosclerosis that occurs in the macrovasculature of nondiabetic persons. Indeed, diabetes, even when treated conventionally with insulin, is said to be characterized by accelerated aging. Many strokes and coronary occlusions and most amputations for gangrene of the toes or feet are diabetes related.

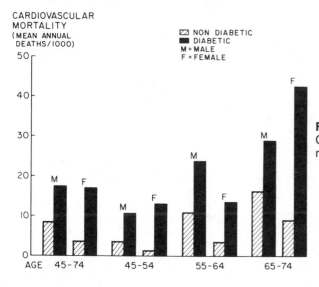

FIG 14–23.
Cardiovascular mortality in diabetic and nondiabetic persons.

Although it is inappropriate here to attempt an essay on the cause of atherosclerosis, it is instructive to reflect on recent ideas about the pathogenesis of the condition and to attempt to explain, at least in part, how diabetes may accelerate it.

Figure 14–24 is a diagrammatic outline of the pathogenesis of atherosclerosis, based largely on the ideas of Ross and Glomset, Colwell et al. (role of platelets), Ledet (growth hormone) and Lopes-Virella et al. (role of lipoproteins). Endothelial injury causes increased permeability of the endothelium of arteries. Platelet adhesion to injured endothelium causes a localized release of a mitogenic stimulus, which stimulates smooth muscle cells to proliferate and migrate. These cells, as well as nacrophages, accumulate lipid, including cholesterol, because low-density lipoprotein (LDL) concentration is elevated, i.e., a high concentration of cholesterol is present in the blood. The deleterious effects of LDL are attenuated by high-density lipoprotein (HDL), which facilitates the removal of cholesterol from the blood. Lipid accumulates subendothelially, and lumina of vessels narrow and eventually become occluded.

Diabetes may accelerate this process in at least three ways: (1) inappropriately high levels of growth hormone may contribute to smooth muscle cell proliferation (Ledet); (2) increased thromboxane synthesis may promote platelet adhesion and mitogen release (Halushka et al.; Waitzman et al.); and (3) in diabetes LDL is elevated as part of the characteristic hyperlipemia of diabetes and the HDL is in short supply (Lopes-Virella). The net result is an amplification of the deleterious effect of LDL. (See upcoming section on glycosylated proteins.)

All of the mechanisms we have suggested may be insufficient to account for the susceptibility of diabetics to atherosclerosis. A 2,500 base pair DNA region (U allele) has been found, adjacent to the insulin gene, which is a strong genetic marker for susceptibility to atherosclerosis not only in Type II diabetics but also in Type I and in nondiabetic subjects as well. Thus, there may be a genetic component (function not known) associated with atherosclerosis susceptibility that may be expressed more frequently in diabetics than in nondiabetics; or, if it is expressed no more frequently, some of the metabolic alterations caused by diabetes may amplify its effect (Mandrup-Poulsen et al.).

Microvascular Disease (Microangiopathy)

Disease of the microvessels—capillaries and their connecting vessels—most frequently expresses itself in diabetes as either kidney or retinal disease. Kidney disease, the result of both macro- and microvascular involvement, is now the leading cause of death in young diabetic patients (Kimmelstiel-Wilson disease). Diabetes is now one of the most frequent causes of blindness. This subject has been studied intensively and imaginatively during the past two decades, both morphologically and biochemically.

BIOCHEMICAL APPROACH TO MICROANGIOPATHY.—The basement membrane of the glomerulus may be obtained in relatively pure form by differential centrifugation and subjected to chemical analysis. The major constituent in glomerular basement protein is a collagen-like glycoprotein material. Spiro (see Claude Bernard Lecture) found that glomerular basement membrane (BM) prepared from diabetic rats contained abnormally high amounts of carbohydrate.

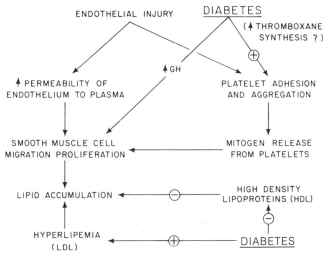

FIG 14–24.
Possible effects of diabetes on atherogenesis. (See chapter 15 for a more detailed discussion of lipoproteins.)

Moreover, one of the enzymes responsible for the posttranslational modification of the glycoprotein, glucosyltransferase, was hyperactive in kidneys of diabetic rats and became progressively more so with increased duration of diabetes from 4 to 20 weeks. Insulin treatment resulted in a return of glucosyltransferase to normal levels. Spiro believes that although insulin deficiency results in decreased glucose utilization by insulin-*dependent* cells, the hyperglycemia resulting from insulin deficiency causes a large increase in glucose utilization over specific pathways in insulin-*in*dependent cells. These pathways may generate products that are important in the pathology of diabetes, or may reflect the quality of control of the diabetes. The pathways are as follows.

1. Synthesis of glycoprotein of *renal* glomerular BM

2. Sorbitol → fructose (*nerve, lens, seminal vesicles*)

3. Glycoprotein synthesis (*vitreous humor* of the eye)

4. Hemoglobin A_{1c} synthesis (see next section)

HYPERGLYCEMIA, HEMOGLOBIN A_{1C}, AND OTHER GLYCOSYLATED PROTEINS.—Hemoglobin A_{1c} is a minor hemoglobin component that is chromatographically separable from HbA, the predominant species. Hb A_{1c} is formed nonenzymatically by covalent binding of glucose to the N terminal valines of the β chains of HbA. Red blood cells normally accumulate Hb A_{1c} as they age over their 120-day lifespan. The main determinant of the extent of Hb A_{1c} formation is the concentration of glucose in the blood. Thus, uncontrolled diabetics have much higher levels of Hb A_{1c} than do normal individuals, and the establishment of control in diabetics results in the return of Hb A_{1c} toward normal values (9.8% of total Hb pigment before versus 5.8% after treatment).

Since spot estimations of blood or urine glucose do not necessarily reflect the fluctuations in blood glucose concentration that may occur over a day, week, or month, and since it is not possible to monitor the blood glucose level day and night in large numbers of diabetic patients, an indirect indicator of the average blood glucose level over a long period would be advantageous. Hb A_{1c} may be such an indicator, since its rate of formation is proportional to concentration of glucose in the RBC × time. In other words, it represents an integration of the area under the curve of hyperglycemia.

Glycosylated albumin may also be used as an indicator of hyperglycemia over a shorter period of time (hemoglobin half-life, about 60 days; albumin half-life, about 20 days). Albumin has the advantage of being obtainable in stored, frozen serum or plasma samples, and therefore may be used in retrospective studies that may not have been designed originally to measure the effects of prolonged hyperglycemia.

Excessive glycosylation of proteins other than hemoglobin and albumin may be involved in a large number of pathophysiologic events associated with some of the long-term complications of diabetes. Nonenzymatic, covalent glycosylation secondary to hyperglycemia occurs in many long-lived structural proteins and enzymes as well as in those, like hemoglobin and albumin, with limited half-lives (Brownlee et al.). Some of these participate in important physiologic functions that may be disrupted by glycosylation, including the following examples:

Protein	*Pathophysiology*
Red cell membrane protein(s)	Red cell deformity
Clotting system proteins	Clotting abnormalities
Endothelial cell membrane protein	Vascular permeability defect
Lens and lens capsule proteins	Visual defects
Glomerular basement membrane	Glomerular pathology
Collagen	Scarring abnormalities
Tubulin and myelin	Neuropathology
Glucose transporters	Insulin resistance

One especially intriguing example of the far-reaching effect of protein glycosylation resulting from hyperglycemia is that of the glycosylation of LDL apoprotein. This impairs LDL binding to its receptor, thereby impairing its receptor-mediated removal from the circulation. This raises serum LDL cholesterol levels. Glycosylation of the apoprotein of *H*DL, which is concerned with the removal of cholesterol from the blood, has the effect of *accelerating* the rate of its abstraction from the blood. The net effect is the high LDL:HDL ratio referred to briefly above. (For more information about lipid transport mechanisms, see Chapter 15.)

Diabetic Neuropathy

Disordered nerve function has long been recognized as a feature of the diabetic condition. Manifestations of diabetic neuropathy can occur in almost every system of the body, and this complication of diabetes can mimic a large catalogue of neurologic diseases. Sensory, motor, and autonomic neurons may be involved in the process. Sensory impairment, in fact, may be an important contributory factor in the development of foot ulcers. Autonomic nervous system dysfunction may take the form of postural hypotension, disturbances in gastrointestinal function or urinary bladder function, impotence and much else. Demyelinization (light microscopy) and more subtle myelin sheath membrane changes (electron microscopy) can be seen in the nerves of many diabetics, but measurable loss of nerve function is demonstrable even in the absence of such changes.

In spite of much work on the problem of diabetic neuropathy, we can present only a tentative catalogue of phenomena that may contribute to its mechanism. *Myelin* is a complex insulating material that consists of triglyceride, cholesterol, phospholipids, glycolipids, and proteins. Alterations in the chemical morphology or amounts of all of these constituents have been described in uncontrolled experimental and clinical diabetes. Many of the abnormalities are correctable with insulin replacement therapy.

The *sorbitol pathway* (referred to above) has been implicated in the pathophysiology of diabetic neuropathy (as well as in that of lens cataract formation and macrovascular disease). It can be described in the following reaction sequence:

$$(1) \quad \text{Glucose} \xrightarrow[\text{NADPH}]{\substack{\text{Aldose} \\ \text{reductase}}} \text{Sorbitol} + \text{NADP}$$

$$(2) \quad \text{Sorbitol} \xrightarrow[\text{NAD}]{\substack{\text{Sorbitol} \\ \text{dehydrogenase}}} \text{Fructose} + \text{NADH}$$

The activity level of the pathway is determined by glucose availability. Thus: hyperglycemia → ↑ activity of the sorbitol pathway → accumulation of sorbitol and fructose → osmotically disturbed intracellular environment → ↓ oxygen consumption (and, presumably, altered function) of nerves. Since this progression is reversible by controlling hyperglycemia, that approach seems to us to be more rational than attempting pharmacologic inhibition of aldose reductase, which has been shown to decrease sorbitol concentration in the nerves of diabetic animals and has been suggested as a possible adjunct to the management of patients with diabetic neuropathy.

Myoinositol is a cyclic hexitol, which is synthesized in nerves from glucose and incorporated into phosphatidylinositol, a precursor of various phospholipid constituents of membranes. Greene et al. found that the concentration of free inositol was low in the nerves of diabetic rats. Moreover, when the rats were fed inositol (1%) in the diet, there was an improvement in nerve conduction velocity to normal levels despite persistence of the diabetes. The investigators concluded that the nerve conduction defect in diabetes was related to an impairment of myoinositol metabolism caused by insulin-deficiency diabetes. The precise mechanism for this was not specified.

Neurones must transport newly synthesized proteins, neurotransmitters, and other materials that are synthesized in the cell body over variably long distances in axons. They do this by the mechanism of *axoplasmic flow,* a complex, energy-requiring, cytoskeleton-dependent, bidirectional movement of some substances from cell body toward the synapse and others in the reverse direction. Axoplasmic flow is demonstrably defective in both directions in uncontrolled diabetes, and the deficiency is corrected when the diabetic state is ameliorated. It is difficult to say which (if any) of the biochemical abnormalities we have mentioned—sorbitol pathway, myoinositol pathway, glycosylation of key proteins, such as tubulin—is primarily responsible for the physiologic disruption. Possibly, they all make a contribution. We are impressed by the fact that *the common denominator among them is the fact that they are corrected by control of hyperglycemia,* at least, before gross morphologic changes, such as demyelinization, occur. This seems to us to reinforce the widely held opinion (belief? impression?) that insulin delivery systems that mimic that of the beta cell as closely as possible promise to prevent or delay the onset of many complications of diabetes (see next section).

Diabetes Control and Experimental Insulin Delivery Systems

Soon after the discovery of insulin, a dialogue began among diabetologists on the advisability of striving for a very strict control of diabetes versus more permissive control. The "strict controllers" attempted to eliminate glycosuria entirely, whereas advocates of the opposing point of view preferred to see a small amount of glucose in the urine of their patients. The rationale for strict control rested on the assumption that normalization of blood glucose regulation over a long time would decrease susceptibility to complications of diabetes. Those who favored less rigid control pointed out that repeated bouts of hypoglycemia caused by overzealous attempts to normalize blood glucose could cause cumulative brain damage, especially in young children.

Actually, what passes for good control—consistently glucose-free urine—is not all that good. When the technology was developed to permit extremely frequent blood glucose samples to be analyzed for long periods (48 hours and longer), it became clear that even those diabetics who appeared to be in good control in a research hospital setting actually showed hyperglycemia during much of the day. This occurred in spite of the availability of many different kinds and combinations of insulin preparations (see Molnar et al.).

It was clear that a more physiologic method of insulin administration was (and is) desirable—one that would prevent hyperglycemia and at the same time protect against hypoglycemia. In brief, investigators wished to duplicate as closely as possible the characteristic features of the normally functioning islet organ, which senses changes in its chemical environment and responds appropriately to them.

Three general strategies have been applied to this important problem: (1) transplantation of the pancreas, isolated islets or cultured β cells; (2) installation of mechanical sensing and pumping equipment ("artificial pancreas"); and (3) insulin injection via a portable, programmable pump.

TRANSPLANTATION STUDIES.—In experimental animals, *islet transplantation*, made possible by Lacy's technique of separating islets from the exocrine pancreas by collagenase digestion (see Kemp et al.), has stimulated hope that this technique may be applicable in human beings. In inbred strains (syngenic) of rats, injection of a suspension of islets into the portal vein normalizes blood glucose concentration for many months in severely diabetic animals. The problem of immunorejection of such grafts by histoincompatible recipients is the major obstacle in applying transplantation techniques.

In 1979, Lacy and colleagues announced a potential breakthrough toward the solution of the rejection problem. They succeeded in producing long-term graft tolerance in genetically *dis*similar rats by culturing the islets for seven days at 24 C and giving the recipient a single injection of antilymphocyte serum. These grafts "cured" diabetes and were effective for over 100 days.

The first pancreas transplant performed in a human was in 1966, but the transplanted pancreatic segment was rejected in a few weeks. Between that time and December, 1982, 337 pancreas transplants were performed. As of December, 1983, 59 were functioning, though 31 of these were producing insulin for 12 months or less. Diabetes was controlled in five patients for 37 months or longer, including one for 65 months. Most of these people had end-stage renal disease and were, therefore, not ideal subjects for testing the efficacy of pancreas transplantation for the control of diabetes. However, the majority of patients selected for the procedure since 1980 in a major center have not been in that category. The availability of cyclosporine as an immunosuppressive agent has generally improved survivability.

Half of a group of 79 patients who received trans-plants of their own islets of Langerhans (following pancreatic resection for cancer or pancreatitis) remained insulin-independent.

An enormous amount of effort and devotion have gone into this pioneering work. We anticipate that, with inevitable advances in the art of immunosuppression, many patients with Type I diabetes will be treated by this method or some modification of it some time in the future. Until then, it will be impossible to compare the relative efficacy of transplantation versus improved insulin delivery systems (next section).

For a detailed summary of the world experience with pancreas transplantation, see Sutherland.

ARTIFICIAL PANCREAS.—Albisser and colleagues have demonstrated that a roomful of equipment, including a glucose analyzer, a computer, suitable pumps and reservoirs of insulin and of glucose can give a reasonably good imitation of the islet organ's ability to control blood glucose. With a knowledge of the distribution volume of injected materials, it is possible to program a computer to deliver corrective doses of either insulin (for rising blood glucose) or glucose (for falling blood glucose) so that the amplitude of fluctuation of blood glucose concentration can be restrained within desired limits.

Considerable progress has been made toward micro-miniaturization of the artificial pancreas. Sensors exist that are able to translate changing blood glucose concentrations into electric signals; microcomputers can translate the signals into demand for insulin; and pump-reservoirs of insulin can respond to the computer's instructions (see Soeldner et al.). The hope is that an implantable device of this sort, about the size of a cardiac pacemaker or smaller, could be commercially produced and implanted for long periods. The chief problem in this approach is the "biocompatibility" of the foreign bodies that must have contact with body fluids over long periods of time.

PROGRAMMABLE, PORTABLE INSULIN DOSAGE-REGULATING APPARATUS (PIDRA).—The physiologic method of regulating blood glucose and the attempts to imitate it with the artificial pancreas approach are "closed loop" information systems, i.e., ↑ blood glucose → insulin secretion → ↓ blood glucose → ↑ insulin counterregulatory hormones → equilibrium level of blood glucose. A variety of programmable, portable insulin infusion pumps are now being tested in many countries for their ability to control blood glucose as part of an "open loop" circuit. A typical pump carries a reservoir of insulin sufficient for many days, delivers small amounts between meals (to mimic the normal pancreas), and is programmed, according to the needs of the individual, to deliver a bolus of insulin just before each meal on demand. The information loop is "closed," not entirely by the recruitment of counterregulatory hormones but by self-monitoring of blood glucose (accomplished by means of a suitable instrument, now widely available), and the intercession of conscious judgment of the individual about the adjustment of insulin dosage to perceived need. It is generally accepted that blood glucose is more nearly normalized by this method, called *C*ontinuous *S*ubcutaneous *I*nsulin *I*nfusion (CSII) than it is by *C*onventional *I*nsulin *T*herapy (CIT).

In the proceedings of a recent conference on this subject (Rodger, ed.), the experience of a multicenter study of the effect of CSII on complications of diabetes was reported. It was clear that, compared with CIT, CSII produced better control of blood glucose, blood lactate, and blood ketones. It also reduced significantly albumin excretion rate in patients with microalbuminuria, suggesting that it had a beneficial effect on developing glomerular basement membrane disease. Unfortunately, however, it either failed to inhibit development of diabetic retinopathy or actually made it worse, suggesting that the progress of diabetic retinopathy is related to factors in addition to uncontrolled blood glucose. The interested reader will find references to most of the accumulated world literature on CSII in the conference report cited.

One of the consequences of more severe Type I diabetes of long duration is *combined deficiency of glucagon and epinephrine counterregulation*. Thus, if insulin causes hypoglycemia, the normal protective response is inadequate. Some insulin-dependent diabetics in this category have experienced unfortunate episodes of hypoglycemia during CSII therapy. In some centers, a favorable test of counterregulatory hormone competence is required to qualify for entry into the pump program.

The counterregulatory deficiency is probably a manifestation of diabetic neuropathy and is therefore secondary to uncontrolled diabetes. Whether the deficiency can be corrected by rigorous control of blood glucose depends on the degree of reversibility of the neuropathy. (See Cryer and Gerich for an extensive review of counterregulation and hypoglycemia; also, see Unger, 1983.)

DIABETES AND EXERCISE

Exercise helps to prevent obesity, improves heart and lung function, normalizes blood lipid patterns (decreases cholesterol and increases HDL), helps to prevent intravascular clotting, increases the feeling of well-being, and is believed by many to prevent or delay such atherosclerotic diseases as myocardial infarction. If one accepts the desirability of maintenance of physical training in nondiabetic persons, exercise can be no less beneficial in diabetic patients, who are particularly susceptible to atherosclerotic disease.

Skeletal muscle is an insulin-sensitive tissue; its cells display insulin receptors on their plasma membranes so that stimulatory effects of insulin on glucose uptake and oxidation, glycogen synthesis, and antilipolysis may be demonstrated readily. Insulin is essential for glucose uptake by resting muscle. Contrary to previously held belief, a very *small* concentration of insulin is also necessary for glucose uptake by working muscle (see Berger, Hagg and Ruderman). However, the sedentary diabetic who changes his/her activity pattern (e.g., as occurs when diabetic children go to summer camp) characteristically requires *less* insulin in spite of consuming *more* food. This paradox can be explained by noting that glucose utilization by working muscle in the presence of permissive concentrations of insulin requires much *less* insulin than would be needed to store the same amount of carbohydrate as glycogen or triglyceride. In other words, working muscle promotes glucose use by an insulin-independent process if membrane competence is sustained by insulin.

Physical exercise, in proportion to its intensity and duration, causes the secretion of all of insulin's physiologic antagonists (glucagon, catecholamines, cortisol, growth hormone) while inhibiting the secretion of insulin. If this pattern of response did not occur, the sudden increased rate of utilization of blood glucose by working muscle would cause hypoglycemia. Suppression of insulin secretion helps to prepare the liver for glycogenolysis and gluconeogenesis, which compensate for the increased peripheral utilization rate of glucose. Furthermore, the ascendancy of the antagonist group over insulin favors FFA mobilization from adipose tissue, as well as triglyceride hydrolysis in muscle cells. Thus, adaptation to exercise resembles adaptation to starvation, but in the case of exercise, the adaptation is apparently anticipatory.

Wahren, Felig, and Hagenfeldt have studied the effect of exercise on fuel homeostasis in normal and diabetic subjects. They found that insulin-treated diabetics without ketonemia and with only mild hyperglycemia showed responses that were entirely similar to those of normal individuals. However, patients with ketonemia and marked hyperglycemia made their diabetes worse by exercising: blood glucose increased and so did blood ketone concentration. Similar results were obtained by Berger, Berchtold, et al.

Poorly controlled diabetics also show exaggerated and sustained increases in circulating glucagon and growth hormone in response to measured exercise.

Therefore, the effects of insulin deficiency are amplified by the countervailing force of antagonistic hormones. The possibility that growth hormone may be involved in the causation of atherosclerosis (and also in ocular complications) suggests that these exercise responses of poorly controlled diabetics may be involved in their susceptibility to macro- and microvascular complications of diabetes.

From this account, one can infer that prescription of exercise as an adjunct to control of diabetes in insulin-deficient (Type I) diabetics is an uncertain business at best. However, for patients who are capable of assuming major responsibility for their own management, it is possible to design exercise programs successfully in cooperation with a therapist-teacher. The advent of suitable instruments for self-monitoring blood glucose and the establishment of consistent patterns of exercise have been crucial in the success of this enterprise (Kemmer and Berger). For obese, Type II diabetics, the benefits of exercise in improving insulin sensitivity, decreasing body fat, decreasing blood pressure, decreasing LDL, and increasing HDL have been amply documented. (Bjorntorp and Krotkiewski and Vranic et al. list many reviews of this subject.)

HYPOGLYCEMIAS

Hypoglycemia, or low blood glucose, occurs when (1) glucose is removed from the blood more rapidly than it can be replaced by intestinal absorption or liver secretion, (2) hepatic glycogenolysis and/or gluconeogenesis are insufficient to compensate for the removal rate or (3) some combination of (1) and (2) occurs. Low blood glucose may cause sweating, weakness, hunger, tachycardia, anxiety and, more rarely, sleepiness, loss of consciousness and convulsions. The symptoms of hypoglycemia, when blood glucose falls rapidly, are due to hyperepinephrinemia and sympathetic nervous system activity. When blood glucose falls more slowly, cerebral events are prominent: headache, blurred vision, diplopia, confusion, incoherent speech, coma and convulsions. Hypoglycemia is an indication that homeostatic regulation of blood glucose is faulty; such a finding is only the beginning of a search for the cause.

There are many ways of classifying hypoglycemias, e.g., "organic" or "functional," depending on whether an anatomical cause for the disorder can be found, or whether the hypoglycemia is fasting or nonfasting.

An enumeration of the causes of hypoglycemia is presented (Table 14–4) because it rests on the preceding discussion of blood glucose regulation.

Identification of the cause of hypoglycemia is often related to the history; i.e., do the episodes occur at specific times (early or late) after eating? Or are they associated with food deprivation? (See Shen and Bressler.) Obviously, history, physical examination, and laboratory data are used to detect hypopituitarism and adrenal insufficiency. When insulinoma is present, the circulating insulin concentration is almost always inappropriately high for the prevailing blood glucose level (another example of a simultaneous hormone measurement and the measurement of a regulated function).

Management of patients with hypoglycemia is beyond the scope of this account. It is only necessary to make the point that rational management depends on ability to ascertain the cause of the hypoglycemia in each individual.

Excesses and Deficiencies of Counterregulatory Hormones

The theme of this chapter has been the control of body fuel metabolism by insulin and by its antago-

TABLE 14–4.

Causes of Hypoglycemia

Excess insulin
    Pancreatic islet cell tumor, benign or malignant
    Other insulin-producing tumors
    Stimulation of inappropriate insulin release
        Postgastric surgery
        Early adult-onset diabetes
        Leucine hypersensitivity in children
        Newborn of diabetic mother
        Drug-induced (factitious)
            Insulin
            Sulfonylureas
Deficient insulin antagonist
    Hypopituitarism (GH and ACTH deficiency)
    Adrenocortical hypofunction (cortisol deficiency)
Deficient hepatic glucose production
    Diffuse liver disease (i.e., cirrhosis)
    Ethyl alcohol plus poor nutrition
    Inborn errors of liver metabolism
        Glycogen storage diseases
            Type I, G-6-Pase deficiency ("von Gierke")
            Type III, amylo-1,6-glucosidase deficiency ("Forbes")
            Type VI, phosphorylase deficiency ("Hers")
        Hereditary fructose intolerance
            F-1-phosphate aldolase deficiency
        Galactosemia (Gal-1-phosphate uridyl transferase deficiency)
        Aglycogenosis (glycogen synthetase deficiency, etc.)
Undetermined etiology
    "Functional" hypoglycemia
    Transient hypoglycemia of low birth weight neonates

nists, or counterregulatory hormones: growth hormone, catecholamines, cortisol, glucagon and somatostatin. Our emphasis has been on disturbances of regulation in which relative insulin deficiency or excess occurs. Even when insulin deficiency is the initiating event, inappropriate excesses of antagonists (glucagon, growth hormone) are features of the regulatory disturbance. Are there any circumstances when control of metabolism is disrupted by a primary excess or deficiency of one or more of the physiologic antagonists of insulin?

Growth hormone excess (acromegaly, Chapter 5) is often associated with hyperglycemia and glycosuria, which is ameliorated if the growth hormone excess is eliminated. Similarly, *human placental lactogen* (hPL) is probably responsible for deterioration of glucose tolerance and signs of diabetes in some pregnant women. On the other hand, *hypopituitarism* is characterized by hypoglycemia following glucose ingestion owing to failure to compensate for a falling blood glucose.

Catecholamine excess (e.g., pheochromocytoma, Chapter 13) may cause hyperglycemia and glycosuria, owing in part to the action of catecholamines and also to the fact that catecholamines stimulate glucagon secretion and inhibit insulin secretion. It is difficult to find descriptions of naturally occurring catecholamine deficiency states, but pharmacologic blockade of catecholamine effects is widely used.

The diabetogenic effects of *cortisol* were discussed in Chapter 11. This is a clear case in which inhibition of glucose utilization in the periphery and overproduction of glucose by the liver cause a compensatory hyperinsulinemia, which in susceptible individuals can result in β cell decompensation. Cortisol deficiency, as in Addison's disease or in inborn errors of cortisol synthesis, can, like hypopituitarism, cause reactive hypoglycemia.

Primary secretory disturbances of *glucagon* are rare, but patients with hyperglucagonemia due to a glucagon-producing tumor have been described (Recant et al.). One individual with a selective glucagon deficiency has also been studied (Vidnes and Oyasaeter).

Somatostatin, though only recently discovered, has its own hypersecretion state. Patients with somatostatin-producing tumors have been described (Ganda et al.). There is also a strong possibility that somatostatin deficiency may cause disordered function of the islet organ, since in mice with hereditary obesity-diabetes syndrome, somatostatin-secreting cells are virtually absent from the islets (Patel et al.). These animals show hyperinsulinemia and excessively high circulating insulin levels following stimuli of insulin secretion.

In a word, if something can go wrong, it will. Moreover, as soon as an astute observer recognizes a previously unrecognized condition, its "incidence" usually increases sharply.

Chemical Agents and Islet Cell Function

BETACYTOTOXIC AGENTS

Alloxan

Certain chemical compounds, such as *alloxan*, uric acid, dialuric acid, and others seek out the β cells of the pancreatic islets and destroy them, as if the molecules are equipped with some sort of guidance system that directs them to the vulnerable cells. In fact, alloxan is not as selective in its effect as it seems to be, for it is not difficult to demonstrate acute effects of alloxan intoxication in other tissues, e.g., liver and kidney. But the effects in these tissues are generally transitory, whereas the chemical blow dealt to the β cells is a mortal one.

When alloxan is injected into a suitably prepared animal, a serial response occurs: (1) hyperglycemia, which is believed to be due to epinephrinemia, and also (possibly) to a direct effect of alloxan on the liver; (2) hypoglycemia, which probably represents a response to the sudden release of stored insulin into the blood from damaged β cells; and (3) chronic hyperglycemia, presumably due to irreversible β cell damage.

The advantage of such a chemical tool is obvious. Indeed, countless animals of many species have been rendered diabetic in this way as investigators have studied many of the problems of diabetes and insulin deficiency. There is some reason to believe that an alloxan diabetic animal is not the physiologic equivalent of a depancreatized one, for it has been found that the insulin requirement of the alloxan diabetic is decreased by subsequent pancreatectomy. This result could be due either to the removal of a blood sugar-raising material with the alloxan-treated pancreas (i.e., glucagon) or to a diminished spontaneous food intake postoperatively.

Since alloxan is chemically related to uric acid, a naturally occurring metabolite, it has been suggested that diabetogenic substances may be produced in the body and may be of some importance in the cause of human diabetes, but there is no proof that such is the case. It is interesting to note that glutathione, cysteine, British anti-lewisite (dimercaprol, which is a dithiol) and other –SH -containing substances protect the β cell from damage by alloxan. This suggests that alloxan exerts its toxic effect by combining with –SH groups of vital β cell proteins and that –SH enzymes may be centrally important in the highly specialized function of β cells, which is to synthesize and release insulin.

Streptozotocin

In 1963 Rakieten et al. discovered that the antibiotic streptozotocin, which had been shown to exert some growth inhibition of certain experimental tumors, was diabetogenic in dogs and rats. Histologic evidence of β cell damage can be seen within one hour after an intravenous injection, and selective necrotic destruction of these cells is evident at seven hours. The early β cell damage is accompanied by release of insulin into the circulation. Although these effects are similar to those of alloxan, streptozotocin appears to be much less toxic to other tissues than is alloxan. This is especially true of kidney toxicity. Thus, streptozotocin offers a much wider margin between efficacy and general toxicity and therefore produces a more "pure" diabetes than that induced by alloxan.

Oral Hypoglycemic Agents

Soon after the sulfonamide drugs were introduced (c. 1935), the observation was made that certain patients with typhoid fever exhibited hypoglycemia after one of these drugs had been given. Between 1942 and 1946, the hypoglycemic effect of sulfonamides was studied by Loubatières, and in 1955 it was demonstrated that a sulfonamide drug could function as an "insulin substitute" in certain diabetic patients when it was given orally. This finding stimulated a vast amount of research in this field, both experimental and clinical. The original drug used in the German clinical trials in 1955 was called *carbutamide*, but this compound (although it is still extensively used in Europe) was largely replaced in the United States by a closely related substance, *tolbutamide* (Fig 14–25).

Six oral hypoglycemic compounds have been used extensively in treatment of adult-onset diabetics:

Drug	Duration of action (hours)
Tolbutamide (Orinase)	6–10
Chlorpropamide (Diabinese)	36–60
Acetohexamide (Dymelor)	10–20
Tolazamide (Tolinase)	12–24
Glipizide	10–16
Glyburide	12–24

The first four are called first generation agents; the last two, approved for use in the U.S.A. only in 1984, are known as second generation drugs. They

TOLBUTAMIDE

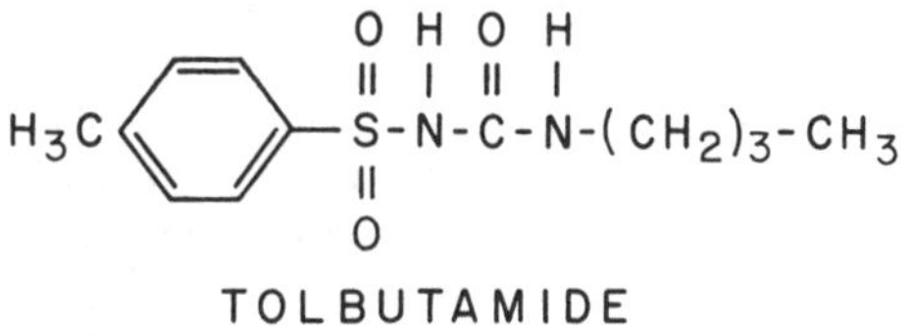

FIG 14–25.
Tolbutamide, a prototype of the sulfonyurea oral hypoglycemic drugs.

differ from first generation drugs mainly in their potency. They show a variety of patterns of metabolic alteration and excretion, which accounts for differences in duration of action. Chlorpropamide is most resistant to metabolism and also is reabsorbed by the renal tubule—reasons enough for its long duration of action. The common structural feature of these drugs is the following configuration:

$$SO_2 \cdot NH \cdot CO \cdot NH$$

It is this structure that is associated with the most prominent aspect of the action of these drugs, i.e., their sensitization of the β cell to its usual stimuli so that insulin secretion is enhanced. It is for this reason that the drugs are ineffective in insulin-deficient, ketosis-prone diabetics.

Almost from the beginning of investigations of the sulfonylureas, peripheral effects were claimed for them in addition to their stimulatory effect on β cell secretion. Recently, Olefsky and Reaven described decreased binding of insulin by circulating monocytes of diabetic patients (in many other studies by Kahn, Roth, et al., monocyte binding reflected binding to adipocyte and liver membranes). When these patients were treated with chlorpropamide, insulin binding improved. In some target cells, postbinding steps in insulin's response are also enhanced by sulfonylurea drugs. Thus, the drug not only improves insulin secretory responses but also may affect insulin sensitivity of peripheral insulin-responsive cells.

Interest in this class of agents has spread beyond the field of diabetes mellitus. Following the serendipitous discovery that chlorpropamide (but not other sulfonylurea drugs) has an ADH-like effect in diabetes insipidus, the drug has been found to enhance or attenuate the biologic effects of a number of hormones, for example: (1) it potentiates the effect of ADH on free water retention in the renal medulla (see Miller and Moses); (2) it antagonizes the action of parathyroid hormone effect on the renal cortical tubules (see Coulson and Moses); and (3) it antagonizes the stimulatory effect of glucagon in the isolated perfused liver (see Blumenthal). It is also reputed to increase the positive inotropic effect of epinephrine on the heart.

All of these hormone effects have one thing in common: they all involve cyclic AMP and its protein kinase. Why some effects are potentiated and others are inhibited is not known with certainty, but one possible explanation is that chlorpropamide has been shown to inhibit both adenylate cyclase *and* phosphodiesterase. Whether potentiation or inhibition results might depend on which of these two enzymes is inhibited to the greater extent (Leichter and Chase).

For many years oral hypoglycemic drugs were used widely, but in some instances uncritically. (Many patients who received the drugs were obese and their diabetes might have been brought under control simply by weight reduction.) In 1970 a report was published by a multiclinic investigative group (University Diabetes Group Program, or UDGP) in which patients taking tolbutamide (see Fig 14–25) showed a statistically significant increase in cardiovascular disease mortality compared with placebo groups or groups taking fixed or variable doses of insulin. The findings of the UDGP study have been subjected to rigorous reexamination by both protagonists and antagonists of the group's conclusions. Although the controversy does not seem to abate, the UDGP report has had the effect of stimulating physicians to select candidates for sulfonylurea treatment with more care and to monitor their responses more closely.

BIBLIOGRAPHY

Abumrad NA, Perry PR, Whitesell RR: Stimulation by epinephrine of the membrane transport of long chain fatty acid in the adipocyte. *J Biol Chem* 1985; 260:9969.

Albisser WD, Leibel BS, Zinman B, et al: Studies with an artificial endocrine pancreas. *Arch Intern Med* 1977; 137:639.

Bell GI, Pictet RL, Rutter WJ, et al: Sequence of human insulin gene. *Nature* 1980; 284:26.

Bergeron JJM, Cruz J, Khan MN, et al: Uptake of insulin and other ligands into receptor-rich endocytotic components of target cells: The endosomal apparatus. *Ann Rev Physiol* 1985; 47:383.

Bjorntorp P, Krotkiewski M: Exercise treatment in diabetes mellitus. *Acta Med Scand* 1985; 217:3.

Blumenthal SA: Potentiation of the hepatic action of insulin by chlorpropamide. *Diabetes* 1977; 26:485.

Boyd ME, Albright EB, Foster DW, et al: In vitro reversal of the fasting state of liver metabolism in the rat. Reevaluation of the roles of insulin and glucose. *J Clin Invest* 1981; 68:142.

Bressler R, Galloway JA: The insulins. *Ration Drug Ther* 1971; 5:May.

Brownlee M: Microvascular disease and related abnormalities: Their relation to the control of diabetes, in Marble A, et al (eds): *Joslin's Diabetes Mellitus*, ed 12. 1984, pp 185–216.

Brownlee M, Vlassara H, Cerami A: Nonenzymatic glyco-

sylation and the pathogenesis of diabetic complications. *Ann Intern Med* 1984; 101:527.

Burkhard SJ, Traugh JA: Changes in ribosome function by cAMP - dependent and cAMP-independent phosphorylation of ribosomal protein S6. *J Biol Chem* 1983; 258:14003.

Campbell IL, Hellquist LNB, Taylor KW: Insulin biosynthesis and its regulation. *Clin Sci* 1982; 62:449.

Cerasi E: A la recherche du temps perdu—epilogue to the Minkowski Award lecture 1974. *Diabetologia* 1985; 28:547.

Cheng K, Larner J: Intracellular mediators of insulin action. *Ann Rev Physiol* 1985; 47:405.

Chick WL, Like AA, Lauris V: Beta cell culture on synthetic capillaries: An artificial endocrine pancreas. *Science* 1975; 187:847.

Clements RS, Jr, Reynertson R: Myoinositol metabolism in diabetes mellitus: Effect of insulin treatment. *Diabetes* 1977; 26:215.

Cohen P: The role of protein phosphorylation in neural and hormonal control of cellular activity. *Nature* 1982; 296:613.

Colwell JA, Sagel J, Crook L, et al: Correlation of platelet aggregation, plasma factor activity, and megathrombocytes in diabetic subjects with and without diabetic vascular disease. *Metabolism* 1977; 26:279.

Coulson R, Moses AM: Effect of chlorpropamide on renal response to parathyroid hormones in normal subjects and in patients with hypoparathyroidism and pseudohypoparathyroidism. *J Pharmacol Exp Ther* 1975; 194:603.

Craighead JE: The role of viruses in the pathogenesis of pancreatic disease and diabetes mellitus. *Prog Med Virol* 1975; 19:161.

Creutzfeldt W, Ebert R: New developments in the incretin concept. *Diabetologia* 1985; 28:565.

Cryer PE, Gerich JE: Glucose counterregulation, hypoglycemia, and intensive insulin therapy in diabetes mellitus. *N Engl J Med* 1985; 313:232.

Cushman SW, Wardzala LJ: Potential mechanism of insulin action on glucose transport in the isolated rat adipose cell: Apparent translocation of the intracellular transport systems to the plasma membrane. *J Biol Chem* 1980; 255:4758.

Czech MP: The nature and regulation of the insulin receptor: Structure and function. *Ann Rev Physiol* 1985; 47:357.

Czech MP (ed): *Molecular Basis of Insulin Action.* New York, Plenum Publishing Corp, 1985.

Ditzel J, Standl E: The oxygen transport system of red blood cells during diabetic ketoacidosis and recovery. *Diabetologia* 1975; 11:255.

Docherty K, Carroll RJ, Steiner DF: Conversion of proinsulin to insulin: Involvement of a 31,500 molecular weight thiol protease. *Proc Natl Acad Sci USA* 1982; 79:4613.

Duncan BB, Heiss G: Nonenzymatic glycosylation of proteins—a new tool for assessment of cumulative hyperglycemia in epidemiologic studies, past and future. *Am J Epidemiol* 1984; 120:169.

Ebina Y, Ellis L, Jarnagin K, et al: The human insulin receptor cDNA: The structural basis for hormone-activated transmembrane signalling. *Cell* 1985; 40:747.

Efendić S, Luft R, Wajngot A: Aspects of the pathogenesis of Type 2 diabetes. *Endocrine Rev* 1984; 5:395.

Ellenberg M, Rifkin H: *Diabetes Mellitus: Theory and Practice,* ed 3. New Hyde Park, New York, Medical Examination Publishing Co, 1983.

El-Maghrabi MR, Claus TH, Pilkis J, et al: Regulation of rat liver fructose 2,6 bisphosphatase. *J Biol Chem* 1982; 257:7603.

Fain JN: Insulin secretion and action. *Metabolism* 1984; 33:672.

Felig P, Saudek CD: The metabolic events in starvation. *Am J Med* 1976; 60:117.

Foster DW: From glycogen to ketones—and back (Banting Lecture). *Diabetes* 1984; 33:1188.

Fujita T (ed): *Endocrine Gut and Pancreas*. New York, Elsevier North-Holland, Inc. 1976.

Gabbay KH, DeLuca K, Fisher JN, et al: Familial hypoinsulinemia—and autosomal defect. *N Engl J Med* 1976; 294:911.

Gammeltoft S: Insulin receptors: Binding kinetics and structure-function relationships of insulin. *Physiol Rev* 1984; 64:1321.

Ganda OP, Weir GC, Soeldner JS, et al: Somatostatinoma: A somatostatin-containing tumor of endocrine pancreas. *N Engl J Med* 1977; 296:963.

Gerich JE, Charles MA, Grodsky G: Regulation of pancreatic insulin and glucagon secretion. *Ann Rev Physiol* 1976; 38:353.

Goeddel DV, Kleid DG, Bolivar F, et al: Expression in *E. coli* of chemically synthesized genes for human insulin. *Proc Natl Acad Sci USA* 1979; 76:106.

Goldberg AL, Griffin GE, Dice JF, Jr: Regulation of protein turnover in normal and dystrophic muscle, in *Pathogenesis of Human Muscular Dystrophy*. Amsterdam, Excerpta Medica, 1976.

Goodkin G: Mortality factors in diabetes: A 20-year mortality study. *J Occup Med* 1975; 17:176.

Gottschalk WK, Jarett L: Intracellular mediators of insulin action in DeFronzo (ed): *Diabetes Metabolism Reviews*. New York, John Willy and Sons, 1985, pp. 228–259.

Greene DA, DeJesus PV, Jr, Winegrad AI: Effects of insulin and dietary inositol on impaired peripheral motor nerve conduction velocity in acute streptozotocin diabetes. *J Clin Invest* 1975; 55:1326.

Griffey MA, Conaway HH, Harshfield DL, et al: Effect of somatostatin on insulin secretion induced by ionophore. *Proc Soc Exp Biol Med* 1977; 154:198.

Halushka PV, Lurie D, Colwell JA: Increased synthesis of prostaglandin E-like material by platelets from patients with diabetes mellitus. *N Engl J Med* 1977; 297:1306.

Haneda M, Polonsky KS, et al: Familial hyperinsulinemia due to a structurally abnormal insulin: Definition of an emerging new clinical syndrome. *N Engl J Med* 1984; 310:1288.

Hansson A, Ingelman-Sundberg M: Insulin stimulated protein synthesis in adipocytes (initiation and ribosomal protein S6). *Eur J Biochem* 1985; 151:97.

Harper ME, Ullrich A, Saunders GF: Localization of the human insulin gene to the distal end of the short arm of chromosome 11. *Proc Natl Acad Sci USA* 1981; 78:4458.

Hedeskov CJ: Mechanism of glucose-induced insulin secretion. *Physiol Rev* 1980; 60:442.

Hers H-G: The discovery and biological role of fructose 2,6 bisphosphate (10th Jubilee Lecture). *Biochem Soc Trans* 1984; 12:729.

Hodgkin DC, Dodson E, Dodson G, et al: Insulin: Three-dimensional structure. *Biochem Soc Trans* 1983; 11:411.

Howell SL: The mechanism of insulin secretion. *Diabetologia* 1984; 26:319.

Johnson IS: Human insulin from recombinant DNA technology. *Science* 1983; 219:632.

Kahn CR, Flier JS, Bar RS, et al: The syndromes of insulin resistance and acanthosis nigricans: Insulin receptor disorders in man. *N Engl J Med* 1976; 294:739.

Kasuga M, Zizk Y, Blithe DL, et al: Insulin stimulation of phosphorylation of the β subunit of the insulin receptor. *J Biol Chem* 1982; 257:9891.

Kemmer FW, Berger M: Exercise in therapy and the life of diabetic patients. *Clin Sci* 1984; 67:279.

King GL, Kahn CR, Samuels B: Synthesis and characterization of molecular hybrids of insulin and insulin-like growth factor. *J Biol Chem* 1982; 257:10869.

Kohen E, Kohen C, Thorell B, et al: Intercellular communication in pancreatic islet monolayer cultures: A microfluorometric study. *Science* 1979; 204:863.

Kono T, Robinson FW, Sarver JA: Insulin-sensitive phosphodiesterase: Its localization, hormonal stimulation, and oxidative stabilization. *J Biol Chem* 1975; 250:7826.

Lacy PE, Davie JM, Finke EH: Prolongation of islet allograft survival following in vitro culture (24° C) and a single injection of ALS. *Science* 1979; 204:312.

Larner J: Insulin and oral hypoglycemic drugs: Glucagon, in Gilman AG, Goodman LS, Rall TW, et al (eds): *Goodman and Gilman's Pharmacological Basis of Therapeutics*, ed 7. New York, Macmillan Publishing Co, 1985, pp 1504–07.

Ledet T: Growth hormone stimulating the growth of arterial medial cells in vitro: Absence of effect of insulin. *Diabetes* 1976; 25:1011.

Lefebvre PJ: *Glucagon*, Vols 1 and 2, *Handbook of Experimental Pharmacology*, Vols 66/1 and 66/2. New York,Springer-Verlag 1983.

Leichter SB, Chase LR: Differential effects of chlorpropamide on adenylate cyclase and phosphodiesterase activity in renal cortex and medulla. *Endocrinology* 1976; 98(*Suppl* 1):71.

Lenmark A, Freedman ZR, Hofman AH, et al: Islet-cell-surface antibodies in juvenile diabetes mellitus. *N Engl J Med* 1978; 299:375.

Livingston JN, Einarsson K, Backman L, et al: Glucagon receptor of human liver. *J Clin Invest* 1985; 75:397.

Lopes-Virella MFL, Stone PG, Colwell JA: Serum high-density lipoprotein in diabetic patients. *Diabetologia* 1977; 13:285.

Malaisse WJ (ed): Stimulus-secretion coupling in the pancreatic B cell (15 review articles). *Experientia* 1984; 40:10–1164.

Mallison CN, Bloom SR, Warin AP, et al: A glucagonoma syndrome. *Lancet* 1974; 2:1.

Mandrup-Poulsen T, Owerbach D, Nerup J, et al: Insulin gene flanking sequences, diabetes mellitus, and atherosclerosis: A review. *Diabetologia* 1985; 28:556.

Marble A, Krall LP, Bradley RF, et al (eds): *Joslin's Diabetes Mellitus*, ed 12. Philadelphia, Lea & Febiger, 1985.

Miller M, Moses AM: Mechanism of chlorpropamide action in diabetes insipidus. *J Clin Endocrinol Metab* 1970; 30:488.

Molnar GD, Taylor WF, Ho MM: Day-to-day variation of continuously monitored glycemia. *Diabetologia* 1972; 8:342.

Moore RD: The case for intracellular pH in insulin action, in Czech MP (ed): *Molecular Basis of Insulin Action*. New York, Plenum Publishing Corp, 1985, p. 145.

Morgan HE, Jefferson LS, Wolpert EB, et al: Regulation of protein synthesis in heart muscle, II: Effect of amino acid levels and insulin on ribosomal aggregation. *J Biol Chem* 1971; 246:2163.

Morgan NG, Rumford GM, Montague W: Studies on the role of inositol triphosphate in the regulation of insulin secretion from isolated rat islets of Langerhans. *Biochem J* 1985; 228:713.

Olefsky JM, Reaven GM: Effects of sulfonylurea therapy on insulin binding to mononuclear leukocytes of diabetic patients. *Am J Med* 1976; 60:89.

Orci L: The insulin factory: A tour of the plant surroundings and a visit to the assembly line. *Diabetologia* 1985; 28:528.

Orci L, Ravazzola M, Amherdt M, et al: Direct identification of prohormone conversion site in insulin-secreting cells. *Cell* 1985; 42:671.

Raskin P: Diabetic regulation and its relation to microangiopathy. *Metabolism* 1978; 27:235.

Robbins DC, Tager HS, Rubenstein AH: Biologic and clinical importance of proinsulin. *N Engl J Med* 1984; 310:1165.

Rodger NW (ed): Proceedings of a conference on insulin pump therapy in diabetes. *Diabetes* 1985; 34(Suppl 3):1–91.

Rossini AA, Like A, Chick WL, et al: Studies of streptozotocin-induced insulinitis and diabetes. *Proc Natl Acad Sci USA* 1977; 74:2485.

Roth J, Le Roith D, Shiloach J, et al: The evolutionary origins of hormones, neurotransmitters and other extracellular chemical messengers. *N Engl J Med* 1982; 306:523.

Roth J, Grunfeld C: Mechanism of action of peptide hormones and catecholamines, Chapter 4 in Wilson JD, Foster DW (eds): *Williams Textbook of Endocrinology,* ed 7. Philadelphia, WB Saunders Co, 1985, pp 76-122.

Sasaki K, Cripe TP, Kock SR, et al: Multihormonal regulation of phosphoenolpyruvate carboxykinase gene transcription: The dominant role of insulin. *J Biol Chem* 1984; 259:15242.

Soeldner JS, Chang KW, Aisenberg S, et al: Progress toward an implantable glucose sensor and an artificial beta cell, in Urquhart J, Yates FE (eds): *Temporal Aspects of Therapeutics.* New York, Plenum Publishing Corp, 1973.

Spiro RG: Search for a biochemical basis of diabetic microangiopathy (Claude Bernard Lecture). *Diabetologia* 1976; 12:1.

Steiner DF: Insulin today (Banting Lecture). *Diabetes* 1977; 26:322.

Straus DS: Growth-stimulating actions of insulin in vitro and in vivo. *Endocrine Rev* 1984; 5:356.

Sutherland DER: Pancreas and islet transplantation I: Experimental studies. *Diabetologia* 1981; 20:161.

Sutherland DER: Pancreas and islet transplant registry data. *World J Surg* 1984; 8:270.

Suzuki K, Kono T: Evidence that insulin causes translocation of glucose transport activity to the plasma membrane from an intracellular storage site. *Proc Natl Acad Sci USA* 1980; 77:2542.

Thim L, Moody AJ: The primary structure of porcine glicentin (proglucagon). *Regul Pept* 1981; 2:139.

Ullrich A, Bell JR, Chen EY, et al: Human insulin receptor and its relation to the tyrosine kinase family of oncogenes. *Nature* 1985; 313:756.

Unger RH: Insulin:glucagon relationships in the defense against hypoglycemia (Berson Memorial Lecture). *Diabetes* 1983; 32:575.

Unger RH, Eisentraut AM: Entero-insular axis. *Arch Intern Med* 1969; 123:261.

Unger RH, Orci L (eds): *Glucagon: Physiology, Pathophysiology, and Morphology of the Pancreatic A Cell.* New York, Elsevier North-Holland, Inc, 1981.

Vidnes J, Oyasaeter S: Glucagon deficiency causing severe neonatal hypoglycemia in a patient with normal insulin secretion. *Pediatr Res* 1977; 11:943.

Volk BW, Arquilla ER (eds): *The Diabetic Pancreas,* ed 2. New York, Plenum Publishing Corp, 1985.

Vranic M, Horvath S, Wahren J (eds): Proceedings of a conference on diabetes mellitus and exercise. *Diabetes* 1979; 28(Suppl 1).

Ward JD Barnes CG, Fisher DL, et al: Improvement in nerve conduction following treatment in newly diagnosed diabetics. *Lancet* 1971; 1:428.

Winegrad AI, Greene DA: Diabetic polyneuropathy: The importance of insulin deficiency, hyperglycemia, and alterations in myoinositol metabolism in its pathogenesis. *N Engl J Med* 1976; 295:1416.

Zawalich W, Zawalich K, Rasmussen H: Insulin secretion: Combined tolbutamide, forskolin, and TPA mimic action of glucose. *Cell Calcium* 1984; 5:551.

Zhang Y-S: Studies on insulin structure and function. *Biochem Soc Trans* 1983; 11:417.

15

Triglyceride and Cholesterol Transport and Metabolism: The Origins, Interactions, and Disposition of Lipoproteins

SOME LANDMARKS IN THE HISTORY OF ATHEROGENESIS, CHOLESTEROL, AND LIPID TRANSPORT		
DATE	EVENT	INVESTIGATOR(S)
c. 1500 B.C.	Atherosclerosis in Egyptian mummies	Ancient papyri
c. 1500 C.E.	"vessels in elderly . . . restrict transit of blood"	Leonardo da Vinci
1768	Angina pectoris described: "serum thick like cream"	Heberden
1778	In angina patient who died, "heart laden with fat, vessels concealed in that substance"	Jenner
c. 1785	Intima of arteries "ulcerated and steatomatous"	Scarpa
1833	Term "arteriosclerosis" coined	Lobstein
1905	Sudden obstruction of coronary arteries described	Herrick, Obsastzow, Straschesko
1908	Atherosclerosis in rabbits caused by feeding milk, egg yolks	Ignatovski
1912	Sunflower seed and fish oil feeding did *not* cause atherosclerosis	Stuckey
1913	Pure cholesterol feeding caused atherosclerosis in rabbits	Anitchkov and Chalatov
1930, seq.	Epidemiologic studies associated high serum cholesterol and atherosclerotic diseases	Many
1939	Familial hypercholesterolemia (FH) identified as a genetic disease	Muller
1940s, seq.	Electrophoresis of plasma proteins	E.J. Cohn
1950s, seq.	Electrophoretic, ultracentrifugal separation of lipoproteins	Many
1950s	Biosynthesis of cholesterol	Bloch; Lynen
1960s	Homozygous and heterozygous FH described	Khachadurian and Fredrickson
1973	LDL receptor discovered	Brown and Goldstein

Adapted from Gotto AM, Jr: *Circulation* 1985; 72:8, and Brown MS, Goldstein JL: *Sci Am* 1984; 251:58, and others.

Atherosclerosis, and its attendant cardiac, brain, and renal complications, certainly antedated the Egyptian experience, for it is likely that it occurred in any ancient civilization in which some people had access to a plethora of food, especially animal fat. Many investigators were stimulated to study lipid transport and metabolism by the epidemiologic and experimental evidence that linked abnormally high cholesterol levels with increased incidence of coronary heart disease and stroke. As a result, we now have a lot of information about how the body assimilates, transports, and uses fatty substances. The awarding of the 1985 Nobel Prize to Brown and Goldstein, for their discovery of LDL receptors and subsequent work, honors not only them but many other distinguished investigators who worked on related problems (see Motulsky, 1986). It is probably no accident that the flowering of knowledge about lipoprotein-receptor interactions occurred contemporaneously with the development of peptide hormone receptorology. There are many parallels between the biology of lipoprotein receptors and that of peptide hormone receptors, and advances in the understanding of each were stimulated by new discoveries in the other.

Some Functions of Lipids

Fatty acids and *triglycerides* are used mainly as fuel. As we have seen, the aggregate stores of carbohydrate in the body are meager, so that it is necessary to draw on fat reserves, especially when the gastrointestinal tract is empty. The storage of triglycerides, in association with a minimum of water, enables people to endure starvation for days and weeks. Triglyceride stores in fat depots may also serve as insulation against heat loss.

Phospholipids are major constituents of membranes. They store precursors of many important biologically active substances, including prostaglandins, thromboxane, prostacyclin, diacylglycerol, inositol triphosphate, etc. They may also serve as modulators of the activities of membrane proteins, such as enzymes and transport proteins.

Cholesterol is a prominent constituent of cell membranes. Variations in membrane cholesterol can affect membrane fluidity and therefore influence the function of membrane proteins. Cholesterol also serves as a precursor for bile acids and, as we have seen, as a precursor for steroid hormones in the adrenal, ovary, testis, and placenta. Although all cells have the potential for synthesizing cholesterol de novo from acetyl CoA, most cells (other than the liver and intestinal epithelial cell) get their cholesterol from the circulating pool. One of the major problems of people living in affluent industrial and agricultural societies is getting rid of an *excess* of dietary cholesterol. Since cholesterol is eliminated from the body mainly by the liver, which uses it for bile acid synthesis and secretion into the bile, avoiding an "overdose" of cholesterol must ultimately involve transporting the material to the liver for metabolism and excretion.

Composition, Structure, and Function of Lipoproteins

Fats are ideally suited for storage in fuel depots because they contain more than twice as many calories per gram and are stored with less water than are carbohydrate and protein. However, they are water insoluble, and this awkward fact has resulted in the evolution of a complex system for transporting and distributing them in blood, a watery internal environment. Unesterified or free fatty acids (FFA) are transported as albumin:FFA complexes; it is in this form that they are exported from adipocyte depots to the liver and other tissues.

Cholesterol, esterified cholesterol, phospholipids, and triglycerides are transported in highly specialized micromicellar aggregates called *lipoproteins*. Although there are many kinds of lipoproteins, they share certain characteristics: (1) their surfaces, or "shells," consist of phospholipids with their hydrophilic ends oriented outward toward the blood water, free cholesterol, and a small amount of protein [see (3) below]; (2) their inner "cores" consist of droplets (at body temperature) of triglycerides and cholesterol-fatty acid esters; (3) each has a distinctive complement of surface *apoproteins*, highly specialized proteins whose helical coils are conveniently lipophilic on their inner aspects (directed toward the core) and hydrophilic on their outwardly directed surfaces. The result is an admirable little vehicle for transporting water-insoluble substances in an aqueous medium.

As we shall soon see in greater detail, the apoproteins play essential roles in the *structure* of the particles, in *receptor recognition* in appropriate cells, and as *cofactors for several enzymes* that participate in lipoprotein metabolism.

Both cholesterol *and* individual apoproteins frequently pass from one lipoprotein to another *as they circulate in blood*. Since different cells carry receptors that recognize only specific apoproteins, a tissue destination or address can be stamped on a particle by incorporating a proper apoprotein in its envelope, or shell.

The circulating lipoproteins are divided into six major classes, depending on their size, density (measured by ultracentrifugation), and electrophoretic mobility. In the case of chylomicrons and very low-density lipoproteins (VLDL), there is considerable variation about the mean size and density. In general, the smaller particles, low-density lipoproteins (LDL) and high-density lipoproteins (HDL), although somewhat variable, are more uniform in size and composition. The large particles (chylomicrons, VLDL) contain a high percentage of triglyceride and a small fraction of protein. LDL is the major cholesterol-carrying lipoprotein. The composition of lipoprotein classes in the circulation differs from that of nascent particles when they first enter the circulation because of additions, exchanges, and subtractions of both lipid and apoprotein components that occur in the plasma.

Figure 15–1 is a graphic summary of some of the physical, structural, and compositional features of the major lipoprotein classes. It is an attempt to make a few fundamental points: (1) The lipoproteins vary widely in size from chylomicrons to HDL. The largest particles show the greatest internal variability. (2) The Greek letter designations for VLDL, LDL, and HDL were originally assigned arbitrarily on the basis of electrophoretic mobility. We do not show intermediate-density lipoproteins (IDL) because we had no readily available composition data for them. As the name implies, they are intermediate in composition between VLDL and LDL and carry the electrophoretic designation prebeta. (3) Lipoproteins with the highest amounts of triglyceride in their cores (chylomicrons, VLDL) are the least dense (i.e., have the lowest specific gravities). (4) LDL is the major cholesterol carrier. (5) HDL is the only lipoprotein that contains more shell components than core components. (6) The tissue or lipoprotein source(s) of the nascent particles (i.e., before they are modified in the circulation by contact with other lipoproteins) are given in parentheses.

In the following discussion, we describe the individual lipoproteins and their relationships in greater detail.

CHYLOMICRONS AND CHYLOMICRON REMNANTS

Triglyceride-rich lipoproteins can enter the circulation from the intestinal epithelium (as chylomicrons) or from the liver (as VLDL). Ingested triglycerides are broken down to FFA or monoglycerides in the

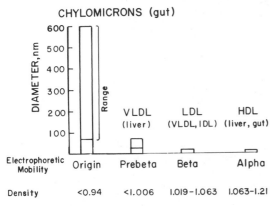

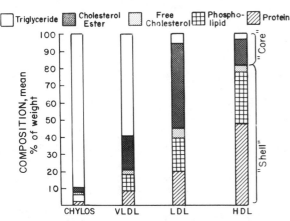

FIG 15–1.
A summary of size, source and composition of major lipoproteins. (For more detailed information, see Bierman and Glomset, Brown and Goldstein (1985), and Schaefer and Levy in bibliography.)

intestinal lumen and absorbed in those forms by the intestinal epithelial cell. Short chain fatty acids (up to 12 carbons in length) may go directly to the liver via the portal circulation. Long chain fatty acids (greater than 14 carbons) are reesterified in the intestinal cell to triglycerides and incorporated into chylomicrons, along with appropriate shell phospholipids and proteins. Absorbed free cholesterol may be used by the intestinal cell for its own purposes, incorporated into the chylomicron shell, or, after esterification, added to its core.

The apoprotein B 48 is synthesized only in the intestinal cell. In the absence of B 48, chylomicrons cannot be formed. Several subtypes of apo A are also added to the chylomicron surface during its assembly, so that the nascent chylomicron, which is secreted into the terminal lymphatics of the thoracic duct, displays only apo B 48 and an assortment of apo A's as the protein components of its surface.

When the nascent chylomicrons enter the blood from the thoracic duct, they encounter HDL particles that carry apoproteins C and E. Chylomicrons and HDL then trade apoproteins according to the following transaction:

$$\text{Chylomicron} \underset{\text{some apo A}}{\overset{\text{apo C, apo E}}{\rightleftharpoons}} \text{HDL}$$

This trade is a crucial one, for apo C II is a cofactor for the tissue enzyme *lipoprotein lipase* (LPL), an enzyme that abstracts triglycerides from chylomicrons and VLDL and hydrolyzes them to FFA and glycerol. The FFA can enter cells either for use as fuel or for reesterification to triglyceride.

It is necessary here to pause and reflect about the enzyme LPL, which is synthesized and secreted by adipocytes, cardiac and skeletal muscle cells, and mammary gland cells. The secreted enzyme attaches to the endothelial cell plasma membranes in the microvessels associated with each of its tissue sources. The regulation of the enzyme (in this case, a reflection of the total number of enzyme units) is not uniform from one tissue to another; a physiologic determinant may, in fact, have *opposite* effects on LPL in two different tissues. The following scheme, in which arrows indicate increase or decrease in LPL activity, illustrates this point:

	Starvation (or diabetes)	Refeeding (or insulin)	Lactation
Adipose tissue	↓	↑	
Heart muscle	↑	↓	
Mammary gland in pregnancy	—	—	↑ ↑ ↑

The activity of the enzyme is affected by the insulin:glucagon ratio (in starvation and refeeding, diabetes and insulin replacement) and by other hormones (in pregnancy and lactation). Adaptive fluctuations in LPL activity in various tissues can affect the localized fate of triglyceride-rich lipoproteins. In diabetes, failure to synthesize LPL due to lack of insulin or insulin resistance is one of the causes of the observed hyperlipidemia. Inborn errors in LPL can also cause hypertriglyceridemia (see below).

As a result of the action of LPL (in partnership with apo C II), the chylomicron particle is greatly diminished in size and fragmented into redundant shell components (including apo C) and a remnant (apo E and apo B containing). The redundant shell components are captured by HDL particles that can then donate apo E and apo C to incoming, virgin chylomicrons. The remnant, having been provident enough to acquire apo E from HDL in a previous trade, is now equipped with just the right apoproteins (B48 and E) to fit the hepatocyte apo E receptor. The remnant:receptor complex is then endocytosed, incorporated into phagolysosomes, and the core contents, mainly cholesterol ester and a small amount of triglyceride, are hydrolyzed. The liver cell may use the cholesterol for its own membrane maintenance, synthesize bile acids from it, or incorporate it into newly synthesized VLDL. Some free cholesterol is excreted into bile, where it is prevented from aggregating into crystals and stones by the combined detergent action of bile acids and lecithin; but that is another very long story. The cholesterol that enters the GI tract in the bile may be reabsorbed or it may undergo metabolism by enteric organisms and excretion in the feces. This and the desquamation of cholesterol-containing intestinal epithelial cells are the only exit routes for cholesterol from the body, a matter we will return to later.

VERY LOW-DENSITY LIPOPROTEINS AND INTERMEDIATE-DENSITY LIPOPROTEINS

VLDL, synthesized in the liver, are the major vehicles for transporting triglyceride to adipose tissue for storage or to cardiac and skeletal muscle cells for use as fuel or storage. VLDL also carries cholesterol in the circulation for distribution to other lipoproteins or to tissues for their specialized needs. VLDL *acquires* cholesterol ester in the circulation from HDL via a cholesterol ester exchange glycoprotein that happens to be present in plasma.

Just as apo B 48 is a specific marker for chylomicrons, apo B 100 (larger than B 48) is distinctively part of VLDL and lipoprotein particles derived from them. VLDL also have apo E and apo C built into their shells, along with free cholesterol. Together, chylomicrons and VLDL carry most of the plasma triglyceride. In the postabsorptive state, when sampling is most frequently done, practically all of the measured triglyceride is normally in VLDL.

As we have seen, VLDL particles are born with apo C and, as in the case of chylomicrons, triglyceride is extracted from them by the LPL-apo C II team. Also like chylomicrons, some of their redundant phospholipid-protein-cholesterol shell fragments are scavenged by HDL in a process accomplished by a plasma phospholipid transfer protein (see Tall et al.). The major remnant is IDL, which contains all of the apo B 100 of the pristine VLDL and a certain amount of triglyceride. IDL may either combine with hepatocyte apo B 100-E receptors (also known as LDL receptors, see below), and undergo endocytosis and metabolism, or be acted upon by a hepatic lipase that extracts most of its remaining triglyceride and, in the process, transforms IDL into LDL.

Low-Density Lipoproteins

LDL carries 60%–70% of the plasma cholesterol, mostly esterified. The major function of LDL is to deliver cholesterol to peripheral cells to meet their needs for membrane biosynthesis, steroid hormone synthesis or, in hepatocytes, bile acid production. In humans, most LDL is formed from IDL as described above, but there is some evidence that a small amount of LDL may be secreted directly by the liver.

In 1973, Brown and Goldstein discovered that LDL were taken up by cultured human fibroblasts by combining with a specific plasma membrane receptor. In Figure 15–2, we have attempted to summarize our knowledge of this process as it has evolved over the past 12 years. The encircled numbers in the following description refer to numbers in Figure 15–2.

① LDL, unlike chylomicrons or VLDL, is small enough to gain access to extravascular spaces where it can bind to ② a specific receptor on cell surfaces. Small IDL particles may bind to the same receptor, although most IDL are cleared by the liver. LDL displays mainly apo B 100, while IDL carries both apo B 100 and apo E. The LDL receptor is sometimes called the B 100-E receptor since it recognizes both apoproteins. The structure of the B 100-E receptor gene has now been determined, and its localization on chromosome 19 has been demonstrated (Sudhor et al.). (Parenthetically, the gene for apoprotein E has also been localized to chromosome 19, which suggests the fascinating possibility of coordinated coevolution of a ligand and its receptor.)

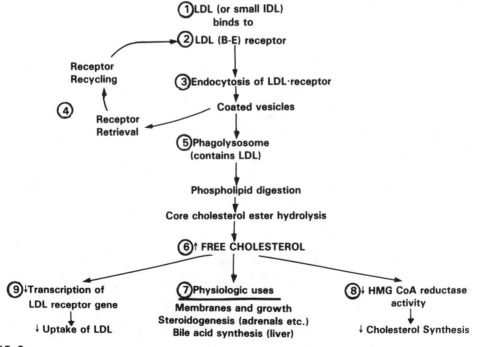

FIG 15–2.
Receptor-mediated metabolism of LDL, mainly according to Brown and Goldstein.

LDL-receptor complexes are aggregated in "coated pits," so called because the plasma membrane in these regions is studded with buttons of the protein clathrin on the cytosol side of the bilayer. The complexes are then endocytosed and appear as coated vesicles ③. Just as we have seen in the case of internalized peptide hormone-receptor complexes, a mechanism exists for retrieving receptors (but not LDL) from the vesicles and recycling them via the Golgi apparatus back to the plasma membrane for reinsertion ④. At an uncertain stage of the process, the vesicle membrane fuses with a lysosome to form ⑤ an LDL-containing phagolysosome. Lysosomal enzymes then proceed to digest the phospholipid shell and hydrolyze the core cholesterol esters, resulting in an increase in the free cholesterol concentration ($[C]_c$) within the cell ⑥.

This increase in $[C]_c$ has several consequences: ⑦ the free cholesterol may be used either directly or stored after esterification to cholesterol ester (CE) via the enzyme acyl CoA:cholesterol acyl transferase (ACAT). Free cholesterol may also be inserted into membranes or used as a precursor for steroid hormones or bile acids.

Another important effect of elevation of $[C]_c$ is to decrease de novo synthesis of cholesterol by the cell ⑧. The high cholesterol concentration inhibits the enzyme hydroxymethyl glutaryl CoA reductase (HMG CoA reductase), which is the enzyme that catalyzes the reduction of HMG CoA to mevalonic acid.

Over a longer time course, the cell has an additional mechanism for protecting itself against a cholesterol overload, for an increase in $[C]_c$ has the effect of *decreasing transcription of the LDL receptor gene* ⑨. This down-regulation drastically decreases the number of LDL receptors in the plasma membrane, thus limiting the amount of LDL that can be ingested by the cell. Indeed, if the whole body is persistently forced to dispose of too much cholesterol, this physiologic protective mechanism may be partly responsible for elevating the concentration of cholesterol in the blood by impairing receptor-mediated removal of LDL. It has been established that the rate of abstraction, or clearance, of radioactively labeled LDL from the blood is directly related to the LDL receptor number on the membranes of peripheral cells.

In normal humans, about two-thirds of plasma LDL are removed from the circulation by receptor-mediated uptake by liver or peripheral cells and tissues. The remaining LDL is removed by processes independent of the B 100-E receptor. One such process involves a receptor that fails to recognize LDL but does bind chemically modified LDL. This receptor has variously been called the *acetyl LDL,* or *scaven-ger cell receptor*, and is found in macrophages and endothelial cells that are unable to bind native LDL. Although the precise chemical nature of the chemical modification of LDL that is presumed to occur in vivo is not known, human cells in culture can transform LDL into a form that can be taken up by macrophages. Macrophages can continue to dispose of large amounts of modified LDL because, apparently, the scavenger receptor, unlike the B-E receptor, is not down-regulated by its ligand. On the other hand, macrophages stimulated to take up excessive amounts of modified LDL by high circulating levels participate prominently in the process of foam cell formation in the atherosclerotic process. Non-receptor-mediated uptake of LDL also occurs (see Mahley, 1985).

HIGH-DENSITY LIPOPROTEINS

The high-density lipoproteins (HDL) are free cholesterol scavengers that collect excess cholesterol from the surfaces of peripheral cells and transport it back to the liver either for excretion or for recycling to the circulation. HDL contains another example of the coenzyme function of an apoprotein (apo C II and LPL was the first). When HDL collects free cholesterol (which, like phospholipids, has a hydrophilic domain), most of it remains in the outer shell at first. However, HDL associates in the circulation with the enzyme lecithin-cholesterol acyl transferase (LCAT). This enzyme catalyzes the esterification of cholesterol with phospholipid-derived fatty acid. Cholesterol ester may then be stored in the core droplet, or it may be transferred to another lipoprotein via plasma cholesteryl ester transport protein.

The concept of *reverse cholesterol transport* (i.e., transport of cholesterol from the periphery to the liver for excretion) in which HDL plays a prominent part, was originally described by Glomset et al. (see Bierman and Glomset). If this process is impaired and an inadequate amount of cholesterol is returned to the liver for excretion, any tendency to accumulate cholesterol carrying lipoproteins in the blood is exaggerated. Some HDL particles that have acquired apo E may themselves be abstracted from the circulation by hepatocytes. Other HDL cholesterol ester may find its way, via a cholesterol ester transport protein, to VLDL or IDL, which display apo B-100 and E, both of which are bound by hepatocyte receptor. It is the ability of HDL to collect cholesterol, esterify it, and transmit it to forms that can be taken up and metabolized by liver cells that is the basis for its reputation as a lipoprotein that inhibits the establishment of hyperlipoproteinemia.

HDL also play a prominent role in the brisk trade in apoproteins, phospholipids, and cholesterol esters that occurs among the various lipoprotein classes. We have already described how HDL donates apo C to incoming chylomicrons, rendering them lipoprotein lipase-sensitive. We have also pointed out that, in the course of LPL's action on chylomicrons and VLDL, shell fragments (phospholipid, apo C, cholesterol, etc.) are generated and incorporated into HDL. Thus, HDL, whose nascent particles are secreted by the liver and intestine, constantly undergo remodelling in the circulation by many additions, subtractions, and exchanges.

A brief review of some features of individual apoproteins is given in Table 15–1.

Modifications of Lipoprotein Metabolism in Health and Disease

Most authorities now agree on the relationship between hyperlipoproteinemia, especially involving LDL, and increased risk for developing the most common complications of atherosclerosis, coronary heart disease, and stroke. The source of accumulated lipids in arteriosclerotic plaques is the circulating pool of lipids, mainly LDL. Concurrent elevations in VLDL may contribute to the risk. Another contributory risk factor is a low level of HDL *when LDL level is elevated*.

Modifications of lipoprotein metabolism can be caused by both environmental and genetic factors. Epidemiologic studies of various population groups and of newborn human infants in atherogenesis-prone societies suggest that what is regarded as a "normal" blood lipid pattern in these societies is, in fact, hyperlipoproteinemia. A sharp increase in risk of macrovascular disease occurs when total cholesterol level (mostly in LDL) rises above 220 mg/dl, a figure usually regarded as within normal limits in industrialized countries. As we have remarked, risk is magnified when there is a concurrent increase in LDL and a *decrease* in HDL.

Blood lipid abnormalities are not the *only* causes of atherosclerosis. The deposition of lipids subintimally and in the walls of arteries is the result of an extremely complex process that may involve (at the very least) abnormalities in platelet aggregation, platelet-derived growth factor and cellular responses to it, growth hormone, arachidonic acid metabolism, and many other factors. Moreover, the ability to tolerate fairly extensive coronary atherosclerosis without lethal consequences may depend on the existence or development of collateral circulation. In other words, individuals may vary in their vascular vulnerability to atherogenic levels of lipoproteins as well as in their capacity to adapt to gradual accretion of lipid deposits in their vessels.

TABLE 15–1.
Some Distinctive Features of Apoproteins*

APOPROTEIN	SOURCE	STRUCTURE	FEATURES
A I	Liver, intestine	243 AA	Binds lipid, structural Main HDL apoprotein Cofactor for LCAT†
A II	Liver	Dimer, known	Binds lipid Second HDL apoprotein
A IV	Liver, intestine	?	Cofactor for LCAT
B 48	Intestine	?	Chylomicron marker
B 100	Liver	Incompletely known	Ligand for B-E receptor VLDL marker
C I	Liver (intestine)	MW 6605	Activates LCAT ? HDL esterification of cholesterol
C II	Liver (intestine)	MW 8824	Activates LPL
C III	Liver (intestine)	MW 8750	Glycoprotein
E (six phenotypes)	Liver	Mostly known	Binds to B-E (LDL) receptor Main ligand for chylomicron remnants in liver

*Modified from Schaefer E, Levy RI: *N Engl J Med* 1985; 312:1300.
†LCAT = lecithin:cholesterol acyl transferase.

SOME EXAMPLES OF GENETIC ABNORMALITIES OF LIPOPROTEIN METABOLISM

Familial Hyperlipidemia (FH)

The pathophysiologic mechanisms in the etiology of FH have been elucidated by Brown and Goldstein and many others. The disease occurs in either homozygous (1 in 1,000,000) or heterozygous (1 in 500) form in the United States. Patients with homozygous FH have heart attacks in childhood or adolescence; those with the heterozygous form often have such attacks in early middle age. The elevated level of LDL in these people is caused by one of several LDL receptor gene abnormalities that interfere with the removal of LDL from the circulation. Since LDL is derived from VLDL via IDL, and since about half of the IDL is taken up in the liver by the LDL receptor, when that receptor is defective, IDL accumulates in the blood. When this happens, LDL is overproduced from IDL; its blood level, already high because its egress route is more or less blocked, increases even more. The disease is much more severe in homozygous individuals because they inherit *two* abnormal LDL receptor genes, while the heterozygous people inherit an abnormal gene and a normal one.

Although all known LDL receptor protein genetic defects have the same consequences (i.e., inadequate binding and internalization of LDL), they may act at different stages in the history of the receptor. In a study of 77 subjects with FH, seven mutations were described (Tolleshaug et al.). In one, no immunoprecipitable receptor precursor was found. In others, precursors were transcribed but failed to be transported to the plasma membrane. In still others, precursors reached the plasma membrane but failed to bind LDL properly. This illustrates the point that mutations at specific amino acid sites may compromise the process of synthesis→transport→insertion→function at different stages. The opportunities for single gene mutations to make mischief are many.

Proteins other than receptors may also undergo mutations and result in abnormal lipoprotein metabolism. From a long list of genetic hyperlipoproteinemias, two examples demonstrate this point. First, there is a rare *genetic deficiency of the enzyme lipoprotein lipase (LPL),* the enzyme mainly responsible for the extraction and hydrolysis of triglyceride from chylomicrons and VLDL. Thus, in this condition, chylomicronemia is contantly present, but serum cholesterol is not notably elevated; it does not carry a risk of early atherosclerosis. Second is an abnormal apoprotein E, which impairs the hepatic removal of chy-

lomicron remnants and IDL from the circulation. (For many references to the genetic hyperlipoproteinemias, see Bierman and Glomset and Brown and Goldstein, 1985.)

DIETARY CHOLESTEROL AND FAT

Environmental influences, particularly diet composition and activity pattern, have striking effects on blood lipid patterns of large populations. For example, as Japanese people moved from Japan to Hawaii and to California, there was a progressive increase in mean serum cholesterol as dietary and life-style acculturation occurred.

It is now generally accepted that a high cholesterol, high saturated fat diet can lead to increased plasma LDL (and cholesterol) concentrations. People react differently to such diets, and some fortunate ones can eat two eggs daily for many decades with comparative impunity. The reasons for these differences are not understood, but some believe in the concept of "latent dyslipoproteinemias," which simply means that some people are less able than others to compensate for excessive dietary intake of cholesterol and saturated fat, most probably on a genetic basis (see DeGennes et al.). Some authorities recommend that entire populations be encouraged to adopt a "prudent" diet (i.e., little red meat, substituting fish and fowl as protein sources, high fiber and complex carbohydrates, low cholesterol, polyunsaturated fat for *some* saturated fat), while others believe that only individuals with appropriately abnormal blood lipid patterns or alarming family histories should be encouraged to change their dietary habits. In any case, there is now evidence that, in the U.S.A., the incidence of heart attacks and strokes has been declining for more than a decade. The reasons for the decline are not known, but indications are that many individuals are consciously decreasing their intake of saturated fat and cholesterol, becoming more physically active, controlling blood pressure, and stopping smoking.

The question "Can the prognosis for individuals with high levels of LDL be improved by cholesterol-lowering maneuvers?" has now been answered in the affirmative according to most of the evidence. (For example, see Lipid Research Clinics Program.)

ENDOCRINE AND OTHER SECONDARY FORMS OF HYPERLIPOPROTEINEMIA

When hyperlipoproteinemia is found to be secondary to endocrine dysfunction or to some other cause, the blood lipid pattern may be restored to normal by attacking the primary pathophysiologic disturbance. Some examples of secondary hyperlipoproteinemia follow.

As we saw in Chapter 14, increased VLDL (and, sometimes, chylomicron levels) are often seen in *diabetes*. This is due both to decreased removal of triglyceride (insulin is necessary for the production of LPL by adipocytes) and to increased VLDL secretion rate (hyperinsulinemia in Type II diabetes exposes the liver to very high portal blood insulin concentrations that stimulate lipogenesis and VLDL secretion). In nondiabetic *obese* individuals, increased VLDL levels are seen for similar reasons, since down-regulation of insulin receptors and assorted postbinding adaptations render cells insulin resistant and, therefore, LPL deficient. Such people are commonly hyperinsulinemic as well. In both diabetes and obesity, correction of the primary problem restores blood lipid patterns toward normal ones.

In *pregnancy* and in women taking *estrogens,* either alone or as constituents of *oral contraceptive pills,* increases in serum VLDL may occur.

HYPOthyroidism and *HYPERadrenocorticism* (Cushing's disease) typically have abnormal lipoprotein patterns that are reversible with appropriate correction of the endocrine dysfunction.

Similarly, some people with a variety of *renal diseases* may show elevations in serum VLDL and/or LDL. *Alcoholics* too may exhibit increased VLDL (and chylomicron) levels that revert toward normal with abstention from ethanol.

A review of some influences that raise and lower LDL and HDL is given in Table 15–2.

Treatment of Hyperlipoproteinemias

We discuss this topic only to reiterate the point that rational therapy in this, as in all of the other subjects we have discussed, is based on understanding of pathophysiologic mechanisms. If hyperlipoproteinemia is judged to be secondary to a primary cause, treatment is directed at correcting the primary disturbance. Similarly, it is important to establish the lipoprotein profile to design an appropriate management strategy.

Hyperlipidemia may occur at any wave length of a broad spectrum, from mild to homozygous familial hyperlipidemia. The less severe types (especially hypertriglyceridemia) may respond to *weight reduction* and/or to the *"prudent diet"* described above (reviewed by Goldberg and Schonfeld). If these conservative measures fail, one or more of a number of *drugs* may be used to modify lipoprotein metabolism in desirable ways. (For documentation, see Brown and Goldstein, 1985). Various *surgical* procedures are being tried experimentally with some hope for future success.

DIET AND EXERCISE

Recommendations for the dietary management of hyperlipoproteinemias have been assembled by a committee of the American Heart Association (Grundy, 1984). The committee suggests (1) that dietary fat be restricted to less than 30% of total caloric intake; (2) that the ratio of polyunsaturated fat:saturated fat (P/S ratio) be approximately 1 (usually accomplished by restricting saturated fat in the diet), and (3) that cholesterol intake be restricted to less than 300 mg/day. Although diets with a high P:S ratio have been found to decrease circulating LDL levels, there is no generally accepted explanation for this phenomenon. Overenthusiastic polyunsaturated fat ingestion is not recommended since the long-term consequences of eating such diets are not yet known.

TABLE 15–2.

Factors That Influence Lipoprotein Levels in Humans

RAISE LDL	LOWER LDL
Sex (M > F pre-, F > M postmenopause)	
Aging	Newborn
Saturated fat diet	Polyunsaturated fat diet
High cholesterol intake	Low cholesterol intake
Low-fiber diet	High-fiber diet
Ethanol ingestion	Abstinence from ethanol
Pregnancy	Delivery
Obesity	Weight loss
Diabetes	Successful treatment
Hypothyroidism	Successful treatment
Cushing's disease	Successful treatment
Uremia	Successful treatment
Nephrosis	Successful treatment
Familial hyperlipidemias	

RAISE HDL	LOWER HDL
Fish protein	Vegetarian, carbohydrate diet
Ethanol	Abstinence from prior ethanol
Exercise	Sedentary lifestyle, obesity
Estrogen	Progestins, androgens
Hypothyroidism	Successful treatment
Beta agonists	Beta blockers
Successful treatment	Diabetes
	Smoking

A similar diet is recommended for obese individuals, but they may need sharper reductions in fat intake to achieve necessary decreases in total diet calories. Sedentary individuals are encouraged to exercise.

DRUGS

Many drugs have been tried as lipid-lowering agents, and a large number have been discarded because of undesirable side effects. A few that are either useful or promising will be described briefly, mainly to illustrate that they act at different stages of lipoprotein metabolism and that no single drug is effective in all hyperlipoproteinemic people.

Bile-acid binding (anion exchange) resins, such as *cholestyramine* and *colestipol,* act by stimulating LDL uptake and cholesterol excretion by the liver. Their effect is based on the fact that the conversion of cholesterol to bile acid is product inhibited, i.e., bile acids prevent their own synthesis. Thus, if the enterohepatic circulation of bile acids back to the liver is prevented by trapping them in the intestinal lumen with a binding, nonabsorbable resin, the cholesterol-bile acid reaction is released from inhibition. This has the effect of lowering the hepatic concentration of cholesterol, which results in the up-regulation of LDL receptors. This increases the rate of removal of LDL from the circulation. In addition, since bile acids are essential for cholesterol absorption, less cholesterol is absorbed when large amounts of bile acids are bound to a nonabsorbable resin. Although these drugs are not pleasant to take and are associated with some side effects, they are the least toxic agents of this group. Prospective studies have demonstrated that hypercholesterolemic men maintained on cholestyramine show significantly less coronary artery disease than do controls on placebo treatment.

All of this, at first glance, seems almost too good to be true. In fact, the resins have one effect that seriously limits their usefulness: decreasing cholesterol levels in tissues removes the inhibitory effect of cholesterol on its own synthesis. Thus, endogenous synthesis, which antagonizes the desired effect of the resin, is stimulated. This has resulted in the testing of two drugs that *inhibit endogenous cholesterol synthesis* at the HMG CoA reductase step: *compactin* and *mevinolin.* Preliminary results suggest that a combination of a bile acid-binding resin and a cholesterol synthesis inhibitor is more effective in lowering serum LDL than is the resin alone.

Another agent of demonstrated usefulness is *nicotinic acid* (in far greater than vitamin doses). This drug decreases both VLDL and LDL by inhibiting adipocyte lipolysis, decreasing hepatic VLDL secre-tion, and stimulating lipoprotein lipase activity; in fact, its effect on lipoprotein lipase resembles that of insulin. As in the case of compactin, resin and nicotinic acid yield additive results. *Clofibrate* has complex effects on blood lipids, including an increase in lipoprotein lipase activity. Although its use is severely limited by its side effects, it was historically important. Recently, a clofibrate analogue, *gemfibrozil,* has been tested with some success. Both of these agents not only lower VLDL and LDL but also increase HDL. (For a detailed discussion and documentation of the pharmacology of lipid-lowering agents, see Brown and Goldstein, 1985.)

SURGERY

The hyperlipoproteinemia that is most refractory to all of the treatment discussed so far is, of course, severe or homozygous familial hyperlipidemia. Several experimental surgical procedures have been tried in a few such individuals with results that warrant further study. These include ileal bypass, portacaval shunt, and periodic plasmapheresis. Since HDL may be removed along with LDL, one team has experimented with the *selective* removal of LDL by a solid-phase anti-LDL antibody and the reinjection of all other plasma constituents.

Another potentially hopeful development is that of a form of surgical-genetic engineering: liver transplantation. We are aware of one report of the transplantation of a genetically normal liver (and heart) into a six-year-old child with homozygous familial hyperlipidemia who had already suffered two heart attacks. There was more than an 80% reduction in serum LDL about 18 months postoperatively. As transplant technology improves, there may be a few individuals who will benefit from this heroic procedure. We commend the report of Bilheimer et al. as an especially elegant example of clinical investigation at its best. It is interesting to see such dramatic confirmation of the importance of functioning LDL receptors in the liver for the drainage of excess cholesterol from the body.

BIBLIOGRAPHY

Bierman EL, Glomset JA: Disorders of lipid metabolism, in Wilson JD, Foster DW (eds): *Williams Textbook of Endocrinology,* ed 7. Philadelphia, WB Saunders Co, 1985, pp 1108–1136.

Bilheimer DW, Goldstein JL, Grundy SM, et al: Liver transplantation to provide low-density-lipoprotein receptors and lower plasma cholesterol in a child with homozygous familial hypercholesterolemia. *N Engl J Med* 1984; 311:1658.

Brown MS, Goldstein JL: How LDL receptors influence cholesterol and atherosclerosis. *Sci Am* 1984; 251:58.

Brown MS, Goldstein JL: Drugs used in the treatment of hyperlipoproteinemias, in Gilman AG, Rall TW, Murad F (eds): *Goodman and Gilman's The Pharmacological Basis of Therapeutics,* ed 7. New York, Macmillan Publishing Co, 1985, pp 827–845.

Cooper AD: Role of the liver in the degradation of lipoproteins. *Gastroenterology* 1985; 88:192.

DeGennes JL, Polonovski J, Paoletti R (eds): *Latent Dyslipoproteinemias and Atherosclerosis.* New York, Raven Press, 1984.

Eisenberg S: High-density lipoprotein metabolism. *J Lipid Res* 1984; 25:1017.

Goldberg AC, Schonfeld G: Effects of diet on lipoprotein metabolism. *Annu Rev Nutr* 1985; 5:195.

Goldstein JL, Brown JS: Progress in understanding the LDL receptor and HMG-CoA reductase: Two membrane proteins that regulate the plasma cholesterol. *J Lipid Res* 1984; 25:1450.

Gotto AM, Jr: Some reflections on arteriosclerosis: Past, present, and future. *Circulation* 1985; 72:8.

Grundy SM: Absorption and metabolism of dietary cholesterol. *Annu Rev Nutr* 1983; 3:71.

Grundy SM: AHA special report: Recommendations for the treatment of hyperlipidemia in adults: A joint statement of the Nutrition Committee and the Council on Arteriosclerosis of the American Heart Association. *Arteriosclerosis* 1984; 4:445A.

Havel RJ: The formation of LDL: Mechanisms and regulation. *J Lipid Res* 1984; 25:1570.

Knott TJ, Rall SC Jr, Innerarity TL, et al: Human apolipoprotein B: Structure of carboxyl-terminal domains, sites of gene expression, and chromosomal localization. *Science* 1985; 230:37.

Lehrman MA, Schneider WJ, Sudhof TC, et al: Mutation in LDL receptor: Alu-Alu recombination deletes exons encoding transmembrane and cytoplasmic domains. *Science* 1985; 227:140.

Lewis B: The lipoproteins: Predictors, protectors, and pathogens. *Br Med J* 1983; 287:1161.

Lipid Research Clinics Program: The lipid research clinics coronary primary prevention trial results: II. The relationship of reduction in incidence of coronary heart disease to cholesterol lowering. *JAMA* 1984; 251:365.

Mahley RW, Innerarity TL, Rak SC, et al: Plasma lipoproteins: Apolipoprotein structure and functions. *J Lipid Res* 1984; 25:1277.

Mahley RW: Atherogenic lipoproteins and coronary artery disease: Concepts derived from recent advances in cellular and molecular biology. *Circulation* 1985; 72:943.

Motulsky AG: The 1985 Nobel prize in physiology or medicine. *Science* 1986; 231:126.

Norum KR, Berg T, Helgerud P, et al: Transport of cholesterol. *Physiol Rev* 1983; 63:1343.

Pittman RC, Steinberg D: Sites and mechanisms of uptake and degradation of high density and low-density lipoproteins. *J Lipid Res* 1984; 25:1577.

Schaefer E, Levy RI: Pathogenesis and management of lipoprotein disorders. *N Engl J Med* 1985; 312:1300.

Stoffel W, Borberg H, Greve V: Application of specific extracorporeal removal of low-density lipoprotein in familial hypercholesterolemia. *Lancet* 1981; 2:1005.

Sudhof TC, Goldstein JL, Brown MS, et al: The LDL receptor gene: A mosaic of exons shared with different proteins. *Science* 1985; 228:815.

Tall AR, Krumholz S, Olivecrona T, et al: Plasma phospholipid transfer protein enhances transfer and exchange of phospholipids between very low density lipoproteins and high density lipoproteins during lipolysis. *J Lipid Res* 1985; 26:842.

Tolleshaug H, Hobgood KK, Brown MS, et al: The LDL receptor locus in familial hypercholesterolemia: Multiple mutations disrupt transport and processing of a membrane receptor. *Cell* 1983; 32:941.

16

Energy Balance

Animals are governed by the same thermodynamic laws that apply to the rest of the physical universe. If the energy content of the food ingested by a man is exactly equal to his total energy expenditure, he is said to be in energy balance. A state of positive energy balance can be produced either by an increase in food intake over energy output or by a diminished output or by a combination of these. Similarly, a decrease in food intake or an increased energy requirement results in negative energy or caloric balance. These facts are so starkly obvious it hardly seems necessary to state them.

The physiologic, medical, and public health importance of the problem of energy balance cannot be overestimated. In many countries of the world, insufficient food is available to large numbers of people, who are therefore forced to become adapted to a chronic state of undernutrition. This may not be merely a quantitative caloric deficit. In many instances, the quality of the food is poor and the accompanying accessory food factors are in short supply. At the other extreme, affluent societies provide a plethora of food and every conceivable chance to avoid physical activity, both of which contribute to a high incidence of obesity. This condition has been called one of our most important public health problems because it predisposes people to many vascular and metabolic diseases. The life expectancy of overweight individuals is substantially less than that of people of average weight, a fact that life insurance companies are not likely to let us forget (Fig 16–1).

There is general agreement that people who remain obese between the ages of 20 and 50 are at greater risk than are older obese individuals (see Fig 16–1). Recently, Andres and colleagues have redrawn height-weight tables so that higher weights (i.e., higher than those in recently upwardly revised life insurance tables) are permitted for ages 55 and above. They did this on the basis of their analysis of the relation between body weight and mortality data in

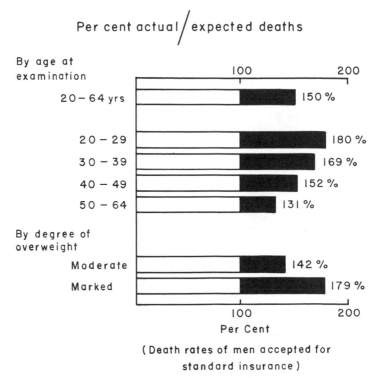

FIG 16–1.
Effect of overweight on life expectancy. *Black bars* represent excess mortality in individuals who were overweight when insurance was issued. (After Marks HH: *Bull NY Acad Med* 1960; 36:15.)

older individuals which suggested that moderately overweight people (according to older standards) had a more favorable prognosis than did thinner individuals. Since there are so many possible variables in addition to body weight that may influence mortality, it is not surprising that other authorities are unwilling to endorse the Andres tables at this time.

Later we will show that the practice of homogenizing all overweight people into a single class, which was done in most epidemiological studies in the past, is no longer permissible. It is now apparent that two people, equally overweight but with differing fat distribution, are not equally vulnerable to the diseases associated with obesity.

Men and women are variably successful in maintaining energy balance. For some, the equation input-outgo is achieved readily and with no conscious effort, whereas others who are successful in maintaining energy equilibrium can do so only by consciously monitoring body weight over a long time. When one considers the extraordinary complexity and variety of the biochemical and physiologic mechanisms that are operative in man and other animals, the precision

with which energy balance is maintained in many individuals is remarkable. It is less remarkable that, with so many forces at work that tend to upset the equilibrium, there is a high incidence of obesity in economically favored countries.

In Figure 16–2, a graphic outline of this chapter is given. It was designed to demonstrate that caloric balance represents a vector of many forces, which operate to displace it in either direction. If these forces tend to cancel one another (e.g., high food intake and high rate of muscle work), balance may still be maintained.

Obesity or Obesities?

Since much of the research on energy balance, both experimental and clinical, is related to the problem of obesity, three important points should be made at the outset.

1. Obesity and overweight are not synonymous, although overweight individuals usually are obese. Some professional athletes with extremely hypertrophic muscles are overweight according to standard

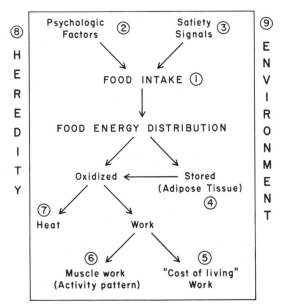

FIG 16–2.
Nine factors that influence energy balance.

tables of weight and height, but they do not have excessively large deposits of fat in their adipose tissue nor are their fat cells enlarged. These people are metabolically similar to people of "normal" weight.

2. Obesity may be defined as an increase in triglyceride deposition in adipocytes. The division between normal and excessive fat deposition is an arbitrary one and varies from one authority to another. Some authorities do not consider people obese unless they are 20% or more above ideal weight, but this is not a universally accepted figure. Indeed, four prominent British authorities on nutrition (see Durnin et al.) have suggested that as much as 30% of the world's population may really be eating too much, and that life insurance tables of ideal weight are skewed toward obesity. By the same reasoning, an unknown number of people who are now regarded as underfed may in fact be adequately nourished quantitatively.

3. Obesity is still considered to be a single entity by many clinicians and epidemiologists. Like anemia and hypertension, "obesity" is a symptom and not a disease. It signals the presence of one or more of a large collection of disturbances in energy balance, which probably have multiple causes. Attempts are now being made (e.g., see Sims) to sort out obesities according to cause, when possible, or according to distinguishing characteristics. Each individual is a composite of all of the genetic, environmental, psychologic, activity pattern and metabolic factors indicated in Figure 16–2. Deposition of fat, or its preven-

tion, can be brought about by many combinations of these factors. In some instances, one factor may predispose to obesity but another may compensate in the other direction (e.g., high food intake and heavy exercise), as noted above.

One of the more important consequences of contemporary behavioral approaches to the problems of obesity (see below) has been reemphasis of the necessity to examine each obese person as an individual functioning in a particular physical and personal environment. This time-consuming analysis sometimes permits assessment of the relative importance of many possible contributory factors to obesity.

Central Nervous Regulation of Food Intake

The study of food intake regulation has been somewhat inhibited by a certain amount of semantic confusion; the following lexicon is therefore in order. *Hunger* is the awareness of the need to ingest food, and it may be accompanied by a complex set of phenomena, including hunger pangs, anticipatory salivation and increased food-searching behavior. In sum, hunger is a malaise, a disagreeable combination of sensations, which, as it progresses, acquires a frantic character. *Appetite* is the desire to ingest food. Unlike hunger, which occurs when the body's store of nutrients becomes depleted below a certain preset maintenance level, appetite may persist even when hunger has been appeased. Appetite is strongly influenced by emotion, by the presence or absence of conditioning or distracting stimuli, and by discriminatory choices of various kinds. *Satiety* is the lack of desire to eat that occurs after ingestion of food. *Anorexia* describes a situation in which the physiologic state that would ordinarily produce a sensation of hunger is present, but all available signals call in vain for resumption of eating behavior.

Cannon's demonstration of the association between the sensation of hunger and the appearance of vigorous, rhythmic gastric contractions led Carlson to the view that the stomach was the organ that communicated the essential hunger and satiety information to the nervous system. Further, he anticipated a widely held modern view that the level of blood glucose has something to do with hunger and satiety, for he was able to amplify hunger contractions by producing insulin hypoglycemia and to cause them to disappear by injecting glucose intravenously.

Antecedent observations on the successful maintenance of caloric balance in gastrectomized animals and later ones on vagotomized (and therefore stomach-denervated) patients failed to sustain Carlson's gastric contraction hypothesis of regulation. Adolph's demonstration that dilution of the diet with inert bulk materials caused rats to increase their food intake to the point at which they were consuming as many calories as in the control period also pointed to extragastrointestinal factors in the regulation of food intake. Recently, there has been a reemphasis on the participation of the mouth and gastrointestinal tract in metering food intake.

EXPERIMENTAL HYPOTHALAMIC OBESITY

Many of the clinical and experimental observations referred to in the chronology had suggested some sort of relationship between structures at the base of the brain and food intake, but recent exploration of the subject began with Hetherington and Ranson's successful induction of experimental obesity in the rat by stereotactic placement of symmetric, bilateral hypothalamic lesions that involved the ventromedial nuclei (VMN). Hetherington's lesions were rather large and his animals were young—circumstances that would tend to obscure changes in food intake and favor the interpretation that the lesions produced obesity by diminishing spontaneous motor activity. Brobeck and his colleagues used smaller lesions and older rats and were impressed by the marked increase in food intake that occurred in their lesioned animals.

It is now generally agreed that effective VMN lesions in young animals at first produce obesity mainly by decreasing spontaneously activity and not by increasing food intake, but that as the young animal matures the usual fall in food intake does not occur and the excessive food intake then becomes an important determinant of the obesity (G. C. Kennedy). In the adult animal, the major cause of the obesity is an increase in food intake, which Brobeck has called "hyperphagia," although there may be a component of hypoactivity in the development of obesity in some animals.

There is a curiously paradoxical aspect of the syndrome of hypothalamic obesity, for although animals with ventromedial lesions overeat when food is readily available in their cages, they will not exert themselves unduly to secure it if they are maintained in circumstances in which they must push a lever or negotiate a maze in order to obtain nourishment.

In addition to its disinclination to press levers in order to obtain food, the hypothalamic obese animal exhibits what has been called "finickiness" when it is offered unpleasantly flavored food. The normal animal tolerates a very much higher concentration of quinine sulfate in the diet than does the animal with an effective VMN lesion. This fact reminds us that there are perceptible effects of many stimuli on food intake in the hypothalamic obese animal and, in fact, such an animal appears to be hypersensitive to some of them. Certain anorexigenic drugs (see below) are actually more effective in reducing food intake in the obese animal than in the lean. In addition, diets very high in protein and those containing unbalanced amino acid mixtures appear to be more anorexigenic in hypothalamic-lesioned animals than in controls.

All of these responses indicate the great complexity of the process of food intake regulation and support the view of Morgane that, although the hypothalamic structures are obviously crucial in regulating food intake behavior, many other parts of the brain are doubtless involved in the process. Some observers have seen hyperphagia in experimental animals after placing lesions in the frontal or temporal lobes, whereas others have observed decreases in food intake after injuring similar parts of the brain. Both aphagia and hyperphagia have been observed following destructive lesions in the amygdalar complex. Clearly, the hypothalamic food intake regulatory structures are only the best studied part of what must be an extraordinarily complex set of interconnected circuits in the brain, which together constitute what we tend to think of as the "appestat." Some of the effects of hypothalamic lesions may be due to the destruction of fibers of passage through the hypothalamus rather than of cell bodies within the hypothalamus.

After establishment of the significance of the VMN, Anand and Brobeck discovered other hypothalamic structures that are of enormous importance in the regulation of feeding behavior. They found that small lesions in the outer part of the lateral hypothalamus, at the same rostrocaudal plane as the VMN, produced a complete absence of food intake behavior. Some of their animals were kept alive by tube feeding. Others would swallow food placed in the mouth, which signified that some eating reflexes were still operative in them, although they did not themselves initiate the eating process even when food was readily available to them. Animals that had been made hyperphagic by lesions placed in the VMN became aphagic when lateral lesions were made.

Morgane (1961) has suggested that there are distinct "feeding" and "hunger motivating" systems in the lateral hypothalamus: stimulation in the midlateral area produces feeding responses in sated animals, but animals will not cross an electrified grill to press a lever for food. Far lateral stimulation, however, produces both eating behavior and the motivation to seek food even in an uncomfortable situation. The latter response depends on the integrity of the median forebrain bundle.

Teitelbaum has stressed the fact that much of the fundamental work on food intake regulation has been done on the rat, a species in which complex encephalization of basic drives has not occurred. In order to appreciate the true character of the hypothalamic structures that have been implicated in the control of food intake, it is necessary to observe results of their destruction in more elaborately encephalized species such as the dog and the monkey. Fonberg, for example, has described not only aphagia and adipsia but also a dramatic change in "personality" of the dog with lateral hypothalamic syndrome. These animals, normally playful, affectionate and interested, seemed sad, indifferent and even depressed. In these studies the important point for physicians is the concept that the hypothalamic structures are not "centers" but rather functional components of intricate, highly encephalized control systems, and that disturbances in higher-center function can cause profound changes in the activity of the food intake-regulating mechanism in both directions. It is, of course, well known that hypothalamic lesions can result in striking changes in behavior.

Many experiments have been done in which the ventromedial and lateral hypothalamic areas have been stimulated in unanesthetized animals, and the effects of such stimulation on food intake behavior have been noted. In general, the results have conformed to a kind of mirror image of the lesion observations. For example, stimulation of the lateral hypothalamic center has been observed to increase food intake in several species, and also to cause such effects as licking, chewing, swallowing, and salivating. Stimulation of the region of the VMN resulted in a small decrease in daily food intake.

Out of these and other experiments, there has grown a tentative conception of the role of the hypothalamic regions in the regulation of food intake. The ventromedial nuclei represent an integrating relay station for satiety information. The destruction of this region results in failure to receive satiety signals, which results in inappropriate overeating and, finally, obesity. The lateral hypothalamic area contains a "facilitatory feeding center," which functions as an integrative communications center for all of the complex visual, auditory, olfactory, tactile, gustatory, and enteroceptive reflexes associated with food intake behavior. These, as Brobeck has suggested, go far beyond the chewing and swallowing reflexes and involve food seeking, examination of food—in fact, the whole complex enterprise of food getting. According to "classic" theory, satiety information reaches the VMN component of the regulating machinery, and this structure in turn acts to inhibit the lateral facili-

tatory feeding centers (Fig 16–3). Experimental proof of the necessity for a direct connection between the medial and lateral centers for effective food intake regulation was obtained in ingenious experiments in which very thin knife cuts were made between the medial and lateral nuclei without much destruction of cellular elements in either. Such "hypothalamic island" rats behaved like ventromedially lesioned animals, i.e., they became obese.

APPESTAT-BAROSTAT HYPOTHESIS

Recent students of food intake regulation (e.g., Morrison) have downgraded the role of the hypothalamus to a modulatory one. It is suggested that extra-hypothalamic mechanisms are more important than hypothalamic ones in determining food intake behavior. For example, the cachexia of cancer, which is associated with a decrease in spontaneous food intake, occurs independently of hypothalamic mechanisms. Others have found that hypothalamic lesion-like syndromes can be produced by destroying fibers of passage, particularly in the lateral hypothalamus. Also, highly selective lesions may produce a dissociation between hyperphagia and finickiness.

Another modification of classic hypotheses occurred when various investigators (e.g., Keesey et al.) pointed out that lesioned animals, whether hyperphagic or hypophagic (i.e., VMN or laterally lesioned) defended a new set-point of body weight either higher or lower than that maintained preoperatively. This led to the set-point, or barostat, hypothesis, which was anticipated by the lipostatic theory of food intake regulation (see below). According to this model, the meal-to-meal and frequency-of-feeding control is wired to a long-range control mechanism, which continuously monitors lipid stores in the adipose tissue. It is uncertain whether the barostat keeps a running inventory of physical activity or whether activity information is fed back to the barostat by depleting fat stores. The meal-to-meal regulator is affected by physiologic hunger as well as by complex sensory signals, which may either positively reinforce feeding behavior (e.g., pleasant taste) or inhibit feeding behavior (e.g., unpleasant taste, distracting work).

Although complicated computer simulations of similar models have been constructed (see Hirsch, in Reichsman), Figure 16–4 is a highly simplified representation of the relationships between and among the many components of maintenance of energy balance. Many aspects of the model are still speculative, especially the nature of the information communicated to the barostat by stored triglyceride, which appears, incidentally, to be more closely correlated with

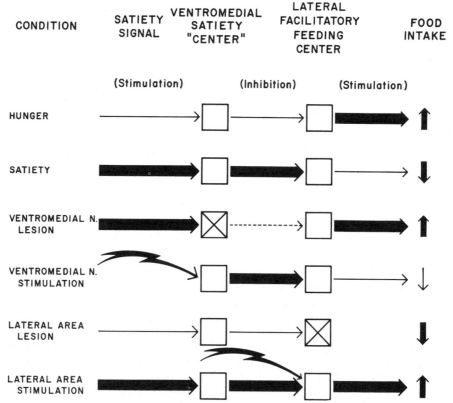

FIG 16–3.
Diagram of classic hypothesis of role of hypothalamus in determination of feeding behavior. These are symmetric, bilateral structures, but only one side is shown in diagram. Width of arrow signifies intensity of stimulation or inhibition. (See review by Anand BK: *Physiol Rev* 1961; 41:677, for documentation. For an account of the limitations of this model, see reviews by Morrison and also Mogenson.)

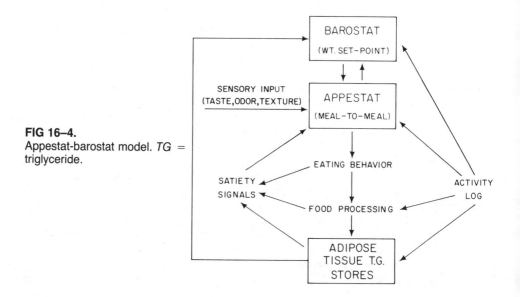

FIG 16–4.
Appestat-barostat model. *TG* = triglyceride.

fat cell size than with fat cell number (see below). Even with this simplified model (which does not specify the anatomical location of appestat and barostat), it is possible to appreciate how complex maintaining a weight set-point can be.

IS HYPOTHALAMIC OBESITY A PURELY "REGULATORY" OBESITY?

Mayer has classified the obesities as "regulatory" (i.e., due to a central disturbance in food intake regulation) and "metabolic" (i.e., due to an inborn metabolic error, which may operate even in the face of adequate regulatory equipment). Recent developments suggest that surgical hypothalamic obesity may have a "metabolic" component. Han has discovered that rats with ventromedial lesions regularly show hypertrophy of the islets of Langerhans and hyperinsulinism. In careful pair-feeding experiments in hypophysectomized animals, he showed that this hyperinsulinism is not secondary to an increase in food intake, nor is it related in any way to a modification in pituitary function by the lesion. Since there is an accumulating body of evidence that implicates the CNS in the modulation of insulin release (Chapter 14), Han's observations relating insulin secretion to the central structures involved in food intake regulation suggest that this function is closely integrated with events that occur after food ingestion.

That insulin secretion is under tonic inhibitory control by the CNS was vividly demonstrated by Jean Renaud, who described a striking increase in the serum insulin response to an intravenous glucose challenge in ventromedially lesioned rats within 10 minutes of placement of the lesions. When he assayed pancreata for content of insulin, glucagon and somatostatin 10 days after the lesions were placed, the concentration of all three pancreatic islet hormones was increased in lesioned rats compared with normals, in spite of the fact that the lesioned animals were food restricted and fed on the same time schedule as were the controls. Thus, placement of obesity-producing hypothalamic lesions has striking effects on islet cell function, which are not mediated by food intake.

In fact, if β cells are destroyed by a betacytotoxic agent, ventromedial hypothalamus (VMH) lesions do not produce obesity. Moreover, Powley and Opsahl have shown that vagotomy (which interrupts a neural connection between hypothalamus and endocrine pancreas) prevents hyperphagia and interrupts the development of obesity in VMH-lesioned animals.

All of these observations suggest that the obesity seen after placement of lesions of the VMH is an extremely complex response that requires intact communication between the brain and the islets of Langerhans.

CHEMICAL AGENTS AND FOOD INTAKE REGULATION

Aurothioglucose

Brecher and Waxler (1949), while doing routine toxicity tests on a potential arthritis remedy called *aurothioglucose* (ATG, or gold thioglucose), discovered that a certain percentage of mice that survived an LD_{50} of the compound (i.e., lethal dose for 50% of the animals) showed very striking obesity (Fig 16–5). The original discoverers of the phenomenon demonstrated that the eating behavior of mice with obesity-producing doses of ATG resembled that of rats with

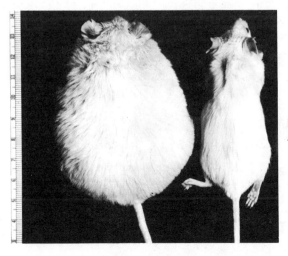

FIG 16–5.
Aurothioglucose (ATG) obesity in the mouse.

VMH lesions. Mayer and colleagues showed that ATG produces destructive lesions of the VMN in the hypothalamus, and it is now generally accepted that ATG obesity represents a chemical form of hypothalamic obesity. Although the VMN lesion is the most prominent one observed, other small lesions, which have no known relation to the process of food intake regulation, are also seen (Perry and Liebelt, 1961). Radioautographic studies with ^{198}Au-labeled ATG have revealed increased concentraions of gold in areas of the brain damaged by the compound. Studies on the distribution of ^{198}Au and ^{35}S suggest that there the gold can be split from the parent molecule; the cytotoxicity of the compound is therefore believed to be due primarily to the heavy metal. It is possible that one of the reasons for the increased vulnerability of certain cells to ATG is the presence in them of a higher activity of a metallic gold-releasing enzyme. A review of the use of gold thioglucose as an experimental tool was written by Deter and Liebelt in 1964.

Neurotransmitters and Food Intake

Many studies have attempted to identify neurotransmitters involved in food intake regulation. For example, the histochemical fluorescence technique for tracing catecholamine pathways in the brain (introduced by Hillarp et al.) may be combined with use of drugs that selectively destroy catecholamine systems. Food intake behavior can then be correlated with the findings at autopsy.

Another way of studying the problem is by microinjection of minute amounts of catecholamine agonists or blocking agents directly into the ventricular system of the brain and observing effects on food intake in either starved or fed animals.

Most observers agree that intracranial injection of *norepinephrine* elicits feeding behavior in fed animals, probably via an α receptor effect. This finding is difficult to reconcile with the well-known inhibition of food intake that is caused by sympathomimetic drugs of the amphetamine series (see next section).

The findings with *dopamine* are more controversial. Ungerstedt, on the basis of experiments with a neurotoxin (6-OH dopamine), which selectively destroys dopaminergic neurons, concluded that the aphagia of the lateral hypothalamic syndrome is due to the destruction of a dopaminergic feeding system. Leibowitz concluded that dopaminergic neurons in the anterolateral hypothalamus *suppress* feeding behavior. The observation that clinical use of dopamine blocking agents is often associated with increased food intake and weight gain is at least consistent with blocking an inhibitory influence.

Another level of complexity was uncovered by Hoebel, who found that intraventricular injection of *para*-chlorophenylalanine, which selectively depletes *serotonin,* causes overeating and obesity (see also Stricker).

The pharmacology of food intake regulation involves (at least) the integration of (1) extremely complex sensory information from environmental stimuli; (2) assessment of the internal metabolic state of the individual; (3) food-seeking and eating behavior; and (4) alleviation of the dysphoria of hunger (some sort of perception of pleasure associated with the feeling of satiety). The complexity of the neural circuits involved in this enterprise is unimaginable. Moreover, a comprehensive theory of central control of food intake must now accommodate the possibility that gastrointestinal hormones in the brain may participate in modulating food intake behavior. For example, Straus and Yalow have found *less* cholecystokinin in the brains of genetically obese mice than in nonobese controls.

Another interesting new development in this field involves the morphine-like peptides (see Chapter 5). Holtzman demonstrated that normal rats, treated with the morphine antagonist naloxone just before feeding, ate less than did controls. Margules et al. measured β endorphin levels in the blood and brain of obese rodents and found them to be elevated. (See Yim et al.)

With the passage of time, the pharmacology of eating behavior, mostly studied in experimental animals, has become more and more difficult to describe succinctly (see Morley and Levine, 1985). The most prominent *enhancers* of feeding behavior are alpha catecholamines and opioid peptides. The list of *inhibitors* of feeding behavior, in addition to beta catecholamines, serotonin, and CCK, includes CRF, TRH, calcitonin gene-related peptide (Chapter 17), and insulin. Feeding behavior can be predictably modified, in one direction or the other, by all of these substances, but the contribution of each to physiologic regulation remains to be established.

Most inhibitors of food intake have been centrally acting substances. There are now a number of peripherally acting appetite suppressants being tested (Sullivan and Gruen).

Sympathomimetic Amines as Anorectics

Certain drugs have profound effects on food intake. Sympathomimetic amines and related compounds are widely used in the clinic as a sort of pharmacologic crutch for patients who have great difficulty in restricting their caloric intake voluntarily. These compounds (of which amphetamine is a prototype) are powerful CNS stimulants, and there is no doubt that they accelerate weight loss for a time. They do so by inhibiting food intake and by increasing spontaneous activity. The mechanism by which they decrease food intake is not known, but it is certainly true that intact ventromedial satiety "centers" are not necessary for the hypophagic effect to occur. In fact, aurothioglucose obese mice and animals with VMN lesions are more sensitive to the anorexigenic effect of amphetamine than are intact controls.

One drug, fenfluramine, is of interest because it is not a central nervous system stimulant in the manner of amphetamine. It has been used extensively as an anorexigenic agent, but its withdrawal may precipitate depression.

In both experimental animals and man, the anorexigenic drugs are effective initially, but tolerance (and, therefore, ineffectiveness) soon appears. Most studies that purport to prove efficacy in man are based on clinical trials that last only a few weeks. Since weight reduction is only meaningful if it persists for years, there is no convincing evidence that the use of anorexigenic drugs has any effect whatever on the natural history of obesity observed over a period of years. In fact, the use of anorexigenic drugs in some circumstances may interfere with the modifications in behavior that are essential for long-term weight reduction. This, coupled with their addictive possibilities, makes the sympathomimetic amines and their congeners extremely unimpressive drugs for the treatment of obesity.

Satiety Signals

We have examined some of the structures in the CNS that are concerned with processing of information related to the metering of food intake. It is pertinent to inquire into the possible nature of the signals that are set up by the ingestion of food and how (or whether) these signals can participate in long-term regulation of energy balance. A growing and perplexing literature on the subject of satiety signals reveals that most experts in this field conclude that food intake regulation by the CNS must represent the results of the processing of many kinds of data. Among the interesting hypotheses, the following have been advanced.

METERING OF FOOD INTAKE IN MOUTH, PHARYNX, AND GASTROINTESTINAL TRACT

Although the presence or absence of gastric hunger contractions does not appear to affect the quantity of food eaten, Janowitz and Grossman have demonstrated that prefed dogs ate less than did animals fed the same amount of food by gastric fistula, and have suggested that gastric distention may constitute a satiety message.

Taste may complicate the regulatory process since sweet-tasting foods or fluids have been observed to cause overweight in animals in spite of a compensatory reduction in the consumption of other diet constituents.

The hormones that control gastrointestinal mobility and secretory processes may affect intestinal emptying and therefore influence feeding behavior. Glucagon has also been implicated in the control of food intake since it has been observed to decrease both the size and length of meals (Geary et al.).

Hepatoreceptors

There is some evidence for the existence of glucoreceptors in the liver (see Niijima). The existence of such receptors has been inferred from neurophysiologic evidence. How or whether such information is used in the regulation of food intake is not known.

Thermostatic Regulation

Brobeck and colleagues have advanced the interesting suggestion that the heat generated by the ingestion of food—the specific dynamic action, or SDA—is one variable that is metered in the CNS and functions as a satiety signal. This theory has the great virtue of including the major foodstuffs—protein, fat, and carbohydrate—as potential contributors to the satiety message.

Metabolite Theories

Mayer has suggested that the cells in the region of the hypothalamic VMN are chemoreceptors ("glucostats"). A good deal of circumstantial evidence supports the view that these cells are somehow capable of reflecting the rate of glucose utilization by peripheral tissues and that, when the peripheral arteriovenous blood glucose difference is small (i.e., when glucose utilization is low), hunger is experienced. Conversely, when the peripheral arteriovenous glucose difference is high (i.e., when glucose oxidation is high), a subjective feeling of satiety supervenes. Recently the glucostatic theory received apparent support from the report by Anand et al. who studied the electric activity of the medial and lateral feeding centers in monkeys and cats in which blood glucose concentration was changed either by glucose infusion or insulin injection. They found increased electric activity in satiety "centers" with elevation of the blood glucose level, but not after infusing protein hydrolysate or fat emulsions. The binding of aurothioglucose to cells in the region of the VMH is considered circumstantial evidence for the existence of glucoreceptors.

Attractive as the glucostatic hypothesis appears to be, there are two reasons for questioning its physiologic importance. (1) Janowitz and Grossman found that prior glucose infusion did not appreciably decrease spontaneous food intake in rats, dogs or human subjects. (2) Van Itallie has demonstrated cycles of hunger and satiety in a subject on a high fat, low carbohydrate diet who showed no fluctuations in arteriovenous glucose difference. In his subjects, the feeling of hunger correlated best with a high level of circulating free fatty acids (FFA), signifying that mobilization of depot fat had occurred.

A variant of this hypothesis has been advanced as the "lipostatic" theory by Kennedy et al., who visualize communication between the aggregate fat depot and the central nervous-regulating structures by way of the bloodstream. Since the quantity of fat mobilized per day may be roughly proportional to the total amount in all the depots, a running inventory of the size of the total fat deposit could be kept by the brain if a critical metabolite were released in association with mobilized FFA. This theory has the great virtue of suggesting how long-range regulation of energy exchange might be achieved in contrast to the acute, single meal regulations possibly accomplished by local gastrointestinal tract metering, or postprandial heat or blood glucose fluctuations.

Both excess protein and imbalanced amino acid mixtures cause anorexia by mechanisms that are presently unknown, but which do not require an intact ventromedial nucleus for their expression (Krauss and Mayer, 1965). Anorexia also is often associated with clinical liver disease, such as hepatitis, but the mechanism of this relationship is also obscure. Possibly these two causes of anorexia may be related, since a sick liver, unable to metabolize amino acids at a sufficiently rapid rate, may lead to accumulation of anorexigenic quantities of amino acids in the body fluids.

In summary, the regulation of food intake represents a kind of rhythmic, recurrent physiologic adjustment such as one sees in respiration, water balance, sleeping and waking and in many other life transactions. The acute or meal-to-meal regulation may be accomplished by a battery of signals, including SDA of ingested food, rate of glucose utilization, metabolic events in the adipose tissue, and local metering in the gastrointestinal tract. Information generated by these signals is processed in the central nervous system by a complex network of adrenergic, serotoninergic, and peptidergic (including endogenous opioid) neurones.

The long-range balance may be achieved by a complicated CNS integration and analysis of many of these processes into which is factored a kind of cumulative work log, for, as we shall see, delayed effects of heavy work on food intake are readily demonstrable in careful studies on human beings.

Adipose Tissue

ITS ROLE IN METABOLISM

The first review article on adipose tissue was published in 1948 by Wertheimer and Shapiro, whose prescient interest in the subject anticipated current developments by decades. The reviewers wrote the following:

Adipose tissue is a tissue with a special structure and a special type of cell. It is supplied by a comparatively dense capillary net and innervated by sympathetic nerve fibers. Deposition and mobilization of fat in adipose tissue is an active process, involving the metabolism of the tissue. Under conditions favoring fat deposition, adipose tissue accumulates glycogen, which is presumably built in the tissue cells themselves. Synthesis of new fatty acids from carbohydrates as well as transformation of one fatty acid into another proceed continuously in this tissue. All of these metabolic activities are regulated by nervous and endocrine factors.

It is unfortunate that fat and adipose tissue are so closely associated with the subject of obesity and are therefore considered to be vaguely pathologic. Actually, in order to exist without the convenience afforded by adipose tissue, it would be necessary to be able to adjust the rate of absorption of food from the gastrointestinal tract to accommodate different rates of energy expenditure. Moreover, fasts of even short duration would be impossible because the total store of tissue and fluid carbohydrate in an adult male is rarely more than 75 gm, or 300 calories, the equivalent of a modest piece of pie. The maneuver of storing both fat and carbohydrate (as fat) in the fat depots postprandially affords a degree of metabolic resiliency and adaptability that must have contributed to the survival advantage of our remote evolutionary ancestors. For the adipose tissue is a sort of energy bank; deposits are made at meal time, and demand notes in the form of fat mobilization signals may be presented any time thereafter. Thus, the fat depots are enormously important in the day-to-day vital economy of people and animals in energy balance. If the deposits exceed withdrawals over a sufficiently long time, obesity occurs. The extent of fat deposition can be unbelievably large—the depot organ appears to be almost infinitely distensible. For example, it is by no means unusual to see a rat with hypothalamic obesity whose carcass contains 50% fat, or 250 gm. This represents 2,150 calories, which would last 43 days at a rate of expenditure of 50 calories per day. Obesity of comparable extent is not rare in the human.

REGULATION OF LIPID STORAGE AND MOBILIZATION IN THE ADIPOCYTE

The fat cell represents a special case of regulation by antagonistic hormones (see Chapter 14).

Figure 16–6,A represents the state of affairs in an insulin-dominated adipocyte. Lipoprotein lipase (*LPL*) is stimulated and the uptake of FFA from circulating *VLDL* (very low-density lipoprotein) is enhanced. Glucose transport is stimulated and glycogen-

esis is promoted. Glucose-6-phosphate metabolism over all of its pathways is stimulated: oxidation to CO_2, fatty acid synthesis and (not shown) oxidation via the pentose phosphate pathway, which provides reducing equivalents for lipogenesis in the form of NADPH. A large supply of α glycerophosphate (α-*GP*) is provided for triglyceride (*TG*) synthesis. This accommodates both incoming fatty acid from *VLDL* and newly synthesized fatty acid. Coordinately with the storage of TG, its hydrolysis by hormone-sensitive lipase (*HSL*) is *actively inhibited* by insulin. As a result, *TG* is sequestered in the adipocyte.

Figure 16–6,B illustrates the poise of a fat cell dominated by insulin antagonists, or when there is a deficiency of insulin. All of the reactions positively stimulated by insulin proceed at a low rate, whereas the antilipolytic effect of insulin is withdrawn. The *HSL*, which is a substrate for cAMP-stimulated protein kinase, becomes phosphorylated and therefore active. Thus, TG storage is markedly depressed and TG hydrolysis is actively promoted.

There is a large and confusing literature on the sub-

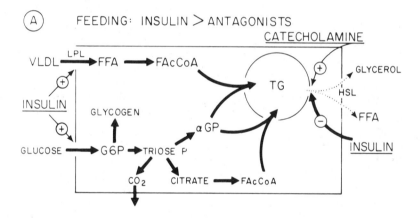

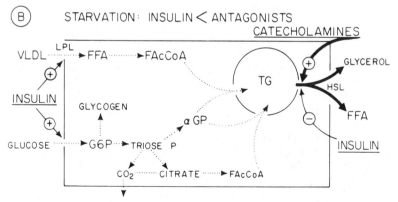

FIG 16–6.
Function of adipocyte in feeding **(A)** and starvation **(B)**.

ject of the role of cAMP in these adjustments. Whereas catecholamines raise cAMP levels and insulin depresses them, biologic effects can be seen without measurable changes in cAMP concentration. This does not rule out participation of the cAMP-protein kinase system beyond the point of cAMP generation. Although the detailed molecular mechanisms of insulin antilipolysis and catecholamine lipolysis remain to be worked out (role of calcium?, role of protein kinase inhibitors and phosphodiesterase activators?), the coordinate nature of the adjustments and their physiologic appropriateness can still be appreciated.

One feature of the coordination that is insufficiently stressed is the inhibition of insulin's effectiveness by lipolysis. The thin sliver of cytoplasm of the adipocyte must be traversed by FFA generated by triglyceride hydrolysis. FFA is a powerful inhibitor of lipogenesis, of G-6-PD and of citrate production and transport by the mitochondria. Insulin resistance is one consequence of lipolysis and high ambient FFA concentrations.

ADIPOCYTE SIZE AND NUMBER: CLASSIFICATION OF OBESITIES

In a series of seminal studies, Hirsch and colleagues (see Stern and Johnson) have added an interesting dimension to the problem of energy balance. Having developed methods for measuring the size of individual fat cells and for estimating the total number of fat cells in an intact animal or person, they demonstrated that overfeeding during the neonatal period (contrasting four nursing rats per mother with 22 per mother) resulted in the development of a significantly larger total number of adipocytes than were present in the underfed group. Moreover, the larger number of fat cells persisted throughout the life of the "privileged" rats.

When human populations were examined, it was found that obese infants and children generally had both an increased size and an increased total number of adipocytes. Sims, Horton et al., who studied obesity in adult human beings who were deliberately overfed, found an increase in adipocyte size but not in total number. Knittle identified two times during the lifetime of human beings when fat cell proliferation occurred: (1) during infancy and (2) in association with the adolescent growth spurt. However, the pocesss is not restricted to those two periods. It is generally agreed that weight reduction results in a decrease in fat cell size, but no significant decrease in fat cell number.

The methods used in making these estimates identify as fat cells only adipocytes that contain enough

triglyceride to float. The method does not detect adipocyte precursor cells or committed adipocytes that may not yet have accumulated a sufficient quantity of triglyceride to be detected. Therefore, it was necessary to devise a method that would distinguish between fat cell replication and recruitment of preexisting fat cells. This was accomplished by measuring the rates of incorporation of radioactive thymidine into DNA under various experimental circumstances. When this was done, it was found that the increases in fat cell number previously observed were associated with periods of accelerated fat cell DNA synthesis.

On the basis of much work in human beings, a tentative classification of obesities based on fat cell size and number has proved useful. An increase in adipocyte size is referred to as *hypertrophic* obesity, whereas an increase in total number of adipocytes is called *hyperplastic* obesity (Fig 16–7). In fact, the fat cells of most of the markedly obese subjects are both hypertrophic and hyperplastic.

All of this implies that, at certain stages of the fat cell's life cycle, a mitogenic influence stimulates the cell, or its immediate precursor, to divide. Or, to put it another way, at other times of the life cycle, fat cells are prevented from dividing. Although no specific stimuli or inhibitors have as yet been identified, these studies suggest a new area in which genetic susceptibility to obesity might operate, since certain experimental genetic models of obesity, notably the Zucker rat, show striking hyperplasia of adipocytes.

Attitudes about adipocyte number being fixed in the neonatal period of the rat are now changing. Stimulation of the appearance of an increased total number

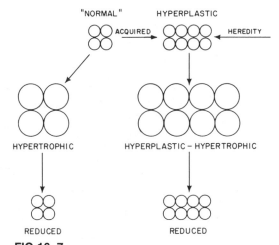

FIG 16–7.
Hypertrophic and hyperplastic-hypertrophic obesities.

of adipocytes in a number of strains of mature rats was accomplished by feeding a highly palatable, high-fat diet instead of a laboratory stock diet. In all fat depots examined, feeding the palatable diet produced first a marked increase in fat cell size and then the appearance of a larger number of cells. Once the new, enlarged number of adipocytes appeared, it was not reduced when the rats were returned to a chow diet. Curiously, the Zucker obese rat (already hypercellular) did not gain an appreciable amount of weight on the rich diet (see Faust et al.).

It is not certain that the neonatal feeding experience has its long-term effect entirely via increased adipocyte number or by way of an increased food intake— or indeed whether the proliferation of adipocytes and the increased food intake are somehow linked. A new demonstration that neonatal hyperphagia fixes hunger at a higher-than-normal level (see Oscai and McGarr) at least suggests the possibility that the neonatal food intake-metering machinery in the brain may be just as imprintable neonatally as are the gonadotropin-regulating and other pituitary-controlling functions.

Effect of Adipocyte Enlargement on Its Metabolism

As fat cells enlarge, they become insulin resistant (see Czech). Also, as fat cells enlarge, they show a diminished number of insulin receptors per cell (see Soll et al.). Insulin receptors decrease not only in fat cells but also in hepatocytes, muscle and, in human beings, in circulating monocytes. When weight reduction is induced by food restriction, fat cells regain their sensitivity to insulin, and insulin receptor number increases in all tissues. Thus, since insulin promotes fat storage in adipocytes, the more storage it promotes the more difficult it becomes for insulin to bring about additional storage. This makes good teleonomic sense, for it effectively inhibits the development of further adiposity and therefore assists the barostat in defending its set-point.

If we look at the reverse situation, i.e., improvement in insulin sensitivity with weight reduction, mobilization of triglyceride fatty acid becomes more and more difficult as adipocytes regain their insulin sensitivity. Thus, if insulin sensitivity is markedly improved while an individual is still obese, further weight loss could be difficult.

It is now generally agreed that the insulin resistance of the enlarged adipocyte cannot be due entirely to loss of insulin receptors; the enlarged cell shows intracellular metabolic adaptations in addition to receptor loss. Since obese animals and people show high resting levels of FFA, we can assume that large tri-

glyceride droplets are associated with high cytosolic FFA or FACoA (fatty acyl CoA) concentrations. Inhibition of lipogenesis and the enzymes of the hexose monophosphate shunt is consistent with this condition. Thus down-regulation of insulin receptors and insulin resistance may be secondary to the intracellular, i.e., postmembrane, adaptations that occur in enlarged cells (see DiGirolamo et al.; Salans and Cushman).

Brown Adipose Tissue (BAT)

Brown adipose tissue, composed of highly specialized adipocytes, has been studied mainly in rodents and in some hibernating species. In humans, it is present in newborns, but its physiologic function in human adults is questionable. The biology of BAT, the only tissue whose main function is the production of heat, has been analyzed imaginatively by many investigators (see Himms-Hagen; Ricquier and Mory for references).

BAT plays an important part in three circumstances: (1) in the human newborn; (2) in adapting to cold environments in some species; and (3) in arousal from hibernation in certain species. (1) and (2) may be manifestations of the same adaptation, since the transition from intrauterine to extrauterine life is often a form of cold exposure.

Brown adipocytes differ from white ones in having a large number of small lipid droplets (instead of one huge one) dispersed through the cell; in being particularly rich in mitochondria which are unique to these cells; and in their luxuriant supply of sympathetic nerve endings and blood vessels.

The sympathetic nerve endings of BAT can be traced back to two regions of the hypothalamus: (1) the preoptic area (POAH), which is involved in temperature adjustments, and (2) the ventromedial nucleus (VMN), which, as we have seen, is associated with food intake regulation. Thus, BAT can be stimulated by cold temperatures, which activate POAH, and by feeding, which operates via VMN. In either case, the result is the local discharge of norepinephrine near the BAT cells and the activation of lipolysis via β_1 receptors.

The distinctive biochemical feature of these cells that makes them microfurnaces is a specific, 32K protein called *thermogenin* which is present on the inner mitochondrial membrane. When fuel is supplied to the mitochondria by lipolysis, or by accelerated carbohydrate metabolism mediated by insulin, *thermogenin* uncouples oxidative phosphorylation so that more heat than ATP is generated. In rodents, stimulation of BAT by cold exposure can account for 30%–

80% of nonshivering thermogenesis. The human newborn uses its BAT for a similar purpose, although it is difficult to estimate the quantitative contribution of BAT to total heat production in the human neonate.

BAT has some interesting endocrine associations. *Hyper*thyroidism indirectly causes atrophy of BAT by stimulating thermogenesis generally. *Hypo*thyroidism, by decreasing heat production, results in hypertrophy of BAT, but the hypertrophic brown adipose tissue is poorly responsive to norepinephrine, and therefore does not generate enough heat to sustain thermogenesis on cold exposure. This is no doubt one of the reasons for cold intolerance in hypothyroid rodents and other animals that depend on BAT for adaptation to cold temperatures.

We have sometimes speculated that some fortunate people who appear to be able to eat very large amounts of food without becoming obese may have some persistent BAT hidden in their lean bodies. We emphasize, however, that a pathophysiologic role for BAT in adult humans has so far only been suggested for patients with catecholamine-producing tumors (pheochromocytoma). Such patients have been shown to have proliferation of BAT which could contribute to their weight loss. Their high catecholamine levels also stimulate thermogenesis in other tissues.

The Metabolic "Cost of Living"

Efficiency of Food Utilization

For many years, there appeared to be a tacit assumption by students of energy balance that the overall efficiency of food utilization was exactly the same in everyone. However, the evidence against this assumption provided by animal breeding experiments was overwhelming. More recently it has become clear that the metabolic "cost of living"—energy expended by the metabolic machinery of the body—is variable from one individual to another and might therefore contribute to establishing obesity or leanness. Moreover, "cost of living" is not static, for it is intimately coupled with food intake, both acutely (i.e., after a single meal) and chronically (i.e., adaptation to over- or underfeeding, or starvation).

The basal metabolic rate, measured as resting oxygen consumption in the postabsorptive state after sleep, represents the minimal energy expenditure for an individual in the waking state. When food is eaten, the energy involved in processing incoming nutrients causes a rise in oxygen consumption, historically called the SDA (specific dynamic action) of foodstuffs. Over and above the energy expended by the

gastrointestinal tract and circulatory systems, it has been estimated that the cost of converting carbohydrate to fat is 11%–20% of ingested carbohydrate calories. The cost of converting amino acids to protein is about 20%. Gluconeogenesis from amino acids requires about 30% of the energy content of the amino acids. Emphasis used to be placed on the high cost of processing amino acids, but the cost of processing carbohydrates is also high. There is some experimental evidence that supports the view that the efficiency of utilization of ingested fat is higher (i.e., energy cost is lower) than for that of an isocaloric amount of carbohydrate.

Although many attempts have been made to detect differences in SDA responses to food intake in obese and lean people and animals, there has been no consistent finding of a *smaller* SDA in the obese that would favor storage of extra energy as triglyceride. In spite of this, it is easy to imagine that subtle differences in food-stimulated thermogenesis might have a cumulative effect over a long period.

Many theories have been suggested to account for possible differences in metabolic efficiency that might contribute to the causes of obesity or leanness. The more efficient (i.e., the less wasteful) type of metabolism could predispose to obesity, whereas the less efficient type could contribute to weight stabilization despite inactivity. For example, genetically determined differences in the operation of what have been called ''futile cycles'' have been suggested as possible loci of differences in energy efficiency (see Stirling and Stock). A futile cycle consists of a pair of metabolites linked by two essentially unidirectional enzymes:

$$\text{Glucose} \rightleftharpoons \text{Glucose-6-P}$$
$$\text{Fructose-6-P} \rightleftharpoons \text{Fructose 1,6 } P_2$$
$$\text{Triglyceride} \rightleftharpoons \text{Fatty acyl CoA}$$

The flow of substrate traffic is determined by the sum of the opposing reactions: when recycling occurs within a pair, ATP is wasted and is therefore unavailable for storage. Although there is no direct evidence that animals or people who are predisposed to obesity differ from controls with respect to the operation of futile cycles, this kind of chemical individuality cannot be ruled out as a potential contributor to differences in energy efficiency.

Other *possible* metabolic differences between obese and lean are in oxidative phosphorylation coupling and in ratio of aerobic:anaerobic metabolism. It is at least conceivable (though never proved) that more tightly coupled mitochondria could contribute to more energy-efficient metabolism in obesity-prone individuals, whereas loose coupling would permit high levels of food consumption without weight gain. Similarly, anaerobic metabolism is less efficient (in terms of ATP yield per mole of glucose) than is aerobic metabolism. There is no compelling reason to assert that everybody in the world operates at the same aerobic:anaerobic ratio.

It is now well established that deliberate overfeeding does not result in deposition of the calculated excess of energy intake as fat (see Sims; Miller et al.). In fact, some deliberately overfed individuals are remarkably resistant to weight gain under laboratory conditions. This phenomenon, which was observed over 80 years ago, has been called "luxus consumption"; it suggests that an adaptive increase in food-induced thermogenesis occurs in response to overfeeding and that this adaptation is one way the body has of defending its weight set-point. The most striking feature of recent descriptions of luxus consumption is the great individual variation in weight gain when a group of subjects is overfed to the same extent.

The sympathetic nervous system is heavily involved in thermogenesis, both in species that have a well-developed apparatus for adapting to cold exposure and in other species, including the human, in which the "set" of sympathetic nervous system activity is determined at least in part by food intake (Landsberg and Young). Fasting suppresses sympathetic nervous activity and overfeeding stimulates it, a possible contributory mechanism to luxus consumption. Incidently, this effect of overeating may be involved in the hypertension of obesity.

When people or animals are deliberately *under*fed, there is a decrease in total energy expenditure, which conserves stored energy. In people of average weight, this response is teleonomically valuable. In obese individuals, however, it may occur while they are still strikingly overweight, and therefore may tend to limit further weight loss. It is possible that variable levels of function of the sympathetic nervous system may participate in these adaptations.

Heat Exchange and Energy Balance

Warm-blooded animals characteristically maintain their internal temperature environment within narrow limits. Temperature regulation involves the bringing into play of heat production and heat conservation mechanisms when temperature begins to fall and of heat-dissipating mechanisms when the environmental temperature rises. Temperature regulation is accomplished in a staged progression of responses: (1) acute reflex changes (e.g., vasodilation or vasoconstriction, shivering, panting, sweating); and (2) longer-range

adaptive changes (e.g., thyroid hypertrophy, increased food intake, change in character of peripheral depot fat on cold exposure). Clearly the problems of temperature regulation and of energy balance are intricately related, and it was this relation that originally suggested to Brobeck the idea of thermostatic regulation of food intake. In his energy balance studies, in which he measured food intake, spontaneous activity, and body weight in the rat over a wide range of ambient air temperatures, he found that high temperatures were associated with decreases in both food intake and locomotor activity, whereas exposure to low temperatures produced hyperphagia and increased activity. Certainly the animal in the cold must "eat to keep warm" (in Brobeck's phrase), for if it did not increase its food intake it would soon go into negative energy balance because of the necessity of stoking its heat production furnace with its own substance.

No energy-converting engine, whether steam engine, diesel engine or people, operates at 100% efficiency levels. People, in fact, are between the other two, for the efficiencies of the three kinds of engines mentioned are 15%, 35%, and 25%, respectively. This should not be regarded as a rigidly set figure, for the efficiencies of all kinds of engines vary with the rate at which they are operated. In humans, for example, efficiency tends to be low when the rate of work is either very low or extremely high, with the most efficient range at the top of a parabolic curve. Moreover, as we have seen, efficiency in people is in part a function of training and skill.

Thyroid Function and Obesity: New Directions

There is a large and confusing literature on the subject of thyroid function and obesity (see Garrow). Since obese people appeared to have normal levels of serum thyroxine, there has been a widespread tendency to belittle the possibility that thyroid hormones could be involved in the obesity problem. Several lines of evidence suggest that a reexamination of this phase of the subject is indicated.

In animals, thyroid hormone is involved in adaptation to cold environments and indeed contributes to the nonshivering thermogenesis that occurs on cold exposure. There may be a similarity between this type of nonshivering thermogenesis and food-induced thermogenesis of hyperphagia. In fact Danforth et al. have described an increase in serum T_3 level and an decrease in rT_3 level in response to deliberate overfeeding. Also, weight reduction in the obese is associated with just the opposite response: decrease in T_3 and increase in rT_3 levels. All of these changes occur without changes in circulating T_4 levels and no doubt reflect peripheral deiodination of T_4. The circulating level of T_3 therefore appears to be correlated with defense of the set-point of body weight when a disturbance occurs in either direction.

There are other ways in which thyroid hormone function and the problem of energy balance converge. For example, the mitochondrial enzyme α GPD (α glycerophosphate dehydrogenase), is a flavin enzyme whose equilibrium level is set by thyroid hormone. Its importance for energy balance may be related to a variety of its effects: (1) if α glycerophosphate (α GP) is metabolized rapidly, less of it is available for esterification of fatty acids (triglyceride synthesis); (2) at high levels of the enzyme, the P:O ratio is lowered, thus increasing food-induced thermogenesis. Conversely, if the enzyme is low, food-induced thermogenesis would be decreased and more energy would therefore be left over for storage. In this connection, Galton and Bray described *low* levels of α GPD obese animals. In this instance we do not know whether the decreased enzyme activity was etiologically involved in establishing obesity or whether it represents an adaptation to the obesity.

The demonstrations by Edelman and colleagues (see Chapter 10) that (1) from 35% to 50% of resting metabolism can be accounted for by the osmotic work performed in pumping Na^+ out of cells and that (2) the level of Na^+K^+ ATPase activity is set by thyroid hormone have stimulated interest in the possibility that ATPase activity may be involved either in susceptibility to obesity or in its perpetuation. Following the findings by York et al. that genetically obese mice (ob/ob) had decreased levels of Na^+K^+ ATPase activity in liver and kidney and that of Lin et al., who showed a decreased population of ATPase molecules in membranes of the obese animals, Guernsey and Moroshige described a decreased number of nuclear T_3 binding sites in liver and lung of ob/ob mice. This is especially interesting because these mice cannot increase thermogenesis on exposure to cold. Thus, in spite of normal circulating levels of thyroid hormones, these mice show decreased end-organ response to thyroid hormone, which helps to explain (1) their low resting oxygen consumption, (2) their apparently "superefficient" metabolism, and (3) their inadequate ability to adapt to cold exposure.

Activity Pattern

Skeletal muscle constitutes about 50% of the weight of the body. It is the one tissue that can vary its energy requirement by a factor of 20 or more. In an exercising person, work is performed not only by the muscles that are active, but also by the heart and respiratory muscles, which must collaborate to deliver sufficient oxygenated blood to meet the increased requirement of the working muscle.

Table 16–1 illustrates some of the changes produced in oxygen consumption and other physiologic parameters by exercise. Many of these changes can be shown to be related to the state of athletic training of the individual under study. Two generalizations can be made about highly trained athletes compared with sedentary people: (1) athletic people show a smaller deviation from the resting level than do the nonathletic in all parameters measured while they are working at similar, moderate work loads; and (2) the more highly trained an athlete is the more nearly can he approach the maximal levels of such parameters as oxygen consumption, blood lactate accumulation, ventilation rate, and cardiac output. In a word, the athlete can work more efficiently (i.e., at a smaller energy cost) at low and moderate work loads, and he can do more work before he is overcome by exhaustion.

Until recently, there was a widespread tendency to belittle the importance of activity pattern as a contributory factor to the maintenance of energy balance. Many students of human energy balance problems are now emphasizing the importance of considering inactivity as an important contributory factor to the cause of obesity in some individuals.

Mayer and colleagues have made careful studies on obese high school girls and have classified them in

TABLE 16–1.

Physiologic Effects of Exercise*

PHYSIOLOGIC EFFECTS	RESTING	DURING EXERCISE	
		AVERAGE	MAXIMAL
Oxygen consumption, ml/min	250	2,500–3,500	5,000
Oxygen debt, L	. . .	4–8	16–19
Lactacidemia, mg/%	10–15	50–100	200
Respiration			
Rate, min	12–16	30	60
Inspiratory vol, ml	350	2,000	2,200
Minute-volume, L	4.5–6	50–70	120
Circulation			
Pulse rate, min	70	120–150	200
Systolic output, ml	60–70	90–110	150
Minute volume, L	4–5	10–20	35
Systolic BP, mm Hg	120	160	180
Temperature, C	. . .	0.5–1	2

*From Houssay BA: *Human Physiology*. New York, McGraw-Hill Book Co, 1955.

two groups: (1) girls who clearly ate too much and (2) extremely inactive girls who did not eat more than did their normally active siblings of average weight. There is experimental evidence to support the view that the food intake-regulating equipment in the CNS was not designed, in a manner of speaking, to cope with the extremely low activity levels that are possible in modern industrial societies. Contrary to a widely held superstition, a change in activity pattern from very low to moderately high does not necessarily stimulate the appetite and therefore cancel out the benefit of the added energy expenditure associated with exercise.

Stunkard and colleagues also have studied the possibility that activity pattern may contribute to the cause of obesity. Even with their crude method of estimating activity by means of the pedometer, an instrument that keeps a cumulative record of distance walked, they were able to show that many obese women (but not obese men) were significantly less active than were their controls of average weight. The food intake of these women was not especially high.

Edholm et al. have explored a most interesting facet of the relation of energy expenditure to caloric balance. These workers studied a group of cadets in training under circumstances that permitted careful estimation of caloric intake and energy expenditure. When they made a correlation plot of many individual daily food intake measurements against daily energy expenditure on any given day, there was an almost perfect *lack* of correlation. But when they plotted energy expenditure on day 0 *versus* food intake two days later, there was an excellent correlation, suggesting that today's level of activity is somehow factored into the spontaneous food intake the day after tomorrow.

Another aspect of the contribution of muscle work to energy balance deserves comment. If a man overeats and becomes progressively more obese, the energy cost of moving his body from place to place becomes greater and greater. Obviously, a 300-pound man does a considerable amount of work when he merely moves across a room. Thus, the increased effort involved in supporting and moving a fat body tends to put limits on the degree of obesity that can be achieved. The absolute oxygen consumption of the obese individual at rest is higher than that of his lean control, but in addition to this, the energy expenditure involved in working may be extremely large. The sad fact is that, just as progressively increasing weight tends to limit weight gain by increasing work load, weight loss tends to limit itself in the opposite way. For as weight is lost, less work is required to support and move the body, and, therefore, the more closely

does the diminished food intake approach the actual requirement for maintenance. Moreover, weight loss results in some reduction in lean body mass ("active metabolic mass"), and therefore in a lower total energy requirement. These may be among the reasons for the difficulty some obese individuals have in attempting to lose weight.

Bjorntorp and colleagues have studied physical training in obese subjects. They discovered that physical training, even when it did not result in measurable weight loss, caused an improvement in glucose tolerance and a decrease in elevated resting insulin levels. Since exercise causes muscle hypertrophy and no weight was lost, adipocyte size decreased. This raises a serious question about weight loss prescription: if obese, sedentary individuals enter a physical training program with metabolic results similar to those found by Bjorntorp et al., does not their risk of complications of obesity diminish? Indeed, Leonhardt et al. (and others) have found that maturity-onset diabetics have smaller numbers of adipocytes than obese nondiabetics; i.e., β cell decompensation correlates with adipocyte size more than it does with adipocyte number. Would obesity carry the penalties of pathology commonly attributed to it if it occurred in hyperplastic form in a physically trained individual? (See section below on long-term repercussions of obesity.)

Experimental Animal Models of Obesity

There are few aspects of biology that have been more dependent on animal models as sources of new ideas than the study of obesity. The usefulness of VMH (ventromedial hypothalamus-lesioned) animals, as well as that of laterally lesioned animals, has already been mentioned. These models continue to yield interesting new information.

In addition, obesity has been produced in rats and mice by *nutritional* manipulations, i.e., feeding a highly palatable, high-fat diet, particularly effective when animals were confined in small cages.

Hyperphagia and obesity can be produced in animals by *chronic insulin injections,* a model analogous to human obesity that occurs in association with insulin-producing tumors. Similarly, insulin resistance, hyperinsulinism and obesity are seen in animals either injected with *glucocorticoids* or implanted with *ACTH-producing tumors.* This type of experimental obesity has its counterpart in human Cushing's syndrome.

From this brief account, it is obvious that obesities may have different causes and may therefore require different kinds of management.

Heredity

EXPERIMENTAL HEREDITARY OBESITIES

There are many different types of genetic obesity in the mouse, the most extensively studied of which is the *ob/ob mouse*, a strain characterized by the co-existence of obesity and hyperglycemia (Fig 16–8). Mice of this strain carry a recessive gene, which manifests itself as extreme obesity in one of four animals. The obesity does not usually become apparent until after the fourth week of life. When food intake is restricted to that of controls, excessive weight gain is prevented, but ob/ob mice contain three times as much fat as do their nonobese siblings.

In spite of their low resting oxygen consumption and hypoactivity, they eat 20%–50% more than do nonobese controls. They have hypertrophic islets of Langerhans and hyperinsulinemia, and all tissues studied show insulin resistance. Their fat cells are resistant to the lipolytic effect of catecholamines and demonstrate hyperlipogenesis even in the fasting state. There is some evidence that they tend to reesterify fatty acids to triglyceride to a greater extent than do normal mice.

Currently, as we have seen, there is great interest in the failure of these animals to institute nonshivering thermogenesis on exposure to cold. Emphasis is now being placed on decreased Na^+K^+ ATPase activity as the basis for both the hypometabolism and the inability to maintain body temperature in a cold environment.

The ob/ob mouse played an important role in studies on insulin receptor regulation by Kahn et al. Adipocytes of ob/ob mice showed decreased numbers of insulin receptors. The number of receptors/cell increased when the animals approached control weight when they were deprived of food. LeMarchand-Brustel has also demonstrated decreased insulin binding to muscle and insulin resistance of that tissue in ob/ob mice. Thus although the fat cell is prominently featured in research on obesity, metabolic aberrations may be found in muscle, liver and other tissues in obese animals.

Another favorite animal model of genetic obesity is the *Zucker* (fa/fa) *rat* (see Bray review). An extensive catalogue of differences between the Zucker rat and the VMH-lesioned animal has been compiled. One of the distinguishing features of the Zucker rat is that it has very high levels of serum triglycerides and cholesterol, which remain abnormally high on fasting.

The Zucker rat is an excellent model of hyperplastic obesity, since it contains abnormally large numbers of fat cells at all ages. Fat cell proliferation in this animal appears not to be confined to the neonatal period. It exhibits early hyperinsulinism and insulin resistance, but the nature of the primary defect is not yet known. Recently Gruen et al. have reported an increase in adipocyte lipoprotein lipase activity during the second postnatal week, long before the obesity is detectable.

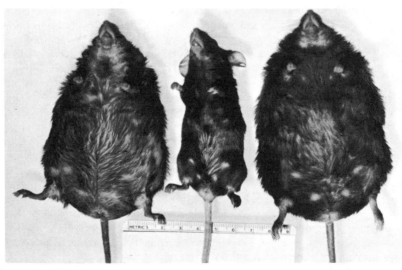

FIG 16–8.
Hereditary obesity-diabetes syndrome in the mouse. These animals have metabolic characteristics that differ from those in the obese mice shown in Figure 16–6.

One observation that illustrates differences in etiology between and among obesities is related to the experiment of Powley and Opsahl, cited above. These investigators showed that vagotomy interrupted the development of obesity in VMH-lesioned rats in a very striking way. When they (Powley and Opsahl) performed a similar experiment on Zucker fat rats, the operation had no effect on the developing obesity. This suggests that an intact connection between the CNS and the endocrine pancreas is an essential feature of VMH lesion obesity but is not required for Zucker obesity. One wonders how long it will be before we are able to perform ethically permissible tests of this sort, which will permit triage of obese people into recognizable categories.

Another interesting study that illustrates the interplay of heredity and environment is that of Hackel et al. (see Brodoff monograph) on the occurrence of *obesity and diabetes in the desert rat*. In its native habitat, this animal eats succulent plants, drinks very little water, and never becomes either obese or diabetic. If it is maintained in a laboratory, it quickly becomes first obese and then diabetic. Obesity and diabetes disappear if the animal is returned to its customary diet. The desert rat's experience duplicates that of certain human populations when they change their life-style drastically. In South Africa, certain Bantu tribe people show a low incidence of obesity and diabetes in their native villages. When they migrate to urban centers, where they eat an energetically dense diet and decrease their energy expenditure, many become both obese and diabetic.

HEREDITY IN HUMANS

There is evidence that supports the view that hereditary factors are at least contributory causes of obesity in man. The finding of a high correlation between the incidence of fatness in parents and children may not be convincing, for children learn food habits from parents very early and may adhere to these habits for many years. But studies on identical twins have revealed a close correspondence of body weight, much closer than that found in fraternal twins or in other siblings. Moreover, when identical twins have been separated in childhood and examined later in life, a striking similarity in body weight is still seen, although the deviation in this case is slightly greater than that observed in the case of twins brought up in the same household.

In 1986, Stunkard et al. presented the most convincing evidence to date not only that obesity has a strong hereditary component but that leanness is equally heritable. In this study of 540 adult Danish adoptees, divided into four categories (lean, median, overweight, and obese), body mass indices of the adoptees correlated closely with those of their natural parents but not at all with those of their adoptive parents. This relation between adoptees and natural parents was observed in all four weight classes.

While this study confirms our impression that there is a strong genetic component in the etiology of human obesity, it would be unfortunate if obese patients and their physicians used it as justification for not attempting to treat obesity. From both animal and human studies, it is obvious that many environmental factors can contribute to the development and maintenance of obesity and that some people are able to limit or even reverse developing obesity. There is also evidence that successful management of obesity can reduce the incidence of serious illness. To students who are interested in the report of Stunkard et al., we recommend the accompanying editorial by Van Itallie.

Metabolic Abnormalities in Obese Human Subjects

Many metabolic abnormalities have been described in obese people. *Impairment of glucose tolerance* was the earliest of these; in the light of more recent findings (to be described), Newburgh and Conn described a return to normal glucose tolerance in obese subjects who successfully lost weight. *Hyperlipidemia* is often seen in obese persons; it may involve both triglycerides and cholesterol, and it often takes the form of a pre-β lipoproteinemia. *Hyperinsulinemia* and exaggerated insulin response to a variety of insulin secretion tests are commonly seen. Much used to be made of increased *urinary glucocorticoid excretion* in the obese, but Streeten and colleagues have demonstrated that obese patients can readily be differentiated from patients with Cushing's disease by referring the glucocorticoid excretion of both to their respective creatinine excretion. With creatinine as a reference standard, glucocorticoid output in the obese subject does not differ from that of the normal subject.

Fluctuations in *plasma growth hormone*, whether they occur after arginine infusion, after exercise or spontaneously during very deep sleep, are very much blunted in obese people.

More recently, the pioneer studies of Hirsch, Salans, Knittle and their colleagues on adipose cell size and number have revealed that many obese patients have an increase in both size and total number of adipocytes, whereas others show only an increase in the size. The large adipocytes of the obese are demonstrably insensitive to insulin in vitro, but after weight reduction causes a marked shrinking in adipocyte size, the smaller cells may actually become comparatively hypersensitive to insulin.

Are these changes secondary to obesity or could any of them have contributed to the etiology of the obesity? Sims, Horton, and Salans (1971) attempted to answer this question in what has become famous as "the Vermont study." These investigators, working with normal male, young adult prisoners in a state penitentiary, made very careful observations on their subjects during a control, or basal, state. Then the men were encouraged to overeat systematically, and when they had gained about 25% above their customary weights, they were restudied. At this point, they resumed ad libitum feeding, lost weight back to their control levels without exception and were studied again. The results of the study are summarized in Table 16–2.

All of these abnormalities reverted to normal when the subjects stopped overeating and resumed their control weights. It is noteworthy that certain subjects were unable to become obese in spite of documented overeating and that there was poor correlation, among those who succeeded in becoming obese, between caloric intake and actual weight gain. One of the most fascinating findings in the study is the last item in Table 16–2: spontaneously obese persons required less than half as many calories to maintain the obese state as did the experimental subjects.

TABLE 16–2.

Findings in "The Vermont Study" (see text)[*]

STRUCTURE	SPONTANEOUS OBESITY	INDUCED OBESITY
Adipose tissue		
Cell size	↑	↑
Cell number	↑ or N	N
Insulin sensitivity		↓
Forearm muscle		
Insulin sensitivity		↓
Blood lipids		
Cholesterol	↑	↑ (trend)
Triglycerides	↑	↑ (trend)
FFA	N or ↑	↓ (trend)
Glucose tolerance	N or ↓	↓ (trend)
Plasma insulin	N or ↑	N or ↑
Plasma GH	↓	↓
Large calories required to maintain obese state	1,300/m²	2,700/m²

[*]From Sims EAH, Horton ES, Salans L: *Annu Rev Med* 1971; 22:235.

Sims properly pointed out that the congruence of the data in spontaneous and induced obesity does not necessarily prove that all of these abnormalities in the spontaneous group were secondary to developing obesity. It simply shows that reversible metabolic changes can occur in previously nonobese people.

The studies on adipocyte size and number may reveal much of the basis for the difficulty many obese people have when they attempt weight reduction. Hypercellularity of adipose tissue represents an enormous caloric sink, which becomes ever more vast as the large cells become smaller and regain their insulin sensitivity. Adipose tissue hyperplasia may be due either to unfortunate genes or to neonatal overfeeding. But among the most important lessons of the Vermont study are these: (1) the subjects spontaneously elected to reduce their food intake back to control levels at the end of the experiment; (2) they required 2,700 calories/m² to maintain the obese state; and (3) they all succeeded in resuming their normal weight. However similar they were to spontaneously obese patients in the parameters studied, they must have differed from them in ways that remain to be discovered.

Obesity is often associated with hyperlipidemia (hypercholesterolemia and hypertriglyceridemia) and, indeed, blood-lipid patterns can often be restored toward normal in people with familial hyperlipidemias by weight reduction. The coexistence of obesity and impaired glucose tolerance has been mentioned, as has the connection between obesity and maturity-onset diabetes mellitus. Since each member of this triad—obesity, hyperlipidemia, impaired glucose tolerance—is itself the product of a complex mosaic of causes and predisposing factors, it is often difficult (especially in epidemiologic studies) to assign single factor significance to one or another. It is mainly for this reason that the importance of "pure" obesity as an authentic risk factor for cardiovascular disease has been questioned (see Mann).

The precise relationship between obesity and hyperlipidemia is not known, nor is it known whether the sequence of events is always the same. Something like the sequence of events depicted in Figure 16–9,A may be inferred from the work of Farquhar et al., who suggest that insulin resistance secondary to obesity is primary and hepatic overproduction of VLDL secondary. Jeanrenaud observes that in most experimental obesities, hyperinsulinism is an early and prominent finding, and may indeed occur when hyperphagia is prevented. Therefore, hyperphagia may be secondary to hyperinsulinism (Fig 16–9,B). In either case, with enlargement of fat cell triglyceride droplets, circulating levels of FFA tend to rise, thereby offering the liver more substrate for VLDL synthesis. Reversal of this state of affairs may be

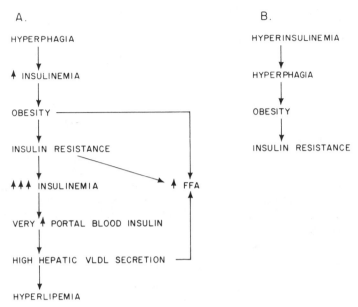

FIG 16–9.
A and **B,** obesity, hyperinsulinemia, hyperlipemia: some possible interrelations.

achieved by weight reduction, which causes restoration of insulin sensitivity in all insulin-sensitive tissues and a decrease in both resting and stimulated serum insulin levels.

Regional Differences in Adipocyte Metabolism and Their Effects on the Metabolic Complications of Obesity

At one time, all of the adipose tissue of the body was presumed to belong to one large dispersed organ. It is now apparent that adipocytes in different fat depots may show consistent differences in size and in response to hormonal stimuli. The earliest hint that all fat cells are not precisely the same was the observation that men tend to accumulate fat in the abdomen and upper body, while women often exhibit lower-body or buttock-thigh obesity. It is widely recognized that metabolic consequences of obesity (impaired glucose tolerance, diabetes, hyperlipidemia, hypertension) are more commonly associated with upper-body (also called abdominal, or android) obesity than with lower-body obesity (femoral, or gynoid). (See Kissebah, also Smith, for documentation.)

It is now possible to explain these differences at the level of cell biology. Following prior demonstrations that human abdominal adipocytes were much more sensitive to lipolytic (beta) stimulation by epinephrine than were femoral fat cells, it was proposed (by Lafontan et al., on the basis of inhibitor analysis) that femoral adipocytes were more responsive to alpha

stimulation than were their abdominal counterparts. Alpha stimulation (like insulin) results in an *anti*lipolytic effect; i.e., it tends to contain lipid in triglyceride droplets. The net effect of these differences in hormonal responsiveness would be to cause a rapid turnover of abdominal adipocyte triglyceride with higher circulating free fatty acid levels and, secondarily, higher levels of VLDL. Higher free fatty acid levels would tend, over time, to cause insulin resistance and secondary portal (and peripheral) hyperinsulinemia. This would stimulate hepatic VLDL secretion even more. The femoral cells, on the other hand, would participate in a slower triglyceride turnover which would not have the consequences we have described.

One of the most interesting examples we have seen of a teleonomically appropriate *change* in function of a specific fat depot was given by Rebuffé-Scrive et al. in their study of regional fat cell responses in pregnancy and lactation. After confirming that the lipolytic response of femoral fat cells to noradrenaline was low in nonpregnant women and in early pregnancy, they demonstrated that the response was a good as that in abdominal cells during lactation. Lipoprotein lipase activity of abdominal cells was unaffected by pregnancy or lactation, but the activity of LPL decreased in femoral cells during lactation, favoring lipolysis. The ultimate beneficiary of this felicitous collaboration between femoral fat cell and secreting mammary gland cell is the suckling infant.

Environment

Obviously, powerful environmental forces interact with physiologic mechanisms and hereditary influences to affect the success or failure of any individual person in achieving energy balance. In order to see the problem in perspective, it is essential to consider a few of the ways in which these forces act.

Energy balance is more compatible with high food intake in cold environments than in warm ones. High temperatures are more tolerable at low humidity than at high humidity. The general availability of food can disturb energy balance in either direction. When, during World War II, whole populations existed on 1,500 calories per day per person, obesity disappeared. In countries that produce an excess of food that is widely distributed, the incidence of positive energy balance is very high, partly due no doubt to the fact that in many of these countries it is possible to live at levels of extremely low energy expenditure.

In addition to the physical environment, there is a complex *psychological environment,* or an environment of interpersonal transactions carried on at many different levels of intimacy. There is no doubt that forces that arise from the interaction of the individual with his environment affect energy balance. The person who is absorbed in his/her job is far less likely to eat inappropriately large amounts of food than is a bored individual who is constantly surrounded by readily available goodies.

A psychological factor that operates in the opposite direction is the standard of beauty that is accepted by large populations. The promotion of the Hollywood starlet ideal of beauty has doubtless stimulated many teen-age girls to make a conscious attempt to keep themselves from getting fat and unattractive, and sometimes this battle is fought at enormous emotional cost (see *Eating Disorders,* below). In other cultures as, for example, among the Banyankole people of East Africa, girls were prepared for marriage by forced feeding and activity restriction, and the more obese they became, the more desirable they were considered as brides.

As the example just cited well illustrates, the psychological environment is inseparable from the *social, political, cultural,* and even *moral* environment. Food habits differ from one culture to another. Industrial civilizations tend to be characterized by low physical activity levels. In many countries, small numbers of people are paid to take exercise for the pleasure of millions who sit and watch them. The effect of the widespread influence of television viewing on the collective energy balance problem of this country is difficult to assess, for this pastime is characterized not only by minimal physical activity but also by maximal temptation in the form of nearly irresistible advertisements for food and beer. This combination taxes the capacity of the best physiologic energy balance-regulating equipment imaginable.

Psychological Factors and Behavior Modification

Although the basic neurophysiologic and metabolic equipment for regulating energy balance in human beings may resemble that in experimental animals, the elaborate encephalization of the process in men and women may veto physiologically appropriate hunger or satiety signals. In most human societies, the eating of food, or abstention from it, is associated with ceremonial, emotional, hedonistic, and even religious practices.

Although psychological disturbances may be initiating factors in the cause of obesity, the vast majority of obese people show no higher incidence of psychiatric malaise than does the general population. However, obese individuals, particularly adolescents, may lose self-esteem and may regard themselves as members of a harassed minority (Mayer), often with considerable justification, for many societies do indeed discriminate against fat people in more or less subtle ways.

The same dilemma—cause or result of obesity?—surrounds the observations of Schachter and others that obese people are more likely to respond to external food cues than to physiologic hunger or satiety messages (see Nisbett). When massively obese people were subjected to ileal bypass operations (see below), psychologic tests showed that they had reverted from the obesity cue-response pattern to that of people of normal weight (Solow et al.). Although eating behavior of obese people resembles that of VMH-lesioned animals, there is no evidence that altered food cue response plays an important part in the cause of human obesity.

Only 10% of obese adults give a history of infantile and childhood obesity, leaving 90% whose obesity occurred in adult life. According to one hypothesis, life-styles that contribute to positive energy balance are largely composed of learned behaviors, which presumably can be unlearned. Acting on this hypothesis, Stuart, a psychologist, devised a strategy for reversing obesity that has come to be known as *behavior modification.* This designation is unfortunate because for many people, behavior modification has a sinister sound. In fact, the procedure involves self-education of the obese person with the assistance of a therapist who assumes the role of teacher. A careful analysis is made, by means of an appropriate diary, of all aspects of the subject's eating and exercise habits. With this information, it is possible systematically to eliminate undesired behaviors and substitute desired ones. The method has the great advantage of individualizing each subject's analysis and prescription. It is also feasible in self-help groups.

Early reports of success rates with this approach were enthusiastic, but follow-up was not long. There is as yet no evidence that the method is valuable in massively obese individuals. However, since conventional methods of managing obesity, even in highly specialized medical centers, have not been impressive, there is hope that this method will fulfill its early promise. Perhaps the high failure rates in most centers can be explained in part by the experience of one diabetes clinic that has achieved some success (see Davidson). In that setting, patients received at least 25 hours of instruction in lieu of the all-too-commonly issued mimeographed diet sheet.

For an example of a behavioral modification program, the reader is referred to the manual by Ferguson.

Surgical Treatment of Massive Obesity

After an obese individual has been unsuccessful in losing weight by diet, exercise, and all other procedures, in some treatment centers, surgery may be attempted. This maneuver is reserved for massively obese people and is treated as an experimental procedure. In many medical centers, candidates are screened by a group consisting of a surgeon, internist, and psychiatrist.

A variety of ileojejunal *bypass operations*, designed to limit the absorbing surface of the jejunum, have been performed on many patients who had to be at least 100% overweight to qualify for the procedure. Many short- and long-term complications have been described, among them fatty infiltration of the liver, outright hepatic decompensation, protein malnutrition, and fluid and electrolyte disturbances. Although some gratifying results have been reported, the current trend is toward one or another form of *gastroplasty*, i.e., mechanically restricting the functional part of the stomach to a small fraction of its former volume. These operations, which are done on people who by definition are poor operative and anesthesia risks, are far from ideal treatment. They will continue to be performed and assessed as long as there are obese people who are desperate enough to sign consent forms even when they are informed of all possible risks. (For a recent review, see Wastell.)

Long-Term Repercussions of Obesity

We have examined the biologic problem of energy balance from a number of points of view and at levels of organization from biochemical to social. Obesity, which can be regarded as the result of prolonged positive caloric balance, has been presented as a result of many contributory forces, and the suggestion has been made that different individuals may become obese for different reasons. Whatever the reasons, obesity—particularly of long duration—carries with it great risks of morbidity and premature mortality. Figure 16–1 shows that the largest penalty for overweight is paid in the currency of premature death in the third, fourth, and fifth decades of life. In Figure 16–10, some of the principal causes for death among men and women, rated by an insurance company as substandard risks for insurance, are shown as percentages of the death rates of persons accepted for standard insurance. Although other data may differ in detail from those shown here, this figure represents a fair estimate of the cost in mortality of overweight. It does not show another estimate, which is practically impossible to make, namely, the cost in serious morbidity or work-days lost due to incapacitating illness in which obesity was a contributory factor. Surely, this cost must be monumental.

The disorders indicated as "principal cardiovascular-renal diseases" include, for the most part, diseases of the heart, brain, and kidneys in which atherosclerotic vascular disease is a common denominator.

As we remarked before, these complications are correlated with the abdominal-android type of obesity and not with the femoral-gynoid type. Since all of the older epidemiologic studies do not make any distinction between the two types, the risks of overweight, particularly in certain obese people under 50–55, may be understated by Figure 16–10. We also pointed out earlier that the risks for obese (or, at any rate, overweight) people over 55 may turn out to be somewhat less than we had previously thought.

Hypertension, a well-known risk factor for atherosclerotic disease, often coexists with obesity. In fact, blood pressure can often be reduced in obese people by weight loss without salt restriction (see Reisin et al.).

A high incidence of gallstones also is associated with obesity because people make lithogenic bile, i.e., bile that contains an inadequate concentration of cholesterol-solubilizing detergents. The statistics in Figure 16–10 are somewhat complicated by the fact that obesity may predispose to gallstone formation, but it also enormously complicates the anesthetic and

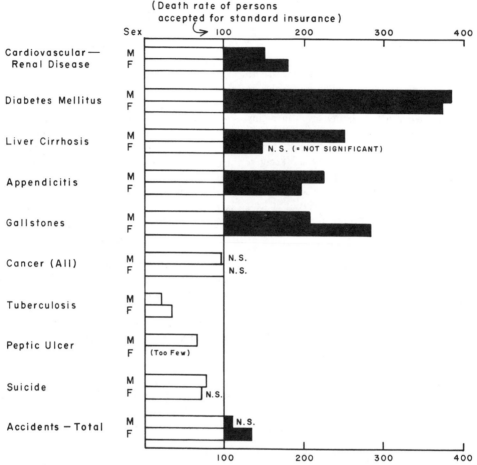

FIG 16–10.
Effects of obesity on susceptibility to various diseases. *Black bars* represent increased susceptibility in overweight individuals. (After Marks HH: *Bull NY Acad Med* 1960; 36:15.)

surgical procedures often demanded by the presence of such stones. The latter complications are probably responsible for the fact that obese patients with appendicitis did poorly in the series cited in Figure 16–10. It is often difficult for the anesthesiologist to maintain an airway in obese patients, and anesthesia induction time and recovery time are likely to be abnormally long in such individuals. Fat deposits and problems of muscle relaxation tax the surgeon's technical skill, and postoperative complications such as thromboembolic phenomena are more likely to occur in the obese.

The high incidence of cirrhosis of the liver among the obese correlates well with the results of animal studies, for all known kinds of experimentally obese

animals that have been examined so far have shown fatty infiltration of the liver—frequently a precursor of cirrhosis.

The cancer problem is complicated by the fact that although there is no clear relationship between obesity and all diseases that are classifiable as cancer, certain experimental and clinical findings suggest that there is a relationship between chronic overnutrition and some specific kinds of cancer. In the laboratory, Waxler has clearly shown that the induction of aurothioglucose obesity not only causes an earlier appearance of mammary cancer in a high incidence strain of mice but also results in larger and faster-growing tumors. He has also made similar observations on the effect of overeating on the development of primary hepatomas. In the clinic, there is evidence to suggest a relationship between obesity and two types of cancer in women, namely, breast cancer and endometrial cancer. Obese women are believed to have more endometrial cancer than do lean women because they have a larger capacity for aromatizing androstenedione to estrone in their adipose tissue. This results in increased stimulation of estrogen-sensitive tissues (see Chapter 9). The high incidence of accidents in overweight women has many conceivable explanations. Whatever the cause, susceptibility to accidents is another penalty of obesity.

A respiratory difficulty has been associated with severe obesity. It is characterized by dyspnea, marked exercise intolerance, somnolence and, in some instances, cyanosis, and it is sometimes referred to as the Pickwickian syndrome because Dickens' description of the Fat Boy appears to some observers to have anticipated the modern recognition of this disorder. The impairment of respiration is due to the fact that the respiratory movements of the thoracic cage are inhibited by the weight of subcutaneous fat deposits while the downward excursion of the diaphragm is limited by large intra-abdominal accumulations of fat. When the difficulties in gas exchange are added to the fact that increased oxygen is required to move and manipulate a heavy body, the relative pulmonary insufficiency becomes even greater. In severe cases, these unfortunate people can manage to do little more than move their tidal air back and forth with rapid, shallow, ineffectual respirations. When this disturbance occurs in elderly people, it may be associated with arteriosclerotic heart disease, contributing an additional component to the dyspnea.

The association between maturity-onset diabetes and obesity is clear, as is the fact that diabetes predisposes people to early death due to cardiovascular disease (see Fig 14–23). Since the incidence of obesity and diabetes in industrialized societies is so high, it is clear that large-scale prevention of obesity, or its successful treatment, would prevent or delay the appearance of an unimaginably vast amount of morbidity. On the other hand, there may be subgroups of overweight people (e.g., those with hyperplastic obesity whose adipocyte size is within normal limits, obese people in good physical training, or those with femoral-gynoid obesity) who are at no greater risk of diabetes than are nonobese controls. With better understanding of obesity, diabetes and atherogenesis, it may be possible one day to identify people at greatest risk and to concentrate preventive and therapeutic efforts on them. At present, every effort should be made to prevent or treat obesity in individuals with a family history of diabetes.

Eating Disorders: Anorexia Nervosa and Bulimia

If the obesities are the major disorders of positive energy balance, insufficient food intake, both in energy and quality, is epidemic among many human populations, mainly in the nonindustrialized countries of the world. It is an ironic fact that, although there are millions of obese people, many more people are undernourished. An analysis of the causes of this global malaise lies more appropriately within the domain of economists, politicians, agronomists, demographers and social scientists than in that of the biologist.

There is one disorder of energy balance that has been called "anorexia nervosa" but seems to be due for renaming. Warren and van de Wiele have called it "puberal starvation-amenorrhea," but that designation may be too narrow.

Anorexia nervosa is a constellation of signs, symptoms, and characteristic laboratory findings that occurs mainly in puberal girls and young women (although it occurs rarely in very young adolescent boys). It is a serious disorder which, if not arrested, may even be lethal. Although every individual may not exhibit all of the features of the syndrome, the following symptoms and signs are common: weight loss, amenorrhea, constipation, bradycardia, low blood pressure, hypothermia, cold sensitivity, hyperactivity, growth of "peach fuzz" hair, yellow palms (hypercarotenemia), and mild diabetes insipidus.

Although many psychiatric theories of the cause of this disorder exist, its victims show little evidence of classic psychiatric disease. Indeed, the typical patient is likely to be the daughter of reasonably well-to-do parents, intelligent, and a successful (even overachieving) student. The word anorexia, which implies a lack of desire for food, is a misnomer, for these young people think about food constantly and develop elaborate food rituals and fantasies as well as compulsive food preferences, which often include eating large amounts of carrots, celery, lettuce, and cabbage. Often periods of low food intake alternate with periods of compulsive gorging and "binge" eating.

It is arresting to reflect on how many manifestations of the disorder involve functions that are prominently represented in the hypothalamus. In addition to food intake regulation, the manifestations of hypotension and bradycardia, hypothermia and intolerance to cold, amenorrhea and evidence of estrogen deficiency all involve integrating mechanisms in the hypothalamus.

Patients with anorexia nervosa may resemble those with hypopituitarism, and, in fact, they have low plasma LH, low plasma FSH, and a poor gonadotropin response to GnRH. However, they have *high* circulating levels of glucocorticoids and may show normal or even supernormal responses to provocative tests for ACTH secretion (i.e., metyrapone test). Thyroxine and T_3 levels tend to be low normal, as does the TSH response to TRH. Thus, the high circulating glucocorticoid levels rule out panhypopituitarism. In individuals who show remission of symptoms with weight gain, gonadotropin secretion resumes or achieves the pattern characteristic for the age of the patient: wide, sleep-related swings in adolescents and the normal adult pattern in sexually mature women. Responses to releasing factors also return to normal. Many of the characteristic features of anorexia nervosa are observed in severely undernourished individuals, which suggests that conscious overriding of physiologic hunger in anorexia nervosa patients is the precipitating event, which entrains the other hypothalamic difficulties.

Bulimia, like anorexia nervosa, is peculiarly a disease of self-image in relation to a perceived estimate of society's perception of one's self. The Hollywood starlet idea of beauty is so pervasive in U.S. society that some overweight adolescent girls learn to control their body weight by self-induced vomiting, frequently after gorging huge amounts of rich food. It is astonishing that reports on the frequency of this behavior vary between 5% and 18% of different populations of high school and college-age females. Some victims of bulimia compound their problems by adding laxatives and/or diuretics to their weight control regimen.

In most cases, bulimia is learned behavior. In some, as we have remarked, it occurs in people who later develop anorexia nervosa. Both anorexia nervosa and bulimia represent conscious attempts to override and deny all of the complex mechanisms that have evolved over eons to regulate food intake to energy need.

For a recent discussion of problems in eating behavior, see Herzog and Copeland.

BIBLIOGRAPHY

Ackerman S: The management of obesity. *Hosp Pract* 1983; March:117.

Ahrens EH, Jr: Obesity and coronary heart disease: New dimensions. *Arteriosclerosis* 1984; 4:177.

Andres R, Elahi D, Tobin JD, et al: Impact of age on weight goals. *Ann Intern Med* 1985; 103:1030.

Björntorp P: Obesity and the risk of cardiovascular disease. *Ann Clin Res* 1985; 17:3.

Björntorp P, de Jounge K, Krotkiewski M, et al: Physical training in human obesity. III: Effects of long-term physical training on body composition. *Metabolism* 1973; 22:1467.

Björntorp P, Vahouny G, Kritchevsky D (eds): *Dietary Fiber and Obesity: Current Topics in Nutrition and Disease,* vol 14. New York, Alan R Liss, 1985.

Bray GA (ed): Symposium on experimental animal models for the study of obesity. *Fed Proc* 1977; 36:137.

Bray GA: The Zucker-fatty rat: A review. *Fed Proc* 1977; 36:148.

Brodoff BN: Adipose tissue metabolism and obesity. *Ann NY Acad Sci* 1965; 131:1.

Curtis-Prior PB (ed): *Biochemical Pharmacology of Obesity.* New York, Elsevier North-Holland, Inc, 1983.

Czech MP, Richardson DK, Smith CJ: Biochemical basis of fat cell insulin resistance in obese rodents and man. *Metabolism* 1977; 26:1057.

Danforth E, Jr, Desilets EH, Horton ES, et al: Reciprocal serum triiodothyronine (T_3) and reverse (rT_3) induced by altering carbohydrate content of the diet. *Clin Res* 1975; 23:573A.

Davidson JK: Educating diabetic patients about diet therapy. *Int Diabetes Fed Bull* 1975; 20:3.

Deter RL, Liebelt RA: Gold thioglucose as an experimental tool. *Texas Rep Biol Med* 1964; 22:229.

DiGirolamo M, Howe MD, Esposito J: Metabolic patterns and insulin responsiveness of enlarging fat cells. *J Lipid Res* 1974; 15:332.

Durnin JVGA, Edholm OG, Miller DS, et al: How much food does man require? *Nature* 1973; 242:418.

Epstein LH, Wing RR, Valoski A: Childhood obesity. *Pediatr Clin North Am* 1985; 32:363.

Farquhar JW, Olefsky J, Stern M, et al: Obesity, insulin, and triglycerides, in Bray GA (ed): *Obesity in Perspective,* vol 2. Fogarty International Center Series on Preventive Medicine. Washington, DC, US Government Printing Office, 1975, part 2, p 313.

Faust IM, Johnson PR, Hirsch J: Adipose tissue regeneration in adult rats. *Proc Soc Exp Biol Med* 1979; 161:111.

Foster DW: Eating disorders: Obesity and anorexia nervosa, in Wilson JD, Foster DW (eds): *Williams Textbook of Endocrinology,* ed 7. Philadelphia, WB Saunders Co, 1985, pp 1081–1107.

Foster WR, Burton BT (eds): The problem of obesity (NIH Symposium). *Ann Intern Med* 1985; 103:983.

Galloway S McL, Farquhar DL, Munro JF: The current status of antiobesity drugs. *Postgrad Med J* 1984; 60(suppl 3):19.

Galton DJ, Bray GA: Metabolism of α glycerol phosphate in human adipose tissue in obesity. *J Clin Endocrinol* 1967; 27:1573.

Geary N, Langhans W, Scharrer E: Metabolic concomitants of glucagon induced suppression of feeding in the rat. *Am J Physiol* 1981; 241:R330.

Gruen R, Hietanen E, Greenwood MRC: Increased adipose tissue lipoprotein lipase activity during development of the genetically obese rat (fa/fa). *Metabolism* 1978; 27(suppl 2):1955.

Herzog DB, Copeland PM: Eating disorders. *N Engl J Med* 1985; 313:295.

Himms-Hagen J: Thermogenesis in brown adipose tissue as an energy buffer. *N Engl J Med* 1984; 311:1549.

Hirsch J: Jejunoileal shunt for obesity. *N Engl J Med* 1974; 290:962.

Hirsch J: Hypothalamic control of appetite. *Hosp Pract* 1984; Feb:131.

Hoebel BG: Brain reward and aversion systems in the control of feeding and sexual behavior, in Jones MR (ed): *Nebraska Symposium on Motivation.* Lincoln, University of Nebraska Press, 1975.

Isaacs AJ, Hoffbrand BI (eds): Obesity management in the 80s. *Postgrad Med J* 1984; (suppl) 3:60.

Jeanrenaud B: An hypothesis on the aetiology of obesity: Dysfunction of the central nervous system as a primary cause. *Diabetologia* 1985; 28:502.

James WPT (ed): Obesity. *Clin Endocrinol Metab* 1984; 13:435.

Keesey RE, Boyle PC, Kemnitz JW, et al: The role of the lateral hypothalamus in determining the body weight set point, in Novin D, Wyrwicka W, Bray G (eds) *Hunger: Basic Mechanisms and Clinical Implications.* New York, Raven Press, 1976.

Khoo C-S (ed): Diet, gastrointestinal function, and eating behavior (symposium). *Am J Clin Nutr* 1985; 42:913.

Kissebah AH: Characteristics of obese patients with hyperinsulinemia: The importance of body fat distribution, in Bjoerntorp P, Vahouny GV, Kritchevsky D (eds): *Dietary Fiber and Obesity.* New York, Alan R Liss, 1985, pp 1–18.

Lafontan M, Dang-Tran L, Berlun M: Alpha-adrenergic antilipolytic effect of adrenaline in human fat cells of the thigh: Comparison with adrenaline responsiveness of different fat deposits. *Eur J Clin Invest* 1979; 9:261.

Landsberg L, Young JB: The role of the sympathoadrenal system in modulating energy expenditure. *Clin Endocrinol Metab* 1984; 13:475.

Leibowitz SF: Brain catecholaminergic mechanisms for control of hunger, in Novin D, Wyrwicka W, Bray G (eds): *Hunger: Basic Mechanisms and Clinical Implications.* New York, Raven Press, 1976, pp 1–18.

LeMarchand-Brustel Y, Freychet P: Studies of insulin insensitivity in soleus muscles of obese mice. *Metabolism* 1978; 27(suppl 2):1982.

Leonhardt W, Hanefeld M, Schneider H, et al: Human adipocyte volumes: Maximum size and correlation to weight index in maturity onset diabetes. *Diabetologia* 1972; 8:287.

Lin MH, Romsos DR, Akera T: Na^+, K^+-ATPase enzyme units in skeletal muscle from lean and obese mice. *Biochem Biophys Res Commun* 1978; 80:398.

Mann GV: The influence of obesity on health. *N Engl J Med* 1974; 291:178.

Mayer J: *Overweight: Causes, Costs, and Control.* Englewood Cliffs, New Jersey, Prentice-Hall, 1968.

Miller DS, Mumford P, Stock MJ: Gluttony: 2. Thermogenesis in overeating man. *Am J Clin Nutr* 1967; 20:1223.

Mogenson GJ: Changing views of the role of the hypothalamus in the control of ingestive behaviors, in Lederis K, Cooper KE (eds): *Recent Studies of Hypothalamic Function.* Basel, S Karger AG, 1974.

Morley JE, Levine AS: The pharmacology of eating behavior. *Annu Rev Pharmacol Toxicol* 1985; 25:127.

Morrison SD: The hypothalamic syndrome in rats. *Fed Proc* 1977; 36:139.

Nestel PJ, Whyte HM: Plasma free fatty acid and triglyceride turnover in obesity. *Metabolism* 1968; 17:1122.

Nicholl CG, Polak JM, Bloom SR: The hormonal regulation of food intake, digestion, and absorption. *Annu Rev Nutr* 1985; 5:213.

Niijima A: Afferent impulse discharges from glucoreceptors in the liver of the guinea pig. *Ann NY Acad Sci* 1969; 157:690.

Nisbett RE: Eating behavior and obesity in men and animals. *Adv Psychosom Med* 1972; 7:173.

Oomura Y: Significance of glucose, insulin, and free fatty acid on the hypothalamic feeding and satiety neurones, in Novin D, Wyrwicka W, Bray G (eds): *Hunger: Basic Mechanisms and Clinical Implications.* New York, Raven Press, 1978.

Opsahl CA, Powley TL: Failure of vagotomy to reverse obesity in genetically obese Zucker rats. *Am J Physiol* 1974; 236:34.

Oscai LB, McGarr JA: Evidence that the amount of food consumed in early life fixes appetite in the rat. *Am J Physiol* 1978; 235:R141.

Para-Covarrubias A, Rivera-Rodriguez I, Almaraz-Ugalde A: Cephalic phase of insulin secretion in obese adolescents. *Diabetes* 1971; 20:800.

Plummer DM, Bray GA, Garrow JS, et al: International symposia on nutrition and obesity: The state of the science. *Med J Aust* 1985; 142:(special supplement): S1–32.

Powley TL, Opsahl CA: Ventromedial hypothalamic obesity abolished by subdiaphragmatic vagotomy. *Am J Physiol* 1974; 226:25.

Rebuffé-Scrive M, Enk L, Crona N, et al: Fat metabolism in different regions in women: Effect of menstrual cycles, pregnancy, and lactation. *J Clin Invest* 1985; 75:1973.

Reisin E, Abel R, Modan M, et al: Effect of weight loss without salt restriction on the reduction of blood pressure in overweight hypertensive patients. *N Engl J Med* 1978; 298:1.

Ricquier D, Mory G: Factors affecting brown adipose tissue activity in animals and man. *Clin Endocrinol Metab* 1984; 13:501.

Salans LB, Cushman SW: Cellular consequences of obesity, in Bray GA (ed): *Obesity in Perspective.* Washington, DC: Dept of Health, Education, and Welfare (75–708), 1976, p 245.

Salans L, Knittle JL II, Hirsch J: Obesity, glucose intolerance, and diabetes mellitus, in Ellenberg M, Rifkin H (eds): *Diabetes Mellitus: Theory and Practice,* ed 3. New Hyde Park, New York, Medical Examination Publishing Co, 1983.

Schachter S: Obesity and eating. *Science* 1968; 161:751.

Simopoulos AP: The health implications of overweight and obesity. *Nutr Rev* 1985; 43:33.

Sims EAH: Syndromes of obesity, in DeGroot LJ (ed): *Endocrinology,* vol 3. New York, Grune & Stratton, 1979, pp 1941–1962.

Smith GP, Gibbs J: Gut peptides and postprandial satiety. *Fed Proc* 1984; 43:2889.

Smith U: The adipose tissue and the metabolic complications of obesity, in Bjoerntorp P, Vahouny GV, Kritchevsky D (eds): *Dietary Fiber and Obesity.* New York, Alan R Liss, pp 33–39.

Soll AH, Kahn CR, Neville D, Jr, et al: Insulin receptor deficiency in genetic and acquired obesity. *J Clin Invest* 1975; 53:582.

Solow C, Silberfarb PM, Swift K: Psychosocial effects of intestinal bypass surgery for severe obesity. *N Engl J Med* 1974; 290:300.

Stern JS, Johnson PR: Size and number of adipocytes and their implications, in Katzen H, Mahler R (eds): *Diabetes, Obesity, and Vascular Disease: Advances in Modern Nutrition,* vol 2. New York, Hemisphere Press, 1978, pp 303–340.

Stirling JL, Stock MJ: Nonconservative mechanisms of energy metabolism in thermogenesis, in Pfelbaum MA (ed): *Energy Balance in Man.* Paris, Masson, 1973, p 219.

Straus E, Yalow RS: Cholecystokinin in brains of obese and nonobese mice. *Science* 1979; 203:68.

Stricker EM: Hyperphagia. *N Engl J Med* 1978; 298:1010.

Stuart RB: Behavioral control of eating: A report, in *Obesity in Perspective: Fogarty International Center Series on Pre-*

ventive Medicine, vol 2. Washington, DC, U.S. Government Printing Office, 1975, p 367.

Stunkard AJ, Sørensen TIA, Harris C, et al: An adoption study of human obesity. *N Engl J Med* 1986; 314:193.

Stunkard AJ, Stellar E (eds): *Eating and Its Disorders: Res Publ Assoc Res Nerv Ment Dis,* vol 62. New York, Raven Press, 1984.

Sullivan AC, Gruen RK: Mechanisms of appetite modulation by drugs. *Fed Proc* 1985; 44:139.

Ungerstedt U: Is interruption of the nigrostriatal dopamine system producing the "lateral hypothalamus syndrome?" *Acta Physiol Scand* 1970; 80:35A.

Van Itallie TB: Bad news and good news about obesity (editorial). *N Engl J Med* 1986; 314:239.

Warren MP, Van de Wiele RL: Clinical and metabolic features of anorexia nervosa. *Am J Obstet Gynecol* 1973; 117:435.

Wastell C: The surgical treatment of obesity. *Postgrad Med J* 1984; 60(suppl 3):27.

Weiner W: Norepinephrine, epinephrine, and the sympathomimetic amines, in Gilman AG, Goodman LS, Rall TW, et al: *Goodman and Gilman's The Pharmacological Basis of Therapeutics.* New York, Macmillan Publishing Co, 1985, pp 145–180.

Woo R, Daniels-Kush R, Horton ES: Regulation of energy balance. *Annu Rev Nutr* 1985; 5:411.

Woods SC, Porte D, Jr: Insulin and the set point regulation of body weight, in Novin D, Wyrwicka W, Bray GA (eds): *Hunger: Basic Mechanisms and Clinical Implications.* New York, Raven Press, 1976.

Woods SC, Porte D, Jr: The role of peptides in the control of food intake. *Excerpta Med ICS* 1984; 655:601.

Yim GKW, Lowy MT: Opioids, feeding, and anorexias. *Fed Proc* 1984; 43:2893.

York DA, Bray GA, Yukimura Y: An enzymatic defect in the obese (ob/ob) mouse: Loss of thyroid-induced sodium and potassium-dependent adenosine triphosphatase. *Proc Natl Acad Sci USA* 1978; 75:477.

PART VIII

Calcium Metabolism

17

Hormonal Regulation of Calcium Homeostasis

Long before the evolution of the bony skeleton, the calcium ion had assumed an important role in biologic processes. In man, maintenance of extracellular calcium ion concentration within narrow limits is essential to the function of many tissues. In *skeletal and cardiac muscle,* Ca^{2+} fluxes between cytosol and sarcoplasmic reticulum are essential to contraction and relaxation (excitation-contraction coupling). If the

Ca^{2+} of the blood is too high, ventricular arrhythmias and ventricular fibrillation may be the result. The excitability of skeletal muscle is increased in low Ca^{2+} media and depressed by an excess of Ca^{2+}. These effects depend on changes in neuromuscular excitability, and they are the basis for the muscle spasms and marked hyperreflexia seen in hypocalcemic tetany. The traditional positive Chvostek sign—a twitching of the facial muscles in response to tapping over the facial nerve at the angle of the mandible—is one manifestation of hypocalcemic tetany. Ca^{2+} is also essential to the *secretory activity* of practically all endocrine and exocrine glandular cells (stimulus-secretion coupling); this was discussed in Chapter 13, on the adrenal medulla, and in the Chapter 14 section on insulin secretion. It is also a key participant in the process of blood clotting. We have emphasized the importance of Ca^{2+} as a second messenger, either with or without the participation of calmodulin. We have also described the role of Ca^{2+} in polyphosphoinositide turnover and its activation of C kinase. Its intracellular messenger effects may either supplement those of cyclic AMP or oppose them. In any case, Ca^{2+} participates centrally in the operation of many hormonal mechanisms, as well as in the function of central and peripheral neurones.

Ca^{2+}, in addition to its regulatory activity, is a *major constituent of the bony skeleton*. This architectural function of Ca^{2+}, which is accomplished by most of the Ca^{2+} present in the body, can be compromised in many ways. The dominant theme of our discussion will be the nature of the dynamic equilibrium that must be maintained among the various organs (GI tract, kidney, bone, and skin) in order to regulate the extracellular fluid Ca^{2+} concentration within narrow limits, at the same time insuring an adequate supply of the ion for its important skeletal function.

Ca^{2+} homeostasis may be disturbed in a variety of disease states. A working knowledge of Ca^{2+} regulation is essential to understanding hyperparathyroidism, hypoparathyroidism, osteoporosis, Paget's disease, osteopetrosis, medullary carcinoma of the thyroid, renal disease, rickets, pancreatitis, and a large number of hypercalcemic states due to many unrelated causes. Obviously, it is not within the province of this chapter to present the pathophysiology of all these disorders; however, selected examples will be given.

Calcium Exchange and Pattern of Its Hormonal Regulation

The plasma concentration of Ca^{2+} is 10 mg/dl, or 5 mEq/L. Of this amount, slightly more than half is ionized; the rest is protein bound, though a small fraction may be chelated to circulating solutes such as citrate. The plasma Ca^{2+} level is tenaciously defended; i.e., changes of as little as 1% in either direction are enough to mobilize homeostatic mechanisms that function to restore the equilibrium concentration.

Figure 17–1 is a graphic description of calcium exchange in an adult person. It is an attempt to demonstrate two main points: (1) quantitative exchange of Ca^{2+} and (2) participation of the major hormones that affect Ca^{2+} exchange. About 1 gm of Ca^{2+} is ingested per day, but of this amount, only about one-third is absorbed from the gastrointestinal tract. The total amount of Ca^{2+} in the extracellular fluid pool of the body also is about 1 gm. Since 0.19 gm is secreted into the intestinal lumen in intestinal secretions, bile and shed epithelial cells, there is a net absorption from the intestine of 0.17 gm. The same amount is excreted in the urine by a person in Ca^{2+} balance.

The skeleton of a 70-kg person contains about 1,000 gm of Ca^{2+}, but only about 0.55 gm of the large amount exchanged daily between bone and body fluid is hormone modulated. In the steady state the amount of Ca^{2+} deposited in bone and the amount resorbed from bone are equal. Obviously in a growing child Ca^{2+} retention would occur in proportion to bone growth. After age 30–40, the bone mass decreases progressively, so that there is a small, constant net Ca^{2+} loss over a period of years.

Figure 17–1 also indicates the three main hormones involved in Ca^{2+} homeostasis: parathyroid hormone (PTH), calcitonin, and the most important metabolite of vitamin D: 1,25 dihydroxycholecalciferol (1,25[OH]$_2$D$_3$). *PTH acts to conserve body Ca^{2+}* and to increase extracellular fluid Ca^{2+} concentration. It does so by promoting resorption of Ca^{2+} from the bony skeleton, by retrieving Ca^{2+} from the glomerular filtrate and by increasing the rate of formation of *1,25(OH)$_2$D$_3$ in the kidney.* This important vitamin D metabolite accelerates the rate of absorption of Ca^{2+} from the gastrointestinal tract. Moreover, it plays a permissive role in the action of PTH on bone (and possibly on the kidney). *Calcitonin* inhibits bone resorption and has other effects that will be described.

Although these are the major hormones of Ca^{2+} homeostasis, many of the hormones discussed in previous chapters have important direct or indirect effects on bone. These include growth hormone and somatomedin, thyroid hormone, estrogens, androgens, and insulin. In addition to these, certain gastrointestinal hormones may participate in controlling secretion of calcitonin.

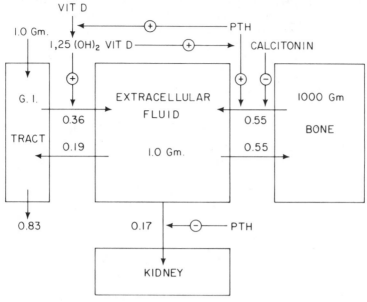

FIG 17–1.
Hormonal control of calcium homeostatis. Not shown are complex effects of PTH on bone formation, which is discussed in text. (Numbers [grams] are from Auerbach GD, Marx SJ, Spiegel AM, in Wilson JD, Foster DW [eds]: *Williams Textbook of Endocrinology,* ed 7. Philadelphia, WB Saunders Co, 1985.)

Coordinate Control of Ca^{2+} Homeostasis

Serum Ca^{2+} is regulated with extraordinary precision within narrow limits. When the circulating level falls, the parathyroid gland is stimulated to release its hormone and the calcitonin-producing cells are inhibited. When Ca^{2+} rises above the equilibrium level, calcitonin is secreted and the parathyroid gland is inhibited. Parathyroid hormone increases the circulating Ca^{2+} level by acting on bone, gut, and kidney. Calcitonin decreases Ca^{2+} in the blood by acting primarily on bone. Figure 17–2 shows that, at the normal

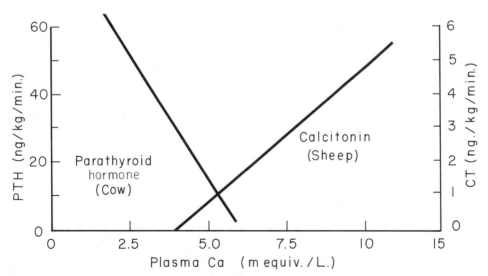

FIG 17–2.
Relationship of production rates of parathyroid hormone and calcitonin to plasma Ca^{2+} concentration. (Adapted from Copp DH: *J Endocrinol* 1969; 43:137.)

concentration of Ca^{2+}, both glands are producing small amounts of their hormones; with increasing levels, there is a positive linear relationship between Ca^{2+} concentration and calcitonin secretion rate. With falling Ca^{2+} levels, there is an inverse linear correlation between Ca^{2+} concentration and PTH secretion rate, i.e., the lower the Ca^{2+}, the higher the secretion rate.

Ca^{2+} itself, that which is being regulated, functions as its own positive (calcitonin) and negative (PTH) signal. The information that is fed back to the controlling glands is in the form of a correction of the Ca^{2+} homeostatic perturbation. That is, when a too-high Ca^{2+} level returns to normal, the stimulus to the calcitonin-secreting cells disappears and so does inhibition of the parathyroid cells. If hypocalcemia is corrected, the reverse effects on the secretory cells occur. The beautiful symmetry of the system is well illustrated in Figure 17–3. Note that there is no known pituitotrophic hormone for either the parathyroid gland or the calcitonin-producing cells. PTH is the major regulatory hormone in this system. The physiologic role of calcitonin within the normal range of serum calcium is questionable (see discussion). It is possible that calcitonin only has an important regulatory role when calcium conservation mechanisms are under stress, e.g., as they are in pregnancy and lactation.

The relationship between serum PTH levels and plasma calcium concentration has been refined by Habener, Potts, et al., who found a gradual linear rise in serum PTH when the serum Ca^{2+} level fell from 10.5 mg/dl to 9. Below 9 mg/dl, there was a steep increase to a maximum, which occurred at 7 mg/dl. (Serum Ca^{2+} is maintained at 7 mg/dl without participation of either PTH or calcitonin.) From 10.5–15

mg/dl, there is a small, steady secretion of PTH, which is not turned off by high calcium concentrations. This calcium nonsuppressible PTH secretion may be due to stimulation of the parathyroid glands by catecholamines. Its existence explains the high PTH levels seen with diffuse hyperplasia of the parathyroids.

Parathyroid Hormone

SYNTHESIS AND SECRETION

Parathyroid hormone is an 84 amino acid protein with a molecular weight of 9,500 daltons (Fig 17–4). The complete amino acid sequence of human PTH has been elucidated, its gene has been isolated. Its structure and its chromosomal location have been determined. The amino acid sequence differs somewhat from those found in other species, but the response to the hormone is not species specific. It is synthesized as follows:

Pre-pro-PTH (115 amino acids)
↓
Pro-PTH (90 amino acids)
↓
PTH (84 amino acids)

Pre-pro-PTH was discovered when mRNA for PTH was translated in a cell-free ribosomal system. In the parathyroid cell, the 25 amino acid *pre* sequence is proteolytically amputated within seconds of the synthesis of the 115 amino acid peptide. Of the 25 extra amino acids of the *pre* sequence, 20 are hydrophobic. Therefore, it is believed that the lipid-soluble *pre* sequence is involved in the transport of the nascent pro-

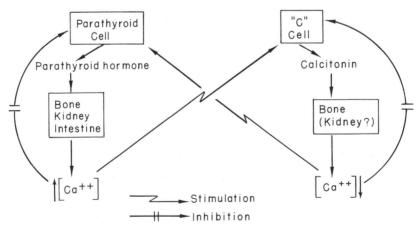

FIG 17–3.
Hormonal control of Ca^{2+} homeostasis.

```
1                               10
Ser Val Ser Glu Ile Gln Leu Met His Asn-

                                20
Leu Gly Lys His Leu Asn Ser Met Glu Arg-

                                30
Val Glu Trp Leu Arg Lys Lys Leu Gln Asp-

                                40
Val His Asn Phe Val Ala Leu Gly Ala Pro-

                                50
Leu Ala Pro Arg Asp Ala Gly Ser Gln Arg-

                                60
Pro Arg Lys Lys Glu Asp Asn Val Leu Val-

                                70
Glu Ser His Glu Lys Ser Leu Gly Glu Ala-

                                80
Asp Lys Ala Asp Val Asn Val Leu Thr Lys-

          84
Ala Lys Ser Gln
```

FIG 17–4.
Amino acid sequence of human parathyroid hormone, showing *(underlined)* a 34 amino acid fragment with full biologic activity. (Modified from Keutmann HT, Sauer MM, Hendy GN, et al: *Biochemistry* 1978: 5723.)

tein across the ER (endoplasmic reticulum) membrane into the lumen of the ER.

The *pro* sequence of 6 amino acids is largely removed within 20 minutes of the completion of the peptide. Some pro-PTH may be secreted by human PTH adenomas and when PTH is produced by other than parathyroid-derived tumors.

REGULATION OF SYNTHESIS AND DEGRADATION

The most important regulator of secretion is the serum Ca^{2+} concentration. The parathyroid cell illustrates a mechanism of control which so far is unusual, i.e., control by regulation of the proportion of synthesized hormone that is channeled into degradative pathways. Figure 17–5 is intended to show that when serum Ca^{2+} level is high, PTH degradation occurs to the extent of about 80% of the total synthesized, leaving 20% for secretion. When serum Ca^{2+} is low, only 60% of the PTH pool is degraded, thus permitting 40% to be secreted. Both low and high calcium levels ultimately have long-range effects on transcription of the pre-pro-PTH mRNA, but the effects of high Ca^{2+} on degradation of synthesized hormone occur over a more acute time scale.

The mechanisms by which Ca^{2+} inhibits PTH secretion are not completely understood. It is likely that intracellular hormone degradation brought about by increased serum Ca^{2+} plays an important part, but this effect cannot account for all of Ca^{2+}'s negative influence on PTH secretion. In the other direction, exposure of parathyroid cells to *low* Ca^{2+} over a longer time increases hormone synthesis, mainly by stimulation mitogenesis and cell proliferation. We do not understand how this is accomplished.

CIRCULATING FORMS AND ASSAY

Although reproducible bioassays for PTH exist, they are not commonly used for measuring circulating

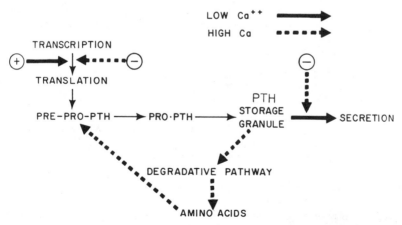

FIG 17–5.
High Ca^{2+} concentration inhibits parathyroid hormone (PTH) secretion and also promotes hormone degradation in the parathyroid cell. (After Habener JF, Rosenblatt M, Potts JT, Jr: *Physiol Rev* 1984; 64:985.)

hormone. Most of our information on circulating PTH levels is based on radioimmunoassay. The heterogeneity of PTH-related peptides was described by Silverman and Yalow, who showed that different antibodies apparently recognized different PTH fragments, and that some of these correlated better with clinical evidence of hyperparathyroidism than did others.

The heterogeneity of PTH immunoreactive material in the circulation is related in part to the fact that some degradation products are released from the gland along with the 84 amino acid hormone. In addition, the intact hormone has a relatively short half-life in the plasma, 10 minutes or less. It is cleaved into fragments of various sizes, mainly in the liver and kidney, some of which appear in the plasma. Among these is a biologically inactive C terminal fragment which has a relatively long half-life in plasma and is detected by many RIAs. Happily, the levels of its radioimmunoreactivity detected by current assays correspond well with clinical states of most patients.

An N terminal peptide of amino acid sequence 1–34 is capable of producing the full biological effect of the intact human hormone, although people are more sensitive (on a molar basis) to the intact, 84 amino acid hormone or to the N terminal 1–38 peptide (Hesch et al.).

CONTROL OF PTH SECRETION

The concentration of Ca^{2+} in extracellular fluid is the main determinant of parathyroid cell secretory activity and hormone synthesis. Mg^{2+} has effects similar to those of Ca^{2+}, but at far higher concentrations. Low Ca^{2+} concentration elicits secretion and hormone synthesis, and high Ca^{2+} inhibits both processes, but not completely (see above).

The hydroxylated metabolites of vitamin D (discussed later) may inhibit PTH secretion, but there are conflicting reports on this point. Although an *acute* inhibitory effect of vitamin D metabolites on PTH secretion is questionable, recent studies have shown that after 24–48 hours of culture in the presence of the most active D metabolite, $1,25(OH)_2D_3$, bovine parathyroid cells produce a decreased amount of mRNA for pre-pro-PTH (Cantley et al.).

Catecholamines stimulate PTH secretion via a beta receptor. This may help to explain the low level of sustained secretion that persists even in the presence of very high serum $[Ca^{2+}]$. It may also account for the frequent finding of hypercalcemia in association with catecholamine-secreting tumors.

Cortisol increases PTH secretion indirectly by inhibiting intestinal Ca^{2+} absorption. The hypocalcemia that ensues results in increased hormone secretion.

Increase in serum phosphate decreases $[Ca^{2+}]$ and therefore indirectly stimulates PTH secretion. It has no direct effect on the PTH cell. This is a mechanism by which failure of renal phosphate excretion, which occurs in renal disease, secondarily stimulates the parathyroid glands to the point of hypertrophy. (For another effect of renal disease on calcium homeostasis, see the section on vitamin D.)

Indeed, any chronic stimulation of the glands results in hypertrophy and hyperplasia. The mechanisms involved in stimulation of cell division are not understood, but the participation of one or more of the growth factors described in connection with adrenal hyperplasia is suspected.

Parathyroid hormone secretion is related to an increase in cAMP in the parathyroid cell. This can be accomplished (1) by a drop in $[Ca^{2+}]$ or (2) by catacholamine (β) stimulation of a plasma membrane receptor. Du Fresne and Gitelman have shown that the adenylate cyclase of parathyroid cells is much more sensitive to inhibition by Ca^{2+} than is the cyclase of other cells in other tissues. This tissue-specific sensitivity of the enzyme conforms beautifully to the inhibitory effect of Ca^{2+} on PTH secretion. There are two pools of PTH within the gland. Cyclic AMP increases secretion from only one of them but low $[Ca^{2+}]$ releases hormone from both.

There is an additional control mechanism of PTH secretion, which operates independently of constantly maintained $[Ca^{2+}]$, i.e., a circadian, sleep-related increase in PTH secretion that occurs during the middle third of sleep (see Jubiz et al.). The mechanism of the sleep-related surge in PTH secretion is not known, but is appears to be teleonomically useful to maintain serum calcium concentration when intestinal absorption of Ca^{2+} is minimal.

EFFECTS OF PTH ON BONE, KIDNEY, AND INTESTINE

The action of PTH on bone, kidney, and intestine can be inferred from the statement that the hormone acts to increase serum Ca^{2+} concentration. Although the quantitative contribution of hormone effects at each of these sites is not clear, the concerted action in bone, kidney, and intestine is striking.

A major $[Ca^{2+}]$-raising effect is that on the *renal tubule*. PTH stimulates reabsorption of Ca^{2+} by the distal renal tubule. At all filtered loads of Ca^{2+}, PTH increases the fractional reabsorption of Ca^{2+}. Thus when PTH is present in excess, as in hyperparathyroidism, it greatly increases the size of the filtered load by mobilizing Ca^{2+} from bone. Therefore, absolutely large amounts of Ca^{2+} appear in the urine *in spite of* the increased fractional reabsorption. This is the basis for the susceptibility of hyperparathyroid people to renal calcium stone formation.

PTH also inhibits PO_4^{2-} reabsorption in the proximal renal tubule and beyond. The resulting decrease in plasma $[PO_4^{2-}]$ facilitates the Ca^{2+} mobilizing effect of the hormone on bone. High levels of $[PO_4^{2-}]$ inhibit bone resorption in vitro and promote bone formation (Raisz, 1983). Thus, PTH, by an action on the renal tubule, increases its own effectiveness in bone.

Another important effect of PTH is on the formation of the most active vitamin D metabolite, $1,25(OH)_2D_3$ (see below).

The effect of PTH on *intestinal Ca^{2+} absorption* is considered to be indirect, by way of its participation in the metabolism of vitamin D to its active hydroxylated derivative. Operationally this is related to the availability of Ca^{2+} in the diet. Ca^{2+} deficiency promotes Ca^{2+} absorption by the following sequence:

$\downarrow$ Serum $Ca^{2+} \longrightarrow \uparrow$ PTH $\longrightarrow$
Conversion of $25(OH)D_3 \longrightarrow \uparrow 1,25(OH)_2D_3$
$\longrightarrow \uparrow$ Intestinal absorption of Ca^{2+}

Another striking effect of PTH—probably via hypercalcemia—is increased gastric acid and pepsin secretion. This could contribute to the association between hyperparathyroidism and peptic ulcer which has sometimes been reported.

The effects of PTH on *bone* are extremely complex and are being reevaluated. Historically, major emphasis was placed on the bone-resorbing effects of PTH, largely as a result of the fact that declared hyperparathyroidism was diagnosed only in its late stages. With the advent and wide use of the multichannel autoanalyzer in many hospital laboratories, it has been possible to recognize many hypercalcemic states, including one that reflects a compensated state of hyperparathyroidism, i.e., increased bone resorption and compensatory increased calcium deposition in the skeleton resulting in no obvious demineralization of bone, although circulating $[Ca^{2+}]$ is abnormally high. As a result, at PTH concentrations that occur when adequate Ca^{2+} is present in the diet, the predominant PTH effect on Ca^{2+} conservation is the renal effect.

When the hormone is present in amounts necessary for decalcification of bone, not only is bone mineral mobilized and excreted, but the organic matrix of bone is also broken down, as is indicated by increased urinary excretion of hydroxyproline, a marker for collagen-like proteins. Excessive PTH therefore causes a net loss of both bone mineral and the organic lattice upon which it is deposited.

In summary, PTH excess results in the following:

$\uparrow$ Plasma Ca^{2+}
$\downarrow$ Plasma PO_4^{2-}
$\uparrow$ Urine Ca^{2+}
$\uparrow$ Urine PO_4^{2-}

Although we are accustomed to think of PTH as a bone catabolic hormone, largely because of the bone resorption that occurs at high levels of PTH, Parsons has emphasized the fact that PTH is in some circumstances a bone growth hormone; i.e., PTH can induce a net increase of bone mass. The mechanism of this effect is not understood.

MECHANISM OF ACTION OF PTH

In spite of much investigative work, there are large gaps in our knowledge of the cellular mechanism of action of PTH. One of the reasons for this is the heterogeneity of target cells on which the hormone exerts its effects: among them, osteocytes, osteoclasts, osteoblasts, stem cells in bone, and renal tubular cells, which reabsorb calcium or phosphorus from the glomerular filtrate.

The general statement may be made that PTH binds to a specific plasma membrane receptor, and that this hormone-receptor interaction stimulates adenylate cyclase to generate cAMP. At the same time, calcium influx into cells is stimulated. Indeed, the very early *lowering* of serum calcium that is seen after PTH administration to intact human beings is probably due to increased calcium uptake by PTH-sensitive cells.

Renal Effects

Specific receptors for PTH, and for PTH-stimulated adenylate cyclase, have been found in both proximal and distal renal tubules. The major effect of PTH on Ca^{2+} excretion is the result of an *increase in its fractional reabsorption in the distal tubule*. (In the proximal tubule, the hormone *decreases* the reabsorption of Ca^{2+}, PO_4^{2+}, and HCO_2^-, but the calcium effect is overridden by the stimulation of reabsorption in the distal tubule.)

Phosphate reabsorption, in contrast, is *inhibited* by PTH in both proximal and distal tubules. This phosphaturic effect, described as early as 1911, is the basis for the lowering of plasma phosphate concentration induced by PTH.

The molecular mechanisms involved in the renal tubular effects are not completely understood, but they certainly involve activation of adenylate cyclase on the basal-lateral (contraluminal) renal tubular cell membrane. The cyclic AMP produced by hormone activation travels across the cell to activate a *luminal* membrane protein kinase. This, in turn, phosphory-lates some luminal membrane protein (or proteins) which is (are) involved in phosphate reabsorption.

Another important renal effect of PTH is to *stimulate the 1-hydroxylation of 25(OH)D₃ to 1,25(OH)₂D₃* (the most active vitamin D metabolite, see detailed discussion below). This has the ultimate effect of stimulating intestinal Ca^{2+} absorption. Since decreased serum PO_4^{2-} facilitates Ca^{2+} mobilization from bone, all three renal actions of PTH collaborate to raise serum $[Ca^{2+}]$.

Bone Effects

Although the mechanism of action of PTH on bone has been studied extensively, it is still only incompletely understood. Perhaps the major obstacle in the path to greater enlightenment is the fact that bone contains a heterogeneous population of highly specialized cells. This makes it difficult to assign observed effects to one cell population or another even when experiments are done in a bone fragment organ culture system. Moreover, bone is in a dynamic equilibrium between formation and resorption. These processes affect one another, so that a primary effect of resorption, for example, may produce a secondary stimulation on bone formation.

When the hormone is administered in vivo there are rapid changes in osteoclasts, osteoblasts, and osteocytes accompanying the release of Ca^{2+} and bone matrix components. Within 30 minutes the surfaces of osteoclasts adjacent to bone show a marked increase in size of their ruffled borders. This is accompanied by an increased release of *hydroxyproline*, a prominent component of matrix collagen, from bone. Since the primary amino acid used in collagen synthesis at the translation level is proline (hydroxylation is a posttranslational modification), hydroxyproline cannot be used for protein synthesis, and therefore it is an indicator of collagen breakdown. In fact, even urinary excretion of hydroxyproline is a useful indicator of collagen catabolism.

With continued stimulation, there is an increase in the *number* of osteoclasts, and eventually, of osteoblasts (bone-forming cells) as well.

Studies of bone fragments treated in vitro with PTH show that PTH increases cyclic AMP and, very early in its action, the uptake of Ca^{2+}. Although PTH receptors are clearly demonstrable on osteoblasts, it is uncertain whether osteoclasts have any in spite of the striking morphologic changes produced in them by hormone administration. In some experiments, PTH effects on isolated osteoclasts cannot be demonstrated unless they are coincubated with osteoblasts (for example, Chambers, 1984).

According to one reasonable though still vague hypothesis, the action of PTH on osteoblasts causes the release of an unidentified osteoclast activator that alters osteoclast morphology and biochemistry so that the powerful phagocyte can attack bone. Proteolytic enzymes (some, probably lysosomal) and organic acids (lactate, citrate) are released from bone in response to PTH. The collaboration between the local high acid environment and enzymes that act optimally at low pH is believed to be responsible for much bone resorption, though osteoclasts are capable of phagocytizing and digesting spicules of bone in addition. The immediate effects of the hormone are independent of RNA and protein synthesis, but the full effect of the administration of a large amount of PTH on bone resorption requires synthesis of new mRNAs and proteins.

The mechanisms involved in the increase in *number* of osteoclasts seen with sustained PTH stimulation are not known, but PTH may stimulate the local production of a mitogenic growth factor.

DISEASES OF PTH DEFICIENCY AND EXCESS

Although it is inappropriate to describe parathyroid disease here, it is important to establish the point that recent advances in our understanding of the biology of the parathyroid system have been applied to the diagnosis and management of parathyroid disease with astonishing speed.

Hyperparathyroidism

Hyperparathyroidism may occur as the result of hypertrophy and hyperplasia of all four parathyroid glands, or it may be produced by a single tumor, usually an adenoma. Not infrequently, people with parathyroid adenomas also show a variety of adenomatous growths in other endocrine glands, particularly the thyroid. Occasionally, excessive parathyroid hormone is produced by a tumor of other-than-parathyroid origin. This is analogous to tumor synthesis and secretion of ADH and ACTH, discussed previously.

Early students of hyperparathyroid patients emphasized severe demineralization of bone and often deformities of long bones. Hyperparathyroidism is now detected often by serum calcium measurements made in the course of automated multichannel analyses, supplemented by appropriate radioimmunoassay.

We now realize that compensated states of hyperparathyroidism can exist in which abnormally high serum calcium can occur without obvious decrease in bone density. As in the previously cited cases of ADH and aldosterone, simultaneous measurement of the hormone and the variable it regulates (in this case, PTH and serum Ca^{2+}) can give more valuable information than a measurement of either alone.

Continuously high levels of calcium in the glomerular filtrate predispose to the formation of renal stones. All individuals who form such stones should be suspected of having hyperparathyroidism. Other conditions that often coexist with hyperparathyroidism are hypertension and peptic ulceration. The latter may be related to increased secretion of gastrin provoked by hypercalcemia.

One of the most striking features of hyperparathyroidism is the frequent occurrence of neuromuscular and neuropsychiatric disorders. Muscle weakness and muscle atrophy are often seen, but sensory abnormalities are not present. In addition, depression, memory impairment, difficulty in concentrating, and personality changes may be seen. Electroencephalographic abnormalities are characteristic of persistent hypercalcemia, whether it is due to hyperparathyroidism or not.

Since the definitive treatment for hyperparathyroidism is surgical, it is important for the surgeon to know the anatomical location of the source of the excess hormone. A new surgical art form of preoperative localization has evolved with the advent of thermography, computerized axial tomography, radioisotope scanning, arteriography and selective venous catheterization and radioimmunoassay for PTH with suitable antibody. The interested reader is referred to the essay by Eisenberg and Pallotta.

Hypoparathyroidism

Parathyroid hormone deficiency may occur (1) as a complication of various kinds of neck surgery or (2) for a variety of idiopathic reasons. Hypocalcemia increases neuromuscular excitability. In milder forms, only paresthesias may be present, but in more severe cases, tetany with muscle cramps or even convulsions can occur. Hypoparathyroidism is only one of literally dozens of conditions in which low serum calcium occurs. In fact, when hypocalcemia is detected as a result of multichannel screening, it is practically never due to hypoparathyroidism. Hypoparathyroidism is diagnosed when circulating PTH is undetectable in the presence of low serum calcium.

Pseudohypoparathyroidism

This condition is characterized by end-organ failure to respond to excessive amounts of endogenous PTH. It is a rare hereditary disorder that is analogous to failure to respond to other hormones. In fact, the hypocalcemia that occurs as a result of the failure of target cells to respond to PTH causes hypertrophy and hyperplasia of the parathyroid glands in a manner reminiscent of the excessive ACTH secretion tht occurs in adrenal virilization syndromes (see Chapter 11).

Several variants of pseudohypoparathyroidism are known. In one, there is a defect in the PTH receptor-adenylate cyclase complex, which results in the failure of the kidney to produce cyclic AMP in response to the hormone. Some patients may have a defect in the PTH receptor itself, while others have a deficiency of normal G_s protein, which couples the hormone receptor to the adenylate cyclase (see Akita et al.). In other patients, cyclic AMP may be produced, but genetic defects distal to its production prevent the biologic response.

Calcitonin

Calcitonin was discovered in 1961 by Copp, who inferred its existence from experiments that suggested that thyroparathyroidectomy (in dogs) not only produced a thyroid hormone deficiency but a deficiency of a serum Ca^{2+}-lowering substance as well. In subsequent experiments, he perfused the thyroid and parathyroid glands of a dog with blood containing a high Ca^{2+} concentration and demonstrated that the effluent had a serum Ca^{2+}-*lowering* effect when perfused into another dog. The active material responsible for the hypocalcemia was soon isolated, purified, and named calcitonin. Determination of its amino acid sequence, its synthesis, and descriptions of its comparative structure in a number of species followed quickly (Copp, 1967, 1969).

The amino acid sequence of calcitonin has been established for five mammalian species, including the human (Fig 17–6), and some nonmammalian species (three types of salmon and the eel). The nonmammalian calcitonins are generally more active in bioassays in the rat and human being than are their respective species-specific hormones. This may reflect the resistance of such calcitonins to degradation. A large literature on the comparative biology of calcitonin suggests that it may have functions other than calcium-regulating ones in older phylogenic forms.

CHEMISTRY

Calcitonin is a 32 amino acid peptide (see Fig 17–6). It is synthesized and secreted by C (parafollicular) cells of the thyroid, cells that belong to Pearse's APUD series, i.e., they are of neural crest origin. In several species, including the human, a few C cells may be found in parathyroid and thymus tissue. It is also secreted by medullary carcinoma of the thyroid cells (C cell adenocarcinoma) as well as by other non-thyroid-derived neoplasms. A recently refined radioimmunoassay procedure (see Parthemore and Deftos) has revealed that calcitonin normally fluctuates between 5 and 100 pg/ml in human beings.

SYNTHESIS AND SECRETION

Like other polypeptide hormones, calcitonin is synthesized originally as a larger molecule that is subsequently cleaved to the 32 amino acid hormone shown in Figure 17–6. The hormone is stored in secretory granules, mainly in thyroid C cells (also known as parafollicular cells, or clear cells). Circulating calcitonin immunoreactive forms include not only the mo-

nomeric hormone, but also a dimer and various other forms that have not been identified precisely.

The calcitonin gene transcription product is noteworthy because it can be processed differently in different tissues. In the C cell, the mRNA for calcitonin is formed, but in the central nervous system, a different mRNA derived from the same primary transcript codes for a substance called *calcitonin gene-related peptide (CGRP)*. Central nervous system and peripheral effects of this peptide are under active investigation (Rosenfeld). The interesting concept illustrated by the calcitonin gene is the fact that, when a cell differentiates, it can alter gene expression by expressing a different array of processing molecules from those expressed by another cell that can transcribe the same gene.

The main stimuli for the secretion of calcitonin are (1) an *elevated serum calcium* and (2) certain gastrointestinal hormones, particularly *gastrin*.

Calcitonin secretion in response to elevation of serum calcium has been seen only when there has been a *large* increase in serum calcium. It is still impossible to assert that serum Ca^{2+} fluctuations in the normal range, which clearly affect PTH secretion, definitely influence the secretion of calcitonin.

The discovery by Cooper et al. that calcitonin secretion could be elicited by oral calcium without a demonstrable change in circulating Ca^{2+} concentration lends credence to the idea that $[Ca^{2+}]$ may not

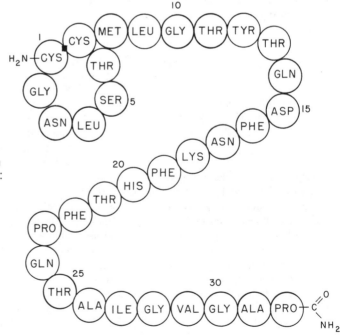

FIG 17–6.
Amino acid sequence of human calcitonin. (From Neher R, et al: *Nature* 1968; 220:984.)

be the main signal for calcitonin release within the normal range of serum calcium. This is another example of the intestinal endocrine cell functioning as an early warning device in the manner described in Chapter 14. In effect, the gastrin-secreting cell senses Ca^{2+} in the intestinal contents and alerts the calcitonin-secreting cell to its imminent absorption. The incoming Ca^{2+} is met by a hormone, which protects against alimentary hypercalcemia. At the same time, PTH secretion is low, and therefore fractional reabsorption of filtered Ca^{2+} in the nephron is also low, thus permitting the kidney to contribute to the maintenance of normal serum Ca^{2+}.

BIOLOGIC EFFECT

The most obvious effect of calcitonin is *inhibition of bone resorption,* which is demonstrable in intact animals and human beings as well as in bone preparations in organ culture. Calcium inhibits the release of organic matrix-derived substances as well as the mineral components of bone. This results in decreased levels of hydroxyproline, calcium, and phosphate. The effect is more readily demonstrable when the rate of bone turnover (resorption *and* formation) is high, as in young, growing animals and humans.

The regulatory importance of these effects in adults has been questioned for a number of reasons:

1. In normal individuals, the effect is transitory.

2. Plasma calcium is well regulated within normal limits after total thyroidectomy.

3. When calcium is present in inappropriately high concentrations (as in medullary carcinoma of the thyroid), it appears to have little effect on bone density.

If authorities disagree about calcitonin's role in minute-to-minute regulation of Ca^{2+} concentration in body fluids, the recent findings of Heath and Sizemore suggest that calcitonin may exert a long-term influence over calcium exchange and bone density. These investigators found that men show higher basal levels of calcitonin than do women and larger increases in serum calcitonin in response to calcium (or pentagastrin) infusion than do women. Since women are more susceptible than men to osteoporosis (decreased bone density) associated with advancing age, it is possible that a relative deficiency of calcitonin could contribute to the cause of that condition. However, although there have been reports of decreased basal and stimulated levels of calcitonin in patients with osteoporosis compared with those of controls, others have not been able to confirm these findings (Tiegs, 1985).

Calcitonin levels increase in pregnant and lactating women, and it has been suggested that the hormone plays a physiologic role in protecting the maternal skeleton from excessive Ca^{2+} loss in these conditions.

Calcitonin also has a small phosphaturic effect that contributes to a decrease in plasma phosphate concentration. It is difficult to reconcile this with calcitonin's effect on bone since, as we have seen in the case of PTH, decreased plasma phosphate favors Ca^{2+} mobilization from bone. Cannon's "wisdom of the body" is occasionally inscrutable.

One intriguing action of calcitonin is *inhibition of gastrin secretion.* Since gastrin stimulates calcitonin secretion and calcitonin inhibits gastrin secretion, it has been suggested that calcitonin may play some as yet undiscovered role in the digestion and assimilation of food. In any case, the gastrin-calcitonin link has proved to be valuable, since gastrin (or preferably its active pentapeptide derivative pentagastrin) is used as a provocative test for calcitonin secretory capacity. Generally, the extent of increase in circulating calcitonin produced by calcium injection or by pentagastrin is similar. Provocative tests of this sort are useful in such studies as those of Heath and Sizemore (cited above) and in detecting the presence of medullary carcinoma of the thyroid (C cell tumor) or of other calcitonin-producing tumors. Measurements of basal and stimulated levels of serum calcitonin are also valuable as indices of the success or failure of treatment of such hormone-producing tumors.

Although the physiologic importance of calcitonin has not been established, it has proved to be useful, especially in Paget's disease. In this condition, which is characterized by an extremely high rate of bone turnover, calcitonin restores the turnover rate toward the normal one.

Although it has not yet proved to be beneficial in patients with osteoporosis, it does have a place in the management of patients with hypercalcemia secondary to a variety of causes.

CELLULAR MODE OF ACTION

The most easily demonstrable cellular effect of calcitonin is upon the multinucleated, bone-eating phagocyte, the osteoclast. Calcitonin is powerfully, if transitorily, inhibitory for osteoclasts, which lose their ruffled borders (indicators of phagocytic activity) within a few minutes after the administration of calcitonin. In patients with Paget's disease, in which *both* bone resorption and bone formation are extremely rapid, calcitonin has a prolonged and markedly inhibitory effect on osteoclasts. This is an important reason for the reported efficacy of calcitonin in the treatment of this disease.

Calcitonin, like so many other peptide hormones, combines with a specific receptor in target cell membranes and activates adenylate cyclase. In the *kidney*, calcitonin receptors and calcitonin-activated adenylate cyclase complexes can be demonstrated in regions of the tubule other than those in which PTH receptors are found. Since the two receptors are in different types of cells, one need not be dismayed by the fact that cyclic AMP is used as a second messenger by the two hormones.

In *bone*, calcitonin receptors are found only in *osteoclasts* (i.e., where PTH receptors are missing). Again, adenylate cyclase is stimulated in a cell population that may be only indirectly responsive to PTH, as we indicated above. Thus, the old dilemma—"How is it possible for PTH and calcitonin to work via cyclic AMP but exert opposite effects on bone?"—appears to be resolved (tentatively) by the likelihood that the two hormones work on different target cells.

In vitro, continued administration of calcitonin, as is the case with other peptide hormones, results in the desensitization of its target cells in bone. Therefore, intermittent administration, in such conditions as Paget's disease and hypercalcemic states, would seem to be an appropriate tactic.

Vitamin D and Its Derivatives

A good clinical description of rickets was given in 1645, but the modern era in our understanding of the disease began when Mellanby discovered an experimental animal model of the human disease, the rachitic dog (see Landmarks). He was able to reproduce the known features of the disease by feeding certain diets and to prevent or cure the disease with cod liver oil. Later, McCollum and his coworkers discovered a fat-soluble, antirachitic material, which they called vitamin D, and Steenbock et al. showed that antirachitic activity could be produced in vitro by irradiating the sterol fraction of food. The active material was purified and identified in 1937 during the golden age of steroid biochemistry. In recent years, new information about vitamin D has blurred the distinction between vitamins and hormones, since the active forms of the vitamin, which are made by serial metabolic alterations of a steroid present in the skin in large quantities, share many of the properties of steroid hormones.

It is remarkable that recent advances in our understanding of the metabolism and action of vitamin D have resulted so promptly in rapid improvements in the diagnosis and management of patients with disordered calcium homeostasis. Clinical investigators have gained new insights not only into vitamin D deficiency but also into the impaired mineralization of bone that occurs in chronic renal disease. Furthermore, it is now possible to explain a number of clinical syndromes, which are collectively designated as vitamin D-resistant rickets.

CHEMISTRY AND METABOLISM

If human beings are exposed to the ultraviolet rays of the sun, dietary vitamin D is not necessary. A large reservoir of provitamin D in the form of 7-dehydrocholesterol is stored in the skin, where it is photoactivated to vitamin D_3, or cholecalciferol. The plant sterol, ergosterol, is transformed into vitamin D_2 (ergocalciferol) by irradiation and has been the main source of vitamin D for addition to foods such as milk. Therapeutic quantities of vitamin D are found in the liver of a number of fishes.

As a result of the imaginative researches of DeLuca, Kodicek, Norman, their colleagues, and many other investigators during the past decade, it is now possible to describe the activation of cholecalciferol, or ergocalciferol, to their biologically effective metabolites. Cholecalciferol is transported to the liver, which avidly concentrates it and hydroxylates it in the 25 position to $25(OH)D_3$. This hydroxylation occurs in the endoplasmic reticulum and requires NADPH, molecular oxygen and Mg^{2+}, and a cytochrome P450 different from those involved in drug metabolism. The reaction is product inhibited, but 25-hydroxylation is not generally regarded as a major control site in the metabolism of vitamin D_3, since the production of large amounts of $25(OH)D_3$ can be forced by giving large doses of D_3. The first hydroxylation product of D_3 is 2–5 times as active as D_3 itself in curing or preventing rickets. It is the principal circulating form of the vitamin, and it is carried in the blood by a carrier protein (MW 51,000), as are the steroid hormones. It is interesting that the α globulin carrier protein for vitamin D binds $25(OH)D_3$ much more avidly than it does either D_3 or subsequent metabolites such as $1,25(OH)_2D_3$.

The amounts of $25(OH)D_3$ that circulate can be considered a secondary reservoir of vitamin D activity. The 25(OH) metabolite is not the active form of the vitamin, for physiologic concentrations will not stimulate Ca^{2+} absorption from the gastrointestinal tract in nephrectomized animals or in human beings with severe chronic renal disease. The kidney has the capability of further hydroxylating 25(OH)D$_3$ to one of three forms (Fig 17–7):

1. 1,25(OH)$_2$D$_3$
2. 24,25(OH)$_2$D$_3$
3. 1,24,25(OH)$_3$D$_3$

The metabolite 1,25(OH)$_2$D$_3$ is the active form of vitamin D. It is about 10 times as active in bioassays as vitamin D$_3$ and it works as well in the absence of the kidneys as in their presence. Hydroxylation of 25(OH)D$_3$ in the 1 position occurs in mitochondria and requires NADPH, molecular oxygen, magnesium ion, cytochrome P450, and an iron-sulfur flavoprotein. Thus, hydroxylation of 25(OH)D$_3$ is entirely analogous to the hydroxylation of steroid intermediates that occurs in the adrenal cortex and in the ovary, corpus luteum, and testis during steroid hormone biosynthesis.

The kidney also has the capability of hydroxylating 25(OH)D$_3$ at the 24 position. This is the preferred route of metabolism of 25(OH)D$_3$ when adequate amounts of Ca^{2+} are being absorbed from the gastrointestinal tract, i.e., when there is no deficiency of vitamin D. Hydroxylation at the 24 position results in production of 24,25(OH)$_2$D$_3$, a metabolite that has little antirachitic activity. No function has yet been clearly demonstrated for the 24,25 hydroxylated compound, although it may play a role in feedback inhibition of PTH secretion (Fig 17–8). Hydroxylation of 24(OH)D$_3$ at the 1 position and at the 24 position is reciprocally related, i.e., when calcium conservation is necessary, 1-hydroxylation predominates, but when there are no indications of calcium deficiency, 24-hydroxylation is dominant. The suggestion has been made that 24-hydroxylation renders the compound more vulnerable to hepatic metabolism and subsequent biliary excretion. Thus the either/or choice of

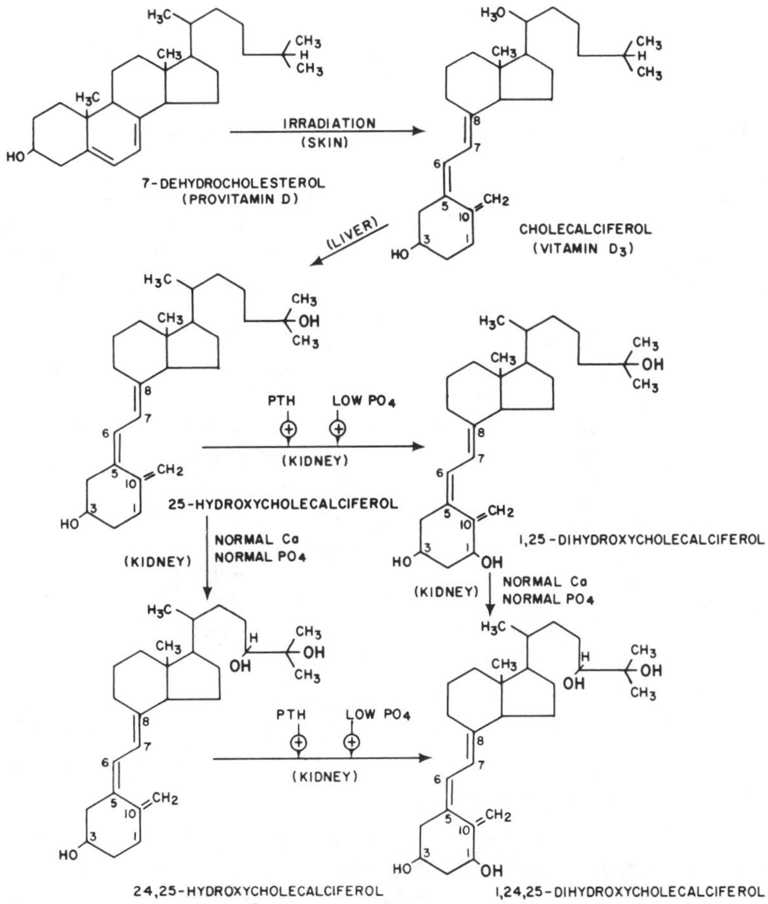

FIG 17–7.
Metabolites of vitamin D and loci of their formation. (Modified from DeLuca HF, in Kumar R [ed]: *Vitamin D: Basic and Clinical Aspects.* Boston, Martinus Nijhoff, 1984, p 1.)

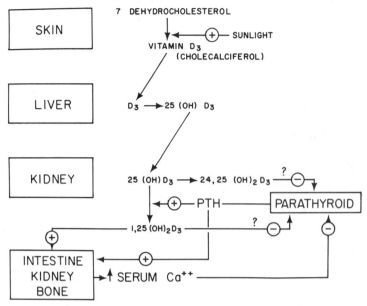

FIG 17–8.
Regulation of vitamin D metabolism by parathyroid hormone (PTH). Note that vitamin D in the diet is vitamin D_2, which is metabolized according to the pattern shown here.

hydroxylation site for $25(OH)D_3$ in the kidney marks the major control switch point in the system. Presently the nature of the controls that operate at this switch point will be discussed.

It was found that $24,25(OH)_2D_3$, which is much less active than $1,25(OH)_2D_3$ in bioassays for vitamin D activity, is completely inactive in the absence of the kidney. This led to the discovery of the triple hydroxylated compound, $1,24,25(OH)_3D_3$. This compound is less active than $1,25(OH)_2D_3$ and may in fact be marked for hepatic inactivation and excretion. In any case, its quantitative significance is probably small.

Like the steroid hormones, the active metabolite of vitamin D is metabolized in the liver, and the inactivated products are conjugated with glucuronide and secreted mainly in the bile. Side chain cleavage occurs in the intact animal and some of the radioactivity in the side chain may appear as expired CO_2.

REGULATION OF RENAL HYDROXYLATION OF $24(OH)D_3$

The major site of control of the fate of $25(OH)D_3$ is on the 1-hydroxylase reaction. When serum calcium concentration is low, 1-hydroxylation is stimulated and 24-hydroxylation is suppressed. At 10 mg/dl of calcium, the reverse is true. Parathyroid hormone (which is elicited in the low-calcium condition) stimulates 1-hydroxylation of $25(OH)D_3$ in the kidney. The control of 1-hydroxylation by PTH may be executed by way of the hypophosphatemic effect of the hormone, for Tanaka and De Luca have found that 1-hydroxylation can be stimulated even in the absence of the parathyroid glands by decreasing phosphate concentration. It is likely that the action of PTH on the renal tubular cell, which is mediated by cAMP, also may involve decreased intracellular phosphate concentrations owing to inhibition of PO_4^{2-} reabsorption.

A role for vitamin D metabolites in the regulation of PTH secretion has been proposed but is still uncertain. It is possible that vitamin D may have a long-term, indirect inhibitory effect on PTH synthesis and secretion by promoting the intestinal absorption of Ca^{2+} and PO_4^{2-}.

CELLULAR EFFECTS AND MECHANISMS OF ACTION OF VITAMIN D_3 METABOLITES

In vitamin D deficiency, there is failure of bone mineralization, owing mainly to inadequate absorption of Ca^{2+} and PO_4^{2-} from the intestine. Vitamin D metabolites also help to raise serum Ca^{2+} by collaborating with PTH in mobilizing bone mineral. Although the quantitative effects of vitamin D on the kidney are not clear, the kidney certainly contains vitamin D receptors and produces a protein—calcium-binding protein—which is inducible by $1,25(OH)_2D_3$ (see below).

In the *intestine*, $1,25(OH)_2D_3$ acts to promote Ca^{2+} absorption by a mechanism that conforms generally to the steroid hormone model described in Chapter 2.

As is the case for estrogens and other steroids, there is no general agreement on whether unoccupied receptors are cytosolic or nuclear. In any case, the *occupied* receptor in the nucleus stimulates the transcription of selected mRNAs together with rRNA and tRNA. Although all agree that the full effect of vitamin D requires RNA and protein synthesis, it now seems likely that there can be an initial stimulation of Ca^{2+} absorption by the intestine *without* new protein synthesis (Wasserman, 1984, 1985). The mechanism of this effect is not known, but it is in the now familiar category of non-transcription-related effects of steroid (or steroid-like) hormones.

Calcium absorption involves at least three steps: (1) uptake of Ca^{2+} at the brush (luminal) border; (2) transcellular transport; and (3) extrusion at the basal lateral (contraluminal) membrane. At least one $1,25(OH)_2D_3$-inducible protein is a brush border membrane protein. The most extensively studied protein inducible by vitamin D is *calcium-binding protein (CaBP)*, a cytosolic protein believed to be the transcellular transport vehicle for Ca^{2+} in the intestinal epithelial cell. Not much information is available about the molecular details of the basal lateral membrane extrusion process. The most parsimonious hypothesis states that vitamin D coordinately induces protein components of all three phases of the Ca^{2+} absorbing complex.

The other major effect of vitamin D in the intestine is *increased phosphate absorption*. Marx et al. have described increases in phosphate absorption by explants of chicken intestine as early as 30 minutes after exposure to $1,25(OH)_2D_3$. The molecular mechanism involved in this effect are not known.

Most authorities now agree that the major effect of vitamin D on *bone* is the provision of Ca^{2+} and PO_4^{2-} for deposition in the skeleton by stimulating their absorption by the intestine. In addition to this indirect effect, the active metabolites of vitamin D have a *direct* effect on bone cells; specifically, on osteoblasts which, unlike osteoclasts, contain receptors for $1,25(OH)_2D_3$ (Raisz, 1984; Bell; also Skjodt). Like PTH, $1,25(OH)_2D_3$ decreases synthesis of collagen by osteoblasts and also stimulates bone resorption by osteoclasts (also like PTH). The latter effect, as it is for PTH, is most probably indirect.

In 1961, Harrison and Harrison discovered that vitamin D *increased renal phosphate reabsorption*. Since then, there has been some uncertainty about whether this effect is direct or indirect (via decreasing PTH levels secondary to stimulated GI uptake of Ca^{2+}). Studies by Costanzo in 1974 and by Kurnik and Hruska (1984) provide evidence that the effect is directly upon the renal tubule. Ca^{2+} reabsorption by the tubule is also stimulated. Thus, the effect of $1,25(OH)_2D_3$ on the kidney, like its effect on the intestinal epithelium, tends to provide and conserve a continuing supply of minerals for deposition in bone.

One of the features of vitamin D deficiency is *muscle weakness*. It has been suggested (see Birge and Haddad) that one metabolite of vitamin D ($25(OH)D_3$, but not $1,25(OH)_2D_3$) may stimulate metabolic processes in skeletal muscle. Whether vitamin D exerts a direct effect on muscle or an indirect one, by way of its effect on electrolyte concentrations in extracellular fluid, remains to be discovered.

Pathophysiology of Some Disorders of Calcium and Phosphorus Metabolism Related to Vitamin D

INBORN ERRORS OF METABOLISM

In temperate zones, the daily vitamin D requirement for prevention of rickets is 400 IU (10 mg). In some individuals, this amount may be inadequate; such people may require pharmacologic doses of the vitamin. Calciopenia, or calcium deficiency, may be the result of vitamin D deficiency, but it may also be caused by defective function of some component of the vitamin D-responsive complex of cells and tissues. For example, the following circumstances are associated with calciopenia:

1. Inadequate metabolism of vitamin D to $1,25(OH)_2D_3$.

2. High rate of destruction or metabolism of vitamin D metabolites.

3. Failure of response of end-organs to normal amounts of vitamin D. The last of these is analogous to other previously discussed conditions characterized by end-organ response failure (testicular feminization, pseudohypoparathyroidism, adrenal virilization).

Rickets also may be caused by phosphate deficiency. A variety of toxic and hereditary disorders of the renal tubule may result in a failure to retrieve phosphate ion from the glomerular fluid and therefore in a net loss of phosphate from the body. In this case, failure of mineralization of bone may occur even in the presence of normal levels of serum calcium, and the hypophosphatemia is said to be primary.

Secondary hypophosphatemia also may occur as a result of primary calciopenia. In the advanced stages of human vitamin D deficiency, the following sequence occurs: hypocalcemia → increased circulating PTH → phosphaturia → decreased plasma phosphate. Thus if hypophosphatemia is associated with high levels of immunoreactive PTH, it is likely to be secondary to hypocalcemia. If PTH is not elevated, the hypophosphatemia is probably of renal origin, i.e., primary phosphatemia.

In the condition known as "hereditary vitamin D dependency" (see Fraser and Scriver), all of the features of rickets are seen, with the exception of a response to the usual doses of vitamin D. The circulating levels of $25(OH)D_3$ are extremely high. The condition is not responsive to $25(OH)D_3$, but it is responsive to $1,25(OH)_2D_3$ in doses of 1 µg/day or less. Therefore, these individuals have a diminished capacity to 1-hydroxylate $25(OH)D_3$. However, if 100–300 times the normal requirement of vitamin D_3 (1,000–3,000 µg/day) is given, evidence of healing of the rickets may be seen. In other words, production of an adequate supply of $1,25(OH)_2D_3$ can be forced by flooding the system with precursor. This condition can be detected within a few weeks after birth, and the expression of the defect can be prevented by adequate treatment.

Hereditary resistance to the effects of $1,25(OH)_2D_3$ occurs in a variety of forms, a finding that is reminiscent of our earlier discussions of testicular feminization and pseudohypoparathyroidism (Marx et al., 1984). In some kindreds, a receptor abnormality permitted a calcemic response to certain calciferol analogues, while in others, such responses could not be elicited. This is to be expected in a complex response system that involves several proteins whose genes could undergo mutation.

ACQUIRED DISORDERS OF VITAMIN D FUNCTION

Osteomalacia Induced by Anticonvulsant Drugs

When epileptic children are treated with anticonvulsant drugs (e.g., diphenylhydantoin), they may develop osteomalacia, which resembles that seen in rickets. These drugs have been found to produce target organ resistance to the action of vitamin D on intestine and bone (Haynes and Murad).

Steroid-Induced Skeletal Mineral Loss

In Chapter 11 we observed that a decrease in bone mass (osteopenia) is a prominent feature of both spontaneously occurring and iatrogenically induced Cushing's syndrome. Steroid-induced osteopenia is most likely to occur in children and in postmenopausal women, and it is most pronounced in trabecular bone, i.e., vertebrae and ribs.

Glucocorticoids in pharmacologic doses exert their effects on the skeleton in various ways: they (1) decrease synthesis of the organic matrix of bone by bone cells, (2) inhibit conversion of precursor bone cells to osteoblasts, (3) antagonize (noncompetitively) the effect of vitamin D on calcium absorption in the intestine and (4) directly increase serum PTH levels by acting on the parathyroid glands.

Thus the net effect of pharmacologic doses of glucocorticoids is to inhibit bone formation and to stimulate bone resorption by inducing a state of hyperparathyroidism indirectly by impairing Ca^{2+} absorption and directly by an effect on PTH secretion by the gland. There are data to suggest that judicious use of vitamin D (in relatively large doses) with supplemental Ca^{2+} can arrest and reverse steroid-induced osteopenia.

Bone Disease Associated with Chronic Kidney Disease

Although the reasons for the thinning of bone that occurs in association with chronic renal disease are extremely complex, recently acquired knowledge about vitamin D metabolism has improved our understanding of the phenomenon. Circulating levels of $1,25(OH)_2D_3$ are low in people with severe, chronic renal disease, whereas levels of $25(OH)D_3$ may be low, normal, or high. The inference is that 1-hydroxylation is impaired, and that intestinal absorption of Ca^{2+} is therefore inadequate. The situation may be made worse by the presence in the circulation of large numbers of D_3 intermediates, which themselves are biologically inactive but may competitively inhibit the action of D_3 metabolites on the intestinal cell. Circulating levels of $1,25(OH)_2D_3$ are low in uremic patients in spite of higher than normal levels of circulating PTH, which occur as a result of hypocalcemia. Both $1,25(OH)_2D_3$ and $1\alpha(OH)D_3$ (which can be 25-hydroxylated in the liver) have shown promise as therapeutic agents in the management of osteodystrophy of uremia (see Brickman et al.; Peacock et al.).

The Liver and Vitamin D

We have already seen (1) that the liver is the site of 25-hydroxylation of cholecalciferol; (2) that it is the major locus of inactivation of D_3 by hydroxylation to inactive intermediates and conjugation to polar metabolites; and (3) that biliary excretion is a major route of elimination of vitamin D metabolites.

Long et al. have reported subnormal circulating levels of $25(OH)D_3$ in patients with a variety of liver diseases. This deficiency of circulating $25(OH)D_3$ is associated with significant osteopenia. It is probably due to mechanisms in addition to failure of hepatic hydroxylation of provitamin D_3. For example, such individuals have a reduced capacity to produce somatomedin. Moreover, in the case of alcoholic cirrhosis of the liver, chronic ingestion of ethanol may result in direct cytotoxic effects on bone and intestine.

Effects of Other Hormones on Bone and Calcium Metabolism

Parathyroid hormone, vitamin D and, to a lesser extent, calcitonin are the major hormones involved in bone metabolism and calcium homeostasis. Almost all of the other hormones, mediators and modulators discussed in earlier chapters are also involved in the regulation of bone growth in one way or another. A brief inventory of some of these will emphasize the point that metabolic processes in the intact human being or animal are controlled by a complex set of intricately interrelated mechanisms.

Prostaglandins

The prostaglandins, particularly PGE_1, inhibit the phosphaturic response of the renal tubular cell to PTH, but not to dibutyryl cyclic AMP; in this respect PTH resembles other cAMP-mediated responses that are antagonized by PGE_1. In cultured bone, however, PGE_1 mimics the action of PTH and causes bone resorption (Raisz). The bone resorption-promoting property of PGE_1 has led to a better understanding of the hypercalcemia that occurs when various types of cancer metastasize to bone; Tashjian and colleagues have discovered that this type of hypercalcemia is due to the production of prostaglandin in the bone-embedded tumor, with consequent bone resorption in the vicinity of the metastasis.

Glucocorticoids

Some of the effects of glucocorticoids on calcium metabolism and bone were discussed above in connection with vitamin D. It should be emphasized that, in low doses, glucocorticoids are necessary for skeletal growth. They are only skeletal growth-inhibiting when they are chronically present in excess, i.e., in naturally occurring or iatrogenic Cushing's disease. In addition to all of the things they do that were enumerated previously, they also inhibit somatomedin generation by the liver.

Estrogens and Androgens

Estrogens and androgens are involved in the puberal growth spurt and in closure of the epiphyses. In childhood and puberty, the steroids of both sexes favor bone formation over resorption but no plausible mechanism for this effect is known. In the adult female, estrogen has a bone resorption-inhibiting effect and it has been credited by some observers with slowing or arresting the progress of postmenopausal osteoporosis.

Thyroid Hormones

The thyroid hormones, as we have seen, are extremely important for development and growth of the skeleton in infancy and childhood. Indeed, retarded bone age, as indicated by ossification center development, is a major feature of hypothyroidism. In excess, as in hyperthyroidism, the thyroid hormones stimulate both bone formation and resorption, the latter more than the former.

Insulin

Insulin deficiency in children is associated with growth retardation. The mechanism of this effect is not well understood but may be an expression of the widespread disturbance in nutrient metabolism that occurs in insulin deficiency. This effect of insulin may have features that resemble the growth failure that is a feature of malnutrition.

Glucagon

Glucagon has curious and, as yet, poorly characterized effects on bone. It can stimulate calcitonin secretion and it also can inhibit bone resorption by direct action on bone in organ culture. The physiologic significance of these observations is uncertain.

Growth Hormone

Growth hormone has striking effects on bone growth by way of *somatomedin,* which is essential for the proliferation and function of chondrocytes. Somatomedin generation is essential for normal growth in children. In adults, excess growth hormone produces striking bony deformities which are associated with accelerated bone formation and resorption, the former process predominating.

All of these interrelated control mechanisms operate in a total environment that is maintained by *nutrition* and importantly influenced by *activity pattern*. Dietary factors involved are calcium and phosphorus, as well as total calories, adequate protein, and accessory food factors. The importance of activity pattern is indicated by the fact that normal people at total bed rest show a preponderance of bone resorption over bone formation and quickly go into negative calcium balance.

BIBLIOGRAPHY

Akita Y, Saito T, Yajima Y, et al: The stimulatory and inhibitory guanine nucleotide-binding proteins of adenylate cyclase in erythrocytes from patients with pseudohypoparathyroidism Type I. *J Clin Endocrinol Metab* 1985; 61:1012.

Auerbach GD, Marx SJ, Spiegel AM: Parathyroid hormone, calcitonin, and the calciferols, in Wilson JD, Foster DW (eds): *Williams Textbook of Endocrinology*, ed 7. Philadelphia, WB Saunders Co, 1985, p 1137.

Auerbach GD, Marx SJ, Spiegel AM: Metabolic bone disease, in Wilson JD, Foster DW (eds): *Williams Textbook of Endocrinology*, ed 7. Philadelphia, WB Saunders Co, 1985, p 1218.

Bell NH: Vitamin D-endocrine system. *J Clin Invest* 1985; 76:1.

Bienkowski RS: Intracellular degradation of newly synthesized proteins. *Biochem J* 1983; 214:1.

Birge SJ, Haddad JG: 25 (OH)D stimulation of muscle metabolism. *J Clin Invest* 1975; 56:1100.

Brickman AS, Coburn JW, Masry SG: 1,25(OH)$_2$D$_3$ in normal man and in patients with renal failure. *Arch Intern Med* 1974; 80:161.

Brommage R, DeLuca HF: Evidence that 1,25-dihydroxyvitamin D$_3$ is the physiologically active metabolite of vitamin D$_3$. *Endocr Rev* 1985; 6:491.

Cantley LK, Russell J, Lettieri D, et al: 1,25-dihydroxy vitamin D$_3$ suppresses parathyroid hormone secretion from bovine parathyroid cells in tissue culture. *Endocrinology* 1985; 117:2114.

Chambers TJ, Athanasou NA, Fuller K: Effect of parathyroid hormone and calcitonin on the cytoplasmic spreading of isolated osteoclasts. *J Endocrinol* 1984; 102:281.

Chambers TJ, McSheehy PMJ, Thomson BM, et al: The effect of calcium-regulating hormones and prostaglandins on bone resorption by osteoclasts disaggregated from neonatal rat bones. *Endocrinology* 1985; 116:234.

Cooper CW, Schwesinger WH, Malgoub AM, et al: Thyrocalcitonin: Stimulation of secretion by gastrin. *Science* 1971; 172:1238.

Copp DH: Endocrine control of calcium homeostasis. *J Endocrinol* 1969; 43:137.

Costanzo LS, Sheehe PR, Weiner IM: Renal actions of vitamin D in D-deficient rats. *Am J Physiol* 1974; 226:1490.

DeLuca HF: The metabolism, function, and physiology of vitamin D, in Kumar R (ed): *Vitamin D: Basic and Clinical Aspects*. Boston, Martinus Nijhoff, 1984, p 1.

Eisenberg H, Pallotta JA: Special localizing techniques for parathyroid disease, in DeGroot LJ, et al (eds): *Endocri-*

nology, vol 2. New York, Grune & Stratton, 1979, pp 717–724.

Fraser D, Scriver CR: Hereditary disorders associated with vitamin D resistance or defective phosphate metabolism, in DeGroot LJ, et al (eds): *Endocrinology*, vol 2. New York, Grune & Stratton, 1979, pp 797–807.

Greenberg PB, Foyle EH, Fisher MT, et al: Treatment of Paget's disease of bone with synthetic human calcitonin. Biochemical and roentgenologic changes. *Am J Med* 1974; 56:867.

Habener JF, Rosenblatt M, Potts JT, Jr: Parathyroid hormone: Biochemical aspects of biosynthesis, secretion, action, and metabolism. *Physiol Rev* 1984; 64:985.

Hahn TJ, Hendin BA, Scharp C, et al: Effect of chronic anticonvulsant therapy on serum 25 hydroxycholecalciferol levels in adults. *N Engl J Med* 1972; 287:900.

Harrison HE, Harrison HC: The interaction of vitamin D and parathyroid hormone on calcium, phosphorus, and magnesium homeostasis in the rat. *Metab Clin Exp* 1964; 13:952.

Haussler MR, McCain TA: Basic and clinical concepts related to vitamin D metabolism and action. *N Engl J Med* 1977; 297:974.

Heath H III, Sizemore GW: Plasma calcitonin in normal man: Difference between men and women. *J Clin Invest* 1977; 60:1135.

Hesch RD, Heck J, Auf'mKolk B, et al: First clinical observations with hPTH (1–38), a more potent human parathyroid hormone peptide. *Horm Metab Res* 1984; 16:559.

Haynes RC, Jr, Murad F: Agents affecting calcification: Calcium, parathyroid hormone, calcitonin, vitamin D, and other compounds, in Gilman AG, Goodman LS, Rall TW, et al (eds): *Goodman and Gilman's Pharmacological Basis of Therapeutics*, ed 7. New York, Macmillan Publishing Co, 1985, p 1517.

Jubiz W, Canterbory JM, Reiss JM: Circadian rhythm in PTH concentration in human subjects: Correlations with serum calcium, phosphate, albumin and growth hormone levels. *J Clin Invest* 1972; 51:2040.

Keutmann HT, Sauer MM, Hendy GN, et al: Complete amino acid sequence of human parathyroid hormone. *Biochemistry* 1978; 5723.

Kleeman KE, Kleeman CR: Parathyroid hormone and calcitonin, in Ingbar SH (ed): *Contemporary Endocrinology*, vol 2. New York, Plenum Publishing Corp, 1985, p 247.

Kronenberg HM, Hellerman J, Igarashi T, et al: Structure and expression of the human parathyroid hormone gene, in Labrie F, Proulx L (eds): *Endocrinology. Excerpta Medica ICS* 655, 1984, p 263.

Kukreja SC, Hargis GK, Rosenthal IM, et al: Pheochromocytoma causing excessive parathyroid hormone production and hypercalcemia. *Ann Intern Med* 1973; 79:838.

Kurnik BRC, Hruska KA: Effects of 1,25-dihydroxycholecalciferol on phosphate transport in vitamin D-deprived rats. *Am J Physiol* 1984; 247:F177.

Leggate J, Farish E, Fletcher CD, et al: Calcitonin and postmenopausal osteoporosis. *Clin Endocrinol (Oxf)* 1984; 20:85.

Marx SJ, Liberman UA, Eil C: Calciferols: Actions and deficiencies in action. *Vitam Horm* 1983; 40:235.

Marx SJ, Liberman UA, Eil C, et al: Hereditary resistance to 1,25-dihydroxy vitamin D. *Recent Prog Horm Res* 1984; 40:589.

Mayer E, Kadiwaki S, Williams G, et al: Mode of action of 1,25 dihydroxy vitamin D, in Kumar R (ed): *Vitamin D:*

Basic and Clinical Aspects. Boston, Martinus Nijhoff, 1984, p 260.

Parsons JA, Neer RM, Potts JT, Jr: Initial fall in plasma calcium after intravenous injection of parathyroid hormone. *Endocrinology* 1971; 89:735.

Peck W, Gennari C, Raisz L, et al: Corticosteroids and bone (roundtable discussion). *Calcif Tissue Int* 1984; 36:4.

Pike JW: Intracellular receptors mediate the biologic action of 1,25-dihydroxy vitamin D_3 *Nutr Rev* 1985; 43:161.

Raisz LG: Mechanisms of parathyroid hormone-mediated bone loss. *Excerpta Medica ICS* 617, 1983.

Raisz LG: Regulation of bone formation. *N Engl J Med* 1983; 309:29 and 83.

Raisz LG: Studies on bone formation and resorption in vitro. *Horm Res* 1984; 20:22.

Rodan GA, Rodan SB, Majeska RJ, et al: The effect of parathyroid hormone on bone cells. *Excerpta Medica ICS* 655, 1984, p 583.

Rosenfeld MG, Amara SG, Evans RM: Tissue specific patterns of RNA processing: Regulation and developmental specificity of neuroendocrine gene expression. *Excerpta Medica ICS* 655, 1984, p 923.

Russell J, Silver J, Sherwood LM: The effects of calcium and vitamin D metabolites on cytoplasmic mRNA coding for pre-proparathyroid hormone in isolated parathyroid cells. *Trans Assoc Am Physicans* 1984; 97:296.

Skjodt H, Gallagher JA, Beresford JN, et al: Vitamin D metabolites regulate osteocalcin synthesis and proliferation of human bone cells in vitro. *J Endocrinol* 1985; 105:391.

Smith DM, Johnston CC, III: Cyclic 3'5' adenosine monophosphate levels in separated bone cells. *Endocrinology* 1975; 96:1261.

Swaminathan R, Bates RFL, Bloom SR, et al: The relationship between food, gastrointestinal hormones, and calcitonin secretion. *J Endocrinol* 1973; 59:217.

Tiegs RD, Body JJ, Wahner HW, et al: Calcitonin secretion in postmenopausal osteoporosis. *N Engl J Med* 1985; 312:1097.

Wasserman RH, Fullmer GS, Shimura F: Calcium absorption and the molecular effects of vitamin D_3, in Kumar R (ed): *Vitamin D: Basic and Clinical Aspects*. Boston, Martinus Nijhoff, 1984, p 233.

Wasserman RH: Vitamin D action. *Nutr Rev* 1985; 43:127.

Index

Numbers in italic represent illustrations; numbers followed by "t" represent material in tables.